Step-Up to USMLE Step 3

Step-Up Series Editors

Samir Mehta, MD
Resident, Department of Orthopaedic Surgery
University of Pennsylvania Health System
Philadelphia, Pennsylvania

Adam J. Mirarchi, MD
Resident, Department of Orthopaedics
Case Western Reserve University
Cleveland, Ohio

Lieutenant Edmund A. Milder, MD
Staff Pediatrician and General Medical Officer
Naval Branch Health Clinic
La Maddalena, Italy

Step-Up to USMLE Step 3

Jonathan P. Van Kleunen, MD
Resident, Department of Orthopaedic Surgery
The Hospital of the University of Pennsylvania
University of Pennsylvania Health System
Philadelphia, PA

Wolters Kluwer | Lippincott Williams & Wilkins
Health
Philadelphia • Baltimore • New York • London
Buenos Aires • Hong Kong • Sydney • Tokyo

Acquisitions Editor: Charley Mitchell
Managing Editor: Kelly Horvath
Marketing Manager: Jennifer Kuklinski
Associate Production Manager: Kevin P. Johnson
Designer: Holly McLaughlin
Compositor: Aptara, Inc.

351 West Camden Street
Baltimore, MD 21201

530 Walnut Street
Philadelphia, PA 19106

Printed in the USA

9 8 7 6 5 4 3 2 1

Library of Congress Cataloging-in-Publication Data

Van Kleunen, Jonathan P.
Step-up to USMLE step 3 / Jonathan P. Van Kleunen.
p. ; cm.
Includes bibliographical references and index.
ISBN 978-0-7817-7963-0 (alk. paper)
1. Physicians—Licenses—United States—Examinations—Study quides. 2. Internal medicine—Case studies. I. Title.
[DNLM: 1. Clinical Medicine—United States—Outlines. WB 18.2 V217s 2009]
R834.5.V36 2009
610.76—dc22

2008035477

DISCLAIMER

Care has been taken to confirm the accuracy of the information present and to describe generally accepted practices. However, the authors, editors, and publisher are not responsible for errors or omissions or for any consequences from application of the information in this book and make no warranty, expressed or implied, with respect to the currency, completeness, or accuracy of the contents of the publication. Application of this information in a particular situation remains the professional responsibility of the practitioner; the clinical treatments described and recommended may not be considered absolute and universal recommendations.

The authors, editors, and publisher have exerted every effort to ensure that drug selection and dosage set forth in this text are in accordance with the current recommendations and practice at the time of publication. However, in view of ongoing research, changes in government regulations, and the constant flow of information relating to drug therapy and drug reactions, the reader is urged to check the package insert for each drug for any change in indications and dosage and for added warnings and precautions. This is particularly important when the recommended agent is a new or infrequently employed drug.

Some drugs and medical devices presented in this publication have Food and Drug Administration (FDA) clearance for limited use in restricted research settings. It is the responsibility of the health care provider to ascertain the FDA status of each drug or device planned for use in their clinical practice.

To purchase additional copies of this book, call our customer service department at **(800) 638-3030** or fax orders to **(301) 223-2320**. International customers should call **(301) 223-2300**.

Visit Lippincott Williams & Wilkins on the Internet: http://www.lww.com. Lippincott Williams & Wilkins customer service representatives are available from 8:30 am to 6:00 pm, EST.

Dedication

To all of the Van Kleunen and Eaton families, here and gone,
I truly appreciate your encouragement through the years.
To Amy, whose constant love and support has made everything possible.

Well done is better than well said.

— Benjamin Franklin

Contents

Preface

The U.S. Medical Licensing Examination (USMLE) Step 3 examination serves as the final hurdle in the transition from medical school to graduate medical education. This test builds on the principles of the Step 1 and Step 2 examinations and places them in a format focused on clinical decision making. The purpose of this test is to determine if the new physician is capable of applying the vast amount of information that he or she has learned from medical school into the treatment of patients. Unlike the prior two components of the USMLE examination, this test not only requires the examinees to recall information that they have learned but also requires them to be able to apply this basic knowledge to realistic clinical scenarios and to make the appropriate decisions based on their knowledge. Also unlike the previous USMLE tests, the Step 3 examination is taken following graduation from medical school and typically during the intern year of residency. This schedule can make preparation for the examination fairly difficult. Unlike during medical school, it is difficult or nearly impossible to block off large amounts of time to study for the test. Test takers must rely on their knowledge gained from the experiences of their intern year, supplemented by a concise, yet high-yield, review of testable information.

Step-Up to USMLE Step 3 has been designed with both the test and the test taker in mind to provide a high-yield review for the USMLE Step 3 examination. Because of the emphasis on patient management in the examination, this book has been designed to provide a realistic clinical scenario for the many tested diagnoses. The organization of this book is unlike other reviews for the USMLE Step 3 in that nearly all of the information is presented in a case-based format. Each case consists of an extensive history and physical for a presenting patient, multiple diagnostic studies performed during the work-up, the diagnosis made due to this work-up, the treatment administered, and the follow-up of the patient following therapy. Following each case, each of the most likely conditions in the differential diagnosis is reviewed, and the reason why each diagnosis is correct or incorrect is explained. This type of review is a better reproduction of the thought processes of the new resident physician than a simple iteration of facts. It seeks to reproduce the clinical decisions that a resident physician is required to make on a daily basis. In addition, the limited amount of time available for test preparation has been considered during the writing of this book. The reviews of each diagnosis are concise and designed to include only the high-yield information that is vital on test day. It is not intended to be a self-assessment of testable information, but rather a presentation of how certain conditions may present and how they are appropriately managed.

Please feel free to forward any comments to me at Step-Up@lww.com. I wish you all the best of luck in taking and passing this final stage of the USMLE examination series. Although the demands of residency are significant, the completion of this test is yet another hurdle that you will have cleared on the road to completing medical education and beginning a complete practice of medicine.

Acknowledgments

I wish to extend thanks to the reviewers whose suggestions helped to shape this book. Special thanks go to Jennifer Clements for her contributions to the artwork in this publication. I would like to especially thank Kelly Horvath and Donna Balado at Lippincott Williams & Wilkins for their planning and editing of this edition and their patience and dedication to bring everything together.

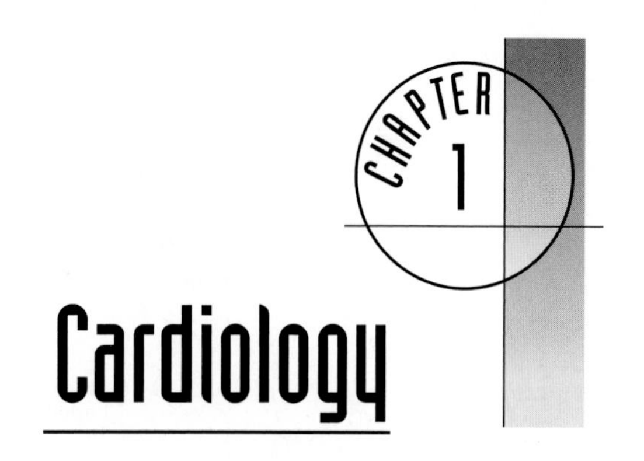

Cardiology

BASIC CLINICAL PRIMER

CARDIAC ANATOMY (FIGURE 1-1)

- Cardiac **ischemia** develops in the distribution of an occluded vessel.

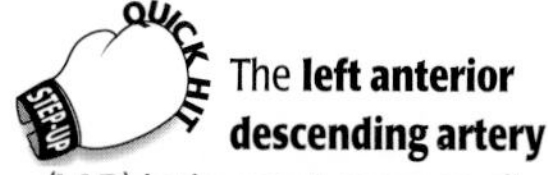

The **left anterior descending artery** (LAD) is the most common site of coronary artery occlusion.

CARDIAC CYCLE (FIGURE 1-2)

- The pressure and volume of each heart chamber vary during the cardiac cycle depending on inflow, outflow, and the activity of contraction
- Pressure is **equal** between two adjacent chambers when the valve between them is **open**

QUICK HIT: Coronary arteries fill during **diastole**, while systemic arteries fill during **systole**. Conditions or drugs that reduce diastolic filling decrease coronary perfusion during a given period of time.

CARDIAC OUTPUT (CO)

- The volume of cardiac outflow to the systemic vasculature over a given period of time
- CO is dependent on the rate of contraction (i.e., heart rate) and the volume of blood forced out of the left ventricle per contraction (i.e., stroke volume)
  - **Heart rate (HR)** is number of contractions per unit of time and is expressed as beats per minute (bpm)
  - **Stroke volume (SV)** is the change in volume from immediately before a contraction to the completion of the contraction
    - SV = (end-diastolic volume) − (end-systolic volume)
    - Dependent on **contractility** (i.e., force of heart's contraction), **preload** (i.e., the amount of stretching force on cardiac muscle fibers at the end of diastole), and **afterload** (i.e., the vascular resistance which ventricles must overcome to produce outflow)
    - Increases with catecholamine release (e.g., epinephrine), increased intracellular calcium, decreased intravascular sodium, digoxin use, and stressful events (e.g., anxiety, exercise)
    - Decreases with β-blocker use, heart failure, and hypoxia with acidosis

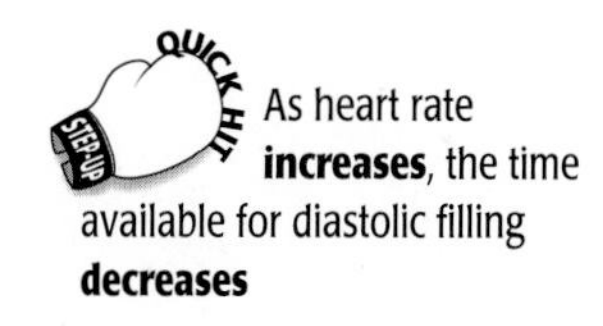

As heart rate **increases**, the time available for diastolic filling **decreases**

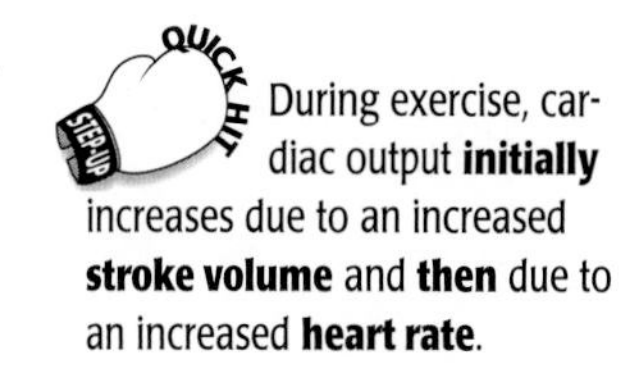

During exercise, cardiac output **initially** increases due to an increased **stroke volume** and **then** due to an increased **heart rate**.

VASCULAR PRESSURES

- **Systolic** blood pressure (SBP) is the maximum vascular pressure experienced during heart contraction; **diastolic** blood pressure (DBP) is the baseline vascular pressure between contractions
- **Pulse pressure** is the increase in blood pressure (BP) attributed to cardiac outflow during contraction
  - Pulse pressure = (SBP) − (DBP)
- **Mean arterial pressure (MAP)** is the average BP considering that unequal amounts of time are spent in systole and diastole
  - MAP = (DBP) + ($^1/_3 \times$ SBP)

FIGURE 1-1 **(A) Anterior and posterior views of the heart. LA, left atrium; LV, left ventricle; RA, right atrium; RV, right ventricle; SVC, superior vena cava. (B) Coronary artery hierarchy and regions of the heart supplied by branches. AV, atrioventricular; SA, sinoatrial.**

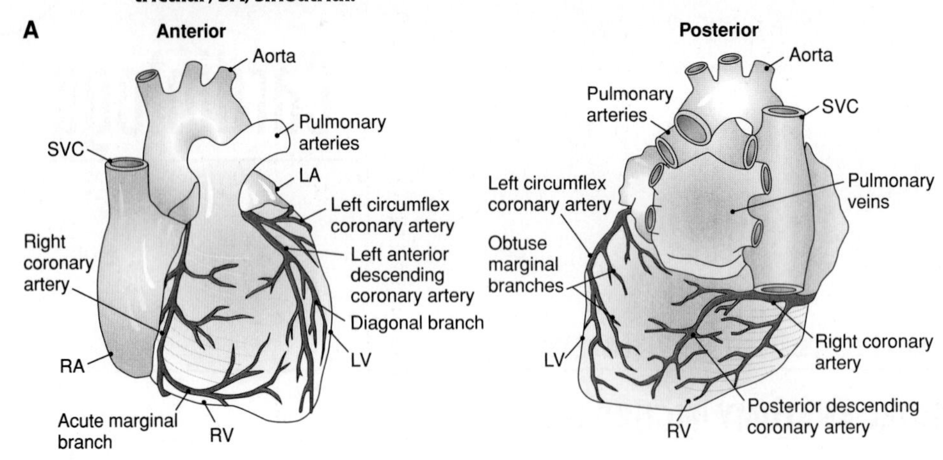

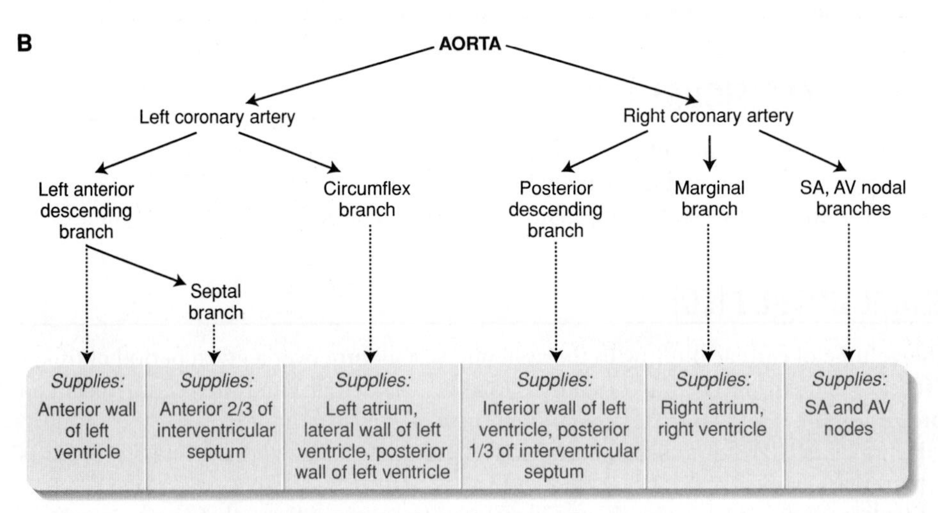

(Modified from Lilly LS. *Pathophysiology of heart disease.* 2nd ed. Baltimore: Williams & Wilkins; 1998. Used with permission of Lippincott Williams & Wilkins.)

PHYSIOLOGY OF HEART CONTRACTION

- Key principles:
  - Increasing the end-diastolic ventricular volume causes an increased stretch on cardiac muscle fibers; this leads to an increase in the force of contraction (i.e., **Frank-Starling relationship**)
  - The end-systolic volume and the pressure generated by the ventricles are dependent on **afterload**
  - Increased **contractility** (i.e., force of contraction independent of preload and afterload) leads to increased muscle fiber tension during isometric contraction

- **Ejection fraction (EF)** $= \dfrac{\text{(stroke volume)}}{\text{(end - diastolic volume)}}$ **(normally 55%–75%)**

- Changes in volume-pressure relationships determine heart compliance; persistent high demands will lead to heart failure
- **Contractile dysfunction**
  - **Systolic** dysfunction is caused by decreased contractility, increased preload, increased afterload, HR abnormalities, or chronic high output conditions (e.g., anemia, hyperthyroidism) and leads to an insufficient cardiac output for the systemic demand

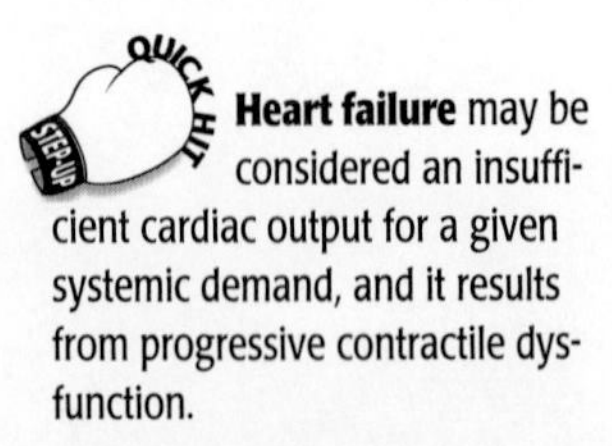

Heart failure may be considered an insufficient cardiac output for a given systemic demand, and it results from progressive contractile dysfunction.

FIGURE 1-2 **(A) Pressure relationships between left-sided heart chambers and the timing between normal heart sounds and the electrocardiogram for one full cardiac cycle. AV, aortic valve; ECG, electrocardiogram; LA, left atrium; LV, left ventricle; MV, mitral valve. (B) Normal left ventricular pressure-volume loop for one full cardiac cycle.**

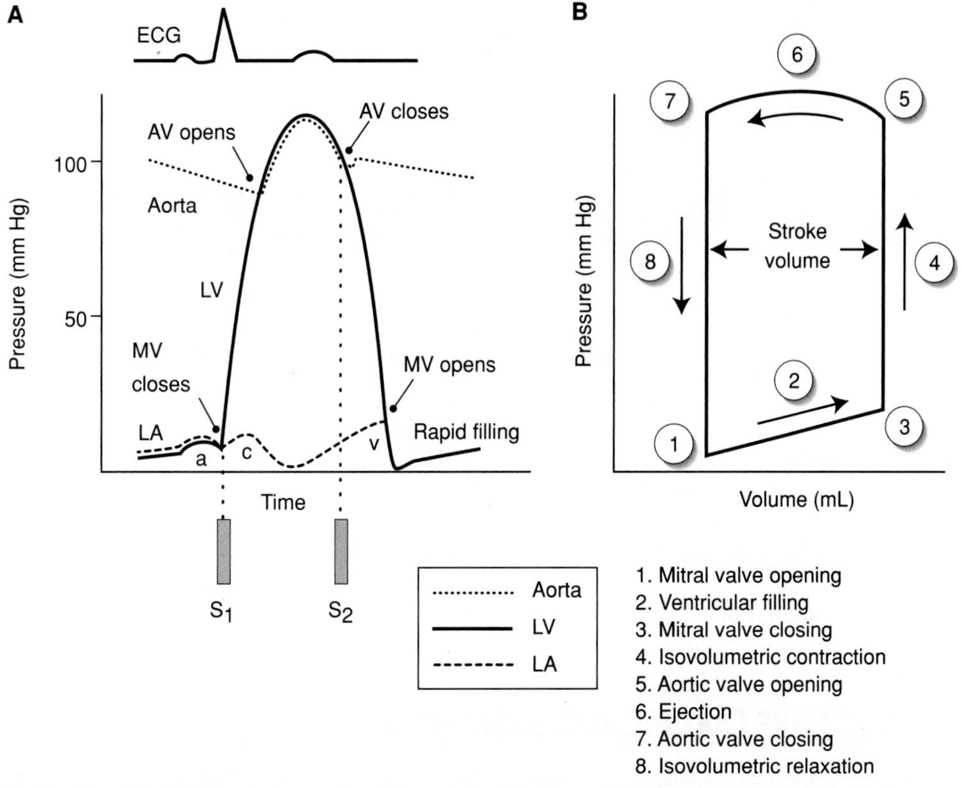

(Modified from Lilly LS. *Pathophysiology of heart disease.* 2nd ed. Baltimore: Williams & Wilkins; 1998. Used with permission of Lippincott Williams & Wilkins.)

- **Diastolic** dysfunction is caused by cardiac hypertrophy or restrictive cardiomyopathy and leads to decreased ventricular compliance, decreased ventricular filling, increased DBP, and decreased cardiac output

ELECTROCARDIOGRAM (ECG)

- Recorded tracing of electrical impulses through the heart that is used to provide information regarding cardiac function (Figure 1-3)
  - A systematic review increases the sensitivity to discerning abnormal patterns
    - Confirm calibration on tracing
    - Rhythm (i.e., regularity, reproduced patterns)
    - Rate
    - Intervals (e.g., PR, QRS, ST)
    - P wave, QRS complex, ST segment, and T wave morphology
  - Normal tracings
    - P wave: atrial depolarization
    - PR interval: conduction through the atrioventricular (AV) node (<0.2 sec)
    - QRS interval: ventricular depolarization (<0.12 sec)
    - ST interval: isoelectric ventricular contraction
    - T wave: ventricular repolarization
    - U wave: relative hypokalemia

NORMAL CHOLESTEROL FUNCTION

- Cholesterols and triglycerides are carried by lipoproteins
  - Increased low-density lipoprotein (LDL) levels lead to an increased coronary artery disease (CAD) risk

FIGURE 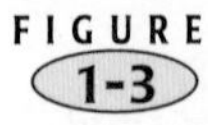 **General structure of the electrocardiogram tracing and the significance of specific regions.**

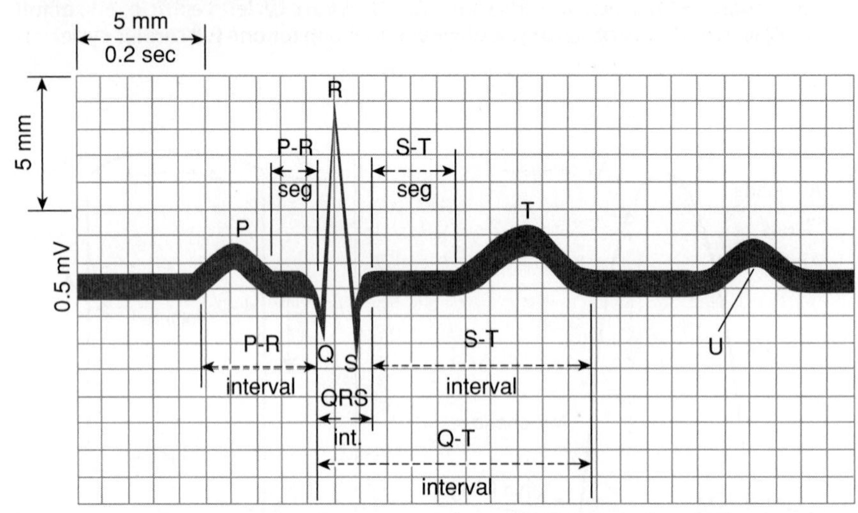

(Modified from Pilliterri A. *Maternal and child nursing*. 4th ed. Philadelphia: Lippincott Williams & Wilkins; 2003. Fig. 41-2. Used with permission of Lippincott Williams & Wilkins.)

- Increased high-density lipoprotein (HDL) is protective
- Increased LDL and decreased HDL result from a diet high in fatty foods, tobacco use, obesity, alcohol use, diabetes mellitus (DM), and certain medications (e.g., oral contraceptive pills [OCPs], diuretics)

PREOPERATIVE CARDIAC RISK ASSESSMENT

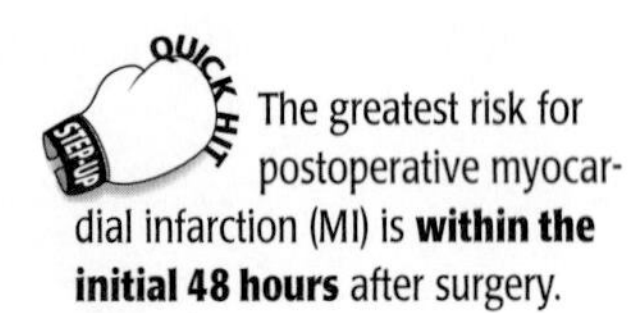

The greatest risk for postoperative myocardial infarction (MI) is **within the initial 48 hours** after surgery.

- **Risk assessment** for a surgical patient estimating the likelihood of an undesired cardiac event occurring as a result of surgery or anesthesia
  - Considers measurable cardiac function, preexisting cardiac disease, age, and important comorbidities
  - Young, healthy patients may be cleared for surgery with a normal ECG
  - Older patients and/or those with comorbidities require a more extensive workup by a cardiologist and/or cardiac function testing
- Factors suggesting an **increased risk of an adverse cardiac event**
  - **Age**: >70 years old
  - **Pulmonary function**: forced expiratory volume in 1 sec/functional vital capacity (FEV_1/FVC) <70% expected, partial pressure of carbon dioxide (pCO_2) >45 mm Hg, pulmonary edema
  - **Cardiac disease**: MI within past 30 days, poorly controlled nonsinus arrhythmia, pathologic Q waves on the preoperative ECG, severe valvular disease, decompensated congestive heart failure with poor ejection fraction
  - **Renal insufficiency**: creatinine (Cr) >2.0 or a 50% increase from baseline
  - **Surgery type**: cardiac/vascular surgery or anticipated high blood loss
- **High-risk** patients should have their cardiac function optimized prior to elective surgery and should be made aware of the increased risks if the surgery is emergent
  - Perioperative β-blockers and postoperative noninvasive cardiac monitoring are frequently recommended for patients determined to have increased cardiac risk

INVASIVE CARDIAC MONITORING

- Arterial line: constant access to artery (e.g., radial, femoral, axillary, brachial, dorsalis pedis) that allows accurate measurement of arterial BP and allows easy access to arterial blood for blood gas measurements
- Pulmonary artery catheter (i.e., Swan-Ganz catheter): catheter inserted through the (usually left) subclavian or (usually right) internal jugular vein that runs through the

heart to the pulmonary artery; a transducer in the catheter allows the measurement of **cardiac output**, mixed venous oxygen (O_2) saturation, systemic vascular resistance, and **pressures** in the **right atrium** and **pulmonary artery**; a balloon may be inflated at the catheter tip to fill the pulmonary artery lumen and to measure the wedge pressure (equivalent to **left atrium pressure**)

FETAL CIRCULATION

- Gas exchange occurs in the uteroplacental circulation
- Fetal hemoglobin (Hgb) has a greater O_2 affinity than adult Hgb and pulls O_2 from maternal blood
- Umbilical arteries carry deoxygenated blood to placenta; umbilical veins carry oxygenated blood from placenta to portal system (Figure 1-4)

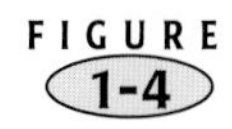

FIGURE 1-4 **Diagram of fetal circulation. Arrows indicate the direction of blood flow; three shunts (ductus venosus, foramen ovale, ductus arteriosus) exist *in utero* but close shortly after birth.**

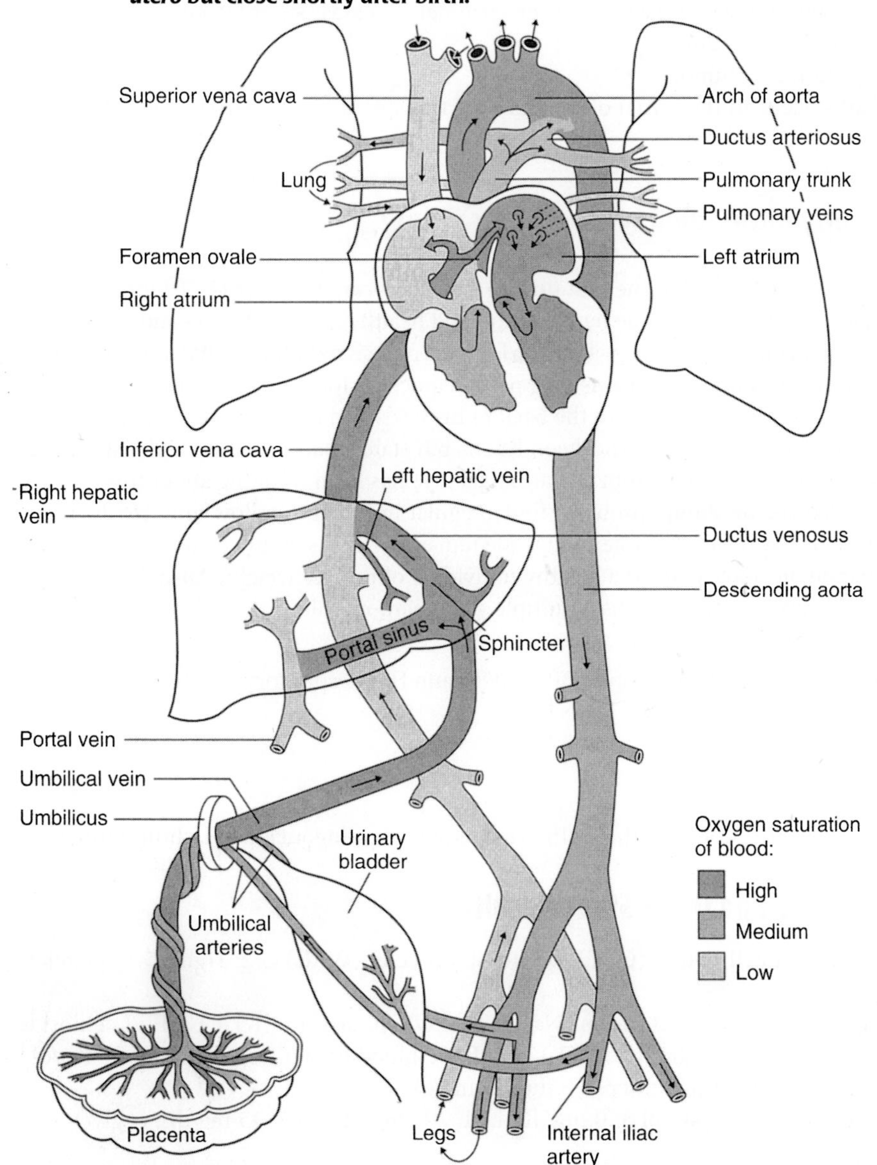

(Taken from Lilly LS. *Pathophysiology of heart disease.* 2nd ed. Baltimore: Williams & Wilkins; 1998. Used with permission of Lippincott Williams & Wilkins.)

- Changes following birth
  - Lung expansion causes an increased pulmonary blood flow leading to an increase in relative blood oxygenation
  - A decreasing serum level of prostaglandin E_2 results in **ductus arteriosus closure**; umbilical cord clamping results in the end of placental circulation and an increase in systemic vascular resistance
  - This increased vascular resistance, in turn, induces **ductus venosus closure** and umbilical artery and vein constriction
  - Left atrial pressure increases (due to increased pulmonary blood flow), and umbilical circulation decreases, causing a decrease in inferior vena cava pressure
  - Decrease in inferior vena cava and right atrial pressures leads to **foramen ovale closure**

CARDIAC TRANSPLANTATION

- Indicated for end-stage cardiac disease (e.g., CAD, congenital disease, cardiomyopathy) with an estimated survival of **<2 years**
- Contraindicated in patients with pulmonary hypertension, renal insufficiency, chronic obstructive pulmonary disease, or other terminal illnesses; smokers and patients >70 years old are also excluded
- Acute rejection is common
- Most deaths occur in the initial 6 months after transplant; 5-year survival is 70%

CASE 1-1 "My father died when he was young"

A 25-year-old man presents for the first time to a primary care provider (PCP) for a wellness check-up. He says that he has been in good health for several years and has only seen a doctor a few times since he was a child for the occasional illness. His only complaint is recurrent Achilles tendon and hamstring pain that occurs following significant exertion. He has noticed some small bumps in the back of his heels and knees in the past year in the regions of pain. He denies any medical conditions but states that his father died last year at a young age (i.e., 50 years old) from a heart attack. He has been thinking about this recently and decided he should probably find a regular internist to follow him. He denies any substance use. A review of systems and the remainder of his family history are negative. On examination, he appears to be a healthy individual of normal weight. Auscultation of his lungs and heart is normal. He has multiple small hard nodules behind his knees and heels. The following vital signs are measured:

Temperature (T): 98.7°F, HR: 90 bpm, BP: 130/85 mm Hg, Respiratory rate (RR): 16 breaths/min

Differential Diagnosis

- Chronic tendonitis, crystal arthropathy (e.g., gout, pseudogout), hypercholesterolemia

Laboratory Data and Other Study Results

- Complete blood cell count (CBC): white blood cells (WBC) 8.2, Hgb 15.1, platelets (Plt) 320
- Chemistry panel (Chem7): sodium (Na) 142 mEq/L, potassium (K) 4.1 mEq/L, chloride (Cl) 107 mEq/L, carbon dioxide (CO_2) 26 mEq/L, blood urea nitrogen (BUN) 20 mg/dL, creatinine (Cr) 0.9 mg/dL, glucose (Glu) 85 mg/dL
- Lipid panel: Total cholesterol 350 mg/dL, LDL 290 mg/dL, HDL 45 mg/dL, triglycerides (Trig) 120 mg/dL
- Coagulation panel (Coags): protime (PT) 12 sec, International normalized ratio (INR) 1.0, partial thromboplastin time (PTT) 40 sec

- Urinalysis (UA): straw-colored, pH 5.0, specific gravity 1.010, no glucose/ketones/nitrites/leukocyte esterase/hematuria/proteinuria

Following these findings, the additional studies are performed:

- ECG: normal sinus rhythm; no abnormal wave morphology
- Biopsy of heel lesion: large collections of cholesterol-laden material

Diagnosis

- Familial hypercholesterolemia (heterozygote)

Treatment Administered

- The patient was placed on a regular exercise regimen and a low-fat, low-cholesterol diet
- The patient was prescribed a regimen of simvastatin and ezetimibe

Follow-up

- A repeat lipid analysis in 1 month found the LDL to be 155 mg/dL
- The tendon xanthomas gradually regressed
- The patient was followed regularly to confirm an adequate reduction of his lipid levels and for cardiac screening

Steps to the Diagnosis

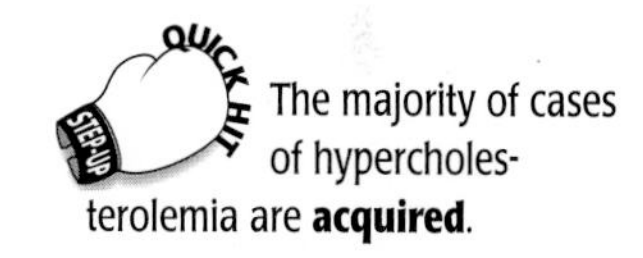

The majority of cases of hypercholesterolemia are **acquired**.

- **Congenital hypercholesterolemia**
  - **Inherited** form of hypercholesterolemia in which a genetic defect causes abnormally high levels of total cholesterol, LDL, and/or triglycerides
    - Patients have a **significantly increased risk of ischemic heart disease**
    - Common types:
- **Familial hypercholesterolemia** (FH): autosomal dominant defect in LDL receptors with an associated increased total cholesterol and LDL; the disease is much more severe in homozygotes than heterozygotes
- Familial combined hyperlipidemia: hypercholesterolemia and hypertriglyceridemia associated with an increased hepatic production of apolipoprotein B-100 protein
- Familial defective apolipoprotein B-100: similar to FH except that the defect is in the LDL particle and not LDL receptor
  - **History**: tendonitis around xanthomas, possible symptoms of ischemic heart disease (homozygotes experience symptoms in childhood, heterozygotes are usually asymptomatic until adulthood)
  - **Physical examination: xanthomas** (i.e., cholesterol deposits in tendon or skin), xanthelasmas (i.e., deposits in eyelids), cholesterol emboli are seen in the retina on funduscopic examination
  - **Tests:**
    - **Total cholesterol** and **LDL** >250 mg/dL in heterozygotes and >600 mg/dL in homozygotes
    - Triglycerides are elevated (>200 mg/dL) in familial combined hyperlipidemia
    - A biopsy of xanthomas will detect collections of cholesterol; genetic testing is available but typically unneeded for the diagnosis
  - **Treatment:**
    - Healthy diet, exercise, and smoking cessation will decrease the risk for an ischemic event
    - Patients should be educated about the role of risk factors
    - **Lipid-lowering agents** are administered (consisting of one statin and at least one other drug) to achieve LDL levels below 160 mg/dL or lower depending on the number of cardiac risk factors (Figure 1-5, Table 1-1)
    - Triglyceride-lowering drugs may be added if required

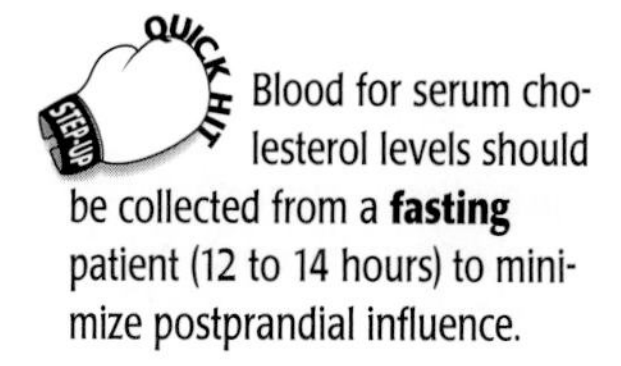

Blood for serum cholesterol levels should be collected from a **fasting** patient (12 to 14 hours) to minimize postprandial influence.

FIGURE 1-5 Decision tree for screening for hypercholesterolemia. BP, blood pressure; CAD, coronary artery disease; DM, diabetes mellitus; HDL, high-density lipoprotein; HTN, hypertension; LDL, low-density lipoprotein; PVD, peripheral vascular disease.

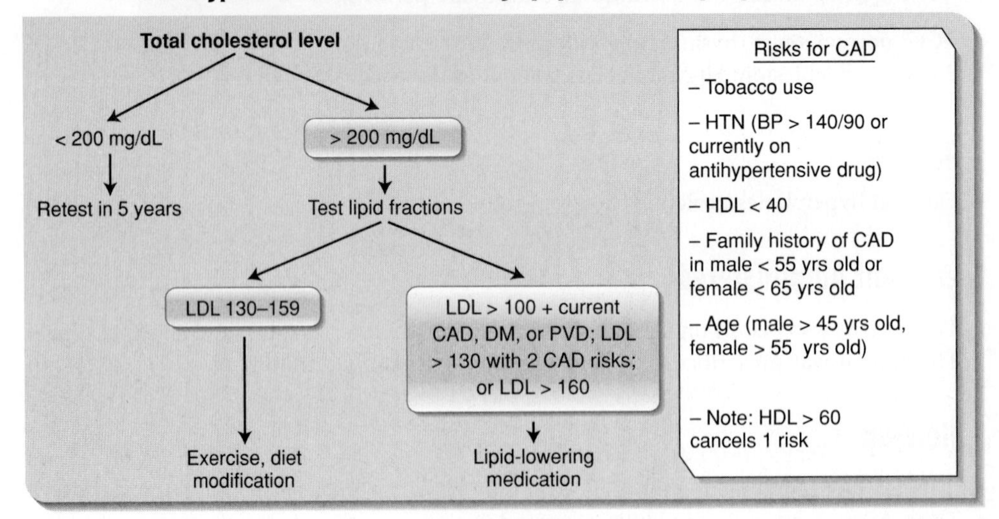

- **Outcomes**:
  - Significantly increased risk for **ischemic heart disease**
  - Prognosis is heavily dependent on the ability to control LDL levels
  - Patients with homozygous disease have poorer prognosis
- **Clues to the diagnosis**:
  - History: death of father at a young age
  - Physical: xanthomatous nodules behind the knee and ankle
  - Tests: increased total cholesterol and LDL, biopsy results
- **Acquired hypercholesterolemia**
  - Most common variant of hypercholesterolemia
    - Typified by **high LDL** levels and/or **low HDL** levels with an associated increased risk of ischemic heart disease
  - **History**: usually **asymptomatic**

TABLE 1-1 Lipid-Lowering Agents

Drug	Site of Action	Effect on LDL	Effect on HDL	Effect on Triglycerides	Side Effects
HMG-CoA reductase inhibitors (e.g., lovastatin, pravastatin, simvastatin)	Liver	↓↓↓	↑	↓	Myositis, increased LFTs (must monitor)
Cholesterol absorption inhibitors (e.g., ezetimibe)	Intestines	↓↓	—	—	Myalgias, possible increased LFTs
Fibric acids (e.g., gemfibrozil, fenofibrate)	Blood (all stimulate lipoprotein lipase)	↓↓	↑	↓↓↓	Myositis, increased LFTs (must monitor)
Bile acid sequestrants (e.g., cholestyramine, colestipol, colesevelam)	GI tract	↓↓	—	—/↑	Bad taste, GI upset
Niacin	Liver	↓↓	↑↑	↓	Facial flushing, nausea, paresthesias, pruritus, increased LFTs, insulin resistance, exacerbates gout

HMG-CoA, 3-hydroxy-3-methyl-glutaryl-CoA; GI, gastrointestinal; HDL, high-density lipoprotein; LDL, low-density lipoprotein; LFTs, liver function tests; ↑, increased; ↑↑, more increased; ↑↑↑, most increased; —/↑, normal or increased.

- **Physical examination**: the xanthomas seen in the congenital form are rare in the acquired form
- Tests: increased total cholesterol and LDL (typically <**300 mg/dL**), decreased HDL
- **Treatment**:
  - Focus is initially on the prevention of cardiac disease and the reduction of cholesterol levels through **exercise**, **low-fat and low-cholesterol diet**, and smoking cessation
  - **Cholesterol-lowering medication** is used in patients with increased cardiac risks or in patients unable to achieve ideal cholesterol levels with nonpharmacologic treatment alone (Table 1-1); the **goal LDL level** should be **below 160 mg/dL** in patients with less than two CAD risk factors, **below 130 mg/dL** in patients with two or more risk factors, and **below 100 mg/dL** in patients at a high risk for CAD (e.g., multiple risk factors, advanced age, very high LDL, peripheral vascular disease, diabetes mellitus, aortic aneurysms)
- **Outcomes:** the prevention of cardiac disease is contingent on the patient's ability to follow nonpharmacologic recommendations and the ability of medications to optimize LDL levels
- **Why eliminated from differential**: the LDL levels and presence of tendon xanthomas seen in this patient are higher than what would be expected for the acquired form and are more consistent with congenital disease

- **Chronic tendonitis**
  - More thorough discussion in Chapter 9
  - **Why eliminated from differential**: the presence of calcified tendon masses may be seen in chronic tendonitis, but this diagnosis cannot explain the patient's cholesterol levels
- **Crystal arthropathy**
  - More thorough discussion in Chapter 9
  - **Why eliminated from differential**: tophi may be confused with xanthomas, but the biopsy confirms the identity of the nodules as xanthomas, and this diagnosis would not explain the patient's cholesterol levels

CASE 1-2 "I get pains in my chest when I work in the yard"

A 61-year-old man presents to his PCP with a complaint of occasional chest pain. He describes the pain as a dull ache near the center of his chest that radiates to his left shoulder. He says that the pain has occurred during the past 2 months when he was cutting down a couple of trees in his yard and chopping them into firewood (about four times). He has a sedentary desk job and denies pain at work or rest. He does not exercise and denies pain with walking or stair climbing. He denies nausea and vomiting and is unsure if the pain tends to follow eating. He says that he has had some mild dyspnea during the episodes that was slightly worse in the most recent episode during the previous weekend. He denies any paresthesias or paralysis. In each case, the pain has resolved within several minutes after resting. He denies any drug use. His past medical history is only significant for hypertension (HTN) that he has controlled with a diuretic. He notes that his brother had a heart attack 2 years ago. On examination, he appears to be comfortable and breathing normally. Chest auscultation finds normal breath sounds bilaterally, no murmurs, and an accentuated second heart sound. He has no abdominal pain on palpation. He remains asymptomatic during walking in the hallway. His neurologic examination is normal. The following vital signs are measured:

T: 98.2°F, HR: 84 bpm, BP: 140/88 mm Hg, RR: 16 breaths/min

Differential Diagnosis

- Angina pectoris, panic disorder, esophagitis/gastritis/reflux disease, pulmonary embolism, pericarditis, aortic dissection

Laboratory Data and Other Study Results

- Pulse oximetry: 99% on room air at rest and during ambulation
- Chem7: Na: 141 mEq/L, K: 4.0 mEq/L, Cl: 105 mEq/L, CO_2: 27 mEq/L, BUN: 20 mg/dL, Cr: 1.0 mg/dL, Glu: 90 mg/dL
- Lipid panel: total cholesterol: 230 mg/dL, LDL: 165 mg/dL, HDL: 40 mg/dL, Trig: 125 mg/dL
- Chest x-ray (CXR): clear lung fields; normal cardiac shape and size
- ECG: normal sinus rhythm; normal wave and interval morphology

Given the benign results above, the following tests are ordered on an outpatient basis:

- Exercise stress test: development of chest pain at 75% predicted maximum heart rate; 1 mm ST interval depression during this time; chest pain and ECG abnormality resolve following cessation of the test and a brief rest
- Nuclear perfusion test: technetium-99m-sestamibi is injected during the exercise stress test; scintigraphy demonstrates a perfusion defect in the distribution of the left anterior descending coronary artery
- Echocardiography: 45% ejection fraction, mildly hypokinetic lateral wall, no effusions

Diagnosis

- Stable angina pectoris subsequent to ischemic heart disease

Treatment Administered

- The patient was placed on low-dose aspirin, atorvastatin, lisinopril, and atenolol
- The patient was prescribed sublingual nitroglycerin to be used as needed during any recurrent chest pain episodes
- The patient was provided education for healthy lifestyles

Follow-up

- Following the initiation of medicines, patient had an improved lipid profile and BP control
- A cardiac catheterization demonstrated a 40% blockage of the left anterior descending coronary artery
- The patient reported rare episodes of chest pain (one to two per year) that responded well to nitroglycerin
- The patient continued his cardiology follow-up to track any worsening of his condition

Steps to the Diagnosis

- **Angina pectoris (stable)**
  - **Temporary myocardial ischemia** during exertion that causes chest pain
    - Most commonly due to **ischemic heart disease** (a.k.a. **CAD**)
- An **inadequate** supply of O_2 for a given myocardial demand leads to **myocardial hypoxia** and an accumulation of waste products
- The vast majority of cases of ischemic heart disease arise from **atherosclerosis of the coronary arteries** (i.e., CAD), but arterial vasospasm (i.e., Prinzmetal angina) or valvular pathology are less common causes
  - **Atherosclerosis**
    - A gradual narrowing of arteries due to endothelial dysfunction, progressive formation of plaques (which consist of lipids and smooth muscle), and the associated inflammatory response
    - Plaques may calcify, rupture, and thrombose, leading to further narrowing of arteries and progressive occlusion of blood flow
    - The workup consists of identifying the associated degree of CAD

MNEMONIC

Common risk factors for atherosclerosis may be remembered by the mnemonic **SHIFT MAID**: **S**moking, **H**TN, **I**nsulin resistance (NIDDM), **F**amily history, **T**riglycerides and cholesterol (high), **M**ale, **A**ge (increased), **I**nactivity, **D**iet.

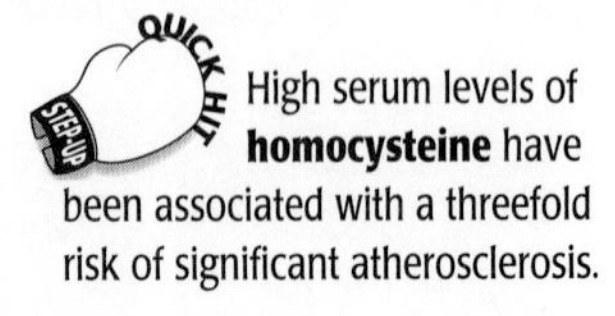

High serum levels of **homocysteine** have been associated with a threefold risk of significant atherosclerosis.

- Treatment focuses on the control of cardiac risk factors (e.g., control of HTN, hyperglycemia, and hypercholesterolemia), healthy diet, exercise, and smoking cessation
- **History**: **substernal chest pain** that may radiate to the left shoulder, arm, jaw, or back and lasts 1 to 5 minutes
- **Physical examination**: may be benign between episodes, an extra heart sound may be heard during episodes
- **Tests**:
  - Severity is determined by quantifying the degree of cardiac ischemia
  - **Exercise stress test**:
    - The patient exercises on an aerobic fitness machine at increasingly strenuous workloads while the heart rate and ECG are constantly monitored
    - The test is continued until the patient achieves 85% of the predicted maximum heart rate (i.e., approximately equal to [220 – patient age]) or the patient develops angina or signs of ischemia as seen on ECG
    - ST segment depression of at least 1 mm is indicative of ischemia
    - ST segment depression of at least 2 mm that is persistent for 5 minutes after cessation of the activity and is accompanied by a minimal increase in BP is indicative of severe disease
    - Ischemic heart disease is diagnosed with signs of **reproducible angina** or obvious signs of **ischemia at low workloads**
  - **Nuclear exercise test**: thallium-201 or technetium-99m-sestamibi is injected during exercise testing, and scintigraphy (planar or single-positron emission computed tomography [SPECT]) is performed to assess myocardial perfusion; it is used in cases of suspected ischemic heart disease in which the results of a regular exercise stress test are equivocal or if the performance of exercise is considered too risky for the patient (Color Figure 1-1)
  - **Exercise stress test with echocardiography**: exercise stress testing is performed in conjunction with echocardiography to increase the sensitivity of detecting myocardial ischemia
  - **Pharmacologic stress testing**: a cardiac inotrope (e.g., adenosine, dobutamine if there is comorbid pulmonary disease) is administered in place of exercise to increase myocardial demand; it is frequently performed in conjunction with a SPECT or performed in patients for whom comorbidities interfere with ability to perform exercise
  - **Positron emission tomography (PET) myocardial imaging**: injection of positron-emitting isotopes with subsequent three-dimensional detection imaging is performed to evaluate the heart for perfusion defects and tissue viability
  - **Cardiac catheterization with coronary angiography**: gold standard for identifying CAD, but more invasive than other techniques
- **Treatment**:
  - Control of comorbid risk factors (e.g., hypercholesterolemia, diabetes mellitus, HTN, smoking) is important to reduce the risk of worsening cardiac ischemia
  - **β-blockers**, **angiotensin-converting enzyme inhibitors** (ACE-I), and **calcium channel blockers** are all useful to decrease the workload of the heart (Table 1-2)
  - **Low-dose ASA** decreases the risk of progressive coronary thrombosis
  - **Sublingual nitroglycerin** may be taken as needed during episodes to reduce symptoms
  - Patients with multiple vessel disease or >50% occlusion of the left main coronary artery may require catheterized or surgical intervention
- **Outcomes**: prognosis is related to the ability to prevent progression of atherosclerosis and to control comorbid factors; left ventricle function and the degree of left coronary artery occlusion are the strongest predictors of long-term survival
- **Clues to the diagnosis**:
  - History: exertion-induced chest pain with radiation to the left side that resolves with rest
  - Physical: noncontributory
  - Tests: increased cholesterol, exercise stress test, and nuclear perfusion test results

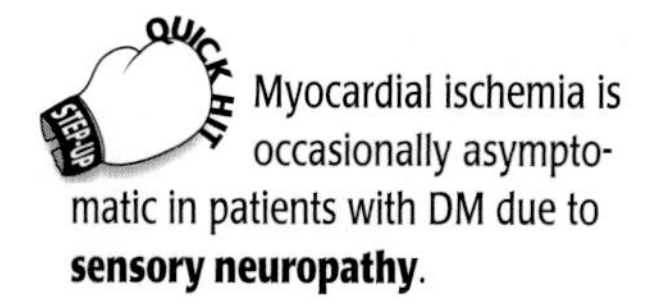

Myocardial ischemia is occasionally asymptomatic in patients with DM due to **sensory neuropathy**.

MNEMONIC

The differential diagnosis for **chest pain** may be remembered by the mnemonic **CHEST PAIN**: **C**ocaine/**C**ostochondritis, **H**yperventilation/**H**erpes zoster, **E**sophagitis/**E**sophageal spasm, **S**tenosis of aorta, **T**rauma, **P**ulmonary embolism/ **P**neumonia/**P**ericarditis/**P**ancreatitis, **A**ngina/**A**ortic dissection/ **A**ortic aneurysm, **I**nfarction (myocardial), **N**europsychiatric disease (depression).

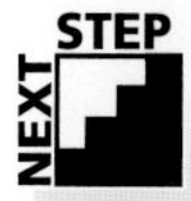

You must rule out a cardiac cause for chest pain with a formal stress test before considering alternative diagnoses.

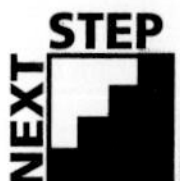

An inconclusive noninvasive perfusion workup in the presence of reversible myocardial ischemia is an indication for **cardiac catheterization**.

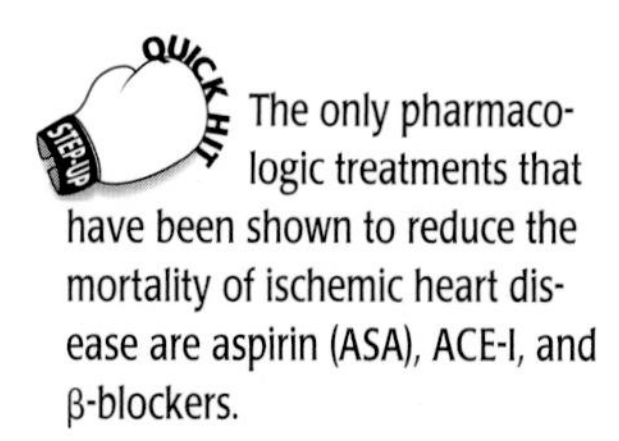

The only pharmacologic treatments that have been shown to reduce the mortality of ischemic heart disease are aspirin (ASA), ACE-I, and β-blockers.

TABLE 1-2 Common Medications Used in Ischemic Disease

Drug	Indications	Cardiovascular Benefits	Contraindications
ASA	MI prevention; during and after MI	Decreases thrombosis risk	High risk of GI bleeding
Clopidogrel	During angina and MI; after PTCA	Decreases thrombosis risk	High risk of GI bleeding
GP IIb/IIIa inhibitor (e.g., abciximab, eptifibatide)	During angina or MI; after PTCA or thrombolysis	Decreases thrombosis risk	High risk of GI bleeding, thrombocytopenia
Nitroglycerin	During angina and MI	Decreases venous pressure causing decrease in preload and end-diastolic volume; as a result, blood pressure, ejection time, and O_2 consumption decrease while contractility and heart rate increase	Significant hypotension
β-Blocker (e.g., metoprolol, atenolol)	MI prevention; during angina; during and post-MI	Decreases blood pressure, contractility, heart rate, and O_2 consumption; increases end-diastolic volume and ejection time; **decreases mortality** following MI	Long-term use with PVD, asthma, COPD, DM (may mask hypoglycemia), and depression (may worsen symptoms)
ACE-I (e.g., lisinopril, enalapril)	Post-MI	Decreases afterload leading to decreased O_2 consumption and blood pressure; **decreases mortality** following MI; particularly helpful with comorbid CHF or DM	Pregnancy
HMG-CoA reductase inhibitors (e.g., simvastatin, atorvastatin)	Post-MI	Decreases risk of atherosclerosis progression by lowering LDL level	Use of multiple lipid-lowering medications
Heparin	Immediately post-MI, inpatient setting	Decreases risk of thrombus formation	Active hemorrhage
Warfarin	Post-MI	Decreases risk of thrombus formation	Pregnancy, active hemorrhage
Morphine	During and immediately post-MI	No direct cardiac benefit, but decreases pain during MI leading to decreased heart rate, blood pressure, and O_2 consumption	Respiratory distress
Thrombolytics (e.g., t-PA, urokinase)	Immediately post-MI, inpatient setting	Breaks up thrombus; **decreases mortality** if used within 12 hr post-MI	High bleeding risk

ACE-I, angiotensin converting enzyme inhibitors; ASA, acetylsalicylic acid; CHF, congestive heart failure; COPD, chronic obstructive pulmonary disease; DM, diabetes mellitus; ECG, electrocardiogram; GI, gastrointestinal; LDL, low-density lipoprotein; MI, myocardial infarction; PTCA, percutaneous transluminal coronary angioplasty; PVD, peripheral vascular disease.

- **Unstable angina pectoris**
  - **Worsening angina** that occurs **at rest** and is due to **plaque rupture**, hemorrhage, or thrombosis in the coronary arteries
  - **History**: angina with any changes from the prior symptoms (e.g., worse pain, increased frequency, **symptoms at rest**, symptoms less responsive to prior treatment regimens)
  - **Physical examination**: tachycardia or bradycardia, extra heart sounds, murmurs, or rales may be heard on auscultation
  - **Tests**:
    - ECG typically demonstrates **ST interval depression** and T wave flattening or inversion (similar to episodes of stable angina but more pronounced)
    - Cardiac enzymes will likely show signs of cardiac distress (Figure 1-6)
    - Creatine phosphokinase myocardial fraction (CK-MB) increases 2 to 12 hours post-MI, peaks in 12 to 40 hours, and decreases in 24 to 72 hours

FIGURE 1-6 **Changes in cardiac enzymes following the onset of chest pain in unstable angina and ST-elevation myocardial infarction. The rise and fall of CK-MB (*solid line*), LDH (*dashed line*), and troponin-I (*dotted line*) follow different patterns. CK-MB, creatine phosphokinase myocardial fraction; LDH, lactate dehydrogenase.**

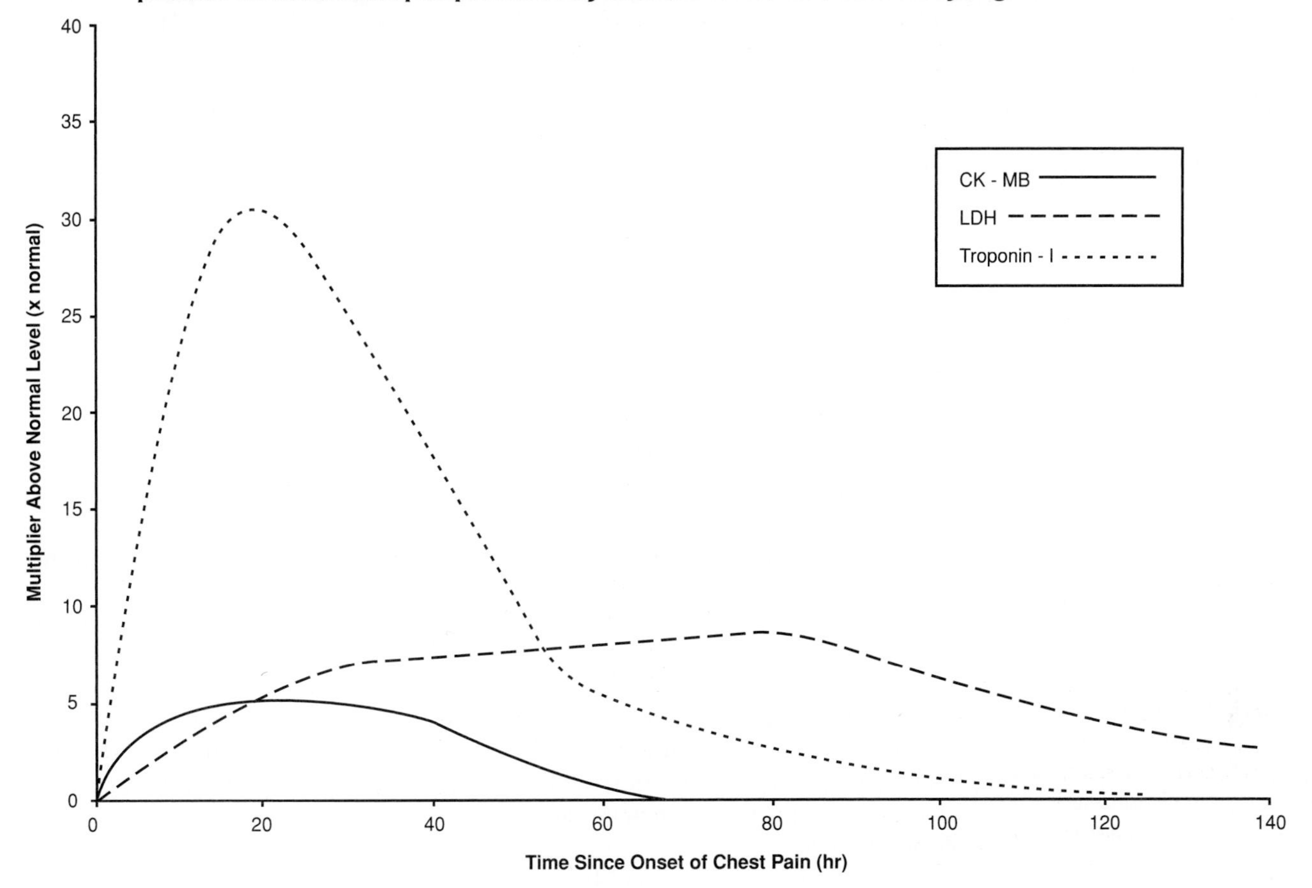

- Lactate dehydrogenase (LDH) increases in 6 to 24 hours and peaks in 3 to 6 days (rarely used for diagnosis)
- Troponin-I increases in 3 hours, peaks in 6 hours, and gradually decreases over 7 days
- Treatment:
  - Unstable angina is an indication for **admission** to the hospital
  - Antiplatelet therapy consisting of **ASA** and either **clopidogrel** (if no intervention is planned) or a glycoprotein **(GP) IIb/IIIA inhibitor** (if catheterized intervention is planned)
  - Heparin or low-molecular-weight heparin (LMWH) should be started to prevent thrombosis
  - O_2, nitroglycerin, β-blockers, ACE-I, and lipid-lowering drugs are administered to reduce cardiac workload
  - **Percutaneous transluminal coronary angioplasty (PTCA)**
    - Suggested in cases that are nonresponsive to medications
    - A catheter is inserted through a femoral or brachial artery and maneuvered through the heart to the stenotic vessel
    - A balloon on the catheter is inflated to dilate the stenosis
    - Catheters may also be used for arthrectomy (i.e., plaque is shaved by a burr on the catheter) or stent placement (i.e., intravascular support structure)
  - **Coronary artery bypass grafting (CABG)**
    - Considered for left main stenosis >50%, three-vessel disease, or a history of CAD and DM
    - A donor vessel is grafted to the coronary artery to bypass the obstruction

Any patient admitted to the hospital with suspected unstable angina or myocardial infarction must be worked up with **serial ECGs** and **cardiac enzymes** to elucidate the evolution of cardiac ischemia or to rule out the process.

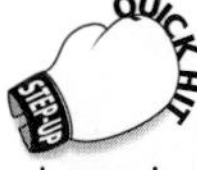

Tight **glycemic control** is important to improving outcomes in **diabetic** patients following unstable angina.

TABLE 1-3 Thrombolysis in Myocardial Infarction (TIMI) Risk Score

Risk Criteria[1]	Cumulative Score	Rate of Adverse Event (%)[2]
• Age ≥65 years	0 or 1	4.7
• 3+ risk factors for CAD (Figure 1-5)	2	8.3
• Prior coronary occlusion ≥50%	3	13.2
• ST interval depression or elevation on admission	4	19.9
• 2+ episodes of angina in past 24 hr	5	26.2
• Elevated cardiac enzymes	6 or 7	40.9
• Use of ASA with past 7 days		

ASA, aspirin; CAD, coronary artery disease.

[1]Value of 1 given if criteria present, 0 if criteria absent.

[2]Defined as death, new or recurrent MI, or recurrent ischemia requiring revascularization.

- The saphenous vein and internal mammary artery are most commonly used
- **Outcomes**:
  - Short-term prognosis is frequently predicted by the thrombolysis in myocardial infarction (TIMI) risk score (Table 1-3)
  - Long-term prognosis is best predicted by EF and the degree of residual ischemia detected on posttherapy stress testing
  - Up to 10% of patients will have a myocardial infarction or will die within 6 months following the onset of new unstable angina
- **Why eliminated from differential**: the reversible nature of symptoms and the ECG changes and the normal cardiac enzymes are most consistent with stable angina and do not meet the definition of unstable angina

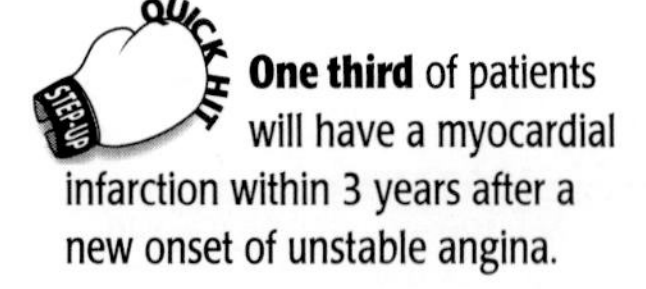

One third of patients will have a myocardial infarction within 3 years after a new onset of unstable angina.

- **Panic disorder**
  - More thorough discussion in Chapter 13
  - **Why eliminated from differential**: the direct relation of symptoms to exertion is more suggestive of a cardiac nature, and stress testing confirms the cardiac cause; the symptomatology does not meet the *Diagnostic and Statistical Manual of Mental Disorders* 4th edition (*DSM-IV*) criteria for panic disorder
- **Esophagitis/gastritis/reflux disease**
  - More thorough discussion in Chapter 3
  - **Why eliminated from differential**: substernal chest pain may be seen in all of these conditions, and reflux may worsen with exertion, but the reversible nature of the symptoms is less consistent with a gastrointestinal (GI) etiology, and the stress test results further rule out these diagnoses

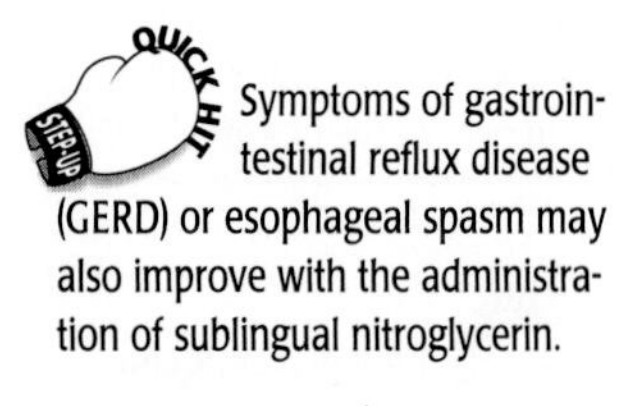

Symptoms of gastrointestinal reflux disease (GERD) or esophageal spasm may also improve with the administration of sublingual nitroglycerin.

- **Pulmonary embolism**
  - More thorough discussion in Chapter 2
  - **Why eliminated from differential**: the normal pulse oximetry, normal CXR, and reversible nature of the symptoms and ECG changes argue against this diagnosis
- **Pericarditis**
  - More thorough discussion in later case
  - **Why eliminated from differential**: although both conditions feature anterior chest pain that may be associated with dyspnea, the absence of diffuse ST elevations (ST **depression** is seen in this case), absence of pericardial effusion on the echocardiogram, absence of pericardial signs (e.g., friction rub, improvement in pain with leaning forward), and the stress test findings all argue against this diagnosis
- **Aortic dissection**
  - More thorough discussion in later case
  - **Why eliminated from differential**: for this diagnosis one would expect to find sudden constant "ripping" chest pain and mediastinal widening on the CXR, neither of which were present in this case

CASE 1-3 "I have severe tightness in my chest!"

A 79-year-old woman is brought to an emergency department by her son with a complaint of significant tightness in her chest for a half hour. The patient says she was watching TV when the tightness started. She says the pain is in the center of her chest and feels like she is being squeezed too tightly. She says the pain radiates into her face. She feels very worried and is having some problems catching her breath. She feels slightly sick to her stomach. She denies any vomiting, syncope, paresthesias, or paralysis. She says that she has a history of high BP and heart disease (diagnosed from pharmacologic stress test 3 years ago) for which she takes an ACE-I and nitroglycerin as needed. She has had a few episodes of milder chest pain in the past month that responded to sublingual nitroglycerin. She has taken three nitroglycerin tablets on this occasion but has had no relief of her symptoms. On examination, she appears to be in moderate distress and is diaphoretic. Auscultation detects tachypneic breathing with faint bibasilar rales, tachycardia, and an extra heart sound. Her abdomen is nontender and soft. Her neurologic examination is normal. The following vital signs are measured:

T: 97.9°F, HR: 110 bpm, BP: 90/70 mm Hg, RR: 24 breaths/min

Differential Diagnosis

- Myocardial infarction, unstable angina, pericarditis, aortic dissection, pneumothorax, pulmonary embolism, upper GI pathology

Laboratory Data and Other Study Results

- Pulse oximetry: 95% on room air, 99% on 2L O_2 via nasal cannula
- CBC: WBC: 9.9, Hgb: 13.1, Plt: 240
- Chem10: Na: 143 mEq/L, K: 3.4 mEq/L, Cl: 103 mEq/L, CO_2: 32 mEq/L, BUN: 25 mg/dL, Cr: 1.1 mg/dL, Glu: 90 mg/dL, magnesium (Mg): 1.9 mg/dL, Calcium (Ca): 10.2 mg/dL, Phosphorus (Phos): 3.0 mg/dL
- Cardiac enzymes: creatine kinase (CK): 290 U/L, CK-MB: 4.5 ng/mL, troponin-I: 0.3 ng/mL
- ECG: sinus tachycardia; 3 mm ST interval elevation, Q waves, and T wave inversions in leads I, aVL, and V_2 to V_6
- CXR: normal heart shadow, slight midlung and bibasilar infiltrates

Diagnosis

- Myocardial infarction, anterolateral wall

Treatment Administered

- O_2 via nasal cannula was continued, and intravenous (IV) fluids with K were initiated
- ASA, eptifibatide (a GP IIb/IIIa inhibitor), metoprolol, captopril, morphine, and IV heparin were administered
- One additional dose of sublingual nitroglycerin was administered
- The patient was rushed to cardiac catheterization and found to have an 80% occlusion of the left anterior descending artery; angioplasty was performed (heparin stopped afterward)

Follow-up

- The patient had symptomatic improvement following intervention
- Repeat cardiac enzymes in 8 and 16 hours demonstrated progressive increases in CK-MB and troponin levels

- Repeat ECGs over several days demonstrated the gradual normalization of ST intervals with maintenance of the abnormal Q waves
- The patient stabilized and gradually was weaned from IV medications
- A nuclear stress test performed prior to her discharge demonstrated a limited irreversible defect in the anterolateral cardiac wall
- The patient's outpatient medication regimen on discharge included ASA, clopidogrel, metoprolol, lisinopril, and atorvastatin
- The patient experienced a recurrent severe episode of chest pain 3 months after the episode described ab1ove, cardiac arrest occurred, and patient was unable to be resuscitated

Steps to the Diagnosis

- Myocardial infarction (MI)
  - Cardiac tissue death resulting from ischemia caused by the **occlusion of coronary arteries** or vasospasm
    - It is often secondary to thrombus formation following plaque rupture
  - **Risk factors**: increased age, HTN, hypercholesterolemia, family history of CAD, DM, and tobacco use, male gender, postmenopausal status
  - **History**: chest pain (tightness or "**elephant on chest**") in the same distribution as prior anginal pain, dyspnea, diaphoresis, nausea, and vomiting
  - **Physical examination**: tachycardia, hypotension, pulmonary rales, new S_4 heart sound, new systolic murmur
  - Tests:
    - **Cardiac enzymes** (typically performed three times, every 6 to 8 hours) will show progressive increases and follow general trends (Figure 1-6)
    - ECG shows **ST elevation**, T wave changes, and possible new arrhythmia, left bundle branch block (LBBB), or pathologic Q waves (Figure 1-7 and Table 1-4)
    - CXR may show pulmonary edema
  - Treatment:
    - Acute

QUICK HIT: **CK-MB** is considered by some to be the first positive test in the initial 24 hours post-MI, but **troponin I** is considered the most overall sensitive test within 7 days following an MI.

QUICK HIT: Because general CK will be increased with significant muscular trauma or degradation, **CK-MB** is a better indicator of cardiac muscle damage.

FIGURE 1-7 **Acute myocardial infarction shown on an electrocardiogram. Note the ST elevation in leads V_2 to V_5 suggesting anterior wall involvement.**

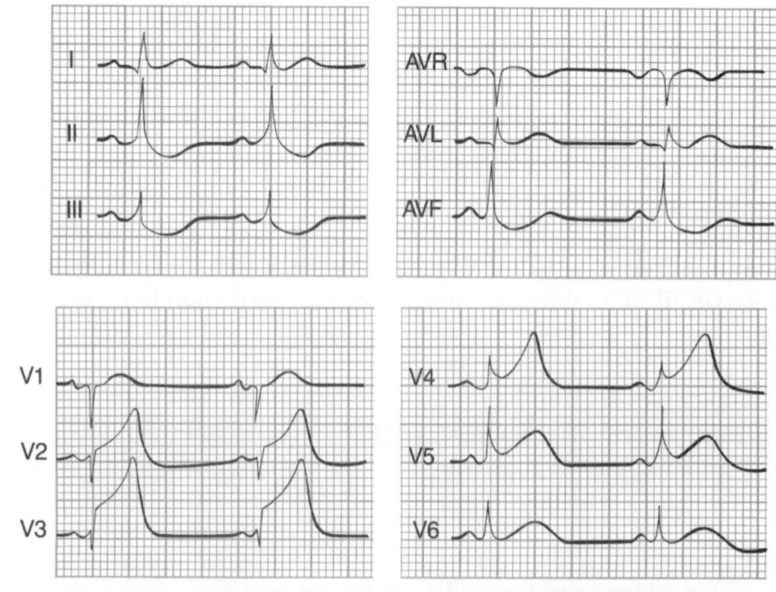

(Taken from Thaler MS. *The only EKG book you'll ever need.* 5th ed. Philadelphia: Lippincott Williams & Wilkins; 2007, p. 242. Used with permission of Lippincott Williams & Wilkins.)

TABLE 1-4 Relation of ECG Changes to Location of Infarct

ECG Leads With Changes	Area of Infarct	Coronary Artery Branch
V_2, V_3, V_4	Anterior	Left anterior descending
V_1, V_2, V_3	Septal	Left anterior descending
II, III, aVF	Inferior	Posterior descending or marginal branch
I, aVL, V_4, V_5, V_6	Lateral	Left anterior descending or circumflex
V_1, V_2 (frequent comorbid inferior MI)	Posterior	Posterior descending

ECG, electrocardiogram; MI, myocardial infarction.

- Give O_2, ASA, clopidogrel or a GP IIb/IIIa inhibitor, **β-blockers**, ACE-I, **nitroglycerin**, **morphine** (pain control may decrease cardiac demand); achieve tight glycemic control in diabetics with insulin; administer potassium and magnesium to keep levels above 4.0 mEq/L and 2.0 mEq/L, respectively
- Consider thrombolysis (e.g., tissue plasminogen activator (t-PA), urokinase) or angioplasty if the patient presents in the initial 12 hours after the start of an MI
- Heparin should be administered for up to 48 hours to reduce thrombus risk (if angioplasty is performed, stop heparin after the procedure)
- If the patient is hypotensive, stop nitroglycerin and give IV fluids
- Give antiarrhythmics for frequent premature ventricular complex (PVCs) contractions or ventricular tachycardia (Vtach)

MNEMONIC

Treatment for MI may be remembered by the mnemonic **BeMOAN**: **Be**ta-blocker, **M**orphine, **O**$_2$, **A**SA/ACE-I, **N**itroglycerin.

- **Subacute**
  - Perform a **stress test** 5 days post-MI to assess future risk; if the test is suggestive of an increased risk for repeat MI, perform cardiac catheterization to measure vessel patency and consider possible PTCA or CABG if significant occlusion is found
- **Long term**
- Risk reduction medications should include **low-dose ASA or clopidogrel, β-blockers, ACE-I**, K-sparing diuretic, and a beta-hydroxy-beta-methylglutaryl-coenzyme A (HMG-CoA) reductase
- Exercise, smoking cessation, and dietary modifications are also important for risk reduction
- **Outcomes**: there is a 30% acute mortality with 50% of survivors being rehospitalized within 1 year and 10% dying within 1 year; complications include infarct extension, arrhythmias, myocardial dysfunction, papillary muscle necrosis, wall rupture, aneurysm, mural thrombus, pericarditis, and **Dressler syndrome** (i.e., fever, pericarditis, and increased erythrocyte sedimentation rate [ESR] 2 to 4 weeks post-MI)
- **Clues to the diagnosis**:
  - History: severe sudden chest pain radiating to the face, history of heart disease
  - Physical: tachycardia, extra heart sound
  - Tests: ECG findings

- **Unstable angina**
  - More thorough discussion in prior case
  - **Why eliminated from differential**: the presentations may be similar, but the greater severity of symptoms, changes in cardiac enzymes and ECG findings (e.g., ST elevation, not depression), and the presence of an irreversible defect on follow-up nuclear stress testing all suggest that MI is the diagnosis
- **Pericarditis**
  - More thorough discussion in later case
  - **Why eliminated from differential**: ST elevation may be seen in both, but the severity of symptoms, positive cardiac enzymes, and nuclear stress test findings are all more consistent with MI

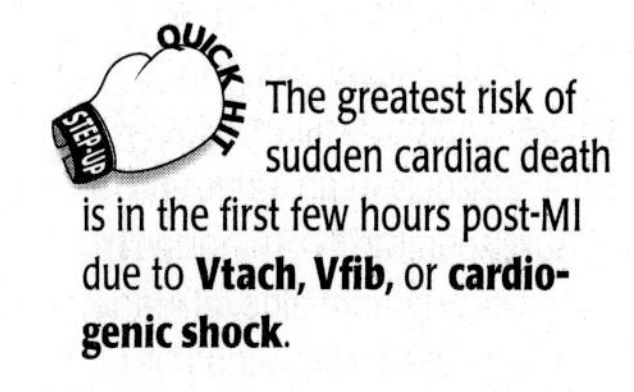

The greatest risk of sudden cardiac death is in the first few hours post-MI due to **Vtach, Vfib,** or **cardiogenic shock**.

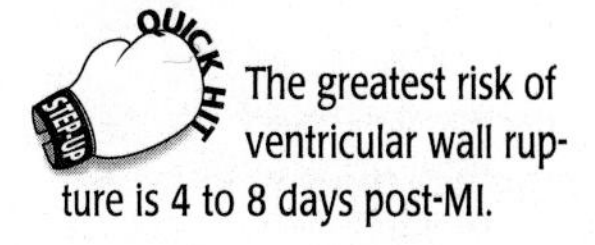

The greatest risk of ventricular wall rupture is 4 to 8 days post-MI.

- **Aortic dissection**
  - More thorough discussion in later case
  - **Why eliminated from differential**: both will have chest pain, but aortic dissection will have a normal ECG and will not feature the cardiac enzyme and stress test changes seen in this case
- **Pneumothorax**
  - More thorough discussion in Chapter 2
  - **Why eliminated from differential**: the CXR in this case does not show collapsed lung fields, and the ECG, cardiac enzyme, and stress test findings in this case would not be expected for this diagnosis
- **Pulmonary embolism**
  - More thorough discussion in Chapter 2
  - **Why eliminated from differential**: some degree of desaturation may be seen in both conditions, but the ECG, cardiac enzyme, and stress test findings would not be expected for this diagnosis
- **Upper GI pathology** (e.g., gastritis, esophagitis)
  - More thorough discussion in Chapter 3
  - **Why eliminated from differential**: chest pain may be common to both, but the ECG, cardiac enzyme, and stress test findings would not be expected for this diagnosis

CASE 1-4 "I'm following up for my heart medication"

A 58-year-old man presents to his cardiologist in follow-up for his ischemic heart disease. He has a history of stable angina that has been treated with a regimen of ASA, atenolol, enalapril, and simvastatin, and nitroglycerin as needed. He had experienced a couple of anginal episodes in the previous month that were treated by increasing the dose of his atenolol. He is following up at this time to make sure that he has had no new episodes since his last appointment. He reports no new episodes of angina and no new problems. On examination, he appears comfortable. His lung fields sound clear. Chest auscultation finds a slightly irregular, slow-sounding heart rate and no extra heart sounds. His peripheral pulses are strong with a similar irregularity. His abdomen is nontender with normal bowel sounds. A neurovascular examination is normal and includes palpable pulses in all four extremities. The following vital signs are measured:

T: 98.6°F, HR: 60 bpm, BP: 105/80 mm Hg, RR: 14 breaths/min

Differential Diagnosis

- Bradycardia, heart block (first, second, third degree)

Laboratory Data and Other Study Results

- Chem10: Na: 142 mEq/L, K: 3.6 mEq/L, Cl: 103 mEq/L, CO_2: 28 mEq/L, BUN: 15 mg/dL, Cr: 0.8 mg/dL, Glu: 90 mg/dL, Mg: 2.1 mg/dL, Ca: 10.0 mg/dL, Phos: 3.0 mg/dL
- ECG: HR 60 bpm; progressive lengthening of PR interval with occasional skipped QRS intervals

Diagnosis

- Second-degree heart block, Mobitz I (i.e., Wenckebach block)

Treatment Administered

- The patient's dose of atenolol was decreased slightly

Follow-up

- The patient was seen 1 week after starting the new dosing of atenolol
- The patient continued to have no symptoms, and a repeat ECG demonstrated normal sinus rhythm

Steps to the Diagnosis

- Heart block
  - Impaired myocardial contraction that occurs when electrical impulses encounter tissue that is electronically unexcitable and result in arrhythmia
  - **Variants**
    - **First degree**: caused by increased vagal tone or functional conduction impairment
    - **Second degree, Mobitz I** (i.e., Wenckebach): caused by **intranodal** or His bundle conduction defect, drug effects (e.g., β-blockers, digoxin, calcium channel blockers), or increased vagal tone
    - **Second degree, Mobitz II**: cause is an **infranodal** conduction problem in the bundle of His or Purkinje fibers
    - **Third degree** (i.e., complete): cause is an **absence** of conduction between the atria and ventricles
  - **History**: all first- and second-degree variants are generally asymptomatic, but patients with third-degree block have syncope and dizziness
  - **Physical examination**: some irregularity in the heart rate may be detected, but third-degree block is more irregular and also is associated with hypotension
  - **Tests**:
    - **First degree** – ECG shows PR longer than 0.2 sec (Figure 1-8A)
    - **Second degree, Mobitz I** (i.e., Wenckebach): **progressive PR lengthening** until a skipped QRS occurs; PR progression then resets and begins again (Figure 1-8B)
    - **Second degree, Mobitz II: randomly skipped QRS** without changes in the PR interval (Figure 1-8C)
    - **Third degree** (i.e., complete): no relationship between P waves and QRS (Figure 1-8D)
  - **Treatment**:
    - **First degree**: none required
    - **Second degree, Mobitz I** (i.e., Wenckebach): adjust doses of medication associated with heart block; no other treatment required unless symptomatic bradycardia (treat with pacemaker)
    - **Second degree, Mobitz II**: ventricular pacemaker
    - **Third degree** (i.e., complete): avoid medications affecting atrioventricular conduction; insert ventricular pacemaker
  - **Outcomes:** reversible first-degree and second-degree block are benign; patients with irreversible second- or third-degree block are at an increased risk of developing ventricular arrhythmias but do very well if treated with a pacemaker
  - **Clues to the diagnosis**:
    - History: recent increase in atenolol dose
    - Physical: slow heart rate
    - Tests: ECG findings
- Sinus bradycardia
  - Heart rate below 50 bpm due to an increased vagal tone or nodal disease
  - **Risk factors**: history of CAD, advanced age
  - **History**: typically asymptomatic with occasional weakness or syncope
  - **Physical examination:** noticeably slow heart rate on auscultation
  - Tests: ECG demonstrates sinus rhythm slower than 50 bpm
  - **Treatment**: stop precipitating medications; pacemaker required if irreversible and symptomatic
  - **Outcomes:** irreversible cases carry a predisposition to the development of other arrhythmias
  - **Why eliminated from differential**: the ECG in this case was pathognomonic for second-degree block Mobitz I and was not a sinus rhythm

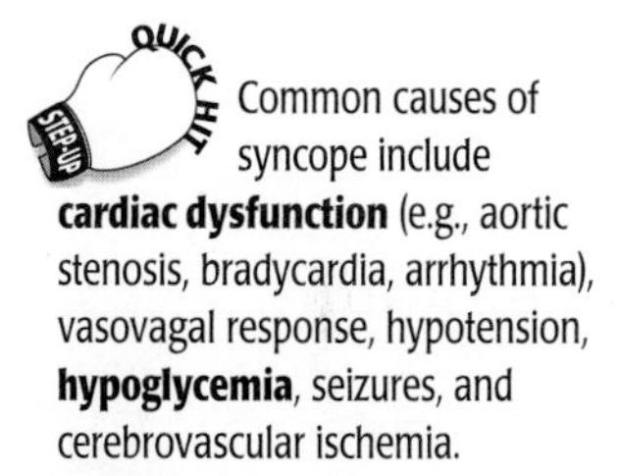

Common causes of syncope include **cardiac dysfunction** (e.g., aortic stenosis, bradycardia, arrhythmia), vasovagal response, hypotension, **hypoglycemia**, seizures, and cerebrovascular ischemia.

MNEMONIC

Common presentations of syncope may be remembered by the mnemonic **SUCH DROPS**: **S**eizures, **U**nexplained (50% presentations), **C**ardiac, **H**ypoglycemia, **D**rugs, **R**eflex mechanisms (vasovagal response), **O**rthostasis (hypotension), **P**sychogenic, **S**troke.

FIGURE 1-8 **(A) Primary heart block: regular PR interval prolongation without skipped QRS. (B) Secondary Mobitz I heart block: progressive lengthening of the PR interval until QRS is skipped. (C) Secondary Mobitz II heart block: regular PR interval with random skipped QRS. (D) Tertiary heart block: no relationship between P waves and QRS.**

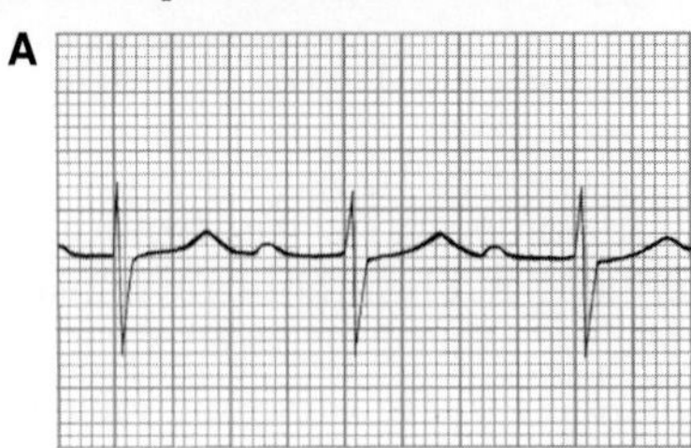

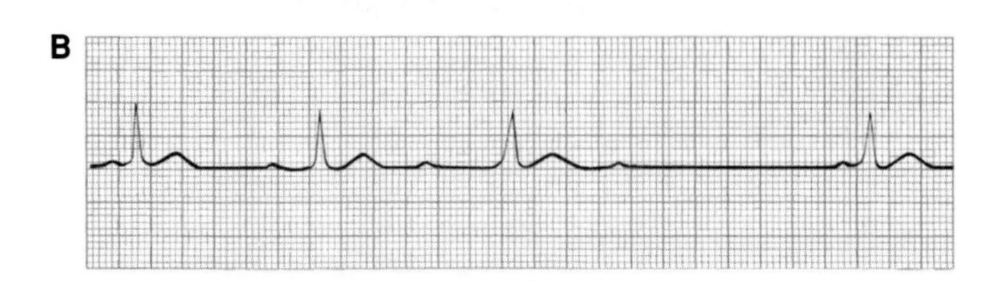

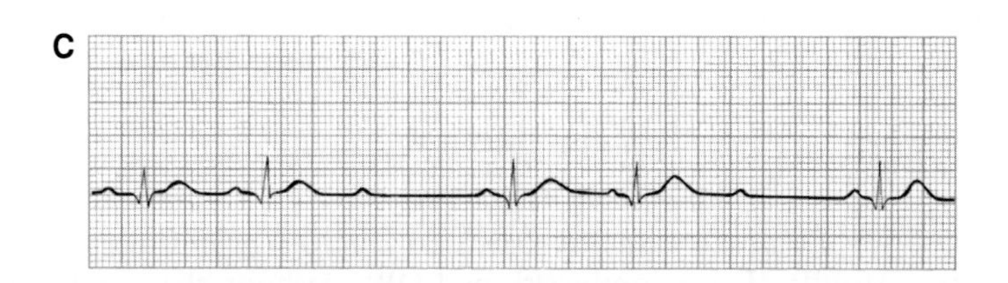

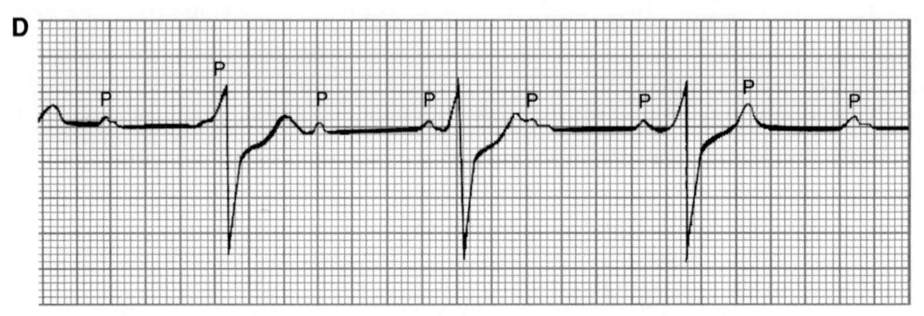

(Taken from Thaler MS. *The only EKG book you'll ever need.* 5th ed. Philadelphia: Lippincott Williams & Wilkins; 2007, pp. 157, 161, 164. Used with permission of Lippincott Williams & Wilkins.)

CASE 1-5 "My mother feels that her heart is racing"

A 75-year-old woman is an inpatient at a hospital 2 days after a successful femoral-popliteal artery bypass. This surgery was performed because of significant atherosclerotic peripheral vascular disease causing severely impeded blood flow to her right leg. The patient has done well since the completion of surgery. While her daughter is visiting her, the patient describes the sudden feeling that her heart is racing. She denies chest pain, dizziness, or difficulty breathing. She says that this experience has never happened previously. She has a history of peripheral vascular disease, HTN, and mild CAD. Her medications include ASA, clopidogrel (started postoperatively), metoprolol, and enalapril. Prior to surgery she was taking pentoxifylline but stopped postoperatively. She was a heavy smoker for several years but quit 2 years ago. On examination, she appears to be slightly nervous. Her lung fields sound clear. Auscultation of the chest reveals a rapid heart beat with significant irregularity; there are no extra heart sounds. The remainder of her examination is normal. The following vital signs are measured:

T: 98.9°F, HR: 120 bpm, BP: 145/83 mm Hg, RR: 18 breaths/min

Differential Diagnosis

- Atrial fibrillation, paroxysmal supraventricular tachycardia, multifocal atrial tachycardia, atrial flutter

Laboratory Data and Other Study Results

- CBC: WBC: 10.1, Hgb: 9.8, Plt: 310
- Chem10: Na: 139 mEq/L, K: 3.8 mEq/L, Cl: 108 mEq/L, CO_2: 24 mEq/L, BUN: 17 mg/dL, Cr: 1.1 mg/dL, Glu: 93 mg/dL, Mg: 1.9 mg/dL, Ca: 10.1 mg/dL, Phos: 3.1 mg/dL
- Coags: PT: 13 sec, INR: 1.1, PTT: 43 sec
- ECG: HR 120 bpm but highly irregular rate; no discernible P waves in tracing

Diagnosis

- Atrial fibrillation

Treatment Administered

- 20 mEq K, 1 mg Mg, and 5 mg metoprolol IV were all administered following review of the ECG
- Transfusion of one unit of packed red blood cells (PRBCs) was started
- An additional 5 mg IV metoprolol was administered when patient failed to convert to sinus rhythm following first dose

Follow-up

- The patient converted into sinus rhythm following the second dose of metoprolol
- The patient's K was maintained at 4.0 mEq/L, Mg was maintained at 2.0 mg/dL, and Hgb was maintained at 10.0
- The patient's dose of metoprolol was titrated to maintain regular sinus rhythm and reduce BP
- The patient remained in sinus rhythm for the remainder of the admission and was discharged home on an appropriate dose of β-blocker
- The patient was followed closely postoperatively to confirm no recurrent episodes of atrial fibrillation

Steps to the Diagnosis

- **Atrial fibrillation (Afib)**
  - A lack of coordinated atrial contractions with independent sporadic ventricular contractions
    - Due to rapid, disorderly firing from a second atrial focus
  - **Risk factors**: left atrial enlargement, **CAD** (particularly MI), **HTN**, **anemia**, valvular disease, pericarditis, chronic obstructive pulmonary disease, pulmonary embolism **hyperthyroidism**, rheumatic heart disease (RHD), sepsis, alcohol use, electrolyte abnormalities (e.g., Mg, phosphorus, K, calcium)
  - **History**: possibly asymptomatic or dyspnea, chest pain, and palpitations
  - **Physical examination: irregularly irregular** pulse and heart beat
  - Tests: ECG shows no discernible P waves and an irregular QRS rate (Figure 1-9)
  - **Treatment**:
    - **Rate control** via calcium channel blockers, β-blockers, or digoxin (Table 1-5)

MNEMONIC

Common risk factors for Afib are remembered by the mnemonic **CHAPTERS**: **C**oronary artery disease, **H**ypertension, **A**nemia, **P**ulmonary disease, hyper**T**hyroid, **E**thanol, **R**heumatic heart disease, and **S**epsis.

FIGURE 1-9 **Atrial fibrillation—irregular QRS rate and no discernible P waves.**

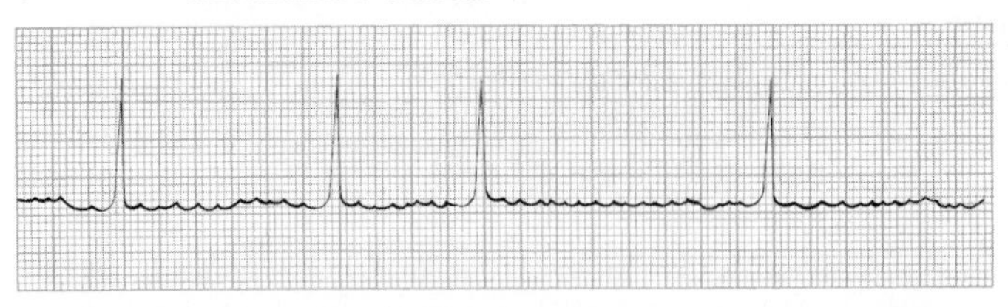

(Taken from Thaler MS. *The only EKG book you'll ever need.* 5th ed. Philadelphia: Lippincott Williams & Wilkins; 2007, p. 128. Used with permission of Lippincott Williams & Wilkins.)

- The initial attempt at rate control and cardioversion is 5 mg IV metoprolol
- IV metoprolol may be repeated twice before attempting to control the rate with IV diltiazem
- **Anticoagulation** (i.e., heparin, then warfarin) is frequently required unless the arrhythmia is identified and treated within 24 hours of onset
- **Electric cardioversion**
  - Electric cardioversion may be performed if the presentation is within the initial 2 days
  - Cardioversion may be performed in delayed presentations if an absence of thrombi is confirmed by transesophageal echocardiogram (TEE)
  - If the patient presents after 2 days or if thrombus is seen on echocardiogram, then anticoagulate and wait 3 to 4 weeks before attempting cardioversion
- AV nodal ablation may be considered for recurrent cases

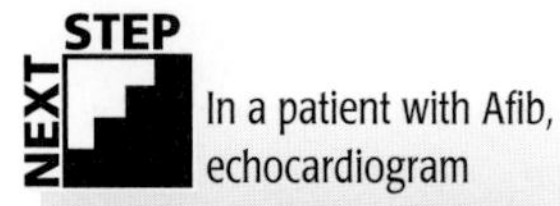

In a patient with Afib, echocardiogram should be performed **before** cardioversion to rule out mural thrombus formation.

- **Outcomes**:
  - Complications include increased risk of MI, heart failure, and mural thrombus formation due to atrial blood stasis
  - Dislodgement of a mural thrombus may cause stroke
  - The risk of complications correlates with the amount of time not spent in normal sinus rhythm
- **Clues to the diagnosis**:
  - History: sudden palpitations
  - Physical: irregularly irregular heart rate
  - Tests: ECG findings

TABLE 1-5 **Classes of Antiarrhythmic Medications**

Class	General Mechanism of Action	Examples	Potential Uses
IA	Na channel blockers (prolong action potential)	Quinidine, procainamide	PSVT, Afib, Aflutter, Vtach
IB	Na channel blockers (shorten action potential)	Lidocaine, tocainide	Vtach
IC	Na channel blockers (no effect on action potential)	Flecainide, propafenone	PSVT, Afib, Aflutter, PSVT
II	β-blockers	Propanolol, esmolol, metoprolol	PVC, PSVT, Afib, Aflutter, Vtach
III	K channel blockers	Amiodarone, sotalol, bretylium	Afib, Aflutter, Vtach (not bretylium)
IV	Calcium-channel blockers	Verapamil, diltiazem	PSVT, MAT, Afib, Aflutter
Other	K channel activation, decrease in intracellular cAMP	Adenosine	PSVT

Afib, atrial fibrillation; Aflutter, atrial flutter; cAMP, cyclicadenosine monophosphate; K, potassium; MAT, multifocal atrial tachycardia; Na, sodium; PSVT, paroxysmal supraventricular tachycardia; PVC, premature ventricular contraction; Vtach, ventricular tachycardia.

FIGURE 1-10 **Mechanism of atrioventricular nodal reentry tachycardia. (A) Action potential reaches division in conduction pathway with both fast and slow fibers. (B) Conduction proceeds quickly down fast pathway to reach distal fibers and also proceeds up slow pathway in retrograde fashion. (C) Impulse returns to original division point after fibers have repolarized allowing a reentry conduction loop and resultant tachycardia. AV, atrioventricular.**

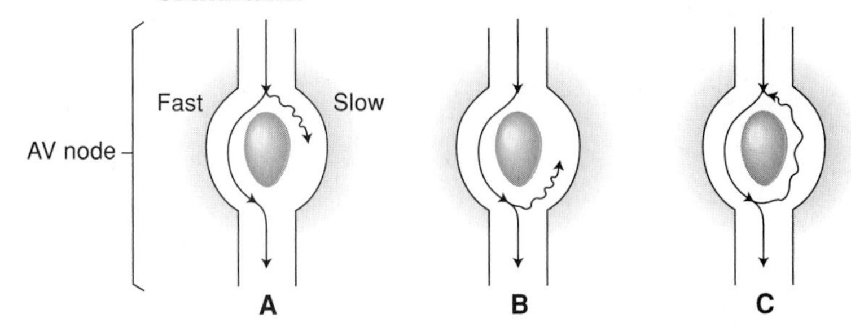

- **Paroxysmal supraventricular tachycardia (PSVT)**
  - Tachycardia (i.e., HR >100 bpm) arising in the atria or atrioventricular (AV) junction
    - Occurs most commonly in **young** patients with otherwise **healthy** hearts
    - Cause frequently is **reentry** anomaly
      - **AV nodal reentry**: presence of both slow and fast conduction pathways in AV node; conduction proceeds quickly through the fast pathway and progresses up slow pathway in retrograde fashion to create a conduction loop and reentrant tachycardia (Figure 1-10)
      - **AV reentry** as found in **Wolff-Parkinson-White (WPW) syndrome**: similar to AV nodal reentry, but instead of fast and slow pathways existing in the AV node, a separate accessory conduction pathway exists between the atria and ventricles that returns a conduction impulse to the AV node to set up a reentry loop (Figure 1-11)
  - **History**: sudden palpitations, possible dyspnea or syncope
  - **Physical examination**: sudden onset of tachycardia
  - **Tests**: ECG shows P waves hidden in T waves, normal QRS morphology, and rate 150 to 250 bpm; ECG shows a delta wave (i.e., slurred upstroke of the QRS) and a shortened PR interval in cases of WPW syndrome (Figure 1-12)
  - **Treatment**: carotid massage or Valsalva maneuver may halt an acute arrhythmia, but cardioversion (frequently using a calcium channel blocker) is required in cases of hemodynamic instability; pharmacologic therapy (e.g., adenosine or calcium channel

FIGURE 1-11 **Mechanism of atrioventricular reentry tachycardia as seen for Wolff-Parkinson-White syndrome. (A) Action potential passes through the AV node and encounters an accessory pathway during conduction to the ventricles. (B) Accessory pathway conducts action potential back to AV node. (C) Return of secondary action potential to AV node completes reentry loop and results in tachycardia. AV, atrioventricular node; AP, accessory pathway.**

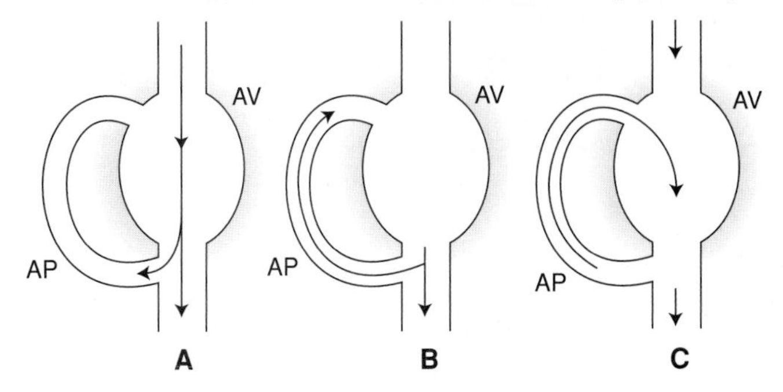

FIGURE 1-12 **Wolff-Parkinson-White syndrome on electrocardiogram. Note the presence of delta waves, slurred upstrokes preceding each QRS that are characteristic of the condition.**

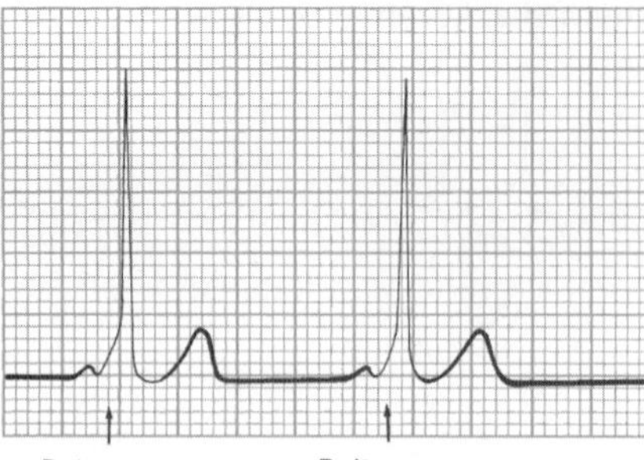

(Taken from Thaler MS. *The only EKG book you'll ever need.* 5th ed. Philadelphia: Lippincott Williams & Wilkins; 2007, p. 197. Used with permission of Lippincott Williams & Wilkins.)

QUICK HIT: Antiarrhythmics other than class IA or IC are contraindicated for WPW syndrome because they may speed up conduction through the accessory pathway.

blocker for AV nodal reentrant tachycardia and adenosine or type IA or IC antiarrhythmic for WPW syndrome) or **catheter ablation** of accessory conduction pathways is frequently used for long-term control in symptomatic patients (Table 1-5)

- **Outcomes**: structural cardiac anomalies may contribute to the development of other arrhythmias; risk of sudden cardiac death is minimal
- **Why eliminated from differential**: the ECG in the case is highly suggestive of Afib, and the clinical scenario (i.e., elderly patient with HTN, anemia, and CAD) is more consistent with AFib than PSVT

- **Multifocal atrial tachycardia (MAT)**
  - Tachycardia caused by several ectopic foci in the atria that discharge automatic impulses (i.e., multiple pacemakers), which causes tachycardia
  - **History**: usually asymptomatic
  - **Physical examination:** tachycardia detected on pulse monitoring and heart auscultation
  - **Tests:** ECG shows tachycardia with a HR >100 bpm and a **variable morphology** of P waves (at least three varieties) (Figure 1-13)
  - **Treatment:** calcium channel blockers or β-blockers acutely; catheter ablation or surgery may be performed to eliminate abnormal pacemakers
  - **Outcomes:** persistent untreated tachycardia may lead to cardiomyopathy
  - **Why eliminated from differential**: the ECG in the case is diagnostic for Afib and does not show the P wave findings expected for MAT

FIGURE 1-13 **Multifocal atrial tachycardia (MAT). Note the variety in the shape of P waves and PR intervals and the irregular ventricular rate.**

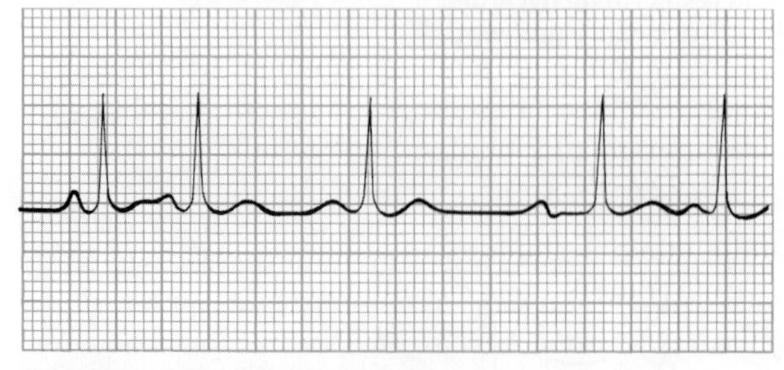

(Taken from Thaler MS. *The only EKG book you'll ever need.* 5th ed. Philadelphia: Lippincott Williams & Wilkins; 2007, p. 129. Used with permission of Lippincott Williams & Wilkins.)

FIGURE 1-14 **Atrial flutter—rapid sawtooth P waves preceding QRS.**

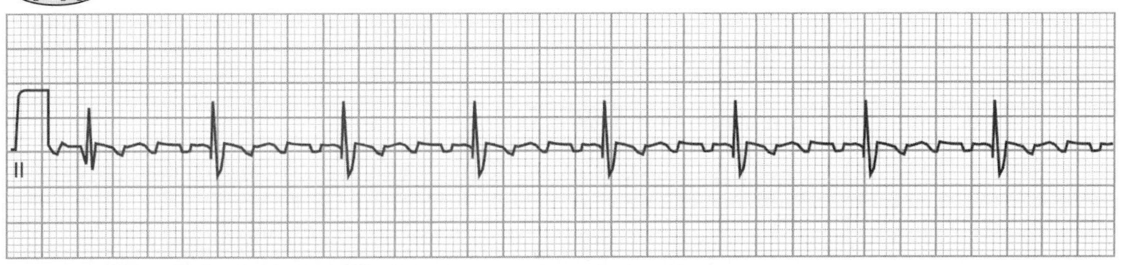

(Taken from Thaler MS. *The only EKG book you'll ever need.* 5th ed. Philadelphia: Lippincott Williams & Wilkins; 2007, p. 303. Used with permission of Lippincott Williams & Wilkins.)

- **Atrial flutter (Aflutter)**
  - Tachycardia due to the rapid firing of an ectopic focus in the atria in a distinct pattern
  - **Risk factors**: CAD, congestive heart failure (CHF), chronic obstructive pulmonary disease (COPD), valvular disease, pericarditis
  - **History**: possibly asymptomatic, possible palpitations or syncope
  - **Physical examination:** rapid regular tachycardia
  - Tests: ECG shows regular tachycardia >150 bpm with a set ratio of P waves to QRS and a **sawtooth pattern of P waves** (Figure 1-14)
  - **Treatment:**
    - **Rate control** with calcium channel blockers or β-blockers
    - Electrical or chemical (class IA, IC, or III antiarrhythmics) cardioversion should be performed if unable to control the rate with medication
    - Catheter ablation may be performed to remove an ectopic focus in some cases
  - **Outcomes:** cases in which successful catheter ablation is performed have rare recurrence; stroke is a possible complication when anticoagulation is not prescribed in cases with delayed treatment
  - **Why eliminated from differential**: ECG in this case is diagnostic for Afib and does not show the characteristics typical of Aflutter

CASE 1-6 "My husband just collapsed!"

A 68-year-old man is an inpatient on the medicine service following a moderate MI. He initially presented to the emergency department with chest pain and was found to have mild ST interval elevation in his anterior ECG leads. He was treated pharmacologically and was stabilized on a regimen of ASA, metoprolol, captopril, and nitroglycerin. A nuclear stress test performed 5 days following admission demonstrated a new area of irreversible ischemia in the anterior cardiac wall. Subsequent cardiac catheterization detected a 65% occlusion of the main left coronary artery that was treated with angioplasty and stenting. His telemetry has been stable for several days, and his cardiac enzymes have begun to trend downward. He was scheduled to be discharged to a cardiac rehabilitation facility today or tomorrow. During a visit, his wife runs to the nurses' station to tell them that her husband had gotten out of bed to go to the bathroom when he suddenly collapsed. When the response team enters the room, they find the patient lying on the ground next to his bed. On examination, he is anxious-appearing, pale, and interacts poorly with the medical team. Chest auscultation detects shallow, rapid breathing and a rapid heart rate. A faint pulse is detectable, and his fingers have minimal capillary refill. Following this initial assessment, the patient becomes unresponsive without respiration or a palpable pulse. The following vital signs are measured:

T: 97.9°F, HR: 150 bpm, BP: 90/60 mm Hg, RR: 24 breaths/min initially then 0 breaths/min

Differential Diagnosis

- Ventricular tachycardia, premature ventricular complexes, ventricular fibrillation, pulseless electrical activity, asystole, PSVT, Afib, Aflutter, MAT

Laboratory Data and Other Study Results

- STAT arterial blood gas with electrolytes (Super Gas): pH: 7.37, partial pressure of oxygen (pO_2): 80 mm Hg, pCO_2: 48 mm Hg, Bicarb: 23 mEq/L, O_2 sat: 86%, Hgb: 13.1, Na: 135 mEq/L, K: 3.4 mEq/L, Cl: 108 mEq/L, Glu: 85 mg/dL, Ca: 9.8 mg/dL
- ECG: HR 150; regular rate; wide QRS intervals; no apparent relation between P waves and QRS intervals

Diagnosis

- Pulseless ventricular tachycardia

Treatment Administered

- The cardiac arrest protocol was initiated, and the patient was intubated and bag ventilated
- Defibrillation was attempted with 200 J shock; no response
- Defibrillation was repeated with 300 J shock leading to the return of spontaneous contractions and circulation
- The patient was transferred to the cardiac intensive care unit (CICU) to continue close cardiac monitoring, K repletion, and titration of antiarrhythmic medications

Follow-up

- Cardiac enzymes demonstrated continued elevation of cardiac enzymes with slow trend downward
- An internal defibrillator was implanted to prevent recurrent episodes of ventricular arrhythmia
- The patient was eventually able to be discharged to cardiac rehabilitation

Steps to the Diagnosis

- **Ventricular tachycardia (Vtach)**
  - Series of **three or more** premature ventricular beats with HR 160 to 240 bpm
  - **Risk factors**: **CAD**, prior MI
  - **History**: possibly asymptomatic if brief or palpitations, syncope, hypotension, impaired consciousness, and dyspnea
  - **Physical examination: tachycardia**, tachypnea, loss of pulse as cardiac output worsens
  - **Tests:** ECG shows series of regular, wide QRS intervals independent of P waves (Figure 1-15)

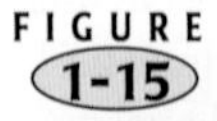

Torsades de pointes is Vtach with a sine wave morphology that carries a poor prognosis and may rapidly convert to Vfib; Mg may be useful in its treatment.

FIGURE 1-15 **Ventricular tachycardia—wide, rapid QRS with no discernible P waves.**

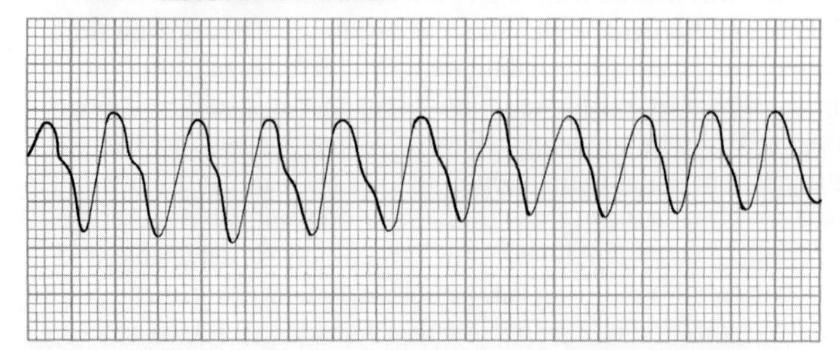

(Taken from Thaler MS. *The only EKG book you'll ever need.* 5th Ed. Philadelphia: Lippincott Williams & Wilkins; 2007, p. 134. Used with permission of Lippincott Williams & Wilkins.)

FIGURE 1-16 **Assessment and initial treatment protocol for the unresponsive patient. CPR, cardiopulmonary resuscitation; EMS, emergency medical services; PEA, pulseless electrical activity; Vfib, ventricular fibrillation; Vtach, ventricular tachycardia.**

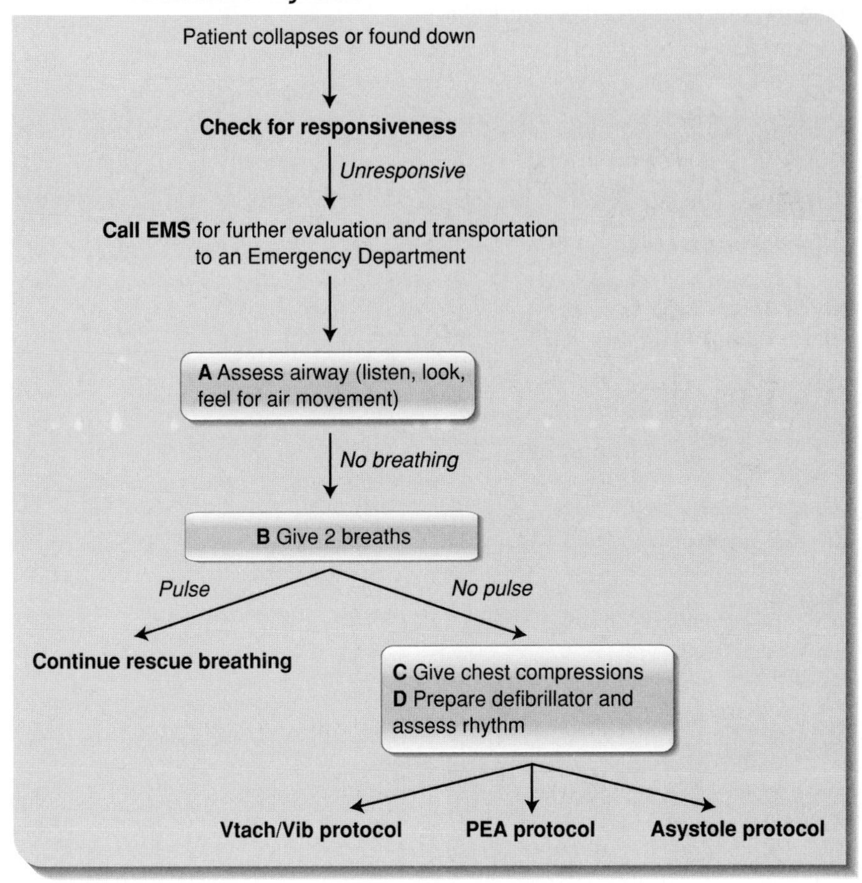

- **Treatment**:
  - Any minimally responsive or unresponsive patient necessitates initiation of the advanced cardiac life support (ACLS) protocol (Figure 1-16)
  - Pulseless Vtach requires defibrillation and/or **antiarrhythmic medications** (Figure 1-17)
  - Vtach **with a pulse** is treated with antiarrhythmic medications alone
  - **Conscious** patients should be treated with **antiarrhythmic medications** (class IA, IB, II, or III)
  - Recurrent Vtach requires ablation of an ectopic focus of signal or the implantation of an **internal defibrillator** (senses ventricular arrhythmia and automatically releases electric pulse to restore normal rhythm)
- **Outcomes**: prognosis correlates with the degree of cardiac infarction at the time of onset; approximately 30% rate of sudden cardiac death within 2 years of onset
- **Clues to the diagnosis**:
  - History: recent MI, sudden collapse
  - Physical: tachycardia, tachypnea progressing to no breathing, pulselessness
  - Tests: ECG findings

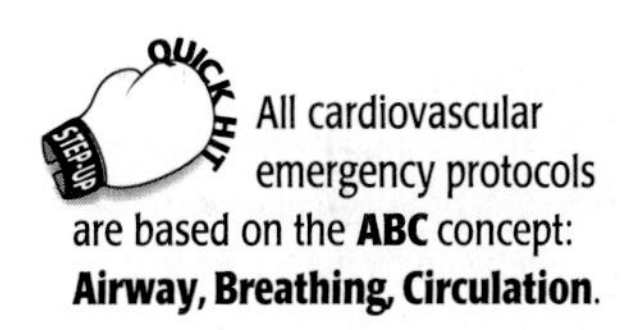

All cardiovascular emergency protocols are based on the **ABC** concept: **Airway, Breathing, Circulation**.

- **Ventricular fibrillation (Vfib)**
  - Lack of ordered ventricular contraction that leads to **no cardiac output** and is rapidly fatal
  - **Risk factors**: CAD, recent MI, recent Vtach
  - **History**: chest pain and palpitations followed by syncope and impaired consciousness
  - **Physical examination**: hypotension, pulselessness, lack of respirations, poorly discernible heart sounds

FIGURE 1-17 **Treatment protocol for ventricular fibrillation or pulseless ventricular tachycardia. ABC, airway, breathing, circulation; CPR, cardiopulmonary resuscitation; IV, intravenous; Vfib, ventricular fibrillation; Vtach, ventricular tachycardia.**

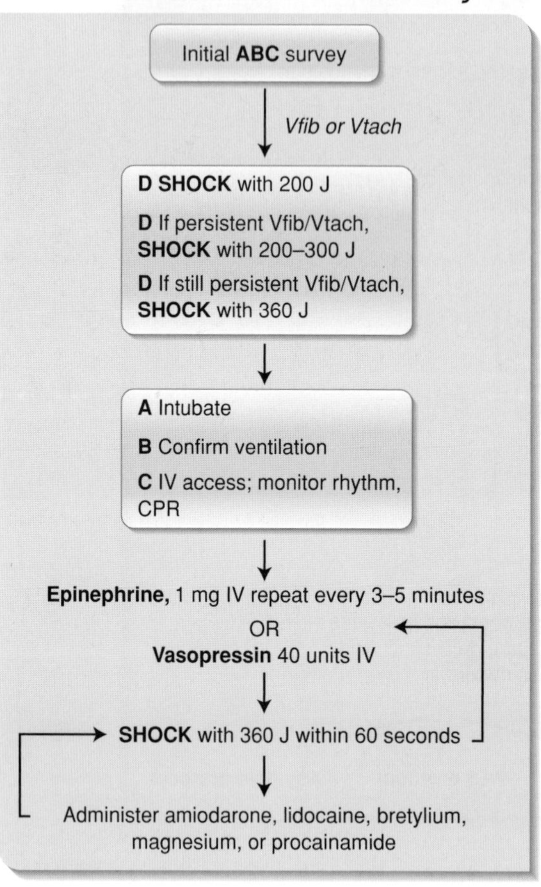

MNEMONIC

The treatment protocol for Vfib or Vtach may be remembered by the mnemonic "**S**hock, **S**hock, **S**hock, **E**verybody **S**hock, **A**nybody **S**hock, **L**ittle **S**hock, **B**ig **S**hock, **M**ama Shock, **P**apa **S**hock, **B**aby **S**hock": **S**hock (200 J)→**S**hock (300 J)→**S**hock (360 J)→**E**pinephrine→**S**hock (360 J)→**A**miodarone→**S**hock→**L**idocaine→**S**hock→**B**retylium→**S**hock→**M**agnesium→**S**hock→**P**rocainamide→**S**hock→**B**icarbonate (sodium)→**S**hock.

- **Tests**: ECG shows **totally erratic tracing with no P waves or QRS intervals** (Figure 1-18)
- **Treatment**: **immediate cardiopulmonary resuscitation** with electric (+/− pharmacologic) defibrillation (Figure 1-17); implantation of an internal defibrillator is needed by patients at a high risk for recurrence
- **Outcomes**: poorer prognosis with high recurrence rate if occurring more than 48 hours after a MI; acute survivorship decreases with delays to treatment or an inability to restore a stable cardiac output

FIGURE 1-18 **Depicts initial torsades de pointes with degeneration into ventricular fibrillation.**

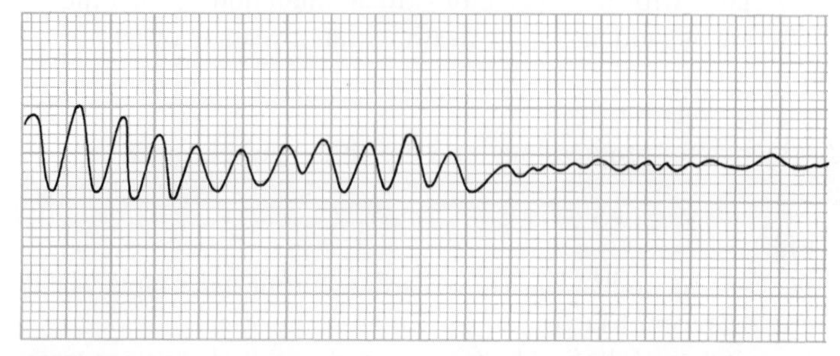

(Taken from Thaler MS. *The only EKG book you'll ever need.* 5th ed. Philadelphia: Lippincott Williams & Wilkins; 2007. p. 135. Used with permission of Lippincott Williams & Wilkins.)

- **Why eliminated from differential**: the ECG in this case demonstrated intact QRS intervals and was not erratic as would be expected for Vfib; given the pulseless nature of the patient in this case, it is quite possible that a transition to Vfib would soon occur
- **Premature ventricular complexes (PVCs)**
  - Isolated ectopic beats from a ventricular origin
    - Frequently benign; may be caused by hypoxia, abnormal serum electrolyte levels, hyperthyroidism, caffeine use
  - **History**: usually asymptomatic, but possible palpitations or syncope
  - **Physical examination:** ectopic beat may be heard if auscultation is performed at time of ectopy
  - **Tests**: ECG shows early and wide QRS without a preceding P wave that is followed by a brief pause in conduction
  - **Treatment:**
    - None is necessary if the patient is healthy
    - Replenish low K or Mg levels
    - Consider β-blockers in patients with CAD
  - **Outcomes:** may be a precursor to more severe arrhythmias in patients with CAD
  - **Why eliminated from differential**: the maintained series of wide QRS intervals seen on the ECG in this case defines the difference between PVCs (only a few isolated ectopic beats) and Vtach (a series of ectopic beats)
- **Pulseless electrical activity (PEA)**
  - Loss of a pulse and no signs of systemic circulation in the presence of recordable cardiac electrical activity
  - **History**: syncope, unresponsiveness
  - **Physical examination**: absent pulse, respiratory arrest, no discernable heart beats, hypotension
  - **Tests**: ECG will demonstrate some form of electrical activity (e.g., several morphologies of QRS intervals and T waves)
  - **Treatment**: pharmacologic cardioversion (Figure 1-19)

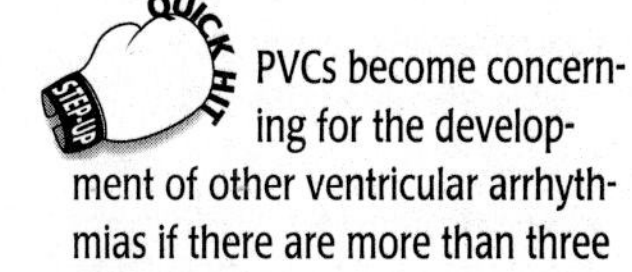

PVCs become concerning for the development of other ventricular arrhythmias if there are more than three PVC/min.

MNEMONIC

Common causes of PEA may be remembered by the **6 Hs** and **4 Ts**: **H**ypovolemia, **H**ypoxia, **H**yperkalemia, **H**ypokalemia, **H**ypomagnesemia, **Hydrogen** ions (acidosis), **T**ension PTX, **T**hrombosis (CAD or PE), **T**ablets (drugs) **T**amponade (cardiac).

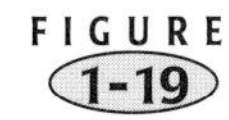

FIGURE 1-19 **Treatment protocol for pulseless electrical activity. ABC, airway, breathing, circulation; CPR, cardiopulmonary resuscitation; IV, intravenous.**

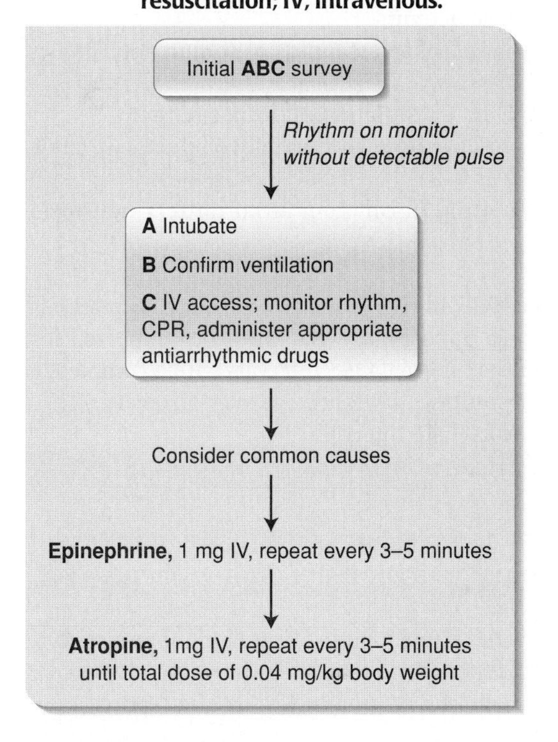

FIGURE 1-20 **Treatment protocol for asystole. ABC, airway, breathing, circulation; CPR, cardiopulmonary resuscitation; IV, intravenous.**

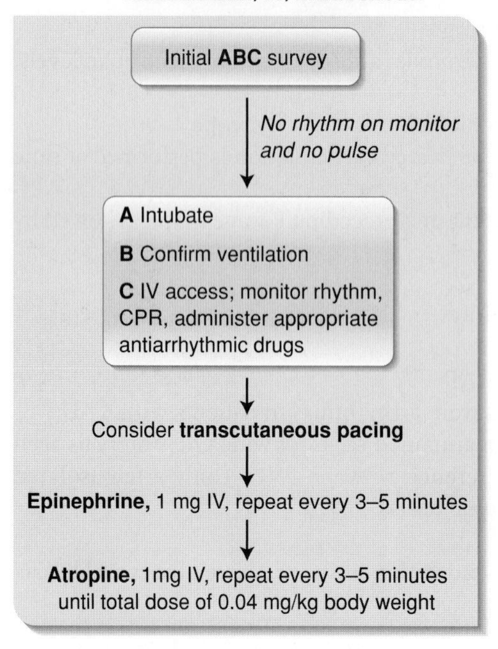

MNEMONIC

For pulseless electrical activity, think **PEA**: **P**ulseless→**E**pinephrine and **A**tropine.

- **Outcomes**: poor prognosis without rapid correction
- **Why eliminated from differential**: despite the pulseless nature of the patient in this case, the ECG displaying regular wide QRS intervals is indicative of Vtach (i.e., more organized than PEA)

- Asystole
  - Absence of any electric cardiac activity
  - **History**: syncope, unresponsiveness
  - **Physical examination**: no signs of circulation, respiratory arrest, no heart sounds, hypotension
  - **Tests**: ECG shows **absence of any electrical activity**
  - **Treatment**: transcutaneous pacing or pharmacologic stimulus of contraction (Figure 1-20)
  - **Outcomes**: poor prognosis without immediate restoration of cardiac output
  - **Why eliminated from differential**: the presence of electric activity on the ECG in this case rules out this diagnosis
- **Paroxysmal supraventricular tachycardia, atrial fibrillation, atrial flutter, multifocal atrial tachycardia**
  - More thorough discussion in prior case
  - **Why eliminated from differential**: the ECG in this case shows wide QRS intervals indicative of a ventricular arrhythmia as opposed to what would be expected for PSVT (i.e., narrow QRS intervals), Afib (i.e., normal QRS intervals with a completely irregular rate), Aflutter (i.e., pattern of multiple sawtooth P waves for every QRS), and MAT (i.e., variable P waves with normal QRS intervals)

QUICK HIT Cardiac arrest lasting more than ten minutes without any cardiac output is generally considered consistent with severe brain injury or brain death.

CASE 1-7 "I've been having a hard time breathing since 2 days ago"

A 63-year-old man presents to the emergency department with a complaint of progressive dyspnea over the past 2 days. He says that he first noticed this symptom at night when trying to sleep and required extra pillows to help him breathe easier. He also reports feeling more tired than usual and coughing frequently. He denies recent illness, fevers, dizziness, chest pain, nausea, vomiting, or neurologic symptoms. He says that he has a "bad heart" for which he takes a couple of medications. He ran out of his medications 1 week ago and did not refill them because "they make [him] go to the bathroom too much." He does not remember the names of his medications. He drinks two alcoholic beverages about 4 days per week. On examination, he is in moderate distress. He pauses often during the history to catch his breath. He has notable distension of his neck veins to the level of his mandibular angle. Auscultation detects decreased breath sounds bilaterally with diffuse rales that are more pronounced in the lung bases. He has an extra heart sound and a palpable impulse near his left axillary line. Slight hepatomegaly is palpable. He has 2+ edema in both legs. His neurologic examination is normal. The following vital signs are measured:

T: 98.4°F, HR: 90 bpm, BP: 160/95 mm Hg, RR: 26 breaths/min

Differential Diagnosis

- Heart failure, unstable angina, MI, chronic obstructive pulmonary disease, pneumonia, idiopathic pulmonary fibrosis

Laboratory Data and Other Study Results

- Pulse oximetry: 92% on room air, 98% on 4L O_2 via nasal cannula
- CBC: WBC: 7.6, Hgb: 13.5, Plt: 320
- Chem10: Na: 137 mEq/L, K: 4.2 mEq/L, Cl: 107 mEq/L, CO_2: 22 mEq/L, BUN: 30 mg/dL, Cr: 1.3 mg/dL, Glu: 102 mg/dL, Mg: 1.9 mg/dL, Ca: 9.5 mg/dL, Phos: 3.3 mg/dL
- Cardiac enzymes: CK: 235 U/L, CK-MB: 2.1 ng/mL, troponin-I: 0.2 ng/mL
- Liver function tests (LFTs): alkaline phosphatase (AlkPhos): 130 U/L, alanine aminotransferase (ALT): 65 U/L, aspartate aminotransferase (AST): 50 U/L, total bilirubin (TBili): 1.3 mg/dL, Direct bilirubin (DBili): 0.3 mg/dL, Indirect bilirubin (IBili): 1.0 mg/dL
- Brain natriuretic peptide (BNP): 610 pg/mL
- ECG: HR: 90 bpm; QRS intervals in I and V_1 to V_5 with >30 mm amplitude; no ST interval changes
- CXR: cardiomegaly; bilateral hilar and basilar fluffy infiltrates; increased marking of pulmonary vessels

Diagnosis

- Congestive heart failure with acute exacerbation due to medical noncompliance

Treatment Administered

- The patient was admitted for respiratory support and diuresis
- O_2 was administered to keep his O_2 saturation above 97%
- Intravenous furosemide was administered to induce diuresis
- A review of medical records notes the current pharmacologic regimen of furosemide, enalapril, atenolol, ASA, and digoxin; the patient was restarted on his outpatient medications

Follow-up

- The patient experienced significant diuresis following the initiation of furosemide and experienced symptomatic improvement
- The patient was discharged to home following symptomatic improvement and improvements in BNP level, CXR appearance, and O_2 saturation
- The patient was educated about the importance of medications, low-salt diet, and recognition of exacerbations

Steps to the Diagnosis

- Congestive heart failure (CHF)
  - Progressive decrease in cardiac output due to systolic and/or diastolic dysfunction
    - Left-sided pathology
      - Left ventricle **unable to produce adequate CO**
      - Blood backs up leading to pulmonary edema that eventually causes pulmonary HTN
      - Progressive **left ventricular hypertrophy (LVH)** to compensate for poor output causes eventual failure because the heart is unable to keep pace with systemic need for CO
    - Right-sided pathology
      - Increased pulmonary vascular resistance leads to **right ventricular hypertrophy (RVH)**, hepatojugular reflux, and systemic venous stasis with associated edema
      - **Most commonly due to left-sided failure** (Eisenmenger syndrome); also may be due to unrelated pulmonary HTN, valvular disease, or congenital defects
      - **Risk factors**: CAD, HTN, valvular disease, cardiomyopathy, COPD, drug toxicity, alcohol use
  - **History**: fatigue, dyspnea on exertion, orthopnea, paroxysmal nocturnal dyspnea, nocturia, cough; symptoms are more severe during exacerbations
  - **Physical examination:** displaced point of maximum impulse, S_3 heart sound, jugular vein distention (JVD), peripheral edema, hepatomegaly
  - **Tests**:
    - **Plasma brain natriuretic peptide (BNP)** and N-terminal pro-BNP will be increased with left ventricle dysfunction
    - Liver enzymes (e.g., ALT, AST) are frequently increased and are a sign of congestive hepatomegaly and cardiac-induced cirrhosis
    - BUN and Cr are slightly elevated with a BUN: Cr ratio >20 and suggest chronic decreased cardiac output and poor renal perfusion
    - ECG may show signs of ventricular hypertrophy (e.g., increased QRS amplitude, heart block, low baseline voltage)
    - CXR shows cardiac enlargement, **Kerley B lines** (i.e., increased marking of lung interlobular septa due to pulmonary edema), and **cephalization of pulmonary vessels** (i.e., increased marking of superior pulmonary vessels due to congestion and stasis)
    - Echocardiogram is useful to assess heart chamber size and function (i.e., can help differentiate systolic and diastolic dysfunction)
  - **Treatment**:
    - CHF due to **systolic** dysfunction
      - First medications given are typically **loop diuretics** (decrease heart preload) and either **ACE-I** or angiotensin receptor blockers (ARB) (decrease preload and afterload and increase cardiac output)
      - β-blockers may be added once a stable ACE-I dose is prescribed and should not be administered during acute exacerbations
      - Digoxin (increases contractility) may be added to the regimen to improve symptoms but has not demonstrated an ability to improve mortality
      - **Spironolactone** or vasodilators may be added for persistent symptoms
    - CHF due to **diastolic** dysfunction
      - BP is controlled with calcium channel blockers, ACE-I, or ARB
      - β-blockers are useful to control the heart rate and to decrease cardiac workload in stabilized patients
      - K-sparing diuretics should be given to reduce cardiac hypertrophy caused by aldosterone
    - Recombinant BNP (i.e., nesiritide) has been shown to improve outcomes during severe acute exacerbations
    - Underlying conditions should be treated
    - The patient should adhere to a low-salt diet
    - Progressive cases may require cardiac transplant or implantation of an assistive device (indicated for an ejection fraction below 35%)

QUICK HIT: COPD may lead to right-side hypertrophy that ends in right-sided failure (i.e., **cor pulmonale**)

QUICK HIT: The presence of an S_3 extra heart sound is the most consistent finding of CHF

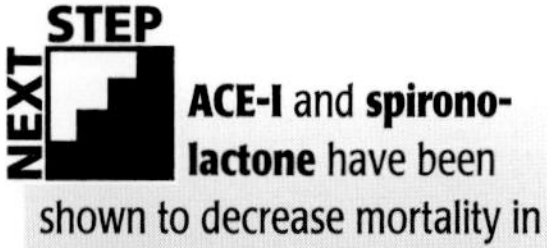

NEXT STEP: **ACE-I** and **spironolactone** have been shown to decrease mortality in CHF and should be incorporated into the treatment plan when appropriate, as other medications have not been proven to reduce mortality.

MNEMONIC: Frequent causes of CHF exacerbations are remembered by the mnemonic **A SMITH PEAR**: **A**nemia, **S**alt, **MI**, **I**nfection, **T**hyroid (high or low), **H**TN, **P**ericarditis, **E**ndocarditis, **A**rrhythmia, **R**x (not taking medications).

- **Outcomes**:
  - Approximately half of patients with CHF will eventually die from a ventricular arrhythmia
  - Hospital admission is associated with up to a 20% mortality rate
  - Mortality increases to 40% in the presence of a comorbid MI and 80% in the presence of hypotension
- **Clues to the diagnosis**:
  - History: dyspnea, nocturnal dyspnea, orthopnea, recent medication noncompliance
  - Physical: tachypnea, rales and decreased breath sounds on auscultation, jugular venous distention, hepatomegaly, peripheral edema
  - Tests: mildly elevated LFTs, increased BNP, CXR appearance, increased lead amplitude on ECG

- **Unstable angina/MI**
  - More thorough discussion in prior case
  - **Why eliminated from differential**: the absence of suggestive ECG changes and normal cardiac enzymes despite the 2-day history of symptoms rules out these diagnoses
- **Chronic obstructive pulmonary disease (COPD)**
  - More thorough discussion in Chapter 2
  - **Why eliminated from differential**: the patient does not have the characteristic appearance of a COPD patient, CXR is not consistent with COPD, and BNP levels suggest a heart failure etiology
- **Pneumonia**
  - More thorough discussion in Chapter 2
  - **Why eliminated from differential**: the lack of fevers or an elevated WBC count argue against this diagnosis, and the BNP level and ECG appearance suggest a cardiac etiology
- **Idiopathic pulmonary fibrosis (IPF)**
  - More thorough discussion in Chapter 2
  - **Why eliminated from differential**: the CXR in the case is less consistent with IPF than CHF, the onset of symptoms is too rapid for progression of IPF, and the BNP level and ECG appearance suggest a cardiac etiology

CASE 1-8 "I was advised to see you by my insurance company"

A 30-year-old woman presents to a cardiologist for assessment of a heart murmur. As part of the application for a life insurance policy, she was required to see a general internist for a history and physical. The only abnormal finding on the examination was the presence of a blowing murmur during chest auscultation. The insurance company doctor advised her to follow-up with her regular physician or a cardiologist. Because she has been in good health and has not seen a physician for several years, she elected to see a cardiologist to assess the cause of the murmur. She describes herself as a healthy individual and has had no medical problems besides an occasional cold for the past 10 years. She sees a gynecologist on a yearly basis but has not seen an internist for over 10 years. She denies any dizziness, syncope, chest pain, palpitations, gastrointestinal symptoms, or neurologic symptoms. She exercises about three times per week and has not noticed any significant dyspnea beyond what she considers normal. She takes no medications besides a multivitamin. She drinks alcohol socially. On examination, she is a healthy appearing, normal weight patient in no distress. Her lung fields are clear bilaterally. Chest auscultation detects an audible blowing holosystolic murmur that radiates from the cardiac apex to the axilla, a faint extra heart sound, and appreciable splitting of her second heart sound. She has no edema or abnormal findings in any of her extremities. Her neurologic examination is normal. The following vital signs are measured:

T: 98.4°F, HR: 72 bpm, BP: 110/80 mm Hg, RR: 14 breaths/min

Differential Diagnosis

- Mitral regurgitation, mitral stenosis, aortic regurgitation, aortic stenosis, pulmonary stenosis

Laboratory Data and Other Study Results

- ECG: normal sinus rhythm; normal wave morphology and amplitude
- CXR: possible left atrial and ventricular enlargement but otherwise normal findings
- Echocardiogram: prolapse of the mitral valve leaflets with associated mild mitral regurgitation; left atrium and ventricle size within upper half of normal range; normal EF (65%)

Diagnosis

- Mitral regurgitation due to mitral valve prolapse

Treatment Administered

- The patient was placed on daily low-dose ASA
- The patient was prescribed prophylactic antibiotics to be taken prior to any intervention with a risk of bleeding (e.g., dental procedures)
- She was permitted unrestricted activity

Follow-up

- The patient was reassessed in 6 months and then every year to follow for any worsening in her condition

Steps to the Diagnosis

- **Mitral regurgitation** (MR)
  - Incompetency of the mitral valve due to degeneration or local myocardial dysfunction that allows **backflow** of blood into the **left atrium**
    - Common causes include mitral valve prolapse (i.e., "floppy" valve), **RHD**, papillary muscle dysfunction, endocarditis, and left ventricle dilation
    - Most commonly a chronic condition
  - **History**: asymptomatic in early and mild cases, palpitations, dyspnea on exertion, orthopnea, and paroxysmal nocturnal dyspnea seen in worse cases
  - **Physical examination**: harsh blowing holosystolic murmur radiating from apex to axilla, S_3, widely split S_2, midsystolic click (Figure 1-21)

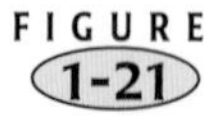

FIGURE 1-21 **Common murmurs associated with valvular diseases.**

Diagram	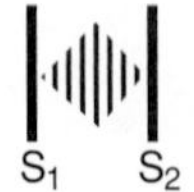 S_1 S_2	S_1 S_2	S_1 S_2	S_2 S_1	S_2 S_1
Murmur Type	Systolic ejection	Pansystolic	Late systolic	Early diastolic	Mid/late diastolic
Examples	Aortic stenosis Pulmonic stenosis	Mitral regurgitation Tricuspid regurgitation	Mitral valve prolapse	Aortic regurgitation Pulmonic regurgitation	Mitral stenosis
Location & Radiation	2nd right interspace→neck (but may radiate widely) 2nd-3rd left interspace	Apex→axilla Left lower sternal border →right lower sternal border	Apex→axilla	Along left side of sternum Upper left side of sternum	Apex

(Modified from Lilly LS. *Pathophysiology of heart disease.* 2nd ed. Baltimore: Williams & Wilkins; 1998. Used with permission of Lippincott Williams & Wilkins.)

FIGURE 1-22 **Apical view echocardiogram demonstrating mitral valve prolapse with associated mitral regurgitation. Both mitral valve leaflets (*arrows*) are prolapsed into the left atrium and are well beyond the normal level of the mitral annulus (*dashed line*). LA, left atrium; LV, left ventricle; RA, right atrium; RV, right ventricle.**

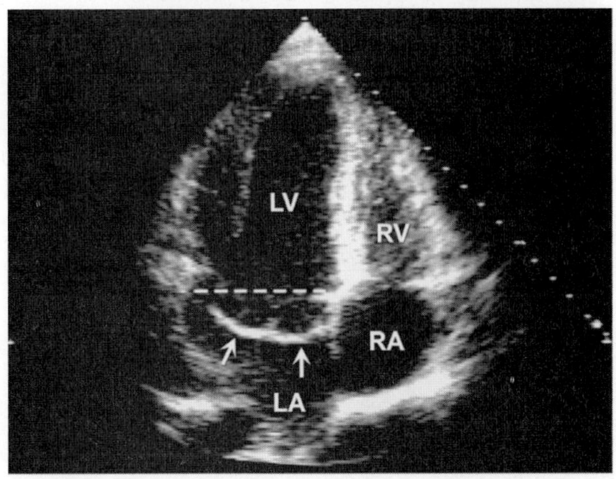

(Taken from Oh JK, Seward JB, Tajik AJ. *The echo manual*. 3rd ed. Philadelphia: Lippincott Williams & Wilkins; 2006. Fig. 12-30B. Used with permission of Lippincott Williams & Wilkins.)

- **Tests**: CXR may detect LVH and left atrial enlargement; echocardiogram demonstrates regurgitation and is useful to determine the cause of MR, the size of the left heart chambers, and the ejection fraction (Figure 1-22)
- **Treatment**:
  - **Prophylactic antibiotics** are given for any intervention with risk of bleeding to reduce risk of accidental valve infection (**risk** is **higher** with any **valvular** disease)
  - **Anticoagulation** is prescribed to reduce the risk of thrombus formation (ASA if healthy, warfarin with a history of Afib or stroke)
  - Vasodilators are given if the patient is symptomatic at rest
  - Severe or acute cases require surgical repair or reconstruction
- **Outcomes**: mild cases have few complications; more severe cases are associated with the development of CHF and pulmonary disease
- **Clues to the diagnosis**:
  - History: history of heart murmur
  - Physical: systolic murmur radiating to the axilla, split S_2, midsystolic click
  - Tests: echocardiogram results

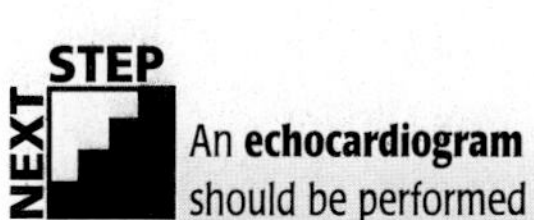

An **echocardiogram** should be performed anytime you suspect a valvular lesion.

- **Mitral stenosis** (MS)
  - Decreased mitral valve motion or inability to open fully resulting in an obstruction of blood flow from the left atrium to the left ventricle
    - Most commonly a result of **RHD**
  - **History**: asymptomatic for initial approximately 10 years of condition followed by dyspnea on exertion, orthopnea, and paroxysmal nocturnal dyspnea
  - **Physical examination**: opening snap after second heart sound, diastolic rumble, loud S_1 heart sound, possible peripheral edema, and hepatomegaly
  - **Tests**: CXR shows RVH, left atrial enlargement, and mitral valve calcifications (Figure 1-23); echocardiogram shows a thickened and calcified mitral valve with decreased mobility and allows measurement of the decreased mitral opening
  - **Treatment**:
    - **Prophylactic antibiotics** are given for any intervention with a risk of bleeding to reduce the risk of accidental valve infection
    - Diuretics are given to reduce preload

FIGURE 1-23 **Chest x-ray in a patient with mitral stenosis due to rheumatic heart disease and secondary tricuspid regurgitation. Note the increased left atrial size (*arrows*) due to mitral regurgitation and the significantly increased right atrial size (*arrow heads*) due to tricuspid regurgitation.**

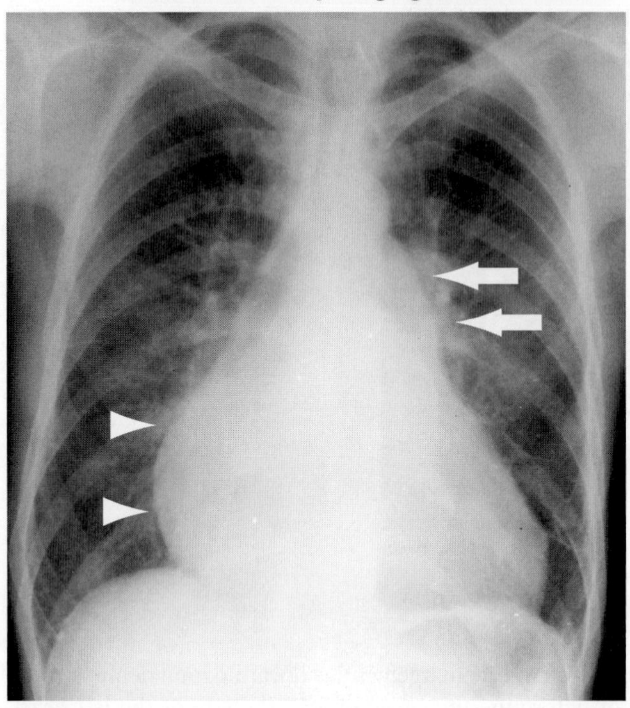

(Taken from Topol EJ, ed. *Textbook of cardiovascular medicine*. 3rd ed. Philadelphia: Lippincott Williams & Wilkins; 2007. Fig. 47-68. Used with permission of Lippincott Williams & Wilkins.)

QUICK HIT: Successful treatment and surgical correction of valvular diseases depend on diagnosing the disorder before severe symptoms develop.

- Antiarrhythmics and anticoagulants are required with the development of Afib
- Surgical repair, replacement, or balloon valvotomy is required prior to progression
- **Outcomes**: progressive CHF and pulmonary disease; poor prognosis without surgical treatment in advanced disease
- **Why eliminated from differential**: the murmur heard in the case is systolic (diastolic murmur expected in MS), and the echocardiogram is diagnostic of mitral valve prolapse

- **Aortic regurgitation (AR)**
  - Aortic valve incompetency causing backflow of blood into the left ventricle
    - Common causes include congenital defects, endocarditis, RHD, tertiary syphilis, aortic root dilation, and aortic dissection
  - **History**: initially asymptomatic with eventual development of dyspnea on exertion, orthopnea, and chest pain
  - **Physical examination**: bounding pulses, widened pulse pressure, **diastolic decrescendo murmur** at right second intercostals space, late diastolic rumble (i.e., **Austin-Flint murmur**), capillary pulsations in the nail beds that become more visible with application of pressure (i.e., Quincke sign)
  - **Tests**: CXR shows aortic dilation and LVH; echocardiogram demonstrates abnormality of aortic valves or root and a backflow of blood
  - **Treatment**:
    - **Prophylactic antibiotics** are given for any intervention with a risk of bleeding to reduce the risk of accidental valve infection
    - ACE-I, calcium channel blockers, or nitroglycerin are used to decrease afterload
    - **Valve replacement** is eventually required

- Outcomes:
  - Increased risk of CHF, arrhythmias, or sudden cardiac death
  - Yearly risk of mortality in symptomatic patients is up to 5%
  - This risk increases to 10% with angina and to 20% with comorbid CHF
- **Why eliminated from differential**: the murmur heard in the case is systolic (diastolic murmur expected in MS), and the echocardiogram is diagnostic of mitral valve prolapse

- Aortic stenosis (AS)
  - Narrowing of the aortic valve causing obstruction of the flow of blood from the left ventricle to the aorta
    - Common causes include **congenital defects**, RHD, and valvular calcification (elderly patients)
  - **History**: **syncope**, chest pain, dyspnea on exertion
  - **Physical examination:** weak prolonged pulse, **systolic crescendo-decrescendo murmur** radiating from the right upper sternal border to the carotid arteries (murmur lessens during Valsalva), weak S_2 heart sound
  - **Tests**: CXR may show calcified valves; echocardiogram shows the valvular abnormality and detects obstruction of blood flow into the aorta (Figure 1-24)
  - **Treatment**:
    - **Prophylactic antibiotics** are given for any intervention with risk of bleeding to reduce risk of accidental valve infection
    - β-blockers help to reduce cardiac workload against the obstruction
    - **Valve replacement** is indicated for severe symptomatic AS or for patients with moderate to severe AS requiring other cardiac or aortic surgery
  - **Outcomes**:
    - The development of symptoms is correlated with an increased risk for CHF, arrhythmias, and sudden cardiac death
    - The development of CHF is a poor prognostic sign
    - Without surgical correction, mortality in symptomatic patients commonly occurs within 3 years
  - **Why eliminated from differential**: the patient's normal exercise tolerance and the echocardiogram findings rule out this diagnosis

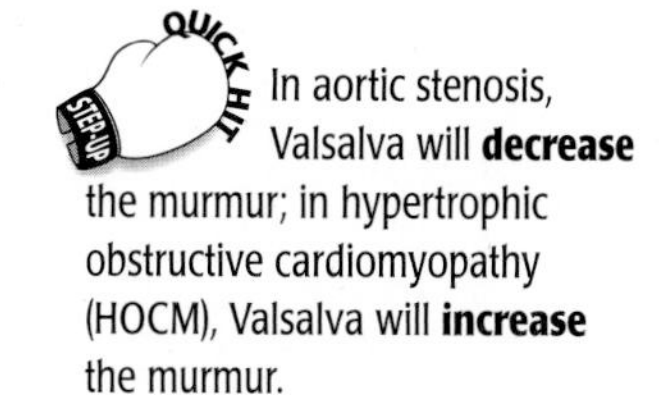

In aortic stenosis, Valsalva will **decrease** the murmur; in hypertrophic obstructive cardiomyopathy (HOCM), Valsalva will **increase** the murmur.

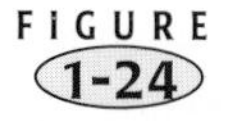

FIGURE 1-24 Parasternal long-axis view echocardiogram in a patient with significant aortic stenosis. Note the thickened, calcified aortic valve with impaired opening. AV, aortic valve; LA, left atrium; LV, left ventricle; RV, right ventricle; VS, ventricular septum.

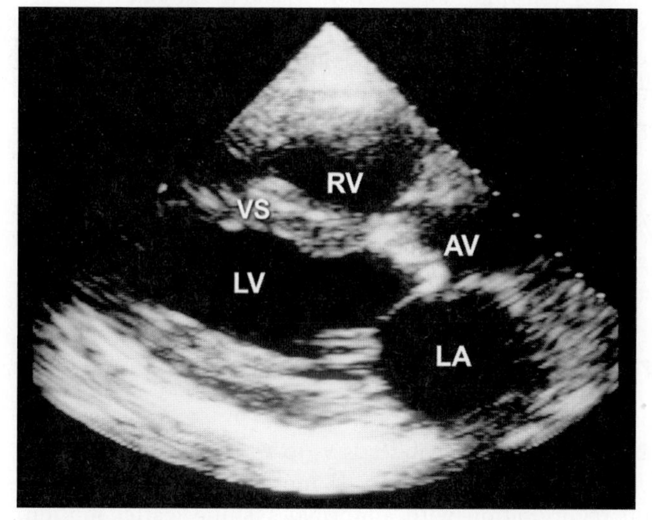

(Taken from Oh JK, Seward JB, Tajik AJ. *The echo manual.* 3rd ed. Philadelphia: Lippincott Williams & Wilkins; 2006. Fig. 12-1. Used with permission of Lippincott Williams & Wilkins.)

- **Pulmonary stenosis**
  - Obstruction of blood flow from the right ventricle to the pulmonary arteries due to a diseased valve
    - Most commonly due to a congenital defect
  - **History**: initially asymptomatic with eventual development of fatigue and dyspnea on exertion
  - **Physical examination:** peripheral edema, cyanosis, **systolic crescendo-decrescendo murmur**, midsystolic click
  - Tests: CXR shows dilation of the pulmonary arteries and RVH; echocardiogram detects an abnormal pulmonary valve with impaired blood flow
  - **Treatment**:
    - **Prophylactic antibiotics** are given for any intervention with a risk of bleeding to reduce the risk of accidental valve infection
    - **Valvuloplasty** is the preferred treatment
  - **Outcomes:** good prognosis unless stenosis is severe (right-sided heart failure develops)
  - **Why eliminated from differential**: the CXR in the case does not display pulmonary dilation; the echocardiogram is confirmatory of a mitral pathology

CASE 1-9 "I get short of breath whenever I exercise"

A 24-year-old man presents to his PCP with a complaint of exertional dyspnea and mild chest pain that has worsened over the past few months. He says that he has become mildly short of breath during exercise for several years, but that this symptom has seemed to worsen over the past few months. He has also started to feel slight chest discomfort during exercise over this time. He states that his childhood pediatrician reasoned that his dyspnea was due to asthma and provided him with an albuterol inhaler. He rarely uses his inhaler because he feels that it does not help his symptoms. He denies any past medical history but says that his brother died a few years ago at the age of 16 when he had a heart attack while playing basketball. Besides the albuterol inhaler, which he does not use, he takes no other medications. He drinks alcohol socially. A review of systems finds a history of dizziness and fainting episodes that have occurred a couple of times each year for several years. On examination, he is found to be in no distress. He has no jugular venous distention. Auscultation reveals clear lung fields, a harsh holosystolic murmur, and both S_3 and S_4 extra heart sounds. He is found to have two apical impulses per heart cycle on chest palpation. Palpation of his carotid pulse finds a similar double pulse. His abdominal and neurologic examinations are normal. The following vital signs are measured:

T: 98.6°F, HR: 80 bpm, BP: 115/80 mm Hg, RR: 16 breaths/min

Differential Diagnosis

- Aortic stenosis, mitral regurgitation, hypertrophic obstructive cardiomyopathy, dilated cardiomyopathy, restrictive cardiomyopathy

Laboratory Data and Other Study Results

- Pulse oximetry: 100% on room air
- ECG: normal sinus rhythm; increased amplitude in leads V_1 to V_4
- CXR: clear lung fields; cardiomegaly with a "boot-shaped" appearance
- Echocardiogram: mild mitral regurgitation with abnormal systolic leaflet motion; increased left ventricular outflow velocity; septal hypertrophy; decreased diastolic ventricular wall motion

Diagnosis

- Hypertrophic obstructive cardiomyopathy

Treatment Administered

- The patient was advised to refrain from strenuous activities
- Metoprolol was prescribed at a low dose
- Partial septal ablation was performed via cardiac catheterization

Follow-up

- The patient experienced improvement in his symptoms following the catheter ablation procedure
- A follow-up echocardiogram demonstrated improved parameters of ventricular outflow
- The patient was allowed to gradually return to physical activities and was followed to observe for signs of recurrent obstruction

Steps to the Diagnosis

- **Hypertrophic obstructive cardiomyopathy (HOCM)**
  - **Septal** and/or ventricular **thickening** causing decreased diastolic filling, **left ventricular outflow obstruction**, and diastolic dysfunction (Figure 1-25A)
    - **Congenital** anomaly due to autosomal dominant genetic defect
  - **History**: dyspnea, orthopnea, palpitations, chest pain, dizziness, or syncope that become **worse with exertion**; **sudden cardiac death** during exertion may be first presentation of disease
  - **Physical examination**: holosystolic murmur, S_3 and S_4 extra heart sounds, **double or triple apical impulse**, double carotid pulse
  - **Tests**: echocardiogram shows **thickening of septum and ventricular wall, increased ventricular outflow velocity**, mitral regurgitation, diastolic dysfunction and decreased wall compliance, and abnormal systolic movement of the anterior leaflet of the mitral valve
  - **Treatment**:
    - Lifestyle adjustment to avoid strenuous activities
    - β-blockers or calcium channel blockers decrease cardiac workload
    - Left ventricular myomectomy or catheter septal ablation is used to decrease the size of outflow obstruction
    - Mitral valve replacement may be required in cases of severe regurgitation
    - Internal defibrillator or pacemaker implantation may be required to prevent fatal arrhythmias
  - **Outcomes**: complications include CHF, arrhythmias, and sudden death; 4% mortality per year (due to sudden death)
  - **Clues to the diagnosis**:
    - History: death of brother at a young age, exertional dyspnea and chest pain, syncopal episodes
    - Physical: holosystolic murmur, extra heart sounds, double apical and carotid pulses
    - Tests: CXR and echocardiogram appearances
- **Dilated cardiomyopathy**
  - Dilation of the ventricles causing valve incompetence and allowing significant regurgitation of blood flow, decreased cardiac output, and pulmonary congestion (Figure 1-25B)
    - May be **idiopathic** or caused by chronic alcohol use, beriberi, coxsackie virus B, cocaine use, doxorubicin administration, human immunodeficiency virus (HIV), or pregnancy
  - **History**: dyspnea, orthopnea, palpitations, chest pain

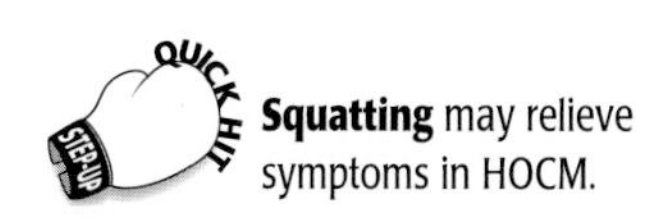

Squatting may relieve symptoms in HOCM.

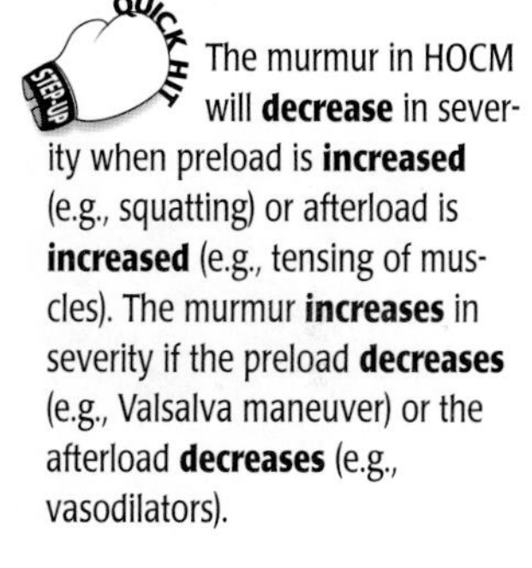

The murmur in HOCM will **decrease** in severity when preload is **increased** (e.g., squatting) or afterload is **increased** (e.g., tensing of muscles). The murmur **increases** in severity if the preload **decreases** (e.g., Valsalva maneuver) or the afterload **decreases** (e.g., vasodilators).

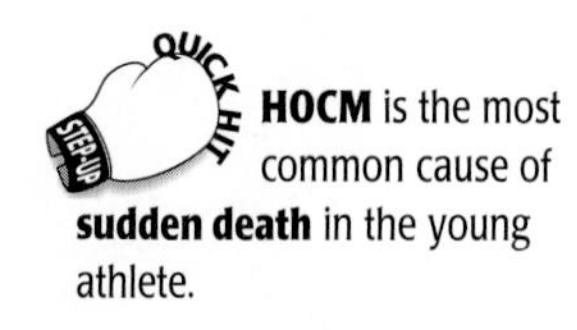

HOCM is the most common cause of **sudden death** in the young athlete.

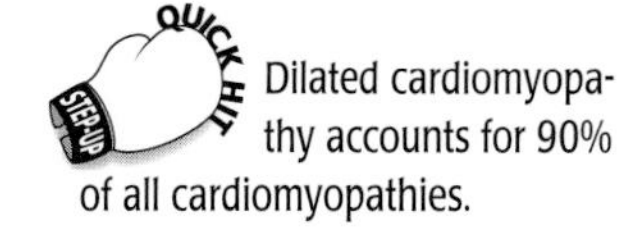

Dilated cardiomyopathy accounts for 90% of all cardiomyopathies.

FIGURE 1-25 **Diagrams of most common variations of cardiomyopathy. (A) Hypertrophic—note the ventricular wall and septal thickening leading to outlet obstruction. (B) Dilated—note the decreased wall thickness and increased ventricular size. (C) Restrictive—note the increased ventricular wall thickness and decreased chamber size.**

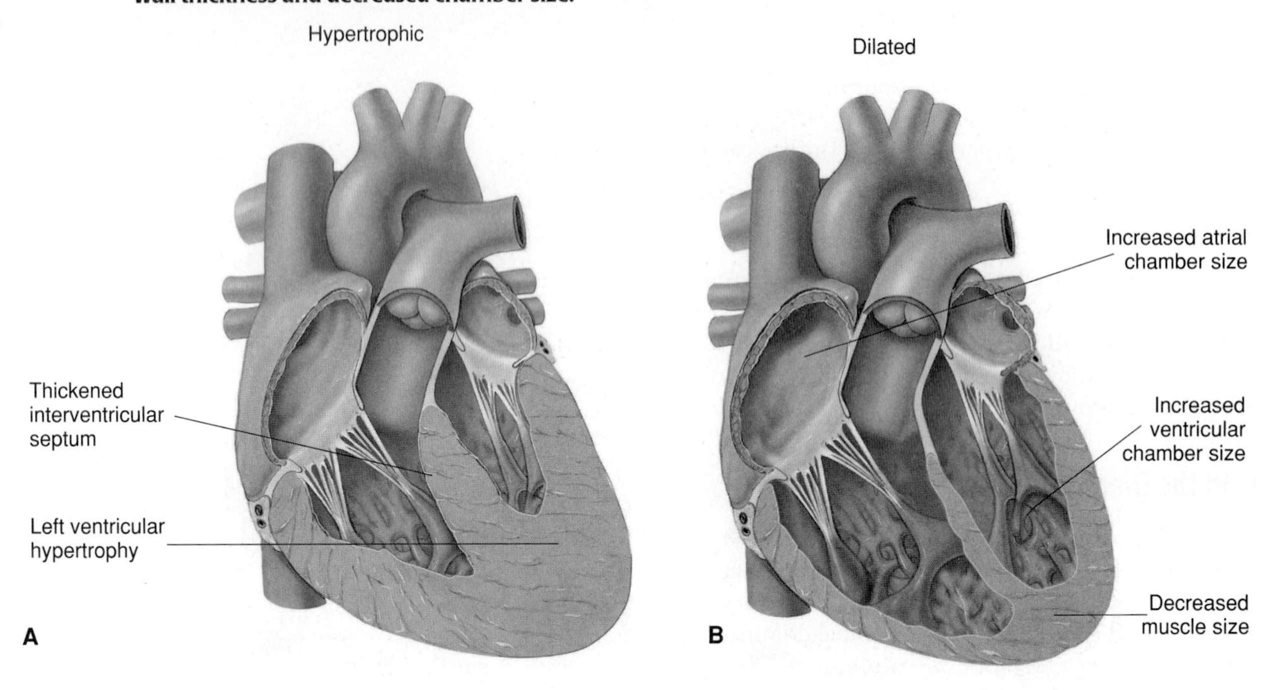

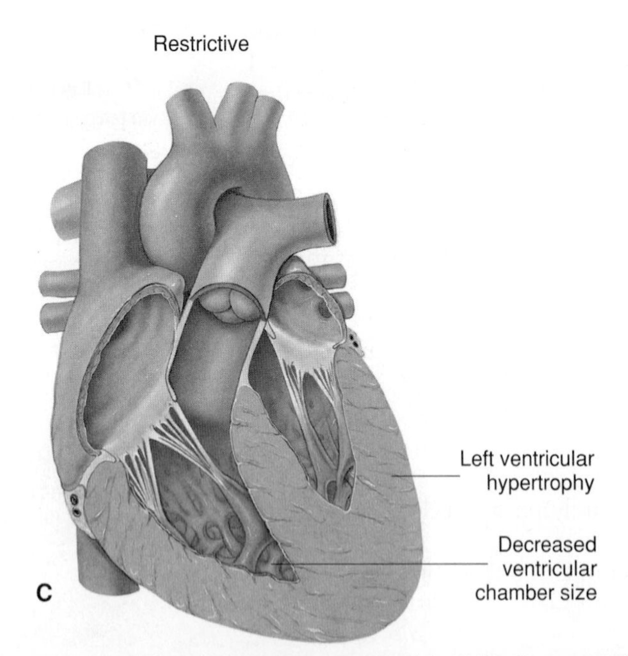

(Taken from Honkonen B. *Atlas of pathophysiology*. 2nd ed. Philadelphia: Lippincott Williams & Wilkins, 2005. Used with permission of Lippincott Williams & Wilkins.)

- **Physical examination**: **jugular venous distention**, hepatomegaly, ascites, decreased breath sounds, rales, displaced point of maximal impulse, holosystolic and diastolic murmurs, S_3 and S_4 extra heart sounds, **peripheral edema**
- **Tests**:
  - Increased creatinine and liver enzymes suggest chronic overload
  - CXR shows cardiomegaly ("water bottle" heart), pulmonary congestion, pulmonary effusions, and Kerley B lines
  - **Echocardiogram** shows dilated ventricular walls, multiple valve regurgitations, and wall motion abnormalities
- **Treatment**:
  - Salt and water restrictions in diet
  - Diuretics, ACE-I, β-blockers, and vasodilators help to reduce preload and afterload and decrease regurgitation
  - Anticoagulants may be required to decrease thrombus risk
  - Implantation of a ventricular assist device or heart transplantation is frequently required for long-term treatment
- **Outcomes**: prognosis is related to underlying cause (i.e., reversible causes carry a better prognosis; patients with severe heart failure due to regurgitation carry a yearly 50% risk of mortality
- **Why eliminated from differential**: the absence of findings suggestive of a right-sided cardiac pathology and the echocardiogram findings argue against this diagnosis

- **Restrictive cardiomyopathy**
  - Uncommon disease of the myocardium in which decreased wall compliance causes impaired diastolic filling (Figure 1-25C)
    - May be due to sarcoidosis or amyloidosis
  - **History**: progressive fatigue, weakness, dyspnea, chest pain, palpitations, or syncope
  - **Physical examination**: jugular venous distension, ascites, peripheral edema, hepatomegaly, holosystolic murmur, loud S_3
  - **Tests**:
    - Eosinophilia may be seen in the CBC
    - CXR may show cardiomegaly and pleural effusions
    - Echocardiogram demonstrates diastolic dysfunction, dilation of both atria, and a **decrease in wall compliance with inspiration**
    - Cardiac catheterization demonstrates increased chamber pressures with a further increase in pressure during diastole
  - **Treatment**: pacemaker implantation may be required to prevent arrhythmias; **heart transplantation** is the only definitive cure
  - **Outcomes**: with few treatment options, long-term prognosis is often poor; complications follow those for the underlying cause and include arrhythmias, mural thrombosis, and sudden death
  - **Why eliminated from differential**: differences between the expected echocardiograms for these diagnoses help differentiate them; the predominance of right-sided heart symptoms (e.g., hepatomegaly, jugular venous distention) would be expected for restrictive cardiomyopathy
- **Aortic stenosis**
  - More thorough discussion in prior case
  - **Why eliminated from differential**: the echocardiogram is able to rule out AS by showing a process involving the myocardium and mitral valve and not limited to the aortic valve
- **Mitral regurgitation**
  - More thorough discussion in prior case
  - **Why eliminated from differential**: although it is apparent that MR is occurring in this patient, the history, physical, and echocardiogram findings are indicative of a more global cardiac process

The following additional Cardiology cases may be found online:

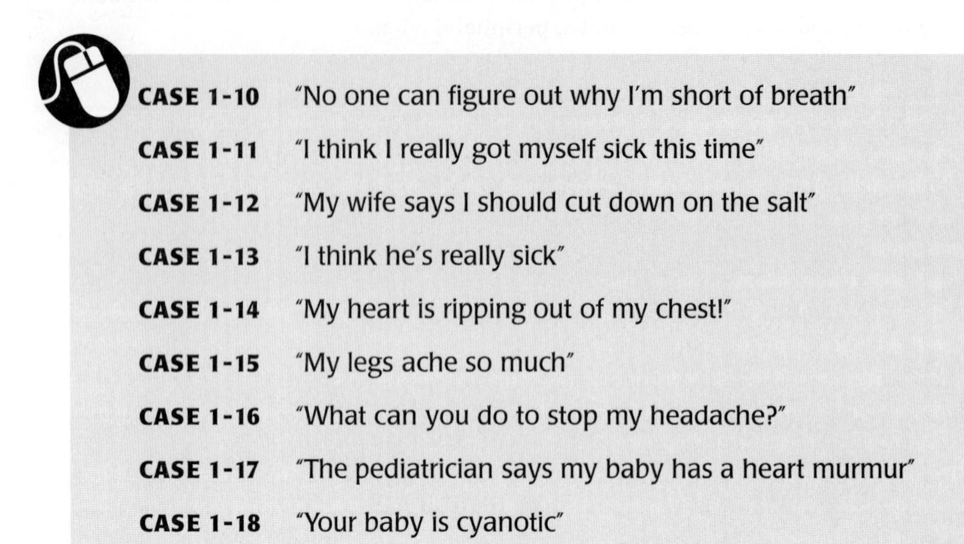

CASE 1-10	"No one can figure out why I'm short of breath"
CASE 1-11	"I think I really got myself sick this time"
CASE 1-12	"My wife says I should cut down on the salt"
CASE 1-13	"I think he's really sick"
CASE 1-14	"My heart is ripping out of my chest!"
CASE 1-15	"My legs ache so much"
CASE 1-16	"What can you do to stop my headache?"
CASE 1-17	"The pediatrician says my baby has a heart murmur"
CASE 1-18	"Your baby is cyanotic"

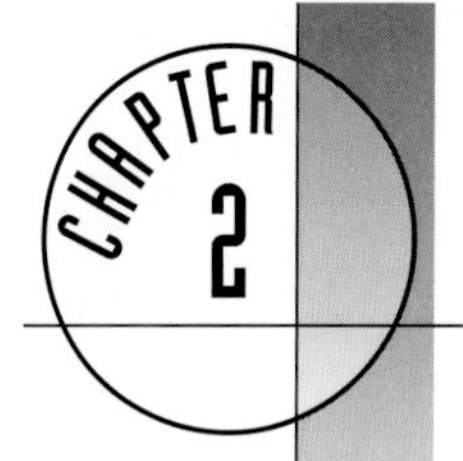

Pulmonary Medicine

BASIC CLINICAL PRIMER

LUNG VOLUMES

- Air volume varies with effort of breathing (Figure 2-1, Table 2-1)

MEASUREMENTS OF AIRFLOW AND AIR EXCHANGE

- Airflow
  - **FEV_1/FVC** is the ratio of forced expiratory volume over 1 second (FEV_1) to functional vital capacity (FVC)
  - **$FEF_{25\%-75\%}$** is the forced expiratory flow rate between 25% and 75% of FVC
  - Quantities describe how much air the lungs are able to expire over a finite period of time
- Air exchange
  - Diffusing capacity of lungs (**D_{Lco}**) measures the relative success of the lungs in transferring gas from the pulmonary alveoli to pulmonary capillaries
  - Expressed as a percentage of the expected value
- Alveolar-arterial gradient (**A-a gradient**)
  - Compares the oxygenation status of alveoli (**PAo_2**) to that for arterial blood (**Pao_2**)
  - **Normal** gradient is **5 to 15 mm Hg**
  - Increases in **pulmonary embolism** (**PE**), **pulmonary edema**, right-to-left cardiac shunting, or in any case in which resistance against right ventricular cardiac outflow increases
  - Facetious normal values may be seen with hypoventilation or at high altitudes
    - PAo_2 is calculated in the following manner:

$$(\text{Atmospheric air pressure}) \times Fio_2 - \left(\frac{Paco_2}{0.8}\right) = PAo_2$$

for room air, this equation becomes:

$$713\ mm\ Hg \times 0.21 - \left(\frac{Paco_2}{0.8}\right) = 150\ mm\ Hg - \left(\frac{Paco_2}{0.8}\right)$$

    - Pao_2 is measured directly from an arterial blood gas (**normal is 90 to 100 mm Hg at room air**)
    - $Paco_2$ is measured directly from an arterial blood gas (**normal is 40 mm Hg at room air**)
    - Fraction of oxygen (O_2) in inspired air (Fio_2) is considered **0.21** for room air
    - A-a gradient is calculated using the variables listed above:

$$713\ \text{mm Hg} \times 0.21 - \left(\frac{Paco_2}{0.8}\right) - Pao_2$$

> QUICK HIT: Normal FEV_1/FVC is 80%; <80% suggests an obstructive pathology; >110% suggests a restrictive pattern.

FIGURE 2-1 **Diagram of healthy lung volumes and their variation with the effort of respiration. ERV, expiratory reserve volume; FRC, functional reserve capacity; FVC, functional vital capacity; IC, inspiratory capacity; IRV, inspiratory reserve volume; RV, residual volume; TV, tidal volume; Vol, volume.**

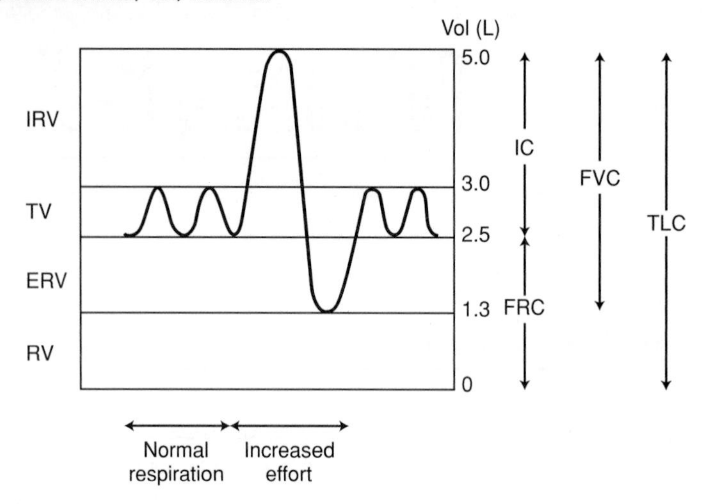

PULMONARY FUNCTION TESTS (PFTs)

- Measure variations in lung volumes and compare them to normal values (Table 2-2)
- Useful to categorize lung processes as obstructive or restrictive
- Useful to assess disease severity and success of treatment

INTUBATION AND MECHANICAL VENTILATION

- **Intubation**
  - Placement of an endotracheal tube to maintain airway patency and to allow mechanical ventilation during general anesthesia and in times of respiratory distress
  - **Tube placement**
    - Nearly all are performed **orally** (nasal intubation is indicated for oral surgery and when vocal cords cannot be visualized by a laryngoscope)

TABLE 2-1 Definitions of Lung Volume Terms and Formulas

Lung Volume	Definition
TV	Inspiratory volume during normal respiration
IRV	Air volume beyond normal tidal volume that is filled during maximum inspiration
IC	Total inspiratory air volume considering both tidal volume and inspiratory reserve volume **(IC = TV + IRV)**
ERV	Air volume beyond tidal volume that can be expired during normal respiration
RV	Remaining air volume left in lung following maximum expiration
FRC	Air volume remaining in lungs after expiration of tidal volume **(FRC = RV + ERV)**
FVC	Maximum air volume that can be inspired and expired **(FVC = IC + ERV)**
TLC	Total air volume of lungs **(TLC = FVC + RV)**

ERV, expiratory reserve volume; FRC, functional reserve capacity; FVC, functional vital capacity; IC, inspiratory capacity; IRV, inspiratory reserve volume; RV, residual volume; TLC, total lung capacity; TV, tidal volume.

TABLE 2-2 Changes in Pulmonary Function Tests from Normal Lung to Obstructive and Restrictive Disease States

Measurement	Obstructive	Restrictive
TLC	↑	↓
FVC	↑	↓
RV	↑	↓
FRC	↓↓	↓
FEV_1	↓	↓
FEV_1/FVC	↓	Normal or ↑

FEV_1, one-second forced expiratory volume; FRC, functional reserve capacity; FVC, functional vital capacity; RV, residual volume; TLC, total lung capacity; ↑, increase; ↓, decrease; ↓↓, large decrease.

- Anesthesia and muscle relaxants are first administered
- The patient is placed into mild cervical flexion while in a supine position
- A laryngoscope is inserted into the mouth to lift the jaw and to visualize the vocal cords (**cricoid pressure** may ease visualization)
- An endotracheal tube is inserted past the vocal cords (**must be visually confirmed!**) to 21- to 23-cm depth (measured at the lips)
- Proper placement is confirmed with **end-tidal carbon dioxide (CO_2) measurement** and by confirming bilateral lung expansion during inspiration
- The endotracheal tube is adjusted as needed, the cuff is inflated, and the tube is secured to the mouth with tape
- Complications of placement include **dental injury**, **esophageal placement**, and increased infection risk

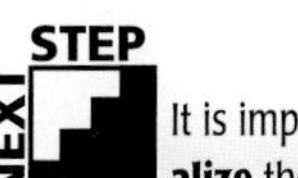

It is important to **visualize** the insertion of the endotracheal tube between the vocal cords to reduce the risk of **esophageal** placement.

- Consider conversion from an endotracheal tube to a **tracheostomy** if ventilation will last **longer than 3 weeks**
- **Ventilation**
  - Assisted respiration is required when a patient is unable to breathe under his or her own power (e.g., anesthesia, respiratory distress or collapse, severe hypoxia, decreased respiratory drive, or neurologic injury) (Table 2-3 presents a description of general settings)

TABLE 2-3 Modes of Mechanical Ventilation

Mode	Machine Actions	Patient Actions	Uses
CMV	Determines and automatically delivers tidal volume and rate	No effort	General anesthesia, overdose
IMV	Determines and automatically delivers tidal volume and rate	Can breathe spontaneously between mechanical breaths	Weaning patient from ventilator
SIMV	Machine tries to synchronize rate with patient-initiated breaths; automatically delivers tidal volume and rate	Can breathe spontaneously between mechanical breaths	More comfortable for patient because of attempted synchronization; frequently used in place of IMV
AC	Machine senses patient's attempt to breathe and delivers full preset tidal volume; backup rate if no spontaneous breaths	Patient driven unless no attempts to breathe (backup rate)	Used when patient is more awake and in progressive weaning
CPAP	Machine maintains airway patency to decrease work of breathing	Patient does all breathing	Used when patient relies less on ventilator; intubation not required

AC, assist-control ventilation; CMV, controlled mechanical ventilation; CPAP, continuous positive airway pressure; IMV, intermittent mandatory ventilation; SIMV, synchronized intermittent mandatory ventilation.

- The ventilator controls inspiration while expiration occurs through natural recoil of the lungs
- Tidal volume, respiratory rate, Fio_2, and inspiratory pressure may be adjusted for variability in respiratory drive, compliance, and oxygenation status
- Positive end-expiratory pressure (PEEP) helps maintain alveolar patency during expiration
- **Ventilator weaning** protocols involve changing modes from patient-independent to more patient-dependent modes; **extubation** is performed when a patient is able to breathe by him- or herself on minimal dependent settings
- Predictors of weaning success
  - Pao_2 >60 mm Hg with an Fio_2 <0.35
  - Pao_2/Fio_2 >200
  - Vital capacity >10 mL/kg
  - Maximum negative inspiratory pressure <30 cm water (H_2O)
  - Minute ventilation <10 L/min

PREOPERATIVE CARDIAC RISK ASSESSMENT

- **Risk assessment** of a preoperative patient to determine the likelihood of pulmonary complications including the **inability to extubate** following surgery
  - **Smoking**
    - Increases the risk of infection and the need for postoperative ventilation
    - Cessation should occur prior to surgery (i.e., preferably 8 weeks)
    - Nicotine replacement may be useful to help patients quit smoking
  - Preoperative testing
    - A **CXR** is routinely performed in any patient older than **50 years** or with a history of pulmonary disease or prior to a surgery with an anticipated length beyond 3 hours
    - **PFTs** are indicated in patients with pulmonary disease or respiratory concerns (e.g., smokers, chronic obstructive pulmonary disease [COPD], myasthenia gravis) to assess their respiratory capacity and to anticipate the need for prolonged ventilation
  - Preoperative antibiotics
    - Given to any patient with a significantly increased risk of developing a respiratory infection following intubation (e.g., COPD)
- Anticipated postoperative care
  - **Incentive spirometry**, deep breathing exercises, pain control, and **physical therapy** are all very important postoperatively to help prevent **atelectasis**, **pneumonia**, and **pulmonary embolism**
  - Bronchodilators and inhaled corticosteroids may be beneficial in postoperative patients with preexisting obstructive disease

LUNG TRANSPLANTATION

- Indicated for **COPD** (particularly patients with α_1-antitrypsin deficiency), primary pulmonary hypertension (HTN), **cystic fibrosis**, or idiopathic pulmonary fibrosis with an estimated survival of **<2 years**
- Contraindicated in patients with poor cardiac function, renal or hepatic insufficiency, or other terminal illnesses; **smokers** (any use within 6 months) and patients older than 65 years are also excluded
- Acute rejection is common, and most patients have at least one episode; chronic rejection is also common
- The risk of **pneumonia** in the postoperative period is fairly high
- Three-year survival is 56%

CASE 2-1 "I have a sore throat and a cold"

A 25-year-old man presents to his primary care provider (PCP) with a 4-day history of fatigue, sore throat, nasal congestion, and a nonproductive cough. He states that he has not taken his temperature at home and has had a few episodes of chills. He is unable to describe any inciting event for his symptoms but describes similar symptoms when he has had a "cold" in the past. He has had some relief of his symptoms with an over-the-counter cold medicine. He denies any past medical history or substance use. On examination, he is found to have pharyngeal erythema without purulent drainage and mild cervical lymphadenopathy. Auscultation detects slightly congested breath sounds and normal heart sounds. The abdominal examination finds no tenderness or masses. The following vital signs are measured:

Temperature (T): 100.2°F, heart rate (HR): 84 beats per minute (bpm), blood pressure (BP): 110/70 mm Hg, respiratory rate (RR) 16 breaths/min

Differential Diagnosis

- Viral pharyngitis, bacterial pharyngitis, tonsillitis, viral rhinitis, influenza

Laboratory Data and Other Study Results

- Complete blood cell count (CBC): white blood cells (WBC): 9.0, hemoglobin (Hgb): 14.5, platelets (Plt): 300
- Rapid streptococcal antigen test: negative
- Throat swab culture: negative (results reported after the initiation of therapy)

Diagnosis

- Viral pharyngitis

Treatment Administered

- Supportive therapy including hydration, expectorant/cough suppression medication, analgesia, and rest was prescribed
- No antibiotics were given

Follow-up

- The patient's symptoms gradually improved and resolved over the next few days

Steps to the Diagnosis

- **Viral pharyngitis**
  - A common viral upper respiratory infection with symptoms due to predominance of inflammation in the oropharynx (Figure 2-2)
  - **History:** sore throat, nasal congestion
  - **Physical examination: pharyngeal erythema**, **absence of tonsillar exudates**, variable degree of lymphadenopathy, possible low-grade temperatures or fever (above 101.5°F)
  - **Tests:** normal WBC; negative rapid streptococcal antigen test and culture
  - **Treatment: supportive therapy** only (e.g., hydration rest, over-the-counter cold medicines, analgesia)
  - **Outcomes:** symptoms should resolve over 7 to 10 days with no long-term effects; usually the diagnosis made and treatment is initiated before study results are reported

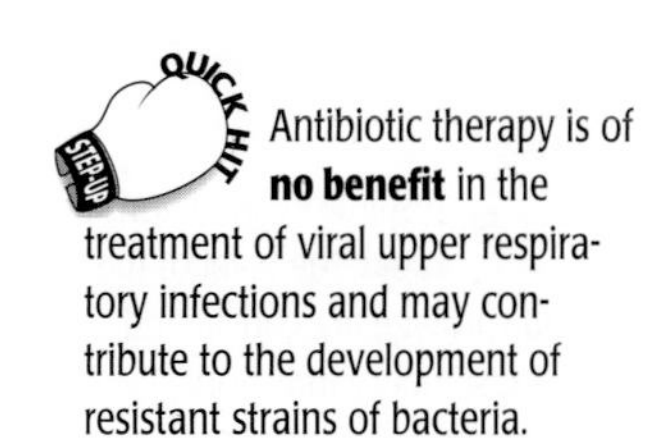

Antibiotic therapy is of **no benefit** in the treatment of viral upper respiratory infections and may contribute to the development of resistant strains of bacteria.

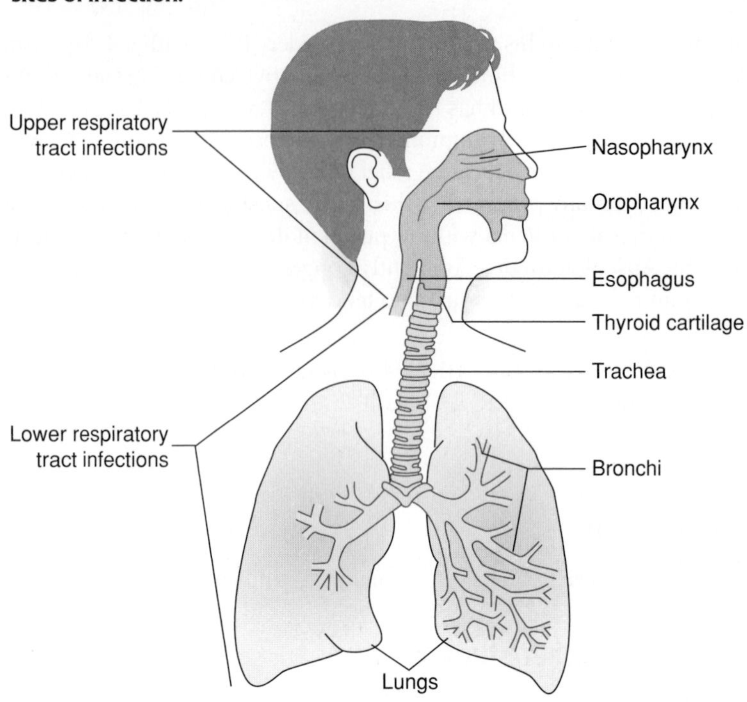

FIGURE 2-2 **Division of the respiratory tree into upper and lower regions and the appropriate sites of infection.**

- **Clues to the diagnosis:**
  - History: fatigue, nasal congestion, nonproductive cough, sore throat
  - Physical: pharyngeal erythema, cervical lymphadenopathy, congested breath sounds
  - Tests: noncontributory
- **Bacterial pharyngitis and tonsillitis**
  - Bacterial infection of the pharynx and possible involvement of the palatine tonsils that is most commonly due to **group A β-hemolytic streptococcus**
  - **History**: sore throat, malaise, headache
  - **Physical examination: pharyngeal erythema**, **tonsillar exudates**, variable lymphadenopathy, fever (more common than in the viral form)
  - **Tests:** normal or mildly increased WBC; rapid streptococcal antigen test and culture will be **positive**
  - **Treatment:**
    - Supportive therapy
    - β-lactam antibiotics reduce the infection length
    - Tonsillectomy may be performed in the case of recurrent infections
  - **Outcomes:**
    - Symptoms will likely self-resolve even without treatment
    - Untreated infection may cause **rheumatic heart disease** (3% of cases) or scarlet fever (i.e., high fevers and a rash during a streptococcal infection)
    - Severe tonsillitis may cause airway obstruction or abscess formation requiring surgical drainage
  - **Why eliminated from differential:** the absence of tonsillar exudates and only a low-grade fever are seen in this case; the presence of a cough and nasal congestion make this diagnosis unlikely
- **Viral rhinitis**
  - Inflammation of the upper airways most commonly caused by rhinovirus, coronavirus, or adenovirus
  - **History:** mild sore throat, prevalent nasal congestion and increased secretions (i.e., **rhinorrhea**), cough

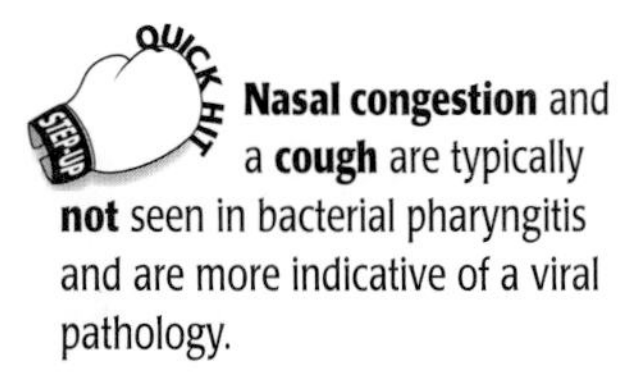

QUICK HIT: **Nasal congestion** and a **cough** are typically **not** seen in bacterial pharyngitis and are more indicative of a viral pathology.

QUICK HIT: Completing a prescribed course of antibiotics for bacterial pharyngitis is important to preventing relapse and the development of **antibiotic resistance**.

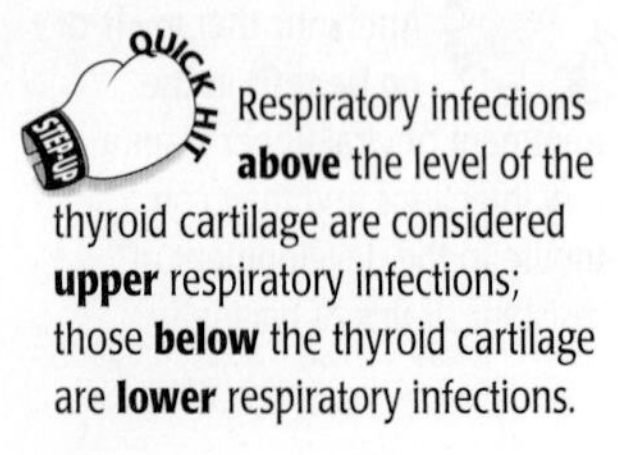

QUICK HIT: Respiratory infections **above** the level of the thyroid cartilage are considered **upper** respiratory infections; those **below** the thyroid cartilage are **lower** respiratory infections.

- **Physical examination:** mild pharyngeal erythema, possible lymphadenopathy, or low-grade fevers
- **Tests:** negative rapid streptococcal antigen test and culture
- **Treatment:** supportive therapy
- **Outcomes:** self-limited
- **Why eliminated from differential:** pharyngeal involvement predominates in this case and is more consistent with pharyngitis

- **Viral influenza**
  - Systemic infection with upper respiratory infection (URI) symptoms caused by one of several influenza viruses
  - **History:** arthralgias, **myalgias**, sore throat, nonproductive cough, nausea, **vomiting and diarrhea**
  - **Physical examination: high fevers**, lymphadenopathy
  - **Tests:** serologic tests are confirmatory of etiology (rarely ordered)
  - **Treatment:**
    - Supportive care (particularly **hydration**)
    - Amantadine may shorten the disease course
    - **Health-care workers,** elderly patients, immunocompromised patients, and patients with respiratory diseases should receive **annual vaccination**
  - **Outcomes:** self-limited; complications may arise from dehydration without an adequate fluid intake
  - **Why eliminated from differential:** the absence of systemic symptoms including myalgias and only low-grade fevers are seen in the case; pharyngeal erythema is more suggestive of a local pharyngeal process

MNEMONIC

Remember the symptoms for viral influenza with the mnemonic **H**aving **F**lu **S**ymptoms **C**an **M**ake **M**oaning **C**hildren **A N**ightmare: **H**eadache, **F**ever, **S**ore throat, **C**hills, **M**yalgias, **M**alaise, **C**ough, **A**norexia, **N**asal congestion.

CASE 2-2 "I have a sore throat and can't eat"

A 19-year-old man presents to the emergency department with a 5-day history of a worsening sore throat. He describes an increasing difficulty with eating because of throat pain and having a "lump in his throat." He feels the pain becomes worse when trying to open his mouth. He says that he has had chills intermittently over the past few days and measured his temperature at home at 102°F. He denies any nasal congestion, nausea, vomiting, or diarrhea. He denies any past medical history or substance use. On examination, he is a moderately sick-appearing individual with a mildly hoarse voice. Examination of his oropharynx finds significant erythema with some streaky whitish material in the posterior pharynx. His pharynx appears slightly asymmetrical with apparent uvular deviation to the right side and a focal area of swelling near the left palatine tonsil. He has palpable lymphadenopathy in his cervical nodes. Auscultation finds mildly rhonchial breath sounds and normal heart sounds. The following vital signs are measured:

T: 102.7°F, HR: 90 bpm, BP: 115/75 mm Hg, RR: 20 breaths/min

Differential Diagnosis

- Viral pharyngitis, bacterial pharyngitis/tonsillitis, peritonsillar abscess, influenza

Laboratory Data and Other Study Results

- CBC: WBC: 13.0, Hgb: 14.0, Plt: 280
- Rapid streptococcal antigen test: positive
- Throat swab culture: positive for group A streptococcus (results reported after initiation of therapy)

Diagnosis

- Peritonsillar abscess

Treatment Administered

- Urgent incision and drainage (I + D) of the peritonsillar abscess was performed; intra-operative cultures were sent to determine the species of bacteria
- Intravenous (IV) ampicillin/sulbactam was initiated

Follow-up

- The patient had a significant improvement in his pain after the I + D
- His symptoms gradually improved after the initiation of treatment
- Group A streptococcus was confirmed in operative cultures with a sensitivity to ampicillin
- A peripheral indwelling catheter was placed that allowed the patient to return home to complete a 14-day course of ampicillin/sulbactam
- The patient was scheduled for elective tonsillectomy

Steps to the Diagnosis

- **Peritonsillar abscess**
  - Progression of bacterial tonsillitis causing the formation of an **abscess** in the peritonsillar or retropharyngeal spaces
  - **History:** sore throat, **difficulty opening mouth** (i.e., **trismus**), hoarseness, chills, drooling, inadequate treatment of a recent case of bacterial pharyngitis
  - **Physical examination:** significantly inflamed pharynx, peritonsillar or retropharyngeal mass, **uvular deviation**, tonsillar exudates
  - **Tests:** increased WBC, positive rapid streptococcal antigen, positive throat culture, positive operative abscess fluid culture (used to confirm pathogen identity); ultrasound (US) may be helpful in locating abscess and measuring its size
  - **Treatment:**
    - IV β-lactam or cephalosporin antibiotics
    - Urgent I + D is performed unless the abscess is extremely small (i.e., microabscess)
    - Planned tonsillectomy is recommended to prevent recurrence
  - **Outcomes:**
    - Respiratory complications and systemic infection can be avoided with prompt drainage
    - Long-term risks are similar to bacterial pharyngitis (e.g., rheumatic heart disease, glomerulonephritis)
    - The recurrence risk argues in favor of tonsillectomy
  - **Clues to the diagnosis:**
    - History: worsening sore throat, trismus, feeling of lump in throat
    - Physical: pharyngeal erythema and purulent exudates, tonsillar mass, uvular deviation, fever, hoarse voice, lymphadenopathy
    - Tests: positive streptococcal screen and culture
- **Viral pharyngitis**
  - More thorough discussion in prior case
  - **Why eliminated from differential:** the signs are consistent with a bacterial infection (e.g., exudates, high fever), and the presence of an abscess eliminates a viral cause from the differential
- **Bacterial pharyngitis/tonsillitis**
  - More thorough discussion in prior case
  - **Why eliminated from differential:** a cellulitic pharyngeal process will precede abscess formation, but the presence of trismus and uvular deviation are highly suggestive of an actual abscess
- **Viral influenza**
  - More thorough discussion in prior case
  - **Why eliminated from differential:** the signs and symptoms seen in the case are not systemic and are limited to the pharynx; abscess formation is not seen in influenza

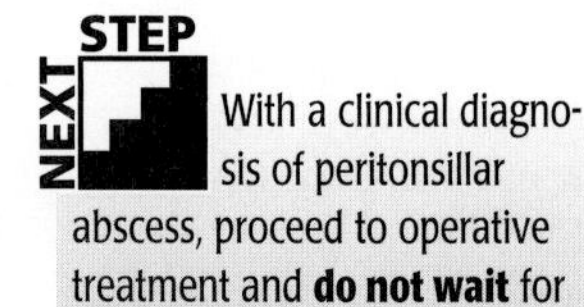

With a clinical diagnosis of peritonsillar abscess, proceed to operative treatment and **do not wait** for culture results to be reported.

CASE 2-3 "I have a cold and a bad toothache"

A 35-year-old woman presents to her PCP's office with 10 days of rhinorrhea and a progressive toothache in the area of both of her upper incisors (with the right side being worse than the left). She feels general malaise and has not taken her temperature. She thought that she was getting better earlier in the week, but her symptoms have been worsening over the past few days. Over the past 3 days she began to notice dark brown discharge when blowing her nose and became concerned. Some of her symptoms have improved after taking a cold medicine containing acetaminophen. She admits to having had "colds" previously, but none have featured this type of toothache pain. She denies any medical problems, and the only medicine she uses is an oral contraceptive. She drinks alcohol and smokes tobacco socially but not on a regular basis. On examination, she is notable for mild tenderness along her "cheek bones" and mild cervical lymphadenopathy. Her pharynx is nonerythematous with no exudates. Auscultation detects minimally rhonchial breathing and normal heart sounds. Her abdominal examination is normal. The following vital signs are measured:

T: 101.2°F, HR: 80 bpm, BP: 113/85 mm Hg, RR: 20 breaths/min

Differential Diagnosis

- Dental abscess, viral rhinitis, acute sinusitis, chronic sinusitis

Laboratory Data and Other Study Results

- CBC: WBC: 11.0, Hgb: 13.0, Plt: 315
- Cranial x-ray: questionable opacification in right maxillary sinus

Diagnosis

- Acute sinusitis, most likely bacterial

Treatment

- A 2-week prescription of oral amoxicillin was provided to the patient
- Supportive therapy was continued to help improve the patient's symptoms

Follow-up

- The patient experienced improvement and resolution of her symptoms and fever over the next few days

Steps to the Diagnosis

- **Acute sinusitis**
  - Sinus infection (most commonly in **maxillary** sinuses) due to viral infection, *Streptococcus pneumoniae*, *Haemophilus influenzae*, or *Moraxella catarrhalis*
    - The bacterial variant is much **less common than viral sinusitis** but most frequently occurs as a complication of the latter
  - **History: pain over the involved sinuses** (one side usually worse than other), thick or purulent nasal discharge (more common with bacterial infection), foul-smelling nasal discharge, **referred toothache pain**; symptoms lasting a week or longer with a brief period of improvement followed by worsening are more consistent with a bacterial infection
  - **Physical examination:** pain on palpation of the involved sinuses, purulent drainage between nasal turbinates on otoscopic examination, illumination test (i.e., light held close to frontal or maxillary sinuses) may detect congestion but is unreliable, possible fever

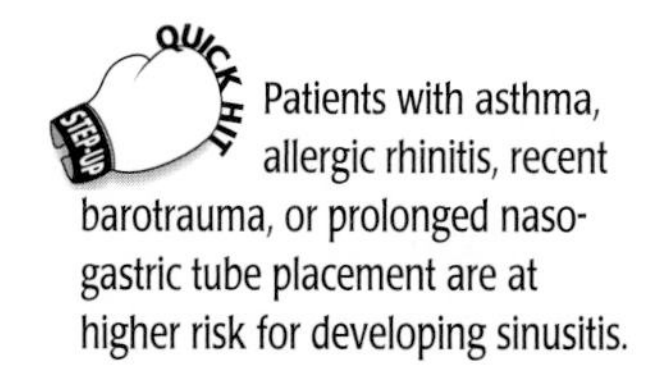

Patients with asthma, allergic rhinitis, recent barotrauma, or prolonged nasogastric tube placement are at higher risk for developing sinusitis.

FIGURE 2-3 **Maxillofacial computed tomography (coronal view) demonstrating complete opacification of the left ethmoid sinuses and congestion of the left maxillary sinus consistent with acute sinusitis.**

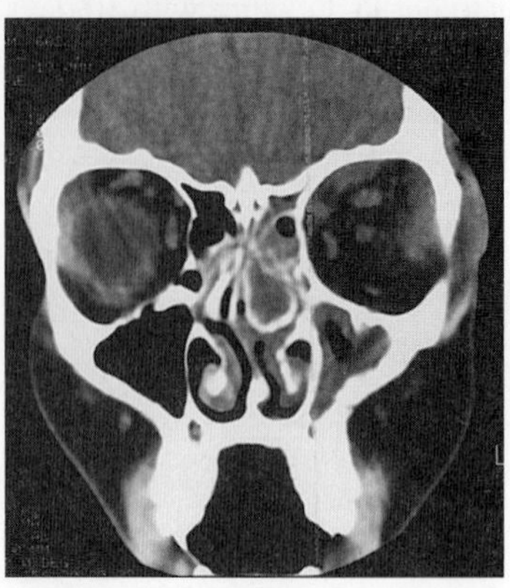

(Taken from Jaeger EA, Tasman W. *Atlas of clinical ophthalmology*. 2nd ed. Philadelphia: Lippincott Williams & Wilkins, 2001. Fig. 10-116B. Used with permission of Lippincott Williams & Wilkins.)

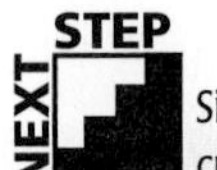

Sinusitis is a common culprit for a persistent fever for which an infectious work-up has found no source. Perform a **sinus CT** to look for sinus opacification if another source has not been detected.

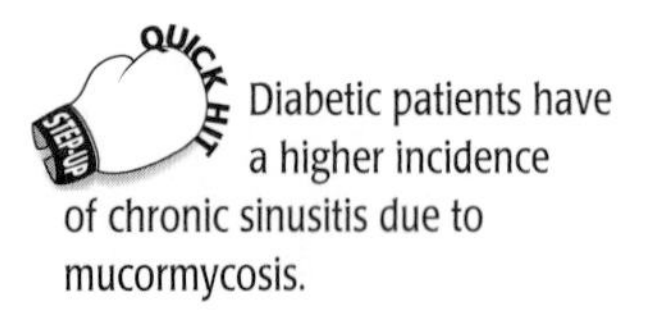

Diabetic patients have a higher incidence of chronic sinusitis due to mucormycosis.

- Tests:
  - Usually a **clinical diagnosis**, so imaging is not recommended unless there is difficulty in making the diagnosis
  - X-ray may show opacification of the sinuses (not highly sensitive)
  - Computed tomography (CT) will detect opacification of the involved sinuses and is superior to x-ray (Figure 2-3)
  - Sinus aspiration and culture is the definitive test but is rarely performed
- **Treatment**: supportive care; a 2-week course of either β-lactam antibiotics, sulfonamide, or erythromycin is indicated if a bacterial cause is suspected
- **Outcomes**:
  - Viral disease will self-resolve
  - Bacterial disease frequently resolves with an adequate antibiotic course
  - Subsequent **meningitis** is a rare complication
- **Clues to the diagnosis**:
  - History: rhinorrhea and toothache pain that initially improved then worsened and has lasted 10 days, dark nasal discharge
  - Physical: sinus tenderness, lymphadenopathy, low-grade fever
  - Tests: appearance of cranial x-ray

- **Chronic sinusitis**
  - Clinical sinusitis lasting >3 months and most commonly related to **sinus obstruction** or anaerobic infection
  - **History**: similar to that for acute sinusitis but symptoms are frequently milder and last >3 months
  - **Physical examination**: similar to that for acute sinusitis; deviated septum or sinus obstruction may be apparent
  - **Tests**: CT is useful to image the sinuses that are likely the source of symptoms; nasal endoscopy may be needed to locate obstructions
  - **Treatment**:
    - Antibiotic therapy for 6 to 12 weeks (may include quinolones in regimen)
    - **Surgical correction** of an obstruction may be required for a definitive cure
    - Prophylactic treatment of allergic rhinitis may help reduce the risk of occurrence
  - **Outcomes**: acute-on-chronic sinusitis is the most frequent complication; cases resolve with adequate antibiotic treatment and removal of obstructions that predispose the patient to recurrences
  - **Why eliminated from differential**: the symptoms in the case were not present for a sufficient time to consider the condition to be a chronic process

- **Dental abscess**
  - The proliferation of bacteria colonized on teeth resulting in extension into gingival tissue or tooth pulp and the development of an abscess
    - Commonly **associated with poor dental hygiene**
  - **History:** significant pain in an affected tooth that may be exacerbated by changes in temperature, general malaise
  - **Physical examination:** pain on palpation of the involved tooth, possible purulent drainage from around tooth, fever
  - **Tests:** usually a clinical diagnosis; dental x-rays may show the degree of tooth destruction
  - **Treatment:** debridement of infected tissue (frequently includes tooth extraction); β-lactamase resistant penicillin or third-generation cephalosporin with or without metronidazole
  - **Outcomes:**
    - Adequate surgical debridement and antibiotics are usually successful to achieve a cure
    - Root canal is usually required in an affected tooth that is not extracted
    - Untreated abscesses may result in the further local extension of infection
  - **Why eliminated from differential:** upper respiratory symptoms (e.g., rhinorrhea) are not typical of dental abscesses
- **Viral rhinitis**
  - More thorough discussion in prior case
  - **Why eliminated from differential:** toothache pain and purulent nasal discharge are more consistent with sinusitis than this diagnosis

CASE 2-4 "Mom is having problems breathing"

A 75-year-old woman is brought to her PCP's office by her daughter who feels that she has been having worsening shortness of breath over the course of the past week. The patient has a significant smoking history, but her respiratory condition has deteriorated rapidly in the afore-mentioned time. The patient reports having frequent chills for several days, and when her daughter took her temperature the morning before the office visit, it was found to be 102.1°F. The patient notes that she has been coughing up copious amounts of thick mucuslike material and has pain on the right side of her chest when coughing. She denies dizziness, syncope, or palpitations. She has a past medical history of uterine fibroids for which she had a hysterectomy 5 years ago. She takes a daily aspirin (ASA), a multivitamin, alendronate, and a calcium supplement. She has smoked close to a pack of cigarettes per day for the past 50 years. On examination, she appears to be an elderly female in mild respiratory distress. She is found to have decreased breath sounds in the base of her right lung field and dullness to percussion in the same region. Her breathing is tachypneic. Auscultation of her heart detects no abnormal sounds and a regular rate. Her abdomen is nontender with no masses. Her neurologic examination is normal. The following vital signs are measured:

T: 101.5°F, HR: 90 bpm, BP: 125/90 mm Hg, RR: 26 breaths/min

Differential Diagnosis

- Pneumonia (viral/bacterial), acute bronchitis, viral rhinitis, chronic obstructive pulmonary disease, pulmonary edema, myocardial ischemia

Laboratory Data and Other Study Results

- Pulse oximetry: 89% on room air, 96% on 4L O_2 via nasal cannula
- CBC: WBC: 17.3, Hgb: 12.3, Plt: 250

- Chest x-ray (CXR): consolidation of right lower lobe; no masses or lymphadenopathy; small right-sided plural effusion at the base of the lung
- Electrocardiogram (ECG): regular rate (90 bpm) and rhythm; no abnormal wave morphology
- Sputum culture: Gram stain demonstrates Gram-positive cocci in pairs; culture pending

Diagnosis

- Bacterial pneumonia, most likely pneumococcal

Treatment Administered

- The patient was admitted to the hospital for respiratory care (e.g., oxygen, pulse oximetry, respiratory therapy), initiation of azithromycin and IV penicillin G, and observation

Follow-up

- The patient began to have gradual improvement in her respiratory function and overall condition following the initiation of treatment
- *Streptococcus pneumoniae* was isolated from the cultures and found to be sensitive to penicillin G; IV penicillin G was continued during her admission
- The patient was eventually able to return home following symptomatic recovery on oral amoxicillin prescribed for a total of 14 days of antibiotic coverage

Steps to the Diagnosis

- **Pneumonia**
  - Infection of the bronchoalveolar tree by host respiratory bacteria (**typical** pneumonia) or bacteria, viruses, or fungi from the surrounding environment (**atypical** pneumonia) (Table 2-4)
    - Common pathogens vary with patient age (Table 2-5)
  - **History**: productive or nonproductive cough, dyspnea, chills, night sweats, **pleuritic chest pain**
  - **Physical examination: tachypnea**, **decreased breath sounds**, rales, wheezing, dullness to percussion, egophony (i.e., change in resonated sound quality over affected region), tactile fremitus
  - **Tests:**
    - Increased serum WBCs (less notable for viral or fungal pneumonia)
    - Positive sputum culture; blood cultures may be positive for respiratory pathogens (Color Figure 2-1)
    - Pulse oximetry will show decreased O_2 saturation
    - **CXR** demonstrates infiltrates or **lobar consolidation** and a possible effusion; similar findings are seen on chest CT (Figure 2-4)
  - **Treatment:**
    - Supportive care (only treatment necessary for viral pneumonia)
    - Appropriate antibiotics for bacterial or fungal cases; β-lactams and macrolides are frequently used for empiric therapy until sensitivities are determined
    - The decision to treat as an outpatient or to admit for inpatient care is based on multiple patient factors
      - Younger, healthy patients with uncomplicated cases are more amenable to outpatient treatment
      - Age >65 years, multiple comorbidities (e.g., respiratory disease, diabetes mellitus, renal failure, cardiac disease, alcoholism, prior stroke, etc.), significant test abnormalities (e.g., significantly abnormal WBC, anemia, hypoxemia, acidosis),

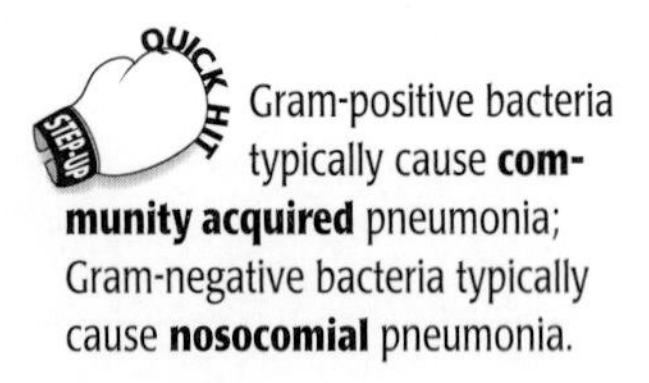

Gram-positive bacteria typically cause **community acquired** pneumonia; Gram-negative bacteria typically cause **nosocomial** pneumonia.

TABLE 2-4 Overview of Etiologies of Pneumonia

Pathogen	Patients Affected	Characteristic Symptoms	Treatment
Viral Pneumonia			
Viral (e.g., influenza, parainfluenza, adenovirus, cytomegalovirus, respiratory syncytial virus)	**Most common pneumonia in children;** common in adults	Classic symptoms[1]; **nonproductive cough**	**Self-limited;** amantadine may be used for influenza A virus
Typical Bacterial Pneumonia			
Streptococcus pneumoniae	**Most common pneumonia in adults;** higher risk of infection in sickle cell patients	Classic symptoms; high fevers, pleuritic pain, **productive cough**	β-lactams, macrolides
Haemophilus influenzae	COPD patients; higher risk of infection in sickle cell patients	Classic symptoms; **slower onset**	β-lactams, TMP-SMX
Staphylococcus aureus	Nosocomial pneumonia, immunocompromised patients	Classic symptoms; abscess formation	β-lactams
Atypical Bacterial Pneumonia			
Klebsiella pneumoniae	Alcoholics, patients with high risk of aspiration, patients staying in the hospital for extended amounts of time, sickle cell patients	**"Currant-jelly"** sputum; classic symptoms	Both cephalosporins and aminoglycosides (e.g., gentamicin, tobramycin)
Mycoplasma pneumoniae	**Young adults**	Less severe symptoms; possible rash; **positive cold-agglutinin test**	Macrolides (e.g., azithromycin, clarithromycin, erythromycin)
Pseudomonas aeruginosa	Chronically ill and immunocompromised **patients, patients with cystic fibrosis,** nosocomial pneumonia	Classic symptoms; rapid onset	Fluoroquinolones (e.g., ciprofloxacin), aminoglycosides, third-generation cephalosporins
Legionella pneumophila	Associated with **aerosolized water** (e.g., air conditioners)	Slow onset of classic symptoms; nausea, diarrhea, confusion, or ataxia	Macrolides, fluoroquinolones
Chlamydia pneumoniae	More common in very young and elderly	Slow onset of classic symptoms; frequent sinusitis	Doxycycline, macrolides
Group B *Streptococcus*	Neonates and infants	Respiratory distress, lethargy	β-lactams
Enterobacter sp.	Nosocomial pneumonia, elderly patients	Classical symptoms	TMP-SMX
Fungal Pneumonia			
Fungi	Travelers to **southwest U.S.** (coccidioidomycosis), **caves** (histoplasmosis), or Central America (blastomycosis)	Less severe symptoms; subacute disease for initial history	Antifungal agents (amphotericin B, ketoconazole)
Pneumocystis carinii (fungi-like)	Immunocompromised patients (e.g., AIDS)	Slow onset of classic symptoms; GI symptoms	TMP-SMX

AIDS, acquired immune deficiency syndrome; COPD, chronic obstructive pulmonary disease; GI, gastrointestinal; TMP-SMX, trimethoprim-sulfamethoxazole.

[1]Classic symptoms are productive or nonproductive cough, dyspnea, chills, night sweats, pleuritic chest pain.

multilobar involvement on x-ray, or signs of sepsis are findings more consistent with a need for inpatient care

- **Outcomes:** risk stratification (considering above factors) is used to determine the need for inpatient treatment; patients able to be treated as **outpatients have less morbidities and mortalities** than those requiring admission
- **Clues to the diagnosis:**
  - History: 1-week history of dyspnea, pleuritic chest pain, productive cough, chills
  - Physical: unilateral decreased breath sounds, dullness to percussion, tachypnea, fever
  - Tests: increased WBCs, CXR appearance, positive sputum Gram stain and culture

TABLE 2-5 Most Common Etiologies of Pneumonia by Age Group

Age Group	Community Acquired	Nosocomial
Neonatal	Group B streptococcus *Escherichia coli* *Klebsiella pneumoniae* *Staphylococcus aureus* *Streptococcus pneumoniae*	*Staphylococcus aureus* Group B streptococcus *Klebsiella pneumoniae* Respiratory syncytial virus
Infant to 5 years of age	Respiratory syncytial virus *Streptococcus pneumoniae* *Staphylococcus aureus* *Mycoplasma pneumoniae* *Chlamydia pneumoniae*	*Staphylococcus aureus* *Klebsiella pneumoniae* Respiratory syncytial virus
5 to 20 years of age	*Streptococcus pneumoniae* *Mycoplasma pneumoniae* *Chlamydia pneumoniae* Respiratory syncytial virus	*Staphylococcus aureus* *Klebsiella pneumoniae* Respiratory syncytial virus
20 to 40 years of age	*Mycoplasma pneumoniae* *Streptococcus pneumoniae* Viruses (various) *Chlamydia pneumoniae*	*Streptococcus pneumoniae* Viruses (various) *Staphylococcus aureus*
40 to 60 years of age	*Streptococcus pneumoniae* *Mycoplasma pneumoniae*	*Streptococcus pneumoniae* *Haemophilus influenzae* *Staphylococcus aureus* *Enterobacter* species
60 + years of age	*Streptococcus pneumoniae* *Haemophilus influenzae* *Chlamydia pneumoniae* *Staphylococcus aureus* Respiratory syncytial virus	*Streptococcus pneumoniae* *Haemophilus influenzae* *Staphylococcus aureus* *Enterobacter* species

(Modified from Mehta S, Milder EA, Mirachi AJ, Milder E. *Step-up: a high-yield, systems-based review for the USMLE step 1.* 2nd ed. Philadelphia: Lippincott Williams & Wilkins, 2003. Used with permission of Lippincott Williams & Wilkins.)

- **Acute bronchitis**
  - Inflammation of the trachea and bronchi by local extension of an URI (usually viral) or from exposure to inhaled irritants
    - The majority of cases are of a **viral** nature, but smokers and patients with other respiratory conditions are at risk for a bacterial infection
  - **History:** sore throat, **productive cough**
  - **Physical examination:** fever, wheezing, rhonchi
  - **Tests:**
    - WBCs are frequently normal
    - CXR does not demonstrate lobar consolidation but may show some mild congestion
    - Sputum culture is usually only performed in persistent cases and is negative except for the uncommon cases with a bacterial cause (typically *Mycoplasma pneumoniae* or *Chlamydia pneumoniae*)
  - **Treatment:** supportive care only if due to a viral cause; antibiotics are given for bacterial cases
  - **Outcomes:** typically self-limited; smokers, elderly patients, or patients with preexisting lung diseases may be at risk for a superimposed secondary respiratory infection
  - **Why eliminated from differential:** the examination findings and x-ray appearance are much more consistent with pneumonia; the positive sputum culture is indicative of pneumonia

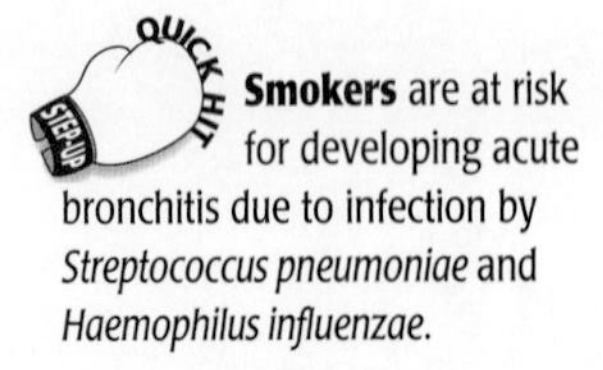

Smokers are at risk for developing acute bronchitis due to infection by *Streptococcus pneumoniae* and *Haemophilus influenzae.*

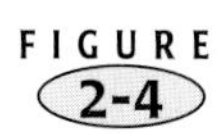

Radiograph demonstrating right upper lobe pneumonia. Note the consolidation of the right upper lobe with an associated volume loss. The division between the right upper and middle and lower lobes is well demarcated by fluid (*white arrows*).

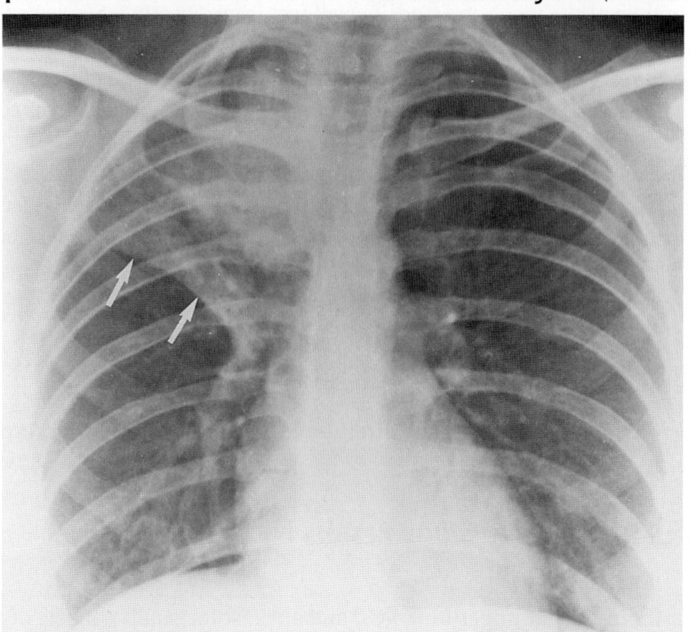

(Taken from Daffner RH. *Clinical radiology: the essentials.* 3rd ed. Philadelphia: Lippincott Williams & Wilkins, 2007. Fig. 4.36 A. Used with permission of Lippincott Williams & Wilkins.)

- **Viral rhinitis**
  - More thorough discussion in prior case
  - **Why eliminated from differential:** the presentation, examination, and tests of the case are indicative of a lower respiratory infection
- **Chronic obstructive pulmonary disease**
  - More thorough discussion in later case
  - **Why eliminated from differential:** the patient would be expected to have more chronic dyspnea and cough for this diagnosis; CXR findings are consistent with an acute lobar process
- **Pulmonary edema**
  - More thorough discussion in later case
  - **Why eliminated from differential:** the CXR in the case demonstrates a lobar process and not diffuse infiltrates as seen in pulmonary edema; the patient also does not have a history of cardiac disease
- **Myocardial ischemia**
  - More thorough discussion in Chapter 1
  - **Why eliminated from differential:** chest pain in the case is more pleuritic in nature than cardiac and the normal ECG decreases the concern for a cardiac cause; cardiac enzymes could be ordered to further rule out cardiac processes if concern still exists

CASE 2-5 "My cousin has had a cough for a very long time"

A 57-year-old woman is brought to an internist's office by her cousin because of a persistent cough. The patient immigrated from Southeast Asia several months ago, and her cousin, who grew up in the United States, reports that she has had a cough ever since she arrived. The patient says that she has had this cough for many months and that while it initially occurred in the morning it now occurs more often. The patient notes that the cough occasionally is productive of yellowish sputum that is also sometimes rusty in appearance. She occasionally

(continued)

CASE 2-5 "My cousin has had a cough for a very long time" Continued

wakes in the middle of the night and finds herself wet from sweating. She feels that she tires easily but denies any fevers or shortness or breath. She says that she is about 10 pounds lighter than she was at this time last year but has not tried to intentionally lose weight. She has never been diagnosed with any medical problems. She does not use any medications or illicit substances. On examination, she does not appear to be in any distress but coughs occasionally. She does not have any significant lymphadenopathy. On auscultation, she has slightly decreased breath sounds in the left upper lung field but no rales or rhonchi. Her heart sounds are normal. Her abdomen is nontender with no masses. She is notable for clubbing of her fingernails. Her neurologic examination is normal. The following vital signs are measured:

T: 99.6°F, HR: 73 bpm, BP: 135/85 mm Hg, RR: 18 breaths/min

Differential Diagnosis

- COPD, lung cancer, gastroesophageal reflux, asthma, chronic lower respiratory infection, avian flu

Laboratory Data and Other Study Results

- CBC: WBC: 8.3, Hgb: 12.2, Plt: 190
- CXR: infiltrates in the left upper lung field and apex; some small pockets of air-fluid levels

Following these findings, the following additional studies are performed:

- PPD: 20 mm induration
- Sputum culture: moderate acid-fact bacilli seen on initial Gram stain

Diagnosis

- Pulmonary tuberculosis, early to intermediate stage of reactivation

Treatment Administered

- The patient was admitted to the hospital and placed in respiratory isolation
- Multidrug chemotherapy was initiated using isoniazid (INH), rifampin, pyrazinamide, and ethambutol
- Close contacts were given purified protein derivatives (PPDs) to rule out infection and were given 6 months prophylactic INH
- The case was reported to local and state health agencies

Follow-up

- The patient was able to be discharged to home after 4 weeks of treatment when her symptoms improved and her sputum no longer displayed acid-fast bacilli
- After the initial 8 weeks of therapy, the regimen was changed to INH and rifampin only for a total of 6 months of therapy
- Human immunodefiency virus (HIV) testing was performed to rule out infection in the patient
- Repeat sputum testing performed at monthly intervals to confirm adequate treatment indicated successful therapy

Steps to the Diagnosis

- **Tuberculosis (TB)**
  - Pulmonary infection caused by *Mycobacterium tuberculosis*
    - There has been a slow increase in the incidence of cases in the United States in the past 20 years due to the HIV epidemic

- Begins as primary infection and typically enters an inactive state
- Untreated infection may enter reactivation (**majority of active cases**) and progress to involve a wider region of the lungs or extrapulmonary sites (i.e., miliary TB)

- **Risk factors:** immunocompromised patients (e.g., **HIV**), alcoholism, preexisting lung disease, diabetes mellitus, homelessness, malnutrition, crowded living conditions, close contact with infected patients (e.g., relatives, **health care workers**), immigrants (much higher incidence in **developing nations**)
- **History:**
  - Primary: rarely chest pain or cough
  - Reactivated: productive (more common) or nonproductive cough, **fatigue**, **night sweats**, weight loss, and possible chest pain, dyspnea, or hemoptysis
- **Physical examination:**
  - Primary: occasional fever
  - Reactivated: decreased breath sounds or rales, fever, clubbing; signs become more prominent as disease progresses
- **Tests:**
  - WBCs are typically normal
  - **PPD** test is useful to screen for exposure (Table 2-6)
  - Acid-fast bacilli are seen on a **sputum acid-fast stain**; culture may take several weeks and is rarely useful in making the diagnosis (Color Figure 2-2)
  - **CXR should be performed in any patient with a positive PPD** and will show lower lobe calcified granulomas (i.e., Ghon complex) or infiltrates in primary or inactive disease and apical infiltrates in reactivated disease (Figure 2-5)
- **Treatment:**
  - Patients requiring admission for respiratory symptoms or current inpatients require **respiratory isolation**
  - All cases must be reported to local and state health agencies
  - For patients with diagnosed infection, multiple drug regimens exist, but all consist of an initial period of **multidrug treatment** (i.e., INH, rifampin, pyrazinamide, and ethambutol) followed by only INH and rifampin for a total of 6 to 9 months
  - High-risk individuals (e.g., close contacts of infected individual, immunocompromised patients, indigents, patients <35 years old, intravenous drug users) with an asymptomatic positive PPD should be given a 6-month course of prophylactic INH
  - Patients should **have monthly sputum acid-fast tests** to confirm adequate treatment
  - Relapse is treated by introducing multiple drugs not utilized in the initial regimen
  - Patients who have received the BCG vaccine should be treated in the same manner as unvaccinated patients if they have been vaccinated more than 1 year prior to presentation or if they have a reactive PPD >10 mm in diameter
- **Outcomes:**
  - Up to 90% of patients respond well to treatment and have a documented cure
  - Recurrent cases are most commonly due to new infection
  - Untreated cases may be complicated by **TB meningitis**, bone involvement (i.e., **Pott disease**), or widespread dissemination to multiple organ systems (i.e., **miliary TB**)

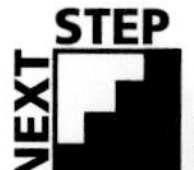

Although patients born in other countries may have received the BCG vaccine and may have a false-positive PPD if they have received the vaccine within the past few years, they should be treated as if they had not been vaccinated unless they have received the vaccine within the past year.

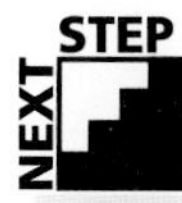

Immunocompromised patients should be given an anergy test (e.g., subcutaneous *Candida* injection) in addition to a PPD to check for an appropriate immune response in TB infection.

MNEMONIC

Remember the multidrug regimen for TB with the acronym **RIPE**: **R**ifampin, **I**NH, **P**yrazinamide, **E**thambutol.

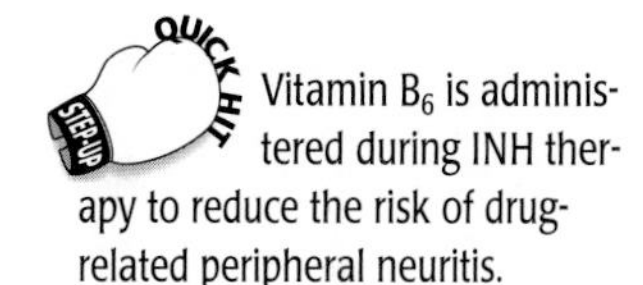

Vitamin B_6 is administered during INH therapy to reduce the risk of drug-related peripheral neuritis.

TABLE 2-6 Criteria Used to Determine Positive Purified Protein Derivative Skin Test for Tuberculosis

Size of Induration[1]	When Considered Positive
5 mm	HIV-positive, close contact with TB-infected patient, signs of TB seen on CXR
10 mm	Homeless patients, immigrants from developing nations, IVDA patients, chronically ill patients, healthcare workers, patients with recent incarceration
15 mm	Always considered positive

CXR, chest x-ray; HIV, human immunodeficiency virus; IVDA, intravenous drug abuse; TB, tuberculosis.

[1]Induration is considered the firm cutaneous region and not the region of erythema.

FIGURE 2-5 **Chest radiograph demonstrating right lung apical infiltrates and cavitation consistent with reactivated pulmonary tuberculosis.**

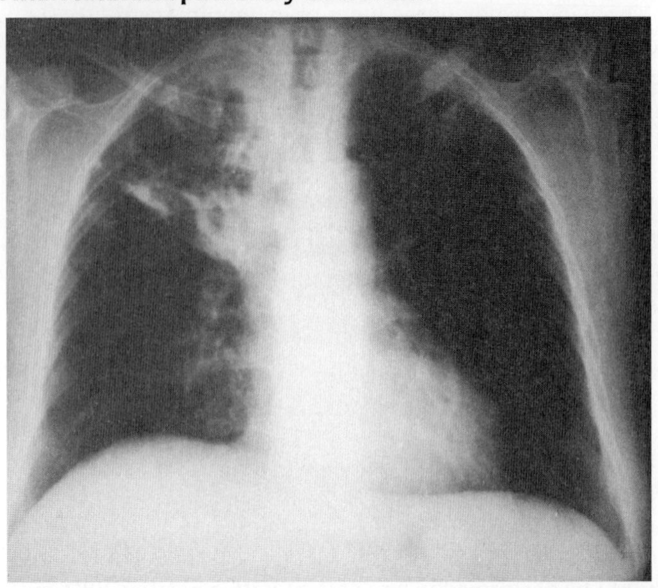

(Taken from Harwood-Nuss A, Wolfson AB, et al. *The clinical practice of emergency medicine*, 3rd ed. Philadelphia: Lippincott Williams & Wilkins, 2001. Fig. 189.1. Used with permission of Lippincott Williams & Wilkins.)

- **Clues to the diagnosis:**
  - History: chronic productive cough with possible hemoptysis, recent immigration from Southeast Asia, weight loss, night sweats
  - Physical: decreased upper lobe breath sounds, digital clubbing
  - Tests: positive PPD, CXR appearance, sputum Gram stain
- **Chronic obstructive pulmonary disease**
  - More thorough discussion in later case
  - **Why eliminated from differential:** although initially a distinct possibility for a diagnosis, the occurrence of night sweats and fever, positive PPD, characteristic appearance on the CXR, and positive acid-fast sputum stain are confirmatory of TB
- **Lung cancer**
  - More thorough discussion in later case
  - **Why eliminated from differential:** should be definitely considered for any case of chronic cough; the sputum findings are confirmatory of TB, but in the absence of this finding, an extensive work-up would be performed to rule out neoplasm
- **Gastroesophageal reflux**
  - More thorough discussion in Chapter 3
  - **Why eliminated from differential:** the absence of a history of heartburn and the presence of night sweats, weight loss, and decreased breath sounds rule out this diagnosis
- **Asthma**
  - More thorough discussion in later case
  - **Why eliminated from differential:** the presence of night sweats, weight loss, and decreased breath sounds are not consistent with this diagnosis, and the characteristic appearance on the CXR and positive acid-fast sputum stain are confirmatory of TB
- **Avian flu**
  - Influenza virus affecting birds that has shown the capacity to undergo genetic reassortment and become transmissible to humans
    - At least one of the severe influenza pandemics in history has been due to transmission of a strain of avian flu to humans
  - **History:** arthralgias, myalgias, sore throat, productive or nonproductive cough, nasal congestion, nausea, vomiting, and diarrhea
  - **Physical examination:** fever, lymphadenopathy, possible conjunctivitis

- **Tests:** CXR may show either patchy or diffuse infiltrates; serologic testing confirms the viral strain but is not useful in the acute setting
- **Treatment:**
  - Supportive care
  - A combination of amantadine or rimantadine with a neuraminidase inhibitor (e.g., oseltamivir, zanamivir) is used as an antiviral regimen
  - Oseltamivir may be given prophylactically to those exposed to an infected individual
- **Outcomes:** significantly higher mortality rate than other strains of influenza (due to severe respiratory infection or encephalopathy)
- **Why eliminated from differential:** the time course of symptoms in the case is much longer than that expected for avian flu; as above, the CXR appearance and positive acid-fast stain confirm the true diagnosis

CASE 2-6 "This intensive care unit (ICU) patient is having more problems breathing"

A 38-year-old man is an inpatient in the ICU due to pneumonia and sepsis associated with end-stage acquired immune deficiency syndrome (AIDS). Overnight the patient becomes increasingly dyspneic and tachypneic. During this time his O_2 requirement has increased, and he is currently on 6L O_2 via nasal cannula. His nurse denies any sudden events in which his condition has worsened and says that this deterioration has been steady but gradual over the past several hours. The critical care team evaluates him in hopes of stopping this downward spiral. On examination, he is stuporous and minimally interactive. He does not have palpable lymphadenopathy. On auscultation he is found to be significantly tachypneic with considerable rales throughout both lung fields. He is tachycardic but lacks any abnormal heart sounds. His abdomen is soft, and no masses are detectable. He is unable to follow commands but withdraws from painful stimuli. He is found to be mildly cyanotic. He has palpable pulses and 2-second capillary refill. The following vital signs are measured:

T: 97.2°F, HR: 110 bpm, BP: 106/70 mm Hg, RR: 26 breaths/min

Differential Diagnosis

- Acute respiratory distress syndrome, pneumonia, pulmonary embolism, septic shock, cardiac pulmonary edema

Laboratory Data and Other Study Results

- ABG (6L O_2): pH: 7.48, pO_2: 68 mm Hg, pCO_2: 23 mm Hg, Bicarb: 20 mEq/L, O_2 sat: 81%
- CBC: WBC: 2.1, Hgb: 10.1, Plt: 130
- Chem7 (7-electrolyte chemistry panel): sodium (Na): 145 mEq/L, potassium (K): 4.5 mEq/L, chloride (Cl): 105 mEq/L, CO_2: 20 mEq/L, blood urea nitrogen (BUN): 30 mg/dL, creatine (Cr): 1.1 mg/dL, glucose (Glu): 85 mg/dL
- Coagulation panel (Coags): protime (PT): 14 s, international normalized ratio (INR): 1.1, partial thromboplastin time (PTT): 40 s, fibrinogen: 190 mg/dL, D-dimer: 0.6 μg/mL
- B-type natriuretic peptide (BNP): 90 pg/mL
- ECG: sinus tachycardia; no abnormal wave morphology
- CXR: diffuse fluffy infiltrates throughout both lungs; no pleural effusions
- Swan-Ganz catheterization: wedge pressure 12 mm Hg

Diagnosis

- Acute respiratory distress syndrome, secondary to sepsis

Treatment Administered

- The patient required intubation and ventilation to improve his respiratory status
- Antibiotic therapy was continued to treat the underlying sepsis

Follow-up

- The patient initially had minimal improvement in his arterial blood gases (ABGs) following intubation
- Over the next 48 hours the patient developed worsening coagulopathy consistent with disseminated intravascular coagulation (DIC), and his respiratory status began to worsen despite the adjustment of ventilatory parameters
- Patient began to exhibit signs of multiorgan dysfunction and died 3 days after the initial decompensation

Steps to the Diagnosis

- **Acute respiratory distress syndrome (ARDS)**
  - Acute respiratory failure secondary to sepsis, trauma, aspiration, near drowning, drug overdose, shock, or lung infection that is characterized by **refractory hypoxemia**, decreased lung compliance, and pulmonary edema
  - **History**: acute dyspnea and general decompensation in the setting of an underlying illness (as listed above), possible cough or chest pain
  - **Physical examination**: cyanosis, **tachypnea**, wheezing, rales, rhonchi
  - **Tests:**
    - ABG demonstrates respiratory alkalosis with low pO_2 (due to impaired alveolar to arterial gas transfer) and low CO_2 (due to hyperventilation)
    - Other lab tests should reflect the underlying pathology (e.g., CBC, toxin screens)
    - CXR will show bilateral infiltrates consistent with pulmonary edema
    - Swan-Ganz catheterization typically shows wedge pressure $<$18 mm Hg
    - Pao_2/Fio_2 ratio will be **$<$200** during mechanical ventilation
  - **Treatment:**
    - **Treatment in the ICU** and **intubation/mechanical ventilation** are frequently required
    - Ventilation should utilize PEEP, increased inspiratory times, and modulation of Fio_2 to aim for a goal O_2 saturation $>$90%
    - The underlying cause must be treated appropriately
    - Extracorporeal membrane oxygenation (ECMO) may be required in severe cases to help maintain an adequate O_2 supply to tissues
  - **Outcomes**: despite improvements in critical care management **mortality remains high** (40%–50%); surviving patients frequently suffer lifelong pulmonary impairment to various degrees
  - Throughout the differential diagnosis, differentiating ARDS from other diagnoses is more of an issue of semantics than clinical differentiation because ARDS incorporates characteristics of several other pulmonary processes; the important keys are realizing that ARDS (and not a single pulmonary process) is developing in a susceptible patient group and that these patients require aggressive intensive treatment
  - **Clues to the diagnosis**:
    - History: existing pneumonia and sepsis, worsening respiratory function, increasing oxygen requirements
    - Physical: cyanosis, tachypnea, diffuse rales
    - Tests: diffuse infiltrates on CXR, hypoxemia and hypocapnia on ABG

MNEMONIC

Common causes of ARDS can be remembered with the mnemonic **ARDS**: **A**spiration/**A**cute pancreatitis/**A**ir or **A**mniotic embolism, **R**adiation, **D**rug overdose/**D**iffuse lung disease/**D**IC/**D**rowning, **S**hock/**S**epsis/**S**moke inhalation.

- **Pneumonia**
  - More thorough discussion in prior case
  - **Why eliminated from differential**: although underlying pneumonia is a large component leading to the development of ARDS in this patient, the patient's hypoxemia that fails to improve despite ventilation indicates the progression to fulminant ARDS and that pneumonia is not the solitary cause of his deterioration

- **Cardiac pulmonary edema**
  - Increased fluid in the lungs caused by increased pulmonary venous pressure and hydrostatic leak of fluid from vessels
    - Most commonly occurs due to **left-sided heart failure**, myocardial infarction (MI), **valvular disease**, arrhythmias, or in association with ARDS
  - **History:** dyspnea, **orthopnea**, **paroxysmal nocturnal dyspnea**
  - **Physical examination:** tachycardia, frothy sputum, wheezing, rhonchi, **rales**, dullness to percussion, **peripheral edema**
  - **Tests:** CXR shows fluid throughout lungs, **cephalization** of vessels (i.e., increased vascular markings in upper lung fields), and **Kerley B lines** (i.e., prominent horizontal interstitial markings in lower lung fields) (Figure 2-6)
  - **Treatment:** treat underlying cause; diuretics, salt restriction, O_2, morphine, vasodilators can decrease fluid overload, improve blood oxygenation, and decrease cardiac workload
  - **Outcomes:**
    - Correction of the underlying cause is the key to long-term resolution
    - Patients with cardiac causes may have repeat exacerbations if optimal control of fluid status and cardiac function is not maintained
    - Patients with pulmonary edema associated with ARDS must have the underlying condition treated to avoid continued pulmonary issues
  - **Why eliminated from differential:** the underlying pneumonia and sepsis is more suggestive of ARDS due to these infectious causes; the normal range BNP and relatively benign ECG rule out sudden cardiac decompensation as an inciting factor
- **Pulmonary embolism**
  - More thorough discussion in later case
  - **Why eliminated from differential:** an increased D-dimer and a sudden onset of hypoxemia would be expected for deep vein thrombosis or pulmonary embolism; if pneumonia/sepsis was not already present and the patient was stable enough to leave the ICU, spiral CT would be a useful study to rule out a suspected pulmonary embolism
- **Septic shock**
  - More thorough discussion in Chapter 1
  - **Why eliminated from differential:** although sepsis is the underlying cause of ARDS in this patient, the patient had not yet entered septic shock at the time of

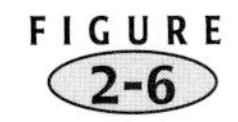

FIGURE 2-6 Chest radiograph demonstrating diffuse pulmonary edema with generalized opacification that is worse near the hilar regions.

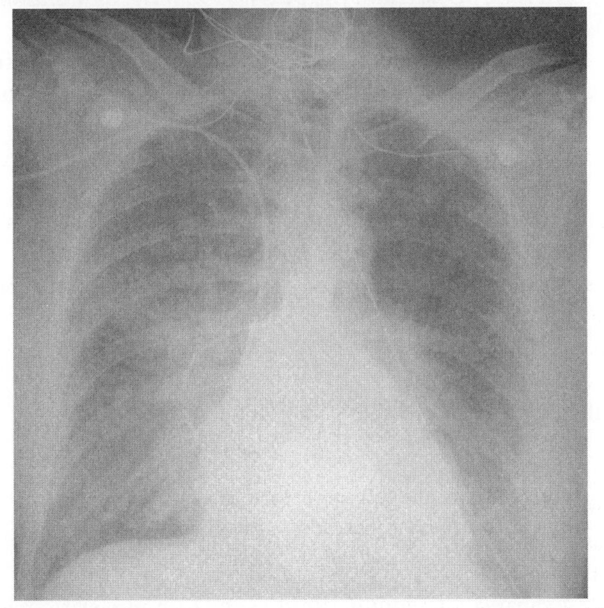

(Taken from Khan GP, Lynch JP. *Pulmonary disease diagnosis and therapy: a practical approach.* Philadelphia: Lippincott Williams & Wilkins, 1997, pp. 66–67. Used with permission of Lippincott Williams & Wilkins.)

initial decompensation (i.e., has mild hypotension and does not require pressors to maintain pressure); although this initial worsening is primarily a pulmonary process, the later development of DIC and the general deterioration of the patient leading to his demise is likely due in part to the eventual development of septic shock

CASE 2-7 "I'm short of breath and don't feel right"

A 64-year-old man is admitted to the surgical floor following an uncomplicated total knee replacement. During his immediate postoperative stay he has inadequate pain control and is resistant to participating in his postoperative physical therapy. He complains of pain in his operative knee radiating to his thigh and calf. On the third postoperative day he experiences sudden shortness of breath and chest pain. He becomes extremely anxious with the onset of these symptoms and exclaims that he has never been through such an experience. He only has a history of HTN, for which he takes lisinopril, and no history of pulmonary disease. He drinks alcohol occasionally but used no other substances prior to his surgery. On examination, he is in moderate distress and is very anxious. He has no swelling in his neck or lymphadenopathy. He is found to be tachypneic and tachycardic. Auscultation of his lungs and heart finds soft rales in his left lung field and a loud second heart sound. His abdomen is soft, nontender, and without masses. His operative leg is painful on palpation of the knee and calf. There is some moderate ecchymoses around his knee. It is swollen to a degree consistent with his recent surgery. All of his pulses are strong and uniform. The following vital signs are measured:

T: 100.6°F, HR: 125 bpm, BP: 145/95 mm Hg, RR: 26 breaths/min

Differential Diagnosis

- Pulmonary embolism, myocardial ischemia, atelectasis, pneumonia, pulmonary hypertension

Laboratory Data and Other Study Results

- CBC: WBC: 8.4, Hgb: 12.5, Plt: 350
- ABG (room air): pH: 7.45, pO_2: 78 mm Hg, pCO_2: 31 mm Hg, Bicarb: 20 mEq/L, O_2 sat: 90%
- BNP: 45 pg/mL
- ECG: sinus tachycardia; T wave and ST segment changes without distinct pattern
- CXR: mild bibasilar infiltrates; no focal consolidation or effusions; no masses or lymphadenopathy

Upon receipt of these results, the following tests are ordered:

- Cardiac enzymes: Creatine kinase (CK) 500 U/L, Creatine kinase myocardial component (CK-MB) 3.4 ng/mL, troponin-I 0.2 ng/mL
- Spiral chest CT: probable occlusion of arterial vessels supplying part of the left lower lobe

Diagnosis

- Pulmonary embolism, likely affecting part of the left lower lobe

Treatment Administered

- The patient was transferred to the ICU for closer observation
- Supplemental O_2 was administered to keep O_2 saturation above 92%
- Subcutaneous enoxaparin was administered every 12 hours started at 1 mg/kg dosing, and he was started on oral warfarin

Follow-up

- The patient was able to return to the surgical floor after remaining stable overnight with no signs of further deterioration
- The patient was discharged to a rehabilitation hospital when he was able to be weaned from oxygen, his pain was adequately controlled, and he was able to participate fully in physical therapy
- The patient remained on enoxaparin therapy until his INR was >2.0; then he was kept on warfarin alone for 6 months without any further complication

QUICK HIT: Ninety-five percent of PEs arise from a deep vein thrombosis (DVT) in the lower extremity.

Steps to the Diagnosis

- Pulmonary embolism
  - Occlusion of the pulmonary vasculature by a dislodged thrombus
    - An increased pulmonary artery pressure due to the occlusion increases the risks for right-sided heart failure and pulmonary infarction
  - **Risk factors: immobilization**, **cancer**, prolonged travel, **recent surgery**, pregnancy, oral contraceptive use, hypercoagulability, obesity, fractures, prior DVT, or severe burns
  - **History: sudden dyspnea**, pleuritic chest pain, nonproductive cough, possible syncope or hemoptysis, feeling of impending doom
  - **Physical examination:** fever, tachypnea, tachycardia, cyanosis, loud S_2 heart sound, rales
  - **Tests:**
    - D-dimer is typically increased with any thrombotic or embolic process
    - ABG is inconsistent as a diagnostic test but may show decreased O_2 and CO_2 and an **increased A-a gradient**
    - ECG shows tachycardia and possible ST segment and T wave abnormalities
    - CXR may be normal or may show a pleural effusion or wedge-shaped infarct
    - Ventilation-perfusion scan (V/Q scan) may demonstrate areas of ventilation-perfusion mismatch and is a fairly specific study
    - **Spiral CT** is a quick and sensitive study that may detect more proximal PEs and has become the standard test at hospitals with good CT experience (Figure 2-7)
    - US is useful for detecting lower extremity DVTs and may be beneficial to making a diagnosis in cases with equivocal results in other studies
    - Pulmonary angiography is the gold standard test but carries higher risks than other diagnostic studies and is used less commonly today
  - **Treatment:**
    - **Supplemental oxygen** is administered to maximize O_2 saturation
    - IV fluids or pressors are used as needed for patients who develop hypotension
    - **Anticoagulate** the patient with either low molecular weight heparin (LMWH, e.g., enoxaparin) or unfractionated heparin (IV infusion titrated for PTT 1.5 to 2.5 times normal)
      - Patients treated with unfractionated heparin will need to be converted to either LMWH or warfarin (dosed to keep INR 2.0 to 3.0) prior to discharge
      - **Anticoagulation is continued 3 to 6 months**
    - An inferior vena cava filter may be placed in patients with contraindications for anticoagulation
    - Thrombolysis may be considered for patients with a massive PE or those with no cardiac contraindications, recent trauma, or surgery
  - **Outcomes:** as long as lung infarction does not occur, the body will gradually breakdown and reorganize the embolus; patients without cardiac arrhythmias or significant pulmonary compromise are more likely to have better outcomes
  - **Clues to the diagnosis:**
    - History: sudden dyspnea and chest pain, recent surgery, immobility, calf pain
    - Physical: tachycardia, tachypnea, rales
    - Tests: hypoxemia and hypocapnia on ABG, spiral CT results

MNEMONIC

Risk factors for PE may be remembered by the **seven H's: H**eredity (genetic hypercoagulability), **H**istory (prior PE or DVT), **H**ypomobility (fracture, surgery, obesity, travel), **H**ypovolemia (dehydration), **H**ypercoagulability (cancer, smoking), **H**ormones (pregnancy, oral contraceptive pills [OCPs]), **H**yperhomocysteinemia.

MNEMONIC

Common causes of dyspnea may be remembered by the mnemonic **AAAAPPPP**: **A**irway obstruction, **A**ngina, **A**nxiety, **A**sthma, **P**neumonia, **P**neumothorax, **P**ulmonary edema, **P**ulmonary embolism.

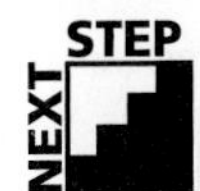

A positive or negative V/Q scan is diagnostic or rules out PE, but an equivocal result indicates a need for additional studies (e.g., CT with contrast, angiography) to provide a definite answer.

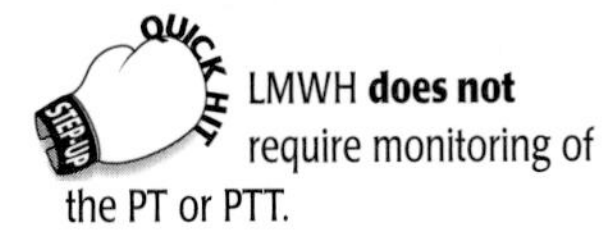

QUICK HIT: LMWH **does not** require monitoring of the PT or PTT.

FIGURE 2-7 **Chest computed tomography with contrast demonstrating multiple sites of pulmonary embolization. (A) Large emboli are present in both pulmonary arteries (*black arrows*) causing intraluminal filling defects. (B) Filling defects are also seen in the left lower lobe pulmonary artery and a right lower lobe segmental arteries indicating further emboli (*white arrows*).**

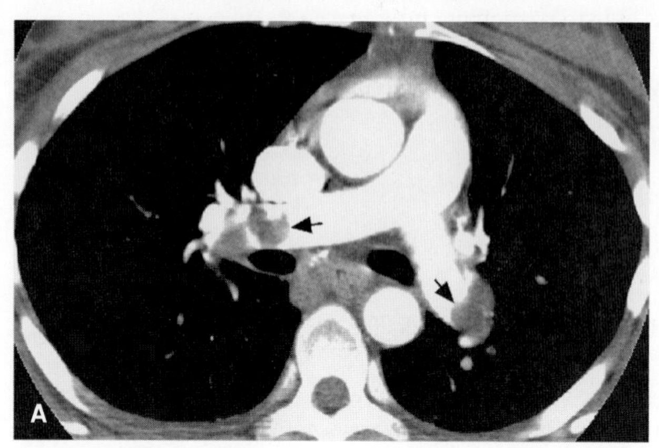

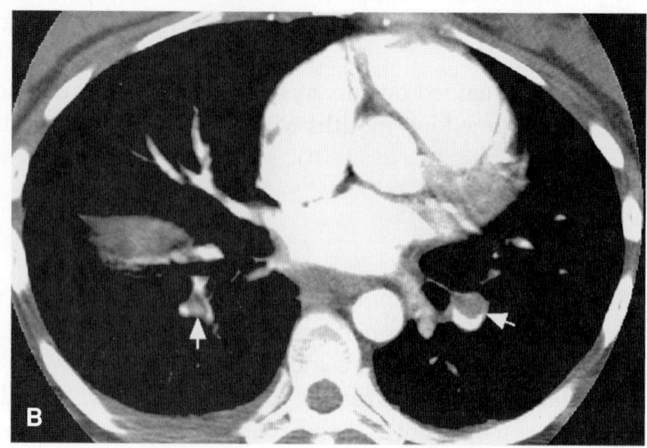

(Taken from Crapo JD, Glassroth J, Karlinsky JB, King TE Jr. *Baum's textbook of pulmonary diseases*. 7th ed. Philadelphia: Lippincott Williams & Wilkins, 2004. Fig. 1-33. Used with permission of Lippincott Williams & Wilkins.)

- Myocardial ischemia
  - More thorough discussion in Chapter 1
  - **Why eliminated from differential:** the ECG is concerning for some type of cardiac processes, but the normal cardiac markers rule out acute myocardial ischemia, and the normal BNP rules out an exacerbation of heart failure
- Pneumonia
  - More thorough discussion in prior case
  - **Why eliminated from differential:** the history of dyspnea and recent hospitalization do create concern for this diagnosis, but the benign appearance of the CXR, lack of fever, and normal WBC rule out this possibility
- Atelectasis
  - Localized alveolar collapse that is common after surgery (particularly abdominal) and anesthesia; also may occur in asthmatics, following foreign body aspiration, or from mass effect (e.g., tumors, pulmonary lesions, lymphadenopathy)
  - **History:** frequently asymptomatic, but possible pleuritic chest pain or dyspnea may occur
  - **Physical examination:** decreased breath sounds, dullness to percussion
  - **Tests:** CXR will show infiltrates in mild cases or lobar collapse in cases of obstruction
  - **Treatment: inspiratory spirometry**, ambulation, and physical therapy are important prophylactic measures used in the hospital and postoperatively; bronchoscopy with suctioning or obstruction relief are required for more severe cases
  - **Outcomes:** generally not clinically serious following surgery; prolonged atelectasis (beyond 72 hours) may predispose patients to developing pneumonia
  - **Why eliminated from differential:** the bibasilar infiltrates seen on the CXR in this case are due to atelectasis, and they may confuse the diagnosis somewhat, but the sudden onset of hypoxemia, dyspnea, tachypnea, and tachycardia suggests a more severe process than what is seen on the CXR
- Pulmonary hypertension
  - Increased pulmonary artery pressure due to **valvular disease**, **PE**, left-to-right cardiac shunts, congestive heart failure (CHF), chronic obstructive pulmonary disease, or idiopathic causes
  - **History:** dyspnea, fatigue, deep chest pain, cough, syncope
  - **Physical examination:** cyanosis, digital clubbing, jugular venous distension, **loud S_2**, hepatomegaly

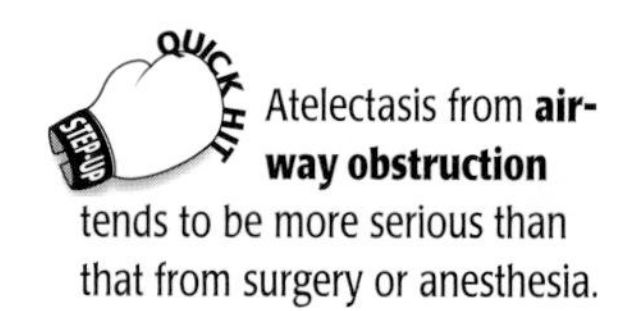

Atelectasis from **airway obstruction** tends to be more serious than that from surgery or anesthesia.

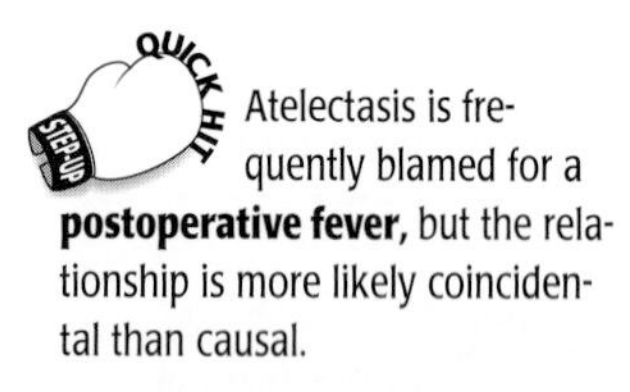

Atelectasis is frequently blamed for a **postoperative fever,** but the relationship is more likely coincidental than causal.

- **Tests:**
  - ECG findings are consistent with right ventricular hypertrophy
  - CXR shows large pulmonary artery and right ventricle
  - Echocardiogram is useful for measuring pulmonary artery pressure noninvasively and detecting any valvular abnormalities
  - Cardiac catheterization is the gold standard test but is riskier than noninvasive studies
- **Treatment:**
  - Treat underlying conditions to lessen pulmonary artery pressure
  - Supplemental O_2 is given if hypoxemia develops
  - Vasodilators decrease pulmonary vascular resistance
  - Anticoagulants may be indicated to reduce the risk of pulmonary thrombus formation
- **Outcomes:** prognosis worsens with development of right-sided heart failure; idiopathic form has a high mortality rate within a few years of diagnosis
- **Why eliminated from differential:** primary pulmonary hypertension is rare, and the condition generally develops secondary to another process; the clinical, laboratory, and radiographic findings suggestive of PE make it a much more likely diagnosis

CASE 2-8 "I get short of breath sometimes"

A 10-year-old boy is brought to his family practitioner by his mother because of a chronic cough and occasional dyspnea. The patient describes episodes of dyspnea that are accompanied by chest tightness that are not constant but last several minutes and occur once or twice a week. He feels that these episodes are worse during "allergy season." His mother describes him as having had "allergy attacks" when he was younger, but the current symptoms have developed over the past few years. He is occasionally forced to take a break during exertional activity because he becomes short of breath. He denies heartburn or symptoms following eating. He has not taken any medications for this problem. He does not have a history of any medical disorders. His mother denies having any allergies besides allergic rhinitis in the fall and spring. His mother denies any similar symptoms in his parents, and he has no siblings. He denies tobacco use. On examination, he appears to be in no distress and is breathing easily. On auscultation of his lungs and heart he is notable for faint wheezing throughout both lung fields. He has normal heart sounds. His abdominal and neurologic examinations are normal. The following vital signs are measured:

T: 98.6°F, HR: 72 bpm, BP: 115/80 mm Hg, RR: 14 breaths/min

Differential Diagnosis

- Asthma, gastroesophageal reflux disease, sarcoidosis, cystic fibrosis

Laboratory Data and Other Study Results

- Height and weight: 5′ 10″, 170 lb, body mass index (BMI) 24.4
- Peak expiratory flow rate (PEFR): 480 L/min
- CXR: clear lung fields; no masses, lymphadenopathy, effusions, or infiltrates
- Chem7: Na: 140 mEq/L, K: 4.0 mEq/L, Cl: 106 mEq/L, CO_2: 30 mEq/L, BUN: 10 mg/dL, Cr: 0.7 mg/dL, Glu: 95 mg/dL
- Sweat test: Cl: 25 mEq/L, Na: 30 mEq/L

Diagnosis

- Asthma

Treatment Administered

- The patient was prescribed a short-acting inhaled β_2-agonist to be used during exacerbations
- The patient was educated regarding common exacerbating factors (e.g., allergens, respiratory irritants), avoidance of precipitating factors, recognition of symptoms, and recognition of a worsening condition requiring emergent care

Follow-up

- The patient was successfully able to use an inhaler during the recurrence of symptoms with a reasonable relief of dyspnea; he noted inhaler use approximately five times per week
- The patient was started on a low-dose corticosteroid inhaler with a continued prescription for a short-acting inhaled β_2-agonist inhaler for breakthrough dyspnea; control improved with minimal exacerbations
- Patient was able to be weaned to a short-acting inhaled β_2-agonist inhaler only as needed over the course of 1 year

Steps to the Diagnosis

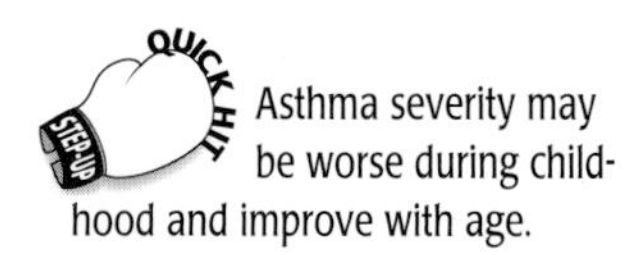

Asthma severity may be worse during childhood and improve with age.

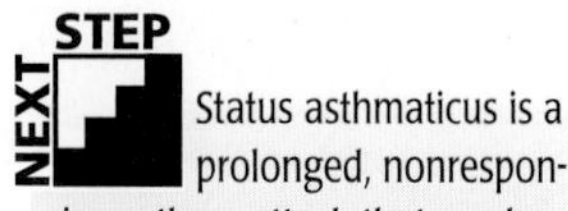

Status asthmaticus is a prolonged, nonresponsive asthma attack that can be fatal and should be treated with **aggressive** bronchodilator therapy, corticosteroids, O_2, and possible intubation.

- Asthma
  - **Reversible** airway obstruction secondary to **bronchial hyperactivity**, acute airway inflammation, mucous plugging, and smooth muscle hypertrophy
    - Characteristic **exacerbations** with sudden airway inflammation and bronchoconstriction may be triggered by allergens (e.g., dust, smoke, pollen, fumes), URIs, exercise, stress, β-antagonistic medicines, and rarely aspirin or sulfites
    - **PEFRs**, clinical symptoms, and frequency of medication use are used to classify the disease as mild intermittent, mild persistent, moderate persistent, or severe
  - **Risk factors:** family history of asthma, allergies, atopic dermatitis, low socioeconomic status
  - **History:** cough, **dyspnea**, chest tightness with a worsening of symptoms during exacerbations
  - **Physical examination:** tachypnea, tachycardia, **wheezing**, **prolonged expiratory duration**, decreased breath sounds, increased accessory respiratory muscle use, possible pulsus paradoxus, cyanosis
  - **Tests:**
    - Decreased O_2 saturation on pulse oximetry
    - **Decreased PEFR**; PFTs also will demonstrate changes consistent with obstructive disease including **decreased FEV_1** (Table 2-2) and normal or increased D_{Lco}
    - ABG less practical except during severe exacerbations (a normalized CO_2 level signals an impending respiratory collapse and indicates need for aggressive treatment)
  - **Treatment:**
    - Treatment follows an algorithm depending on the classification and uses a combination of medications (Tables 2-7 and 2-8)
    - Patients with gradually worsening symptoms will need to be advanced to the next higher treatment level
    - Patients who achieve control of symptoms may have their medications tapered as needed
    - **Patient education** is important in achieving long-term control
  - **Outcomes:** although some patients may have a gradual resolution of symptoms, others may have consistent or worsening disease that requires long-term therapy with possible hospitalization for severe exacerbations
  - **Clues to the diagnosis:**
    - History: chronic cough, dyspnea on exertion, chest tightness
    - Physical: expiratory wheezing
    - Tests: decreased PEFR

TABLE 2-7 Commonly Used Medications for Treatment of Asthma

Medication	Mechanism of Action	Role
Rapid-acting β_2-agonists (e.g., albuterol, pirbuterol, bitolterol)	Bronchodilators that relax airway smooth muscle; have rapid onset of action	First-line therapy in mild intermittent cases and during exacerbations
Long-acting β_2-agonists (e.g., salmeterol, formoterol, sustained-release albuterol)	Bronchodilators that relax airway smooth muscle; have gradual onset and sustained activity	Regular use in patients with moderate persistent or severe asthma
Inhaled corticosteroids (e.g., beclomethasone, flunisolide)	Decrease number and activity of cells involved with airway inflammation	Mild persistent or worse cases; frequently combined with β_2-agonist use
Leukotriene inhibitors (e.g., zafirlukast, zileuton)	Block activity or production of leukotrienes that are involved in inflammation and bronchospasm	Oral agents; adjunctive therapy in mild persistent or worse cases
Mast cell stabilizing agents (e.g., cromolyn, nedocromil)	Stabilizes mast cells; anti-inflammatory prophylaxis	Not useful acutely; anti-inflammatory prophylaxis in mild persistent cases
Theophylline	Bronchodilator	Former first-line therapy but now replaced by β_2-agonists because of side effects and interactions with other drugs; may be useful as adjunct in mild persistent or worse cases
Anticholinergic agents (e.g., ipratropium)	Blocks vagal-mediated smooth muscle contraction	Adjunctive therapy in moderate to severe cases
Systemic steroids (e.g., methylprednisolone, prednisone)	Similar action to inhaled steroids; stronger effect than inhaled preparation	Adjunctive therapy in severe, refractory cases

TABLE 2-8 Classification of Asthma Severity and Treatment Algorithms

Type	Symptoms	PEFR	Treatment of Exacerbations	Long-term Control
Mild intermittent	• ≤2 times/week • Nocturnal awakening ≤2 times/month • May only occur during exercise	• When asymptomatic, >80% predicted value	• Inhaled short-acting β_2-agonist • IV corticosteroids if persistent symptoms	• No daily medications needed • May use mast cell stabilizers if known trigger
Mild persistent	• Bronchodilator use >2 times/week • Nocturnal awakening > every 2 weeks	• >20% fluctuations over time	• Inhaled short-acting β_2-agonist • IV corticosteroids if persistent symptoms	• Inhaled low dose corticosteroid • Consider mast cell stabilizer, leukotriene inhibitor, or theophylline
Moderate persistent	• Daily symptoms • Daily bronchodilator use • Symptoms interfere with activity • Nocturnal awakening >1 time/week	• 60%–80% predicted value	• Inhaled short-acting β_2-agonist • IV corticosteroids if persistent symptoms	• Inhaled low to medium dose corticosteroids and long-acting β_2-agonist • Consider leukotriene inhibitor or theophylline
Severe	• Symptoms with minimal activity • Awake multiple times/night • Require multiple medications on daily basis	• Wide variations • Rarely >70% predicted value • Associated FEV_1 <60% predicted value	• Inhaled short-acting β_2-agonist • IV corticosteroids if persistent symptoms	• Inhaled high dose corticosteroids and long-acting β_2-agonist • Consider systemic corticosteroids

FEV_1, forced expiratory volume in 1 second; IV, intravenous; PEFR, peak expiratory flow rate.

- **Gastroesophageal reflux disease**
  - More discussion in Chapter 3
  - **Why eliminated from differential:** the absence of dyspnea following eating or of symptoms consistent with reflux (e.g., heartburn, dysphagia) make reflux as a cause of dyspnea less likely; the response of symptoms to bronchodilator use also makes a gastric cause of the symptoms less likely
- **Sarcoidosis**
  - Systemic disease of an unknown etiology characterized by **noncaseating granuloma** formation in the lungs
    - Classic patient group is African American females in their 30s or 40s
  - **History:** cough, malaise, weight loss, dyspnea, arthralgias (e.g., knees, ankles), vision loss
  - **Physical examination:** fever, **erythema nodosum** (i.e., tender red nodules on shins and arms), lymphadenopathy, possible cranial nerve palsies
  - **Tests:**
    - Hypercalcemia and hypercalciuria, increased alkaline phosphatase, increased angiotensin-converting enzyme, increased erthrocyte sedimentation rate (ESR), decreased WBC
    - Skin testing (i.e., PPD) frequently demonstrates anergy
    - PFTs show restrictive pattern and decreased D_{Lco}
    - CXR shows **bilateral hilar adenopathy** and ground-glass pulmonary infiltrates
  - **Treatment:** occasionally will self-resolve; systemic corticosteroids, azathioprine, methotrexate, cyclophosphamide, or cyclosporine may be useful in cases with significant pulmonary symptoms
  - **Outcomes:** highly variable disease course; two thirds of patients will have spontaneous resolution, while others have persistent symptoms of variable severity; <5% of patients will have fatal disease
  - **Why eliminated from differential:** sarcoidosis tends to be a diagnosis of exclusion when other processes cannot explain a constellation of symptoms; more systemic symptoms and signs would be expected in sarcoidosis (e.g., malaise, arthralgias, erythema nodosum, neurologic changes, adenopathy apparent on CXR)

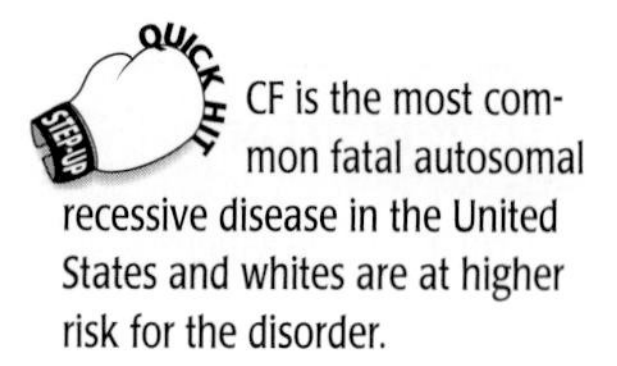

CF is the most common fatal autosomal recessive disease in the United States and whites are at higher risk for the disorder.

- **Cystic fibrosis (CF)**
  - Autosomal recessive disorder due to a defect in the chloride-pumping channels in exocrine glands
    - Ducts of exocrine glands (e.g., lungs, pancreas, reproductive glands) become clogged with thick secretions
    - Causes both pulmonary (e.g., recurrent infections, chronic sinusitis) and gastrointestinal (e.g., malabsorption, pancreatic enzyme deficiency) complications
  - **History: recurrent pulmonary infections** (particularly *Staphylococcus aureus* and *Pseudomonas aeruginosa*), dyspnea, hemoptysis, chronic sinusitis, chronic cough, history of meconium ileus at birth, **steatorrhea**, failure to thrive
  - **Physical examination:** cyanosis, digital clubbing, esophageal varices, rectal prolapse
  - **Tests:**
    - Decreased serum sodium
    - Sweat test shows increased sodium and chloride (>60 mEq/L in children, >80 mEq/L in adults)
    - Genetic testing can locate a mutation in the cystic fibrosis transmembrane conductance regulator (CFTR) gene in affected patients or carriers
  - **Treatment:**
    - DNase aids in decreasing the viscosity of secretions
    - Aggressive chest physical therapy helps in clearing the airways of secretions
    - Bronchodilators, nonsteroidal anti-inflammatory drugs (NSAIDs), and antibiotics frequently are used for pulmonary exacerbations or suspected infections
    - Supplemental pancreatic enzymes and vitamins A, D, E, and K are given for malabsorption
  - **Outcomes:** typically presents in childhood and is universally fatal, but improved therapies allow patients to live into late 20s or 30s

- **Why eliminated from differential:** the patient is older than expected for an initial diagnosis, and there is no failure to thrive; the normal sweat test and electrolyte panel rules out this diagnosis

The following additional Pulmonary Medicine cases may be found online:

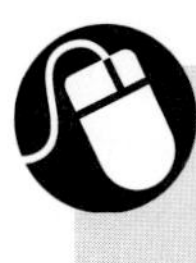

CASE 2-9 "I'm a big smoker"

CASE 2-10 "I'm losing weight and feeling tired"

CASE 2-11 "I was a smoker years ago, and now I'm out of breath"

CASE 2-12 "I keep falling asleep at work"

CASE 2-13 "I can barely breathe , and my chest hurts"

CASE 2-14 "My little boy has a horrible cough"

CASE 2-15 "Newborn in respiratory distress"

CASE 2-16 "Something happened while he was swimming"

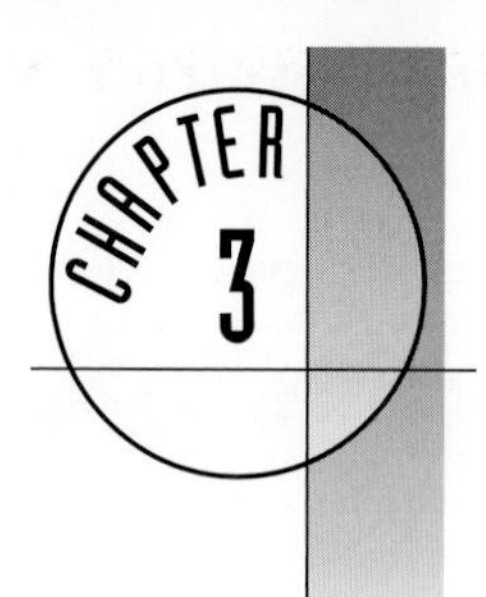

Gastroenterology

BASIC CLINICAL PRIMER

GASTROINTESTINAL ABSORPTION

- Digestion and the absorption of nutrients occurs along the digestive tract from the stomach through the colon (Figure 3-1)
  - Digestion is initiated by saliva in the mouth and esophagus
  - The stomach creates an acidic environment to augment initial digestion and to provide a site for gastrin and pepsin to act
  - The majority of nutrients are absorbed in the small bowel
  - The colon is an important site of water reabsorption

HEPATOBILIARY SYSTEM

- Bile production
  - Bile is produced by the liver and stored in the gallbladder
  - Bile is released from the gallbladder into the duodenum to function as a fat emulsifier
- Bilirubin transport
  - **Unconjugated** bilirubin is a product of red blood cell (RBC) hemolysis and exists in the venous circulation
  - Once unconjugated bilirubin enters the hepatic circulation, it is conjugated by **glucuronosyltransferase** in the hepatocytes
  - Conjugated bilirubin reenters the venous circulation
  - Increases in either or both types of bilirubin depend on the site of pathology

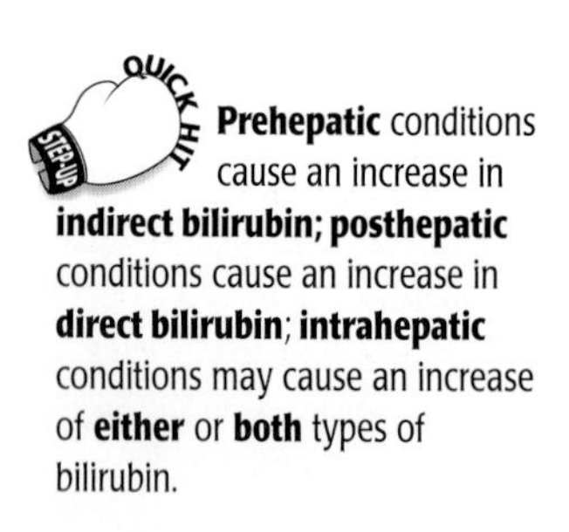

Prehepatic conditions cause an increase in **indirect bilirubin; posthepatic** conditions cause an increase in **direct bilirubin**; **intrahepatic** conditions may cause an increase of **either** or **both** types of bilirubin.

PREOPERATIVE HEPATIC RISK ASSESSMENT

- Perioperative and postoperative mortality are greater with increased levels of bilirubin, decreased albumin, hepatic coagulopathy, and liver-related encephalopathy
- Attempts should be made to correct biliary and hepatic dysfunction prior to the time of surgery
- Surgery should be avoided (unless necessary) in patients with significant hepatitis, cirrhosis, or extrahepatic manifestations of liver disease

LIVER AND PANCREAS TRANSPLANTATION

- **Liver**
  - Indicated for chronic hepatitis B or C, alcoholic cirrhosis, primary biliary cirrhosis, primary sclerosing cholangitis, biliary atresia, and progressive hepatic parenchymal disease (e.g., Wilson disease, hemochromatosis)
  - Contraindicated in **active alcoholism**, multiple suicide attempts, liver cancer, and cirrhosis from chronic hepatitis (uninfected donors)

FIGURE 3-1 **The location of absorption of vitamins, minerals, and nutrients throughout the gastrointestinal tract.**

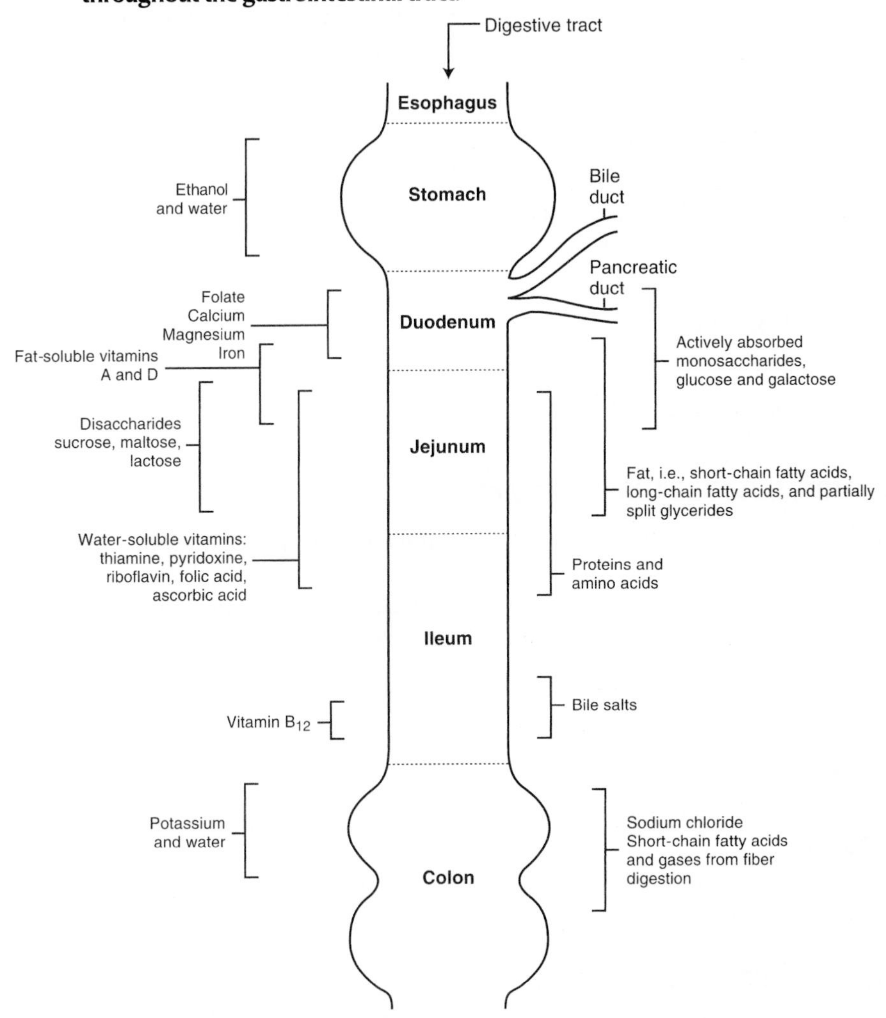

(Modified from Ryan JP. *Physiology.* New York: McGraw Hill 1997. Also see Mehta S, Milder EA, Mirachi AJ, Milder E. *Step-Up: A High-Yield, Systems-Based Review for the USMLE Step 1.* 2nd ed. Philadelphia: Lippincott Williams & Wilkins, 2003. Used with permission of Lippincott Williams & Wilkins.)

- Forty percent of patients experience acute rejection
- Five-year survival is 60% to 70% and correlates with the preoperative health of the recipient
- Pancreas
  - Indicated for severe diabetes mellitus (DM) **type I** or parenchymal pancreatic disease
  - Contraindicated for age >60 years, coronary artery disease (CAD), peripheral vascular disease (PVD), obesity, and **DM type II**
  - Acute rejection is common in most patients
  - Three-year survival is 80%

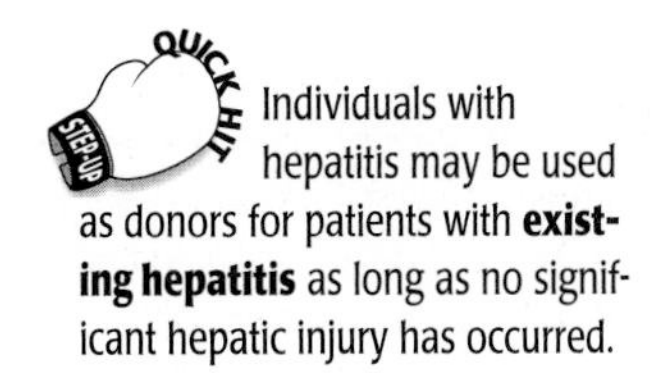

Individuals with hepatitis may be used as donors for patients with **existing hepatitis** as long as no significant hepatic injury has occurred.

CASE 3-1 "I just can't seem to swallow my food"

A 43-year-old woman patient presents to a gastroenterologist on referral for progressive difficulty with swallowing. She says that over the past several years she has experienced progressive difficulty with swallowing both solid food and liquids. More recently, she has had episodes of coughing during eating, and she feels like she is aspirating small amounts of food during these episodes. She occasionally gets heartburn. She feels that she had been losing weight because of the difficulty in consuming food. She denies nausea, vomiting, chest or throat pain, or hoarseness. She had a tubal ligation performed 2 years ago but denies any other medical or surgical history. She takes aspirin (ASA) and a multivitamin daily. She denies any substance use. On examination, she is a thin woman in no distress. No neck masses or lymphadenopathy are detectable. Auscultation detects no abnormal lung or heart sounds. Abdominal examination detects no tenderness or masses. She has normal bowel sounds. Neurologic examination, including commands to swallow, is normal. The following vital signs are measured:

Temperature (T): 98.5°F, heart rate (HR): 72 beats per minute (bpm), blood pressure (BP): 105/74 mm Hg, respiratory rate (RR) 16 breaths/min

Differential Diagnosis

- Esophageal cancer, laryngeal cancer, gastroesophageal reflux disease (GERD), achalasia, diffuse esophageal spasm, Zenker diverticulum, scleroderma

Laboratory Data and Other Study Results

- Barium swallow: dilated esophagus with acute taper at the lower esophageal sphincter (LES)
- Esophagogastroduodenoscopy (EGD): no detectable masses; no evident dysplastic tissue; no gastrointestinal (GI) ulcerations or lesions

Based on these findings, the following test is performed:

- Esophageal manometry: increased LES pressure; decreased LES relaxation during swallowing

Diagnosis

- Achalasia

Treatment Administered

- Nifedipine was prescribed for the patient but discontinued because of hypotension
- Endoscopic pneumatic dilation of LES was performed

Follow-up

- The patient had substantial improvement of her dysphagia and was able to consume solids and liquids with little difficulty

Steps to the Diagnosis

- **Achalasia**
  - Neuromuscular disorder of the esophagus characterized by **impaired peristalsis** and decreased relaxation of the LES resulting in **dysphagia**
    - Due to dysfunction of intramural esophageal neurons
    - Most commonly an idiopathic condition affecting patients 20 to 60 years old
    - **Dysphagia**
      - Difficulty swallowing due to dysfunctional pharyngeal or esophageal transport or pain during swallowing (i.e., odynophagia)
      - Causes include neuromuscular disorders (e.g., achalasia, scleroderma) and obstruction (e.g., peptic strictures, esophageal webs or rings, neoplasm, radiation fibrosis)
      - Obstruction leads to difficulty in swallowing solids only; neuromuscular disorders cause a difficulty in swallowing solids and liquids

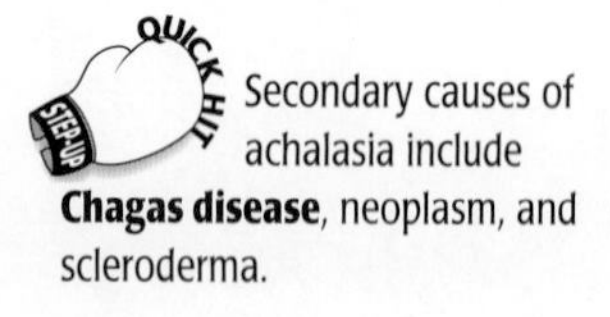

Secondary causes of achalasia include **Chagas disease**, neoplasm, and scleroderma.

- Barium swallow, esophageal manometry, and EGD are useful tools for making a diagnosis
- **History:** progressive dysphagia of solids and liquids, cough, regurgitation, aspiration, heartburn, weight loss from decreased food intake
- **Physical examination:** typically noncontributory
- **Tests:**
  - **Barium swallow** will demonstrate a dilated esophagus with a "bird's **beak**" taper at the site of the LES (Figure 3-2)
  - EGD should be performed to rule out the presence of esophageal masses or obstruction
  - **Esophageal manometry** will demonstrate increased LES pressure, incomplete relaxation of the LES, and impaired peristalsis
- **Treatment:**
  - Nitrates and calcium channel blockers may help to relax the LES but are limited by their vasodilatory effects
  - Endoscopic injection of botulinum toxin or **pneumatic dilation** provides relief for most patients
  - Myotomy may be performed in refractory cases
- **Outcomes:** most patients undergoing pneumatic dilation have good outcomes; esophageal rupture is a risk for EGD or dilation
- **Clues to the diagnosis:**
  - History: difficulty swallowing both solids and liquids, microaspirations
  - Physical: noncontributory
  - Tests: barium swallow and esophageal manometry findings

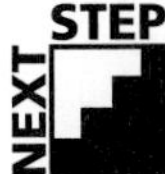

A **barium swallow** is the first study that should be performed in the diagnosis of dysphagia because of its low risk and diagnostic potential.

QUICK HIT

Nitrates and calcium channel blockers are effective in only 10% of patients with achalasia but are safer than esophageal dilation.

FIGURE 3-2 **(A) Barium swallow in a patient with achalasia. Note the distended proximal esophagus with distal tapering and "bird's beak" sign (*white arrow*). (B) Illustration of achalasia demonstrating tapering of the distal esophagus.**

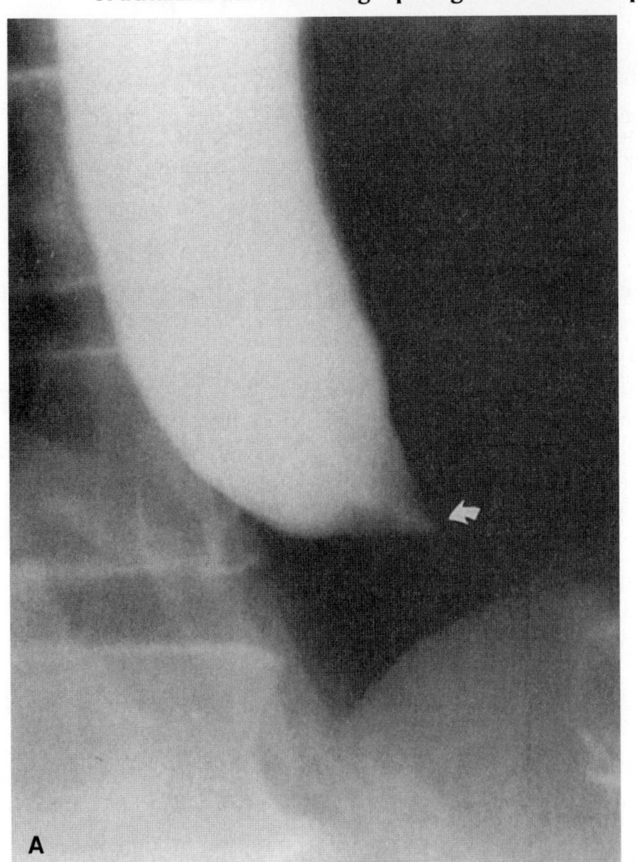

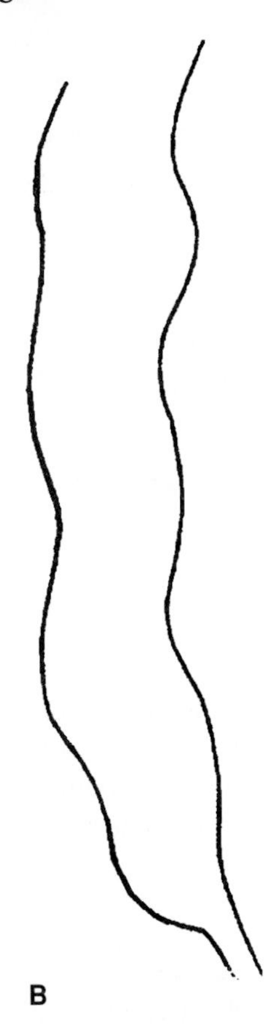

(Taken from Eisenberg RL. *Gastrointestinal radiology: a pattern approach.* 3rd ed. Philadelphia: Lippincott-Raven Publishers, 1996; and Blackbourne LH. *Advanced surgical recall.* 2nd ed. Baltimore: Lippincott Williams & Wilkins, 2004. Used with permission of Lippincott Williams & Wilkins.)

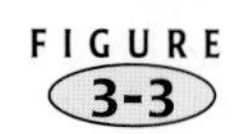

FIGURE 3-3 **(A) Barium swallow in a patient with diffuse esophageal spasm. Note the "corkscrew" pattern throughout the visible esophagus. (B) Illustration of diffuse esophageal spasm demonstrating a twisting "corkscrew" pattern.**

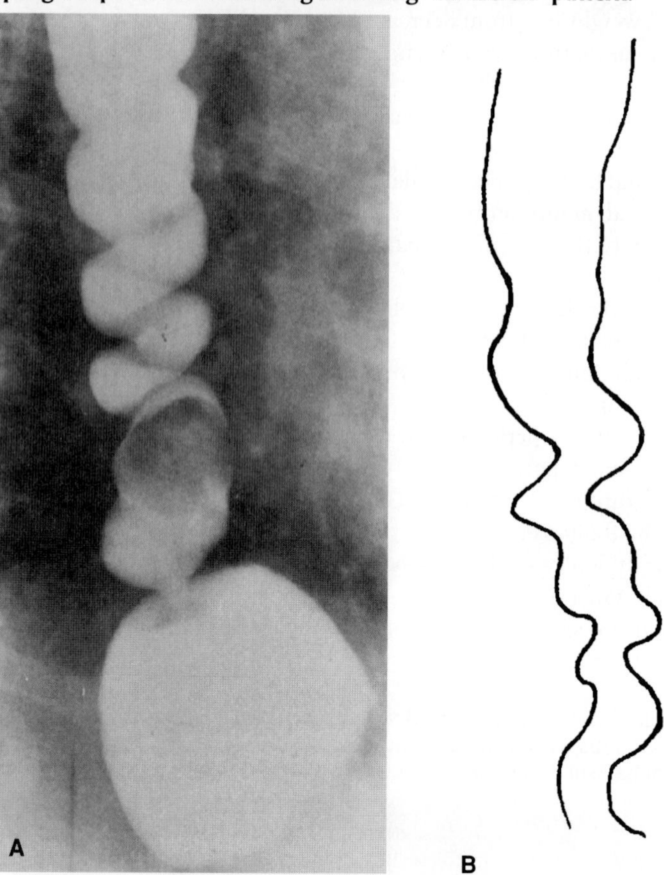

(Taken from Eisenberg RL. *Gastrointestinal radiology: a pattern approach.* 3rd ed. Philadelphia: Lippincott-Raven Publishers, 1996; and Blackbourne LH. *Advanced surgical recall.* 2nd ed. Baltimore: Lippincott Williams & Wilkins, 2004. Used with permission of Lippincott Williams & Wilkins.)

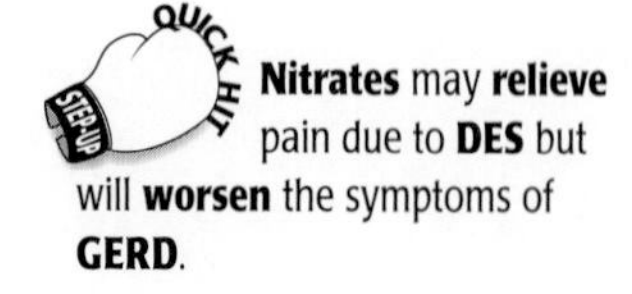

Nitrates may **relieve** pain due to **DES** but will **worsen** the symptoms of **GERD**.

- Diffuse esophageal spasm (DES)
  - Neuromuscular disorder in which the esophagus contracts in a **nonperistaltic** fashion
  - **History**: dysphagia, chest or throat pain
  - **Physical examination**: typically noncontributory
  - **Tests**: barium swallow demonstrates a "**corkscrew**" pattern (Figure 3-3); esophageal manometry demonstrates uncoordinated, nonperistaltic contractions
  - **Treatment**: nitrates, calcium channel blockers, tricyclic antidepressants, and botulinum injections may help reduce dysphagia and chest pain by relaxing esophageal muscles; myotomy may be considered in refractory cases
  - **Outcomes**: prognosis is variable and different patient will respond better to different therapies; esophageal rupture is a risk of myotomy
  - **Why eliminated from differential**: the absence of chest pain and the appearance of the barium swallow help to rule out this diagnosis
- Zenker diverticulum
  - An outpouching in the upper posterior esophagus due a region of smooth muscle weakness
  - **History**: difficulty initiating swallowing, **regurgitation of food hours or days after consumption**, occasional dysphagia, feelings of aspiration, weight loss due to difficulty eating
  - **Physical examination**: bad breath, possible neck fullness
  - **Tests**: barium swallow will demonstrate an outpouching off of the esophagus (Figure 3-4)

FIGURE 3-4 **(A) Barium swallow in a patient with a small Zenker diverticulum (*white arrow*). (B) Illustration of a Zenker diverticulum demonstrating outpouching of the esophagus.**

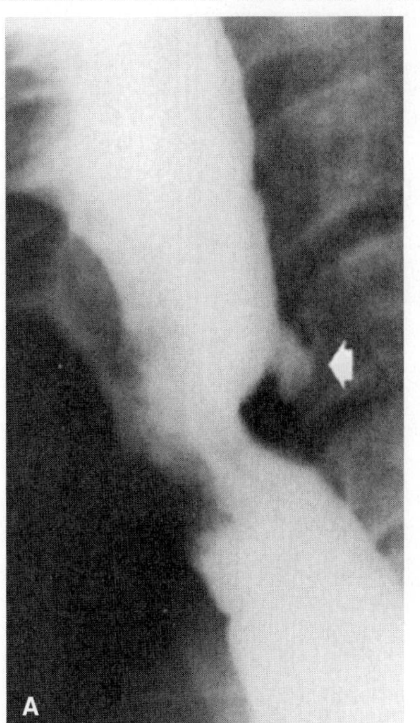

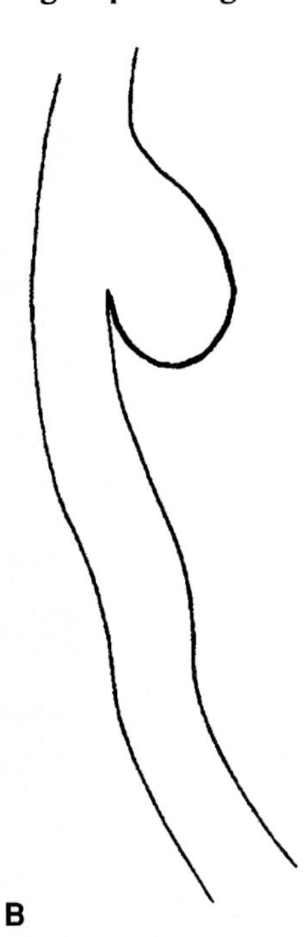

(Taken from Eisenberg RL. *Gastrointestinal radiology: a pattern approach.* 3rd ed. Philadelphia: Lippincott-Raven Publishers, 1996; and Blackbourne LH. *Advanced surgical recall.* 2nd ed. Baltimore: Lippincott Williams & Wilkins, 2004. Used with permission of Lippincott Williams & Wilkins.)

- **Treatment:** surgical cricopharyngeal myotomy or diverticulectomy
- **Outcomes:** surgery has a high rate of successful alleviation of the condition; vocal cord paralysis, mediastinitis, and recurrence are possible complications of surgery
- **Why eliminated from differential:** bad breath and delayed regurgitation are not seen in this case, and the barium swallow did not detect a diverticulum

- Esophageal cancer
  - **Squamous cell carcinoma** (most commonly) or adenocarcinoma (less common) of the esophagus
    - **Adenocarcinoma** is commonly preceded by the development of **Barrett esophagus** (i.e., columnar metaplasia of the distal esophagus secondary to chronic GERD)
  - **Risk factors:** alcohol, tobacco, chronic GERD, obesity (adenocarcinoma only)
  - **History:** progressive dysphagia of solids initially and both solids and liquids later, weight loss, odynophagia, regurgitation, vomiting, weakness, cough, hoarseness, hematemesis
  - **Physical examination:** possible lymphadenopathy
  - **Tests:**
    - Barium swallow will show narrowing of the esophagus and the presence of an abnormal mass (Figure 3-5)
    - Magnetic resonance imaging (MRI), computed tomography (CT), or positron emission tomography (PET) scan may be used to determine the extent of the disease
    - **EGD** is performed to locate the lesion and perform a biopsy
    - **Biopsy** provides a histologic diagnosis of the lesion
  - **Treatment:**
    - Photodynamic therapy with optional laser thermal ablation may be used to treat Barrett esophagus and prevent further progression
    - Total esophagectomy is performed for early stage cancers
    - Radiation therapy and chemotherapy are used as adjuncts to surgery or as primary therapies in unresectable cases

FIGURE 3-5 **Barium swallow in a patient with squamous cell carcinoma of the esophagus. Note the irregularity of the left esophageal wall due to the neoplastic mass.**

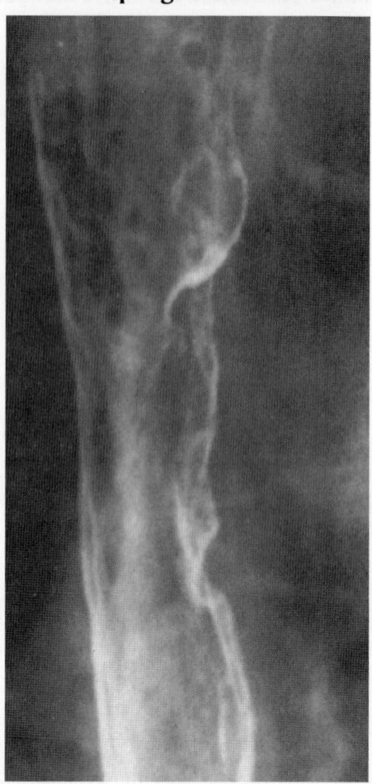

(Taken from Eisenberg RL. *Gastrointestinal radiology: a pattern approach.* 3rd ed. Philadelphia: Lippincott-Raven Publishers, 1996. Used with permission of Lippincott Williams & Wilkins.)

- **Outcomes:** esophageal leakage, myocardial infarction (MI), arrhythmias, atelectasis, and pneumonia are potential surgical complications; nonmetastatic disease is associated with up to a 25% 5-year survival rate, while the 5-year survival for metastatic disease is only 5%
- **Why eliminated from differential:** the presentations of esophageal cancer and achalasia are very similar, but the absence of a lesion on EGD and the esophageal manometry findings help to rule out cancer

- **Laryngeal cancer**
  - Squamous cell cancer of the larynx associated with **tobacco** and **alcohol** use
  - **History: progressive hoarseness**, dysphagia, ear pain, hemoptysis, weight loss
  - **Physical examination:** decreased neck mobility, neck mass
  - **Tests:**
    - Laryngoscopy is used to visualize the lesion
    - Biopsy is used to confirm the histologic diagnosis
    - MRI is used to detect a soft tissue mass and to measure its extent
    - PET scan may be useful to detect early lesions or metastases
  - **Treatment:**
    - Partial or total laryngectomy is performed to remove lesions confined to the larynx
    - Radiation therapy may be used as an adjunct to surgery or as a single therapy in cases of extensive disease
    - Advanced lesions may require surgery, radiation, and chemotherapy
  - **Outcomes:** five-year survival rates are 60% to 85%
  - **Why eliminated from differential:** although the patient has a history of dysphagia and weight loss, the absence of hoarseness decreases the concern for this condition; in the absence of the barium swallow findings a laryngoscopy should be performed
- **Gastroesophageal reflux disease**
  - More thorough discussion in later case
  - **Why eliminated from differential:** although regurgitation, cough, dysphagia, and aspiration may be seen with GERD, the severity of dysphagia seen in this case is typically

not experienced; esophageal manometry demonstrates an increased LES tone instead of insufficient LES tone

- **Scleroderma**
  - More thorough discussion in Chapter 9
  - **Why eliminated from differential:** although esophageal dysmotility is seen in scleroderma, the absence of other systemic sclerosis findings rules out this diagnosis

CASE 3-2 "My heartburn really bothers me"

A 54-year-old man presents to his primary care provider (PCP) with the complaint of chronic heartburn not responding to medication. He says that he has had intermittent heartburn for several years that had previously responded to over-the-counter antacids. These episodes of heartburn had become more frequent over the past year and occasionally were fairly painful, so he was started on omeprazole. He reports that although this medication has helped improve his symptoms somewhat, he is continuing to have occasional moderate heartburn. He describes this sensation as a burning feeling behind his sternum. He says that his symptoms are worse after eating spicy foods, drinking alcohol, or bending over. He denies dysphagia, odynophagia, dyspnea, hematemesis, melena, hematochezia, or radiation of his discomfort away from his sternum. He states that he has a history of hypercholesterolemia and hypertension (HTN) for which he takes ASA, simvastatin, and losartan. He drinks approximately eight beers per week and three cups of coffee every morning. He acknowledges that he has done poorly with following lifestyle recommendations that were made at his previous visit. On examination, he is an obese man in no acute distress. He has no lymphadenopathy and swallows normally. Auscultation detects no abnormal heart or lung sounds. Abdominal examination detects no masses or tenderness. He has normal bowel sounds. The following vital signs are measured:

T: 98.8°F, HR: 86 bpm, BP: 126/85 mm Hg, RR: 17 breaths/min

Differential Diagnosis

- Achalasia, esophageal cancer, gastritis, peptic ulcer disease, GERD, hiatal hernia, MI

Laboratory Data and Other Study Results

- Urea breath test: negative
- Barium swallow: apparent sliding hiatal hernia of moderate size
- EGD: no detectable esophageal masses, erosions, or dysplastic areas; moderate lower esophageal irritation

Diagnosis

- Sliding hiatal hernia with secondary GERD

Treatment Administered

- The patient was encouraged to adopt the lifestyle changes of raising the head of his bed, decreasing his alcohol and caffeine intake, losing weight, and exercising
- The patient was placed on an aggressive twice daily dose of esomeprazole

Follow-up

- The patient had further improvements in his symptoms but not complete resolution of his occasional heartburn
- After 6 months of therapy without complete resolution of his symptoms, the patient underwent a Nissen fundoplication
- The patient responded well to surgical treatment with significantly improved symptoms

QUICK HIT: GERD symptoms are usually absent in patients with **paraesophageal** hiatal hernias.

Steps to the Diagnosis

- **Hiatal hernia**
  - Herniation of a section of the stomach above the level of the diaphragm
    - **Sliding type**: gastroesophageal junction and stomach are displaced above the diaphragm (**95% of cases**)
    - **Paraesophageal type**: stomach protrudes through the diaphragm, but the gastroesophageal junction remains fixed in the correct location
  - **History**: most patients are asymptomatic, but some patients with sliding hernias may have symptoms of GERD that are refractory to normal therapy
  - **Physical examination**: typically noncontributory, but symptoms are more common in obese or pregnant patients
  - **Tests**: chest x-ray (CXR) or barium swallow is useful for detecting the section of the stomach that has herniated through the diaphragm (Figure 3-6)
  - **Treatment**: sliding hernias frequently respond to H_2 antagonists or protein pump inhibitors (PPIs); paraesophageal hernias and sliding hernias with refractory GERD symptoms may be treated with gastropexy or Nissen fundoplication
  - **Outcomes**: complications include incarceration of the stomach with paraesophageal hernias and the sequelae of chronic GERD with sliding hernias
  - **Clues to the diagnosis:**
    - History: heartburn not responding to medication
    - Physical: noncontributory
    - Tests: barium swallow findings
- **Gastroesophageal reflux disease**
  - Insufficiency of the LES leading to an abnormal reflux of gastric contents into the esophagus
  - **Risk factors**: obesity, hiatal hernia, pregnancy, scleroderma, tobacco use, consumption of alcohol, caffeine, or fatty foods

FIGURE 3-6 Detection of a sliding type hiatal hernia with x-ray. (A) Anteroposterior view of a hiatal hernia (*arrows*) with partial protrusion of the stomach above the diaphragm. (B) Lateral view of the same hiatal hernia.

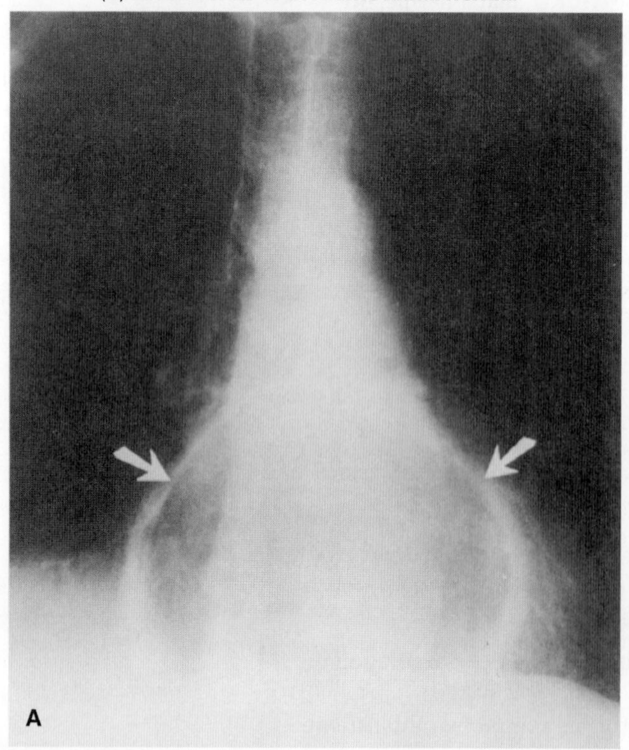

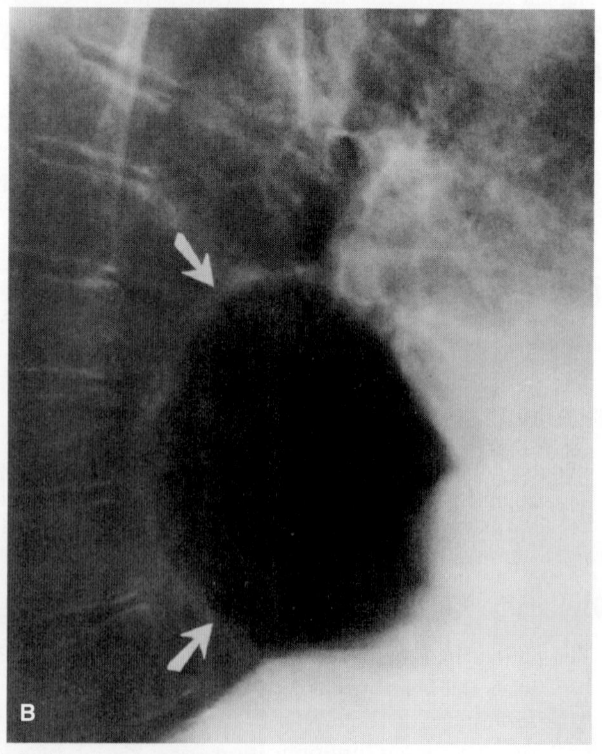

(Taken from Eisenberg RL. *Gastrointestinal radiology: a pattern approach.* 4th ed. Philadelphia: Lippincott Williams & Wilkins, 2003. Fig. 13-9. Used with permission of Lippincott Williams & Wilkins.)

- **History:** burning chest pain ("**heartburn**") approximately 30 minutes after eating, worsening of pain with reclining or bending over, sour taste in the mouth, regurgitation, dysphagia, odynophagia, nausea, cough
- **Physical examination:** typically noncontributory
- **Tests:**
  - The diagnosis is frequently **clinical** and does not require invasive testing
  - Esophageal pH monitoring will detect decreased pH if measured over a 24-hour period
  - Esophageal manometry detects decreased LES tone
  - EGD or barium swallow may be performed to rule out esophageal cancer or Barrett esophagus
- **Treatment:**
  - Elevation of the head of the bed, weight loss, and decreasing the consumption of substances that precipitate symptoms (e.g., alcohol, caffeine, fatty foods) are all recommended lifestyle modifications
  - Antacids are initially used on an as-needed basis (Table 3-1)
  - H_2 antagonists are prescribed if antacids are insufficient to control symptoms and are effective in 70% to 80% of cases of mild esophagitis
  - PPIs are used in more severe cases and are highly effective in most cases
  - Promotility agents may improve symptoms by speeding gastric emptying
  - Refractory disease may be treated surgically with Nissen fundoplication
- **Outcomes:** the vast majority of patients will respond to pharmacologic treatment; complications of chronic disease include esophageal ulceration, esophageal stricture, Barrett esophagus, and adenocarcinoma
- **Why eliminated from differential:** GERD does occur in this patient and explains his collection of symptoms, but the failure of pharmacologic therapy to alleviate his symptoms points to an underlying cause of his GERD

QUICK HIT: Symptoms of GERD may mimic asthma or a MI.

- **Peptic ulcer disease (PUD)**
  - More thorough discussion in later case
  - **Why eliminated from differential:** the predominance of esophageal symptoms, the negative urea breath test, and the negative EGD findings rule out this diagnosis
- **Gastritis**
  - More thorough discussion in later case
  - **Why eliminated from differential:** the predominance of esophageal symptoms, the negative urea breath test, and the negative EGD findings rule out this diagnosis
- **Achalasia**
  - More thorough discussion in prior case

TABLE 3-1 Medications Used in Treatment of Gastroesophageal Reflux Disease

Medication	Mechanism	Adverse Effects	Prescription Strategy
Antacids (e.g., calcium carbonate, aluminum hydroxide)	Neutralize gastric acid	Constipation, nausea, diarrhea	Initial therapy, as needed
H_2 antagonists (e.g., cimetidine, ranitidine)	Reversibly block histamine H_2 receptors to inhibit gastric acid secretion	Headache, diarrhea, rare thrombocytopenia; cimetidine may cause gynecomastia and impotence	Patients not responding to antacids
PPIs (e.g., omeprazole, lansoprazole)	Irreversibly inhibit parietal cell proton pump (H^+/K^+ ATPase) to block gastric acid secretion	Well tolerated; may increase effects of warfarin, benzodiazepines, phenytoin, digoxin, or carbamazepine in some patients	Patients not responding to antacids
Promotility agents (e.g., cisapride)	Promote gastric emptying	Headache, diarrhea, cardiac effects	Patients with poor LES function

GERD, gastroesophageal reflux disease; H^+, hydrogen ion; K^+, potassium ion; LES, lower esophageal sphincter; PPIs, proton pump inhibitors.

- **Why eliminated from differential:** the absence of significant dysphagia makes this diagnosis unlikely, and the barium swallow findings further confirm the true diagnosis
- **Esophageal cancer**
  - More thorough discussion in prior case
  - **Why eliminated from differential:** the negative EGD findings and absence of a mass on barium swallow rule out this diagnosis
- **Myocardial infarction**
  - More thorough discussion in Chapter 1
  - **Why eliminated from differential:** the quality of chest pain in this case is more consistent with reflux than a cardiac cause; the frequent recurrence of heartburn, relation to eating, and response to antacid drugs further help to suggest a GI pathology

CASE 3-3 "I get burning pains every time I eat"

A 63-year-old man presents to his PCP with the complaint of burning epigastric pain that occurs soon after eating on a fairly regular basis. He says that this pain begins within an hour after meals. He also describes mild nausea accompanying this pain. He had two episodes during the prior week in which he vomited due to this nausea and noticed some brown discoloration to his emesis. He says that these symptoms have been occurring for the past 2 months. He denies any gross blood during episodes of emesis, any blood in his stool, or weight loss. He has gotten some relief from over-the-counter antacids and ranitidine. He describes a history of significant osteoarthritis in both of his knees and takes naproxen and ASA as medications. He has approximately four alcoholic drinks per week and denies tobacco use. On examination, he is in no distress. He does not exhibit lymphadenopathy. Auscultation detects no abnormal lung or heart sounds. Abdominal examination detects mild tenderness on epigastric palpation, no masses, no guarding, and no rebound tenderness. The following vital signs are measured:

T: 98.5°F, HR: 78 bpm, BP: 130/85 mm Hg, RR: 16 breaths/min

Differential Diagnosis

- Gastritis, peptic ulcer disease, Zollinger-Ellison syndrome, pancreatitis, GERD, gastric cancer

Laboratory Data and Other Study Results

- Complete blood cell count (CBC): white blood cells (WBC): 7.4, hemoglobin (Hgb): 13.5, platelets (Plt): 290
- 7-electrolyte chemistry panel (Chem7): sodium (Na): 135 mEq/L, potassium (K): 3.9 mEq/L, chloride (Cl): 106 mEq/L, carbon dioxide (CO_2): 26 mEq/L, blood urea nitrogen (BUN): 20 mg/dL, creatine (Cr): 0.5 mg/dL, glucose (Glu): 95 mg/dL
- Coagulation panel (Coags): protime (PT) 10.9, international normalized ratio (INR): 1.0, partial thromboplastin time (PTT) 24.7
- Amylase: 100 U/L
- Lipase: 90 U/L
- Urea breath test: negative
- *Helicobacter pylori* antibody screen: negative
- Barium swallow: small uniform focal pooling of contrast within lesser curvature of stomach; no esophageal or duodenal abnormalities

Following these tests, the additional following studies are ordered:

- EGD: small ulceration on lesser curve of stomach; biopsy of ulcer performed; no active bleeding from ulcer; no esophageal or duodenal abnormalities
- Ulcer biopsy: fibrous tissue with infiltration of monocytes; no dysplastic cells

Diagnosis

- Gastric ulcer (peptic ulcer disease) secondary to nonsteroidal anti-inflamatory drug (NSAID) overuse

Treatment Administered

- The patient was prescribed regular ranitidine and lansoprazole
- Naproxen was discontinued, and the patient was started on celecoxib for arthritis pain

Follow-up

- The patient experienced a gradual improvement in his symptoms with a complete resolution of epigastric pain in 4 months

Steps to the Diagnosis

- **Peptic ulcer disease**
  - Erosion of the gastric or duodenal mucosal surface secondary to impaired endothelial protection and increased gastric acidity (Color Figure 3-1)
    - **Duodenal** ulcers are more common and are most often a result of ***H. pylori*** infection (Table 3-2)
    - **Gastric** ulcers are less common and are commonly due to **NSAID overuse** or *H. pylori* infection (Table 3-2)
  - **Risk factors:** ***H. pylori infection, NSAIDs***, tobacco, alcohol, corticosteroids
  - **History**: periodic **burning epigastric pain** that may vary in intensity following meals, nausea, hematemesis, melena, hematochezia
  - **Physical examination:** epigastric tenderness, and acute perforation of an ulcer is associated with abdominal rigidity and rebound tenderness
  - **Tests:**
    - CBC is useful for detecting anemia due to active bleeding
    - A positive urea breath test or positive immunoglobulin G (IgG) antibodies to *H. pylori* helps diagnose the respective infection
    - Abdominal x-ray (AXR) will detect free abdominal air in cases of perforation; a barium swallow may detect collections of barium within ulcerations
    - EGD is performed to visualize ulcers, assess bleeding, and perform biopsies to rule out cancer
  - **Treatment:**
    - **PPIs** and **H_2 antagonists** are used to decrease gastric acid levels and prevent further mucosal damage

TABLE 3-2 Distinguishing between Gastric and Duodenal Ulcers

Characteristic	Gastric Ulcer	Duodenal Ulcer
Patients	Age >50 years, *Helicobacter pylori* infection, NSAID users	Younger, *H. pylori* infection
Frequency	25% cases	75% cases
Timing of pain	**Soon after** eating	**2–4 hours after** eating
Gastric acid level	Normal/low	High
Gastrin level	High	Normal
Effect of eating	May **worsen** symptoms and cause nausea and vomiting	**Initial improvement** in symptoms, with **later worsening**

NSAIDs, nonsteroidal anti-inflammatory drugs.

MNEMONIC

Causes of peptic ulcer disease may be remembered by the mnemonic **ANGST HAM**: **A**spirin, **N**SAIDs, **G**astrinoma (ZES), **S**teroids, **T**obacco, ***H.** pylori*, **A**lcohol, **M**EN type I.

NEXT STEP

Peptic ulcers may develop secondary to the systemic inflammatory response seen with severe burns (i.e., **Curling ulcers**), intracranial injuries (i.e., **Cushing ulcers**), or multisystem trauma, so all trauma patients with significant injuries should receive prophylactic **ranitidine**.

QUICK HIT

Barium swallow radiographic findings that suggest the presence of a malignant lesion associated with an ulcer include **abnormal-appearing mucosal folds** in the region of the ulcer, the presence of a **mass** near the ulcer, and irregular **filling defects** in the base of the ulcer.

NEXT STEP

Patients younger than 40 years with symptoms suggestive of PUD for a short duration of time may be worked-up with noninvasive testing; an EGD is required to rule out gastric malignancy in older individuals or those with symptoms lasting longer than 2 months.

- Sucralfate, bismuth subsalicylate, and misoprostol may be useful to aid in mucosal protection
- *H. pylori* infection is eliminated by **multidrug regimens** (e.g., clarithromycin, amoxicillin, and a PPI and metronidazole, tetracycline, bismuth, and a PPI for 14 days are two common regimens)
- Partial gastrectomy may be required for severe hemorrhage due to erosion of an ulcer into the gastric vasculature; parietal cell vagotomy or antrectomy may be considered in refractory cases

NEXT STEP: Patients with refractory PUD that does not respond to PPI therapy should undergo **fasting gastrin** and **secretin-stimulation** testing to determine if they have **Zollinger-Ellison syndrome**.

- **Outcomes:** complications include significant **hemorrhage** (the gastroduodenal artery in particular with posterior ulcers), **perforation** (most common in anterior ulcers), and lymphoproliferative disease; uncomplicated ulcers typically respond very well to medical therapy
- **Clues to the diagnosis:**
  - History: epigastric pain and nausea following eating, clotted blood in emesis, response to antacid medication, frequent use of NSAIDs and ASA
  - Physical: epigastric tenderness
  - Tests: low normal Hgb, barium swallow findings, EGD, and biopsy findings

- **Gastritis**
  - Inflammation of the gastric mucosa without full mucosal penetration
    - **Acute** variant: rapidly developing superficially erosive lesions in any region of the stomach that are related to **NSAID** use, alcohol, corrosive substance ingestion, or stress from severe illness
    - **Chronic** variant: nonerosive lesions most common in the antrum or fundus of the stomach (Table 3-3)
  - **History:** possibly asymptomatic or epigastric pain, indigestion, nausea, vomiting, hematemesis, or melena
  - **Physical examination:** frequently normal with occasional epigastric tenderness and bad breath
  - **Tests:**
    - A positive urea breath test or positive IgG antibodies to *H. pylori* help diagnose this infection
    - Analysis of pepsinogen isoenzymes is useful to the detection of autoimmune disease (decreased pepsinogen I/pepsinogen II ratio in disease)
    - EGD allows visualization of the mucosa and biopsy
    - Gastric biopsy may help differentiate causes of chronic disease
  - **Treatment:**
    - Acute disease is treated in a similar fashion to PUD (e.g., stopping offending medications, prescribing PPIs and H_2 antagonists)

QUICK HIT: In **pernicious anemia**, autoantibodies destroy parietal cells, leading to low levels of intrinsic factor, vitamin B_{12} malabsorption, and megaloblastic anemia.

TABLE 3-3 Variants of Chronic Gastritis

Characteristic	Type A (Autoimmune)	Type B (*Helicobacter pylori*)	Type C (Chemical)
Site	**Fundus**	**Antrum**	**Antrum**
Pathology	Autoantibodies for parietal cells induce gastric atrophy	*H. pylori* infection	Chronic chemical irritation (e.g., NSAIDs) or biliary reflux
Labs	Decreased gastric acid level, decreased gastrin	Increased gastric acid level, increased gastrin	May be normal
Associated conditions	Pernicious anemia, achlorhydria, thyroiditis	Peptic ulcer disease, gastric cancer	Peptic ulcer disease, incompetent pyloric sphincter, abnormal intestinal motility

NSAIDs, nonsteroidal anti-inflammatory drugs.

- Chronic gastritis due to *H. pylori* is treated with regimen similar to that for PUD
- Chemical chronic gastritis is treated by identifying and stopping use of the offending agent
- Autoimmune chronic gastritis requires vitamin B_{12} replacement
- Sucralfate, bismuth subsalicylate, and misoprostol may be useful for mucosal protection

- **Outcomes:** complications include PUD, hemorrhage, pernicious anemia (autoimmune gastritis), and gastric cancer (*H. pylori* gastritis)
- **Why eliminated from differential:** although gastritis and PUD may have similar presentations, the barium swallow and EGD findings are confirmatory of the presence of an ulcer

- Zollinger-Ellison syndrome
  - Syndrome of refractory PUD and malabsorption due to the presence of a gastrin-producing tumor
  - **History: refractory PUD**, abdominal pain, nausea, vomiting, indigestion, diarrhea, steatorrhea
  - **Physical examination:** possible epigastric tenderness, hepatomegaly, jaundice
  - **Tests:**
    - **Increased fasting gastrin**
    - Administration of secretin causes an excessive increase in serum gastrin levels (i.e., secretin-stimulation test)
    - Venous gastrin sampling may be useful to localize the tumor
    - Single-positron emission computed tomography (SPECT) with somatostatin receptor imaging may be useful for tumor localization
    - Angiography may detect tumor hypervascularity
  - **Treatment:**
    - Surgical resection is indicated for nonmetastatic disease (easiest for extrapancreatic lesions)
    - PPIs and H_2 antagonists may help mollify symptoms
    - Octreotide is used to improve symptoms in metastatic disease
  - **Outcomes:**
    - Occasionally associated with other endocrine tumors (e.g., multiple endocrine neoplasia 1 [MEN1])
    - Sixty percent of tumors are malignant
    - Hemorrhage and perforation due to severe PUD
    - Nonmetastatic disease has an excellent prognosis
  - **Why eliminated from differential:** the good response of the patient to a regimen of lansoprazole and ranitidine without recurrence make this diagnosis unlikely

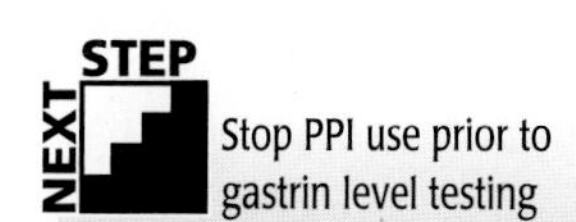

Stop PPI use prior to gastrin level testing to ensure an accurate measurement.

- Gastric cancer
  - **Adenocarcinoma** (more common) or squamous cell carcinoma (rare, due to esophageal invasion) involving the stomach
    - **Ulcerating:** dysplastic irregular ulcers that may be confused for PUD
    - **Polypoid:** large intraluminal neoplasms
    - **Superficial spreading:** mucosal and submucosal involvement only
    - **Linitis plastica:** all layers of the stomach are involved; impaired stomach elasticity
  - **Risk factors:** *H. pylori* infection, family history, Japanese heritage and living in Japan, tobacco, alcohol, vitamin C deficiency, high consumption of preserved foods, male gender
  - **History:** weight loss, anorexia, early satiety, vomiting, dysphagia, epigastric pain
  - **Physical examination:** abdominal mass, left supraclavicular lymphadenopathy (i.e., **Virchow node**), periumbilical lymphadenopathy (i.e., **Sister Mary Joseph node**)
  - **Tests:**
    - Increased carcinoembryonic antigen (CEA)
    - Increased 2-glucuronidase in gastric secretion analysis
    - Barium swallow may show a mass or a thickened "leather bottle" stomach in the case of linitis plastica

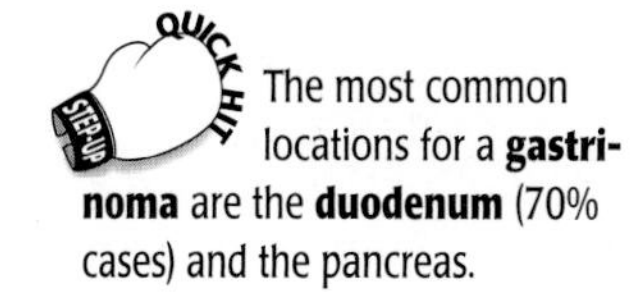

The most common locations for a **gastrinoma** are the **duodenum** (70% cases) and the pancreas.

  - EGD is used to visualize ulcerations and masses and to perform biopsies
  - Biopsy is required to provide a histologic diagnosis
- **Treatment:** subtotal gastrectomy is performed for tumors in the distal third of the stomach, and total gastrectomy is performed for more proximal or invasive tumors; chemotherapy and radiation therapy are performed as adjuncts to surgery or alone for extensive disease
- **Outcomes:**
  - Superficial spreading type has the best prognosis, linitis plastica has the worst
  - Early detection has cure rates up to 70%, but prognosis is poor for any delays in detection (<15% 5-year survival)
- **Why eliminated from differential:** the results of the biopsy indicate that the ulcer in this patient is not cancerous

- **Gastroesophageal reflux disease**
  - More thorough discussion in prior case
  - **Why eliminated from differential:** epigastric pain and a response to antacid drugs may be seen in both conditions, but the barium swallow and EGD results are confirmatory of PUD
- **Pancreatitis**
  - More thorough discussion in later case
  - **Why eliminated from differential:** both conditions may cause epigastric pain, but the normal amylase and lipase levels and barium swallow and EGD findings rule out this diagnosis

CASE 3-4 "This diarrhea is driving me crazy!"

A 43-year-old man presents to his PCP with a complaint of six episodes of bloody diarrhea since the previous evening. He also describes achy abdominal pain. He denies any dizziness, syncope, weakness, numbness, arthralgias, vision symptoms, or hematemesis. He says that he went to a picnic 5 days ago and believes that he must have eaten something that caused these symptoms because some of the other people who attended the picnic have been having the same complaints. He denies previous episodes of bloody diarrhea and any past medical history. He denies any medication or illicit substance use. On examination, he appears to be uncomfortable but not in any distress. He has a pink skin color. He has no palpable lymphadenopathy. Auscultation detects hyperactive bowel sounds but no abnormal lung or heart sounds. He has mild abdominal pain on deep palpation and no masses, rebound tenderness, or rigidity. His neurologic examination is normal. His pulses are bounding, and he has quick capillary refill. The following vital signs are measured:

T: 100.2°F, HR: 90 bpm, BP: 110/78 mm Hg, RR: 17 breaths/min

Differential Diagnosis

- Bacterial gastroenteritis, viral gastroenteritis, parasitic gastroenteritis, celiac sprue, inflammatory bowel disease (IBD), diverticulitis

Laboratory Data and Other Study Results

- CBC: WBC: 11.2, Hgb: 15.9, Plt: 290
- Fecal leukocytes: positive
- Stool culture: no parasites visible in microscopic examination; culture pending
- *Clostridium difficile* stool assay: negative

Diagnosis

- Bacterial gastroenteritis

Treatment Administered

- The patient was strongly encouraged to drink liquids to maintain his hydration
- The patient was started on empiric ciprofloxacin

Follow-up

- The patient experienced some improvement in the degree of diarrhea after the initiation of antibiotics
- Stool culture grew *Campylobacter jejuni*, so the prescribed antibiotic was changed to erythromycin
- The patient experienced a further improvement in his symptoms, and the diarrhea stopped by two days after beginning treatment

Steps to the Diagnosis

- **Bacterial gastroenteritis**
  - Infection of the GI tract due to a bacterial cause that results in some type of GI disturbance (e.g., vomiting, diarrhea) (Table 3-4)

TABLE 3-4 Common Pathogens in Bacterial Gastroenteritis

Pathogen	Source	Signs and Symptoms	Treatment
Bacillus cereus	Fried rice	**Vomiting** within several hours of eating, diarrhea later	Self-limited; hydration
Campylobacter jejuni	Poultry (second most common food-bourne bacterial GI infection)	**Bloody** diarrhea, abdominal pain, fever; rare Guillain-Barré syndrome	Hydration, erythromycin; generally self-limited
Clostridium botulinum	Honey, home-canned foods	Nausea, vomiting, diarrhea, **flaccid paralysis**	Botulism antitoxin (not given to infants); self-limited
Clostridium difficile	**Antibiotic-induced suppression** of normal colonic flora	**Watery** diarrhea; gray pseudomembranes seen on colonic mucosa	Metronidazole, vancomycin
Escherichia coli (enterotoxigenic)	Food/water (i.e., **travelers'** diarrhea)	**Watery** diarrhea, vomiting, fever	Hydration; self-limited
E. coli type **O157:H7** (enterohemorrhagic)	Ground beef, indirect fecal contamination	**Bloody** diarrhea, vomiting, fever, abdominal pain, risk of HUS	Hydration; self-limited; antibiotics may actually worsen symptoms due to toxin release
Staphylococcus aureus	Room-temperature food	**Vomiting,** within several hours of eating, diarrhea later	Self-limited; hydration
Salmonella species	Eggs, poultry, milk, fresh produce **(most common food-bourne bacterial GI infection)**	Nausea, abdominal pain, **bloody** diarrhea, fever, vomiting	Hydration; self-limited; treat immunocompromised patients with fluoroquinolone
Shigella species	Food/water; associated with overcrowding	Fever, nausea, vomiting, **severe bloody** diarrhea, abdominal pain, risk of HUS	Hydration; self-limited; ciprofloxacin, TMP-SMX in severe cases
Vibrio cholerae	Water, seafood	**Copious watery** diarrhea, signs of dehydration	**Hydration**; tetracycline or doxycycline decrease disease length
Vibrio parahaemolyticus	Seafood (e.g., oysters)	Abdominal pain, **watery** diarrhea within 24 hours of eating	Hydration; self-limited
Yersinia enterocolitica	Pork, produce	Abdominal pain, **bloody** diarrhea, right lower quadrant pain, fever	Hydration; self-limited

GI, gastrointestinal; HUS, hemolytic uremic syndrome; TMP-SMX, trimethoprim-sulfamethoxazole.

FIGURE 3-7 Diagnostic and treatment pathways for acute diarrhea.

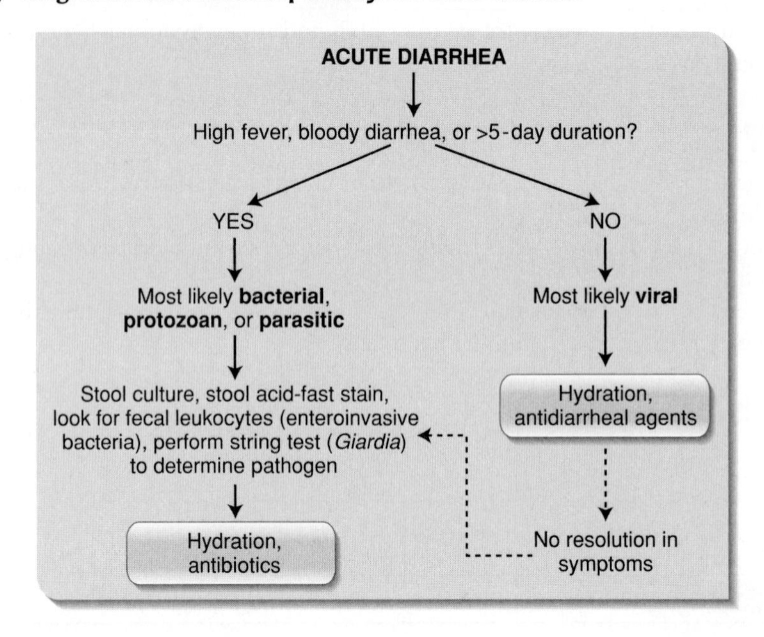

MNEMONIC

Common pathogens involved in food poisoning are remembered by the mnemonic "**E**ating **C**ontaminated **S**tuff **S**ometimes **C**auses **V**ery **B**ig **S**melly **V**omit": ***E**scherichia coli* (enterotoxigenic, enterohemorrhagic), ***C**ampylobacter jejuni*, ***S**taphylococcus aureus*, **S**almonella, ***C**lostridium botulinum*, **V**ibrio cholerae, **B**acillus cereus, **S**higella, **V**ibrio parahaemolyticus.

QUICK HIT

Rotavirus is the most common cause of acute diarrhea in children.

- Contaminated food and water are the most common source of infection
- **Diarrhea**
  - Frequency of bowel movements (stool production >200 g/day) and increased stool liquidity
  - **Acute** diarrhea lasts <2 weeks and is usually due to infection (Figure 3-7)
  - **Chronic** diarrhea lasts longer than 2 weeks and may be due to chronic infection, malabsorption, or dysfunctional GI motility (Figure 3-8)

FIGURE 3-8 Diagnostic pathway for chronic diarrhea.

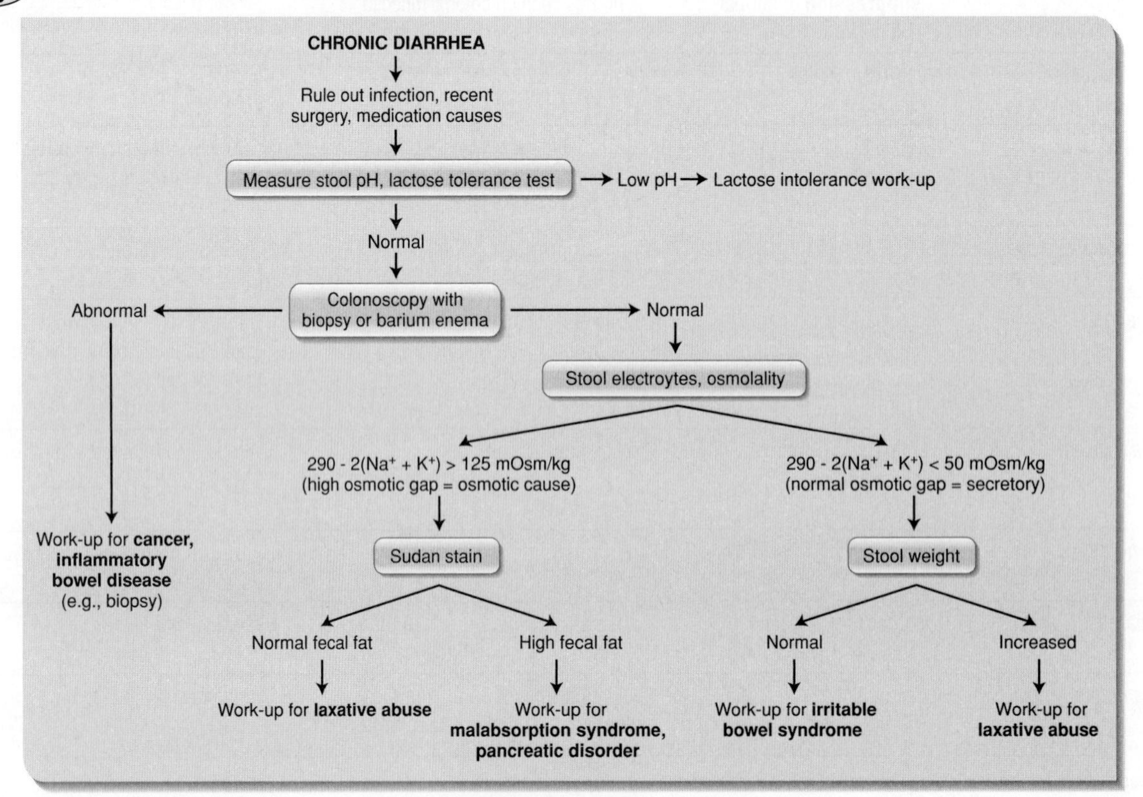

    - **Secretory** diarrheas are usually **hormone mediated** or due to enterotoxic bacterial infections
    - **Osmotic** diarrheas are due to an increased intraluminal solute concentration that leads to a decreased reabsorption of water
    - **Inflammatory** diarrheas are due to an autoimmune process or chronic infection
    - Diarrhea is common in immunocompromised patients (e.g., human immunodeficiency virus [HIV], chronic corticosteroid use) and is typically due to opportunistic pathogens
  - **History:** nausea, **diarrhea** (watery or bloody), abdominal pain, possible vomiting,
  - **Physical examination:** perianal erythema, signs of dehydration (e.g., decreased skin turgor, dry mucous membranes), increased bowel sounds, rare neurologic deficits
  - **Tests:**
    - **Fecal leukocytes** are present on stool analysis
    - Stool assays exist for the detection of *C. difficile*
    - Culture will provide an identification of the causative organism
    - Colonoscopy may be useful to visualize pseudomembrane formation in *C. difficile* colitis
  - **Treatment:**
    - The majority of cases are self-limited and only require supportive care (particularly **rehydration**)
    - Patients who are immunosuppressed, significantly dehydrated, have bloody diarrhea, or are very young or old are treated with empiric antibiotics pending culture results (typically fluoroquinolones)
    - Species-appropriate antibiotics are prescribed when the pathogen is identified (14 days of therapy)
  - **Outcomes:** prognosis is good with administration of the proper therapy; uncommon complications include chronic malabsorption, hepatic damage, and spread of infection to non-GI sites
  - **Clues to the diagnosis:**
    - History: acute bloody diarrhea, similar symptoms in other picnic attendees
    - Physical: abdominal tenderness, hyperactive bowel sounds
    - Tests: mildly increased WBC, positive stool leukocytes

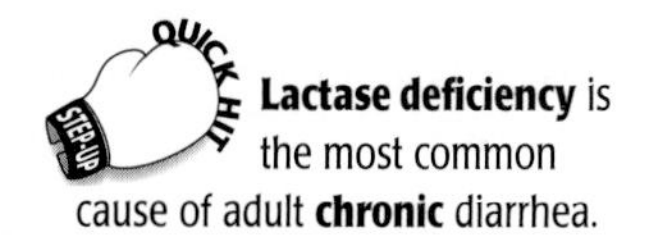

Lactase deficiency is the most common cause of adult **chronic** diarrhea.

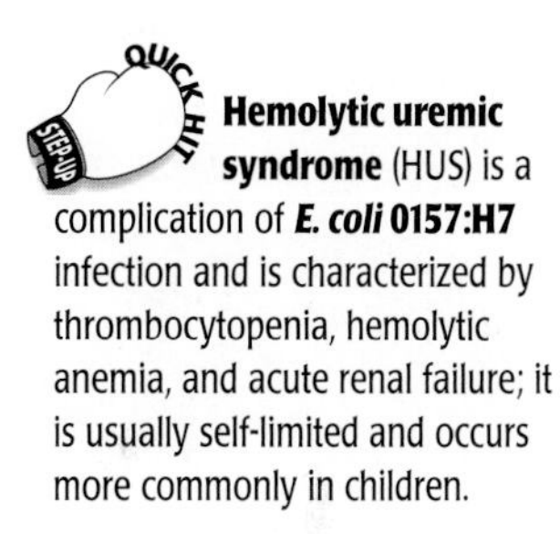

Hemolytic uremic syndrome (HUS) is a complication of ***E. coli*** **0157:H7** infection and is characterized by thrombocytopenia, hemolytic anemia, and acute renal failure; it is usually self-limited and occurs more commonly in children.

- **Viral gastroenteritis**
  - Infection of the GI tract by a viral pathogen resulting in GI disturbance
    - Common pathogens include **Norwalk virus**, Coxsackie virus A1, echovirus, adenovirus, and rotavirus
  - **History:** nausea, vomiting, diarrhea, abdominal pain, myalgias
  - **Physical examination:** low-grade fever, mild abdominal tenderness
  - **Tests: no fecal leukocytes** are present in stool analysis; viral cultures may be performed but are rarely necessary
  - **Treatment:** supportive care only
  - **Outcomes:** self-limited
  - **Why eliminated from differential:** the presence of fecal leukocytes in the stool analysis rules out this diagnosis
- **Parasitic gastroenteritis**
  - Infection of the GI tract by a protozoan or parasitic organism (Table 3-5)
  - **History:** abdominal pain, **diarrhea** (watery, greasy, or bloody), malaise, myalgias
  - **Physical examination:** fever, abdominal tenderness, signs of dehydration, rare neurologic deficits
  - **Tests:** parasites are visualized in a stool sample; antibody tests exist for several pathogens
  - **Treatment:**
    - Supportive care (especially rehydration)
    - Species-specific antiparasitic therapy (e.g., metronidazole, paromomycin)
    - Surgical decompression and resection of necrotizing colitis or hepatic abscesses
  - **Outcomes:** excellent prognosis with the appropriate treatment; possible complications include hepatic abscesses, intestinal obstruction, necrotizing colitis, and neurologic infection

TABLE 3-5 Common Pathogens in Parasitic and Protozoan Gastrointestinal Infections

Pathogen	Source	Signs and Symptoms	Treatment
Giardia lamblia (Color Figure 3-2)	Surface water (usually limited to wilderness or other countries)	**Greasy**, foul-smelling diarrhea; abdominal pain, malaise; cysts and trophozoites seen in stool sample	Metronidazole; hydration
Entamoeba histolytica	Water, areas of poor sanitation	Mild to severe **bloody** diarrhea, abdominal pain; cysts and trophozoites seen in stool sample	Metronidazole, paromomycin
Cryptosporidium parvum	Food/water; immunocompromised patients	**Watery** diarrhea, abdominal pain, malaise; acid-fast stain of stool shows parasites	Control immune suppression; nitazoxanide
Trichinella spiralis	Undercooked pork	Fever, **myalgias**, periorbital edema; eosinophilia	Albendazole, mebendazole if CNS or cardiac symptoms
Taenia solium	Undercooked pork	Mild diarrhea, **CNS symptoms**	Praziquantel, corticosteroids if more than five cysts

CNS, central nervous system.

- **Why eliminated from differential:** the absence of visible parasites on microscopic examination makes this diagnosis less likely
- **Celiac sprue**
  - More thorough discussion in later case
  - **Why eliminated from differential:** diarrhea in this condition would be a more chronic condition, so this diagnosis is less likely for the given case presentation; the diagnosis could be further ruled out by performing testing for antiendomysial and antigliadin antibodies
- **Inflammatory bowel disease**
  - More thorough discussion in later case
  - **Why eliminated from differential:** this diagnosis would be expected to be a more chronic process, to have presented earlier in the patient's life, and also to feature multiple extraintestinal symptoms; colonoscopy and biopsy could be performed to aid in the diagnosis if concern for this condition existed
- **Diverticulitis**
  - More thorough discussion in later case
  - **Why eliminated from differential:** left lower quadrant pain and lower GI bleeding would predominate in this presentation, and diarrhea would not be common; CT could be performed to look for free air, diverticuli, and possible rupture if a strong clinical suspicion remained

CASE 3-5 "My bowels just aren't right"

A 37-year-old woman presents to a gastroenterologist on referral from her PCP for the work-up of chronic diarrhea and multiple other GI symptoms. The patient says that she has had frequent bouts of loose stools or watery diarrhea for the past 5 years and has become increasingly frustrated with attempts to change her diet in order to improve these symptoms. She also describes frequent abdominal cramping, flatulence, bloating, fatigue, and an itchy rash on her trunk. She has occasionally had problems maintaining her weight. She denies bloody diarrhea, rectal bleeding, nausea, vomiting, or arthralgias. She believes that her symptoms have stemmed from an intolerance of meat and tries to be a strict vegetarian. However, she says that her symptoms have not improved and actually have worsened with some vegetarian meals. She has a history of depression for which she takes fluoxetine but no other known medical conditions. She has undergone allergy testing that detected no apparent allergies. She denies tobacco, alcohol, and illicit substance use. She traveled to Mexico last year but was forced to cut her trip short because of her symptoms. On examination, she is a thin-appearing white woman in no distress. Chest auscultation detects no abnormal sounds. Her abdomen is mildly distended and hypertympanic, and auscultation detects hyperactive bowel sounds. No masses or organomegaly are present. She has a faint papular rash on her abdomen and anterior legs. A rectal examination detects no gross blood or masses. She has mild weakness on all strength testing but no paresthesias. The following vital signs are measured:

T: 98.4°F, HR: 80 bpm, BP: 108/76 mm Hg, RR: 15 breaths/min

Differential Diagnosis

- Irritable bowel syndrome, celiac sprue, tropical sprue, lactose intolerance, IBD, gastroenteritis, laxative abuse, Whipple disease, pancreatitis

Laboratory Data and Other Study Results

- CBC: WBC: 6.5, Hgb: 11.5, Plt: 260
- 10-electrolyte chemistry panel (Chem10): Na: 142 mEq/L, K: 3.7 mEq/L, Cl: 106 mEq/L, CO_2: 27 mEq/L, BUN: 20 mg/dL, Cr: 1.1 mg/dL, Glu: 80 mg/dL, magnesium (Mg): 1.7 mg/dL, calcium (Ca): 8.4 mg/dL, phosphorus (Phos): 3.0 mg/dL
- Parathyroid hormone (PTH): 6.7 pmol/L
- Amylase: 100 U/L
- Lipase: 210 U/L
- Nutrition panel: albumin: 3.6 g/dL, iron (Fe): 34 μg/dL, transferrin: 220 mg/dL, ferritin: 50 ng/mL
- Lactose tolerance and breath tests: negative
- D-xylose tolerance test: positive (decreased urinary excretion)
- Stool pH: 7.1
- Stool microscopy: no fecal leukocytes; no parasites

Based on these results, the following additional studies are performed:

- Barium enema: no abnormal masses or defects in colon
- Stool osmolality gap: 136 mOsm/kg
- Stool Sudan stain: positive for high fecal fat content
- Antigliadin antibodies: positive
- Antiendomysial antibodies: positive

Diagnosis

- Celiac sprue

Treatment Administered

- The patient was placed on a gluten-free diet
- The patient was referred to a nutritionist to help guide her diet planning

Follow-up

- The patient experienced a significant improvement in her symptoms with institution of the gluten-free diet and had resolution of her GI symptoms and fatigue

Steps to the Diagnosis

- **Celiac sprue**
  - Genetic disorder of gluten (e.g., wheat, barley, rye) intolerance in which antiendomysial and antigliadin antibodies cause jejunal mucosal damage

- Occurs in a bimodal distribution with presentations within the 1st year or third decade of life
- **Risk factors:** European heritage (white)
- **History:** failure to thrive, bloating, loose stools or watery diarrhea, steatorrhea, weight loss, flatulence, fatigue, depression, anxiety
- **Physical examination:** weakness, abdominal distention, peripheral edema, papular rash on trunk and extensor surfaces, orthostatic hypotension, possible Chovstek or Trousseau sign
- **Tests:**
  - Decreased K, Mg, and Ca
  - Albumin may be decreased
  - Iron is frequently low with an associated decreased Hgb
  - Sudan stain detects fat in stool (Figure 3-9)
  - D-xylose tolerance test will show decreased urinary excretion
  - Presence of antiendomysial and antigliadin antibodies in serum
  - Jejunal biopsy demonstrates loss of duodenal and jejunal villi
  - Small bowel follow through after barium swallow shows dilation of the jejunum and loss of the normal mucosal surface (will not be apparent on barium enema)
- **Treatment:** a gluten-free diet is the key to treatment and may be all that is needed to eliminate symptoms; corticosteroids may be required to decrease bowel inflammation in refractory cases
- **Outcomes:** patients who respond to a gluten-free diet have an excellent prognosis; patients with refractory disease tend to have chronic symptoms
- **Clues to the diagnosis:**
  - History: chronic loose stools and diarrhea, flatulence, bloating, cramping, fatigue
  - Physical: abdominal distention, hyperactive bowel sounds, papular rash
  - Tests: mildly decreased electrolytes, low normal albumin, low iron, positive D-xylose test, anemia, increased stool osmolality gap, positive fecal fat, positive antigliadin, and antiendomysial antibodies

- **Tropical sprue**
  - Malabsorption syndrome similar to celiac sprue with a likely infectious etiology
    - Acquired disorder in patients spending time in the **tropics**
    - **Folate** deficiency likely plays some role in the pathology

QUICK HIT: Classic symptoms of malabsorption syndromes include weight loss, bloating, diarrhea, steatorrhea, glossitis, dermatitis, and edema.

QUICK HIT: Celiac and tropical sprue exhibit the same symptoms, but only celiac sprue responds to removal of gluten from diet, and tropical sprue occurs in patients who have spent time in the tropics.

FIGURE 3-9 **Diagnostic pathway for suspected malabsorption syndrome.**

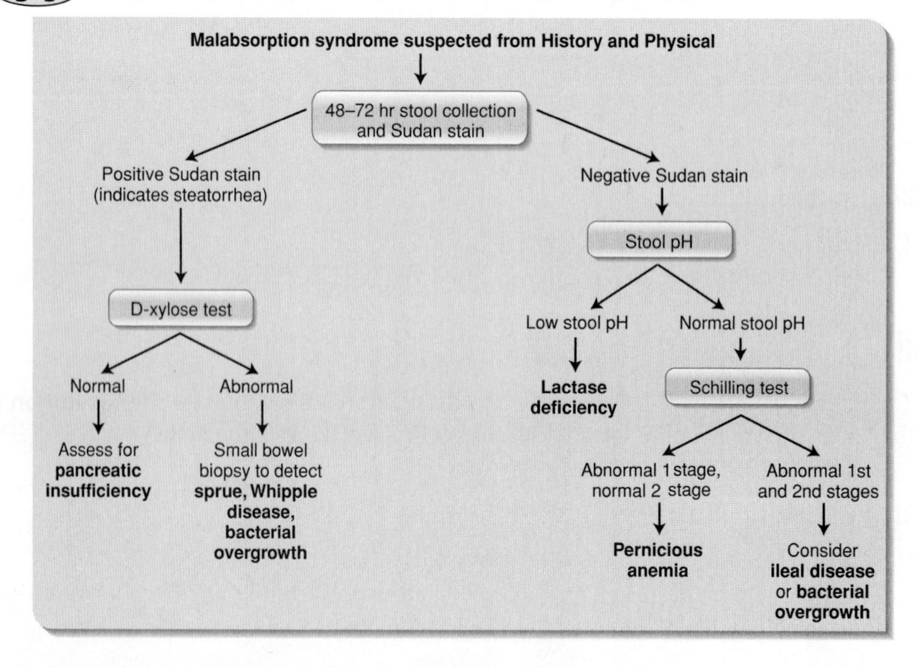

- **History:** bloating, loose stools or diarrhea, fatigue, weight loss, steatorrhea, flatulence
- **Physical examination:** weakness, abdominal distention, peripheral edema, papular rash on trunk and extensor surfaces, orthostatic hypotension, possible Chovstek or Trousseau sign
- **Tests:** test profile similar to celiac sprue except **no antiendomysial and antigliadin antibodies** are detected
- **Treatment:** folate replacement and tetracycline for 6 months; gluten-free diet has no effect
- **Outcomes:** with folate and antibiotic therapy prognosis is generally good
- **Why eliminated from differential:** the patient in the case had symptoms prior to her trip to Mexico; the presence of antiendomysial and antigliadin antibodies confirms celiac sprue as the diagnosis

- **Lactose intolerance**
  - Malabsorption syndrome resulting from a deficiency of **lactase**
    - Undigested lactose causes an osmotic diarrhea
    - A similar syndrome may also occur secondary to bacterial overgrowth or Crohn disease
  - **History:** abdominal pain, flatulence, diarrhea, and bloating following dairy consumption
  - **Physical examination:** typically noncontributory
  - **Tests:** positive lactose breath test (i.e., increased hydrogen concentration in expired air following a lactose meal); positive lactose tolerance test (i.e., minimal increase in serum glucose concentration following a lactose meal)
  - **Treatment:** lactose-free or lactose-restricted diet with adequate nutrients; lactase replacement may be beneficial in some patients
  - **Outcomes:** patients do very well when following the prescribed diet
  - **Why eliminated from differential:** the negative lactose breath and tolerance tests rule out this diagnosis
- **Irritable bowel syndrome (IBS)**
  - Idiopathic disorder of **irregular bowel habits** and chronic abdominal pain
    - Most common in **female** patients during the second and third decades of life
  - **History:**
    - Abdominal pain, diarrhea or loose stools alternating with constipation, bloating, nausea, possible vomiting, and weight loss
    - **Manning criteria:** the likelihood of a diagnosis of IBS increases with the number of satisfied criteria
      - Abdominal pain relieved with defecation
      - Stool frequency increases following onset of abdominal pain
      - Stools become looser following the onset of abdominal pain
      - Visible abdominal distention
      - Passage of mucus with stool
      - Feeling of incomplete defecation
  - **Physical examination:** mild abdominal tenderness, abdominal distention
  - **Tests:** no tests are diagnostic for IBS, but tests should be ordered to rule out other causes of chronic diarrhea and GI distress (e.g., malabsorption, neoplasms, IBD, infection)
  - **Treatment:**
    - Reassurance from the physician that a serious condition is not the cause of the symptoms
    - A diet high in fiber and low in caffeine, lactose, and legumes may help to improve the symptoms
    - Psychotherapy may be beneficial in patients with comorbid psychiatric conditions
    - Antispasmodics, antidepressants, and serotonin receptor antagonists have demonstrated benefit in some patients
  - **Outcomes:** IBS is frequently a chronic condition with multiple relapses, but associated with no significant complications
  - **Why eliminated from differential:** evidence of a malabsorptive process (e.g., increased stool osmolality and presence of fecal fat) and the presence of antiendomysial and antigliadin antibodies rule out this condition

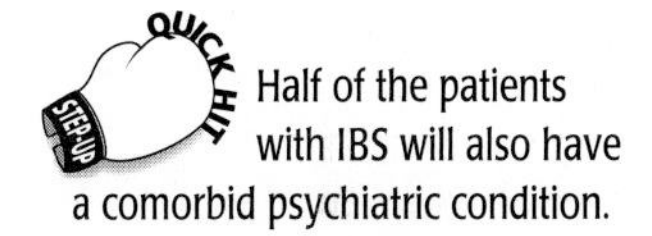

Half of the patients with IBS will also have a comorbid psychiatric condition.

- **Whipple disease**
  - A malabsorption disorder due to ***Tropheryma whippelli* infection** and an associated immunodeficiency that also effects several other organ systems
  - **Risk factors:** white males with European ancestry
  - **History:** weight loss, joint pain, abdominal pain, diarrhea, dementia, cough, bloating, steatorrhea
  - **Physical examination:** fever, vision abnormalities, lymphadenopathy, new heart murmur, progressive wasting
  - **Tests:** jejunal biopsy will show villous atrophy and **foamy macrophages** on periodic acid-Schiff stain
  - **Treatment:** trimethoprim-sulfamethoxazole (TMP-SMX) or ceftriaxone for 12 months
  - **Outcomes:** seventy percent of patients will have complete resolution of symptoms if treated (30% will have relapses); mortality is 100% within 1 year if untreated
  - **Why eliminated from differential:** the absence of cardiac, central nervous system (CNS), and visual symptoms and the presence of antiendomysial and antigliadin antibodies rule out this condition

MNEMONIC

The characteristic features of Whipple disease may be remembered by the mnemonic **WAD TAMP**: **W**eight loss, **A**rthralgias, **D**iarrhea, ***T**ropheryma whippelli*, **A**bdominal pain, **M**ultiple systems involved, **P**eriodic acid-Schiff used for diagnosis.

- **Inflammatory bowel disease**
  - More thorough discussion in later case
  - **Why eliminated from differential:** the presentations for IBD and sprue may be similar, but the presence of antiendomysial and antigliadin antibodies is pathognomonic for celiac sprue; the normal barium enema also makes IBD an unlikely diagnosis
- **Gastroenteritis**
  - More thorough discussion in prior case
  - **Why eliminated from differential:** the chronicity of the symptoms, normal WBC count, and absence of leukocytes or organisms on microscopy make this diagnosis unlikely
- **Laxative abuse**
  - Excessive use of laxatives in the attempt to prevent weight gain or to induce weight loss
  - **History:** significant concerns over weight and body image, possible bingeing history, frequent stools or diarrhea, depression
  - **Physical examination:** possible edema
  - **Tests:** stool pH, osmolality, and fat content will be normal, but 24-hour stool weight will be increased
  - **Treatment:** cessation of laxative use; psychotherapy or antidepressants may be useful to modify self-image and weight compensation behaviors
  - **Outcomes:** long-term abuse may lead to chronic constipation, steatorrhea, and protein loss
  - **Why eliminated from differential:** the increased stool osmolality and presence of fecal fat rule out this diagnosis
- **Pancreatitis**
  - More thorough discussion in later case
  - **Why eliminated from differential:** although malabsorptive diarrhea may be present in chronic pancreatitis, the normal amylase and lipase levels seen in the case make this diagnosis unlikely

CASE 3-6 "Can drinking give you diarrhea?"

An 18-year-old man presents to a gastroenterologist on referral from an internist at his college's student health center for the work-up of bloody diarrhea. The patient is a freshman college student who initially sought treatment at the student health center for recurrent bouts of bloody diarrhea, abdominal pain, and painful bowel movements. He is worried that his heavy drinking during weekend parties has caused these symptoms. He says that the abdominal pain is crampy in nature and has occurred occasionally over the past 8 months. The diarrhea has been bloody in nature and occurs three or four times per week.

He has formed bowel movements between these episodes, but they are frequently painful. This altered bowel behavior has developed over the past 6 months. Prior to the past 8 months he never exhibited any of these symptoms. He denies vomiting, constipation, or urinary symptoms. He denies any past medical history or medication use. He denies any similar history in family members. He drinks more than five alcoholic beverages on two to three nights per week but denies tobacco or illicit drug use. On examination, he appears to be a thin, white male in no acute distress. Auscultation of his heart and lungs finds no abnormal sounds. He has diffuse mild abdominal tenderness and no organomegaly. His bowel sounds are normal. A rectal examination detects occult blood. Neurologic examination is normal. The patient has multiple painful nodules on his anterior lower legs. The following vital signs are measured:

T: 99.3°F, HR: 90 bpm, BP: 120/75 mm Hg, RR: 16 breaths/min

Differential Diagnosis

- Ulcerative colitis, Crohn disease, bacterial or parasitic gastroenteritis, celiac sprue, lactose intolerance, Whipple disease, IBD, carcinoid tumor

Laboratory Data and Other Study Results

- CBC: WBC: 12.5, Hgb: 13.0, Plt: 450
- Chem7: Na: 139 mEq/L, K: 3.6 mEq/L, Cl: 106 mEq/L, CO_2: 27 mEq/L, BUN: 18 mg/dL, Cr: 0.7 mg/dL, Glu: 84 mg/dL
- Erythrocyte sedimentation rate (ESR): 33 mm/hr
- C-reactive protein (CRP): 2.1 mg/dL
- Liver function tests (LFTs): alkaline phosphatase (AlkPhos): 120 U/L, alanine aminotransferase (ALT): 40 U/L, aspartate aminotransferase (AST): 20 U/L, total bilirubin (TBili): 1.0 mg/dL, direct bilirubin (DBili) 0.3 mg/dL
- Nutrition panel: albumin: 3.2 g/dL, Fe: 33 μg/dL, transferrin: 432 mg/dL, ferritin: 16 ng/mL
- Lactose tolerance and breath tests: negative
- D-xylose tolerance test: negative
- Stool microscopy: several polymorphonuclear cells (PMNs); no parasites or bacteria

Following receipt of these results, the following tests are performed:

- Abdominal CT: no abscesses, fistulas, masses, or hemorrhage; mild colonic wall thickening
- Colonoscopy: highly friable colonic mucosa involving the full length of the colon without interruption; no pseudomembranes; biopsy performed
- Colonic wall biopsy: inflammation of colonic mucosa with no extension to deeper layers of the bowel wall

Diagnosis

- Ulcerative colitis

Treatment Administered

- The patient was prescribed supplemental iron, mesalamine, and a short course of prednisone

Follow-up

- The patient had a gradual improvement in his symptoms after the initial treatment regimen
- The patient experienced one to two exacerbations per year requiring short-term corticosteroid therapy

- The patient continued to be followed closely for the development of disease sequelae
- The patient was counseled on responsible alcohol consumption

Steps to the Diagnosis

- Ulcerative colitis (UC)
  - Variant of **inflammatory bowel disease (IBD)** characterized by **continuous** involvement of a region of the colon (Table 3-6)
    - Disease begins at the rectum and extends to a proximal end point within the colon
    - Only the **mucosal** layer of the bowel is involved
    - Typically begins in second or third decade of life
    - Extraintestinal manifestations include arthritis, uveitis, ankylosing spondylitis, primary sclerosing cholangitis, erythema nodosum, and pyoderma gangrenosum
  - **Risk factors:** white, Ashkenazi Jewish heritage
  - **History:** abdominal pain, urgency of bowels, **bloody diarrhea**, painful bowel movements (i.e., tenesmus), nausea, vomiting, weight loss
  - **Physical examination:** fever, abdominal tenderness, tachycardia, **occult blood on rectal examination**, orthostatic hypotension
  - **Tests:**
    - Serum WBCs are mildly increased, mild anemia, increased ESR and CRP, decreased albumin and iron, decreased K, **positive** perinuclear antineutrophil cytoplasmic antibodies (pANCA), antisaccharomyces cerevisiae antibodies (ASCA) **rarely present**
    - Stool analysis will frequently detect PMNs
    - Barium enema shows a "**lead pipe**" colon without haustral markings and generalized shortening of the colonic length (Figure 3-10)

MNEMONIC

Characteristics of ulcerative colitis can be remembered by the mnemonic **CECAL PLUMB**: **C**ontinuous involvement, **E**xtraintestinal symptoms (e.g., eyes, joints, skin, liver), **C**ancer risk, **A**bscesses in crypts, **L**arge bowel only, **P**seudopolyps, "**L**ead pipe" colon, **U**lcerations, **M**ucosa depth, **B**loody diarrhea.

TABLE 3-6 Comparison of Crohn Disease and Ulcerative Colitis

	Crohn Disease	Ulcerative Colitis
Site of involvement	**Entire GI tract may be involved** with multiple **"skipped"** areas; distal ileum most commonly involved; **entire bowel wall affected**	**Continuous disease beginning at rectum** and **extending possibly as far as distal ileum**; only mucosa and submucosa affected
Symptoms	Abdominal pain, weight loss, **watery** diarrhea	Abdominal pain, urgency, **bloody** diarrhea, tenesmus, nausea, vomiting, weight loss
Physical examination	Fever, right lower quadrant **abdominal mass**, abdominal tenderness, **perianal fissures and fistulas**, oral ulcers	Fever, abdominal tenderness, orthostatic hypotension, tachycardia, gross blood on rectal examination
Extraintestinal manifestations	Arthritis, ankylosing spondylitis, uveitis, primary sclerosing cholangitis, nephrolithiasis	Arthritis, uveitis, ankylosing spondylitis, primary sclerosing cholangitis, erythema nodosum, pyoderma gangrenosum
Labs	ASCA frequently positive, pANCA rarely positive; fecal occult blood test positive stool; biopsy diagnostic	ASCA rarely positive, pANCA frequently positive; biopsy diagnostic
Radiology	Colonoscopy shows colonic ulcers, strictures, "**cobble-stoning**," fissures, and "**skipped**" areas of bowel; barium enema shows fissures, ulcers, and bowel edema	Colonoscopy shows **continuous involvement**, pseudopolyps, friable mucosa; barium enema shows "**lead pipe**" colon without haustra and colon shortening
Treatment	Mesalamine, broad-spectrum antibiotics, corticosteroids, immunosuppressives; surgical resections of severely affected areas, fistulas, or strictures	Mesalamine, supplemental iron, corticosteroids, immunosuppressives; total **colectomy is curative**
Complications	Abscess formation, fistulas, fissures, malabsorption, toxic megacolon	**Significantly increased risk of colon cancer**, hemorrhage, toxic megacolon, bowel obstruction

ASCA, antiyeast *Saccharomyces cerevisiae* antibodies; GI, gastrointestinal; pANCA, perinuclear antineutrophil cytoplasmic antibodies.

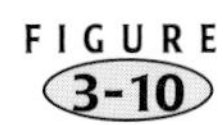

Barium enema in a patient with ulcerative colitis. Complete loss of haustra is seen in the descending colon, sigmoid colon, and rectum (i.e., "lead pipe" colon). Haustra are maintained in the ascending and transverse colon.

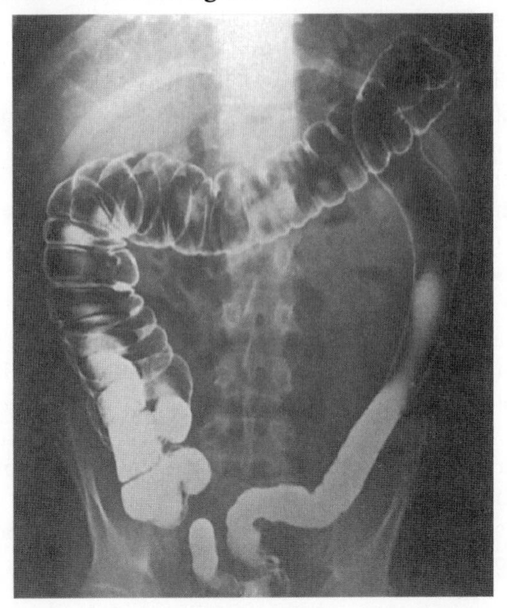

(Taken from Eisenberg RL. *Gastrointestinal radiology: a pattern approach.* 4th ed. Philadelphia: Lippincott Williams & Wilkins, 2003. Fig. 51-31. Used with permission of Lippincott Williams & Wilkins.)

- Colonoscopy demonstrates a friable mucosa and pseudopolyps in **continuous** fashion
- Biopsy demonstrates inflammation limited to the mucosal layer of the bowel wall

- **Treatment:**
  - **Aminosalicylates** (e.g., mesalamine, sulfasalazine) are the first line of therapy to suppress disease activity
  - Corticosteroids may be used in patients with disease that is not responsive to aminosalicylates alone
  - Patients not responding to the drugs listed above may benefit from immunomodulators (e.g., mercaptopurine, azathioprine, infliximab)
  - Total colectomy is curative and may be performed in patients with disease that does not respond to medical treatments
- **Outcomes:**
  - Exacerbations are common with 50% of patients having such an episode within 2 years of diagnosis
  - Patients with limited disease tend to have progression of the bowel involvement over time
  - After the initial decade of the disease, the risk of developing **colon cancer** increases by 1% per year
  - Complications include the several extraintestinal manifestations, colon cancer, bowel obstruction, severe hemorrhage, and toxic megacolon
- **Clues to the diagnosis:**
  - History: bloody diarrhea, abdominal pain, age
  - Physical: abdominal tenderness, occult blood on rectal examination, erythema nodosum
  - Tests: mildly increased WBC, anemia, mild hypokalemia, increased ESR and CRP, decreased albumin, colonoscopy results

- **Crohn disease**
  - Variant of IBD characterized by multiple sites of involvement throughout the gastrointestinal tract (Table 3-6)

MNEMONIC

Characteristics of Crohn disease can be remembered by the mnemonic **CHRISTMAS**: **C**obble-stoning, **H**igh temperature (fever), **R**educed lumen size, **I**ntestinal fistulae, **S**kip lesions, **T**ransmural involvement, **M**alabsorption, **A**bdominal pain, **S**ubmucosal fibrosis.

    - **Entire GI tract** may be involved with multiple **skipped** regions (i.e., intermittent normal bowel)
    - The **distal ileum** is the most commonly involved region
    - The **entire bowel wall** thickness is involved
    - The disease has a bimodal distribution and typically begins in either the second or third decade of life or the seventh or eighth decade of life
    - Extraintestinal manifestations include arthritis, uveitis, ankylosing spondylitis, primary sclerosing cholangitis, and nephrolithiasis
  - **Risk factors**: white, Ashkenazi Jewish heritage
  - **History**: abdominal pain, weight loss, **watery diarrhea**
  - **Physical examination**: fever, abdominal pain (worse in the right lower quadrant), perianal fissure and fistulas, oral ulcers
  - **Tests**:
    - Serum WBCs are mildly increased, mild anemia, increased ESR and CRP, decreased albumin and iron, decreased K, **rarely positive** pANCA, **positive** ASCA
    - Fecal occult blood testing of stool is frequently positive
    - Stool analysis will frequently detect PMNs
    - Barium enema displays fissures, ulcers, and edema of the bowel wall in an incomplete distribution (Figure 3-11)
    - Colonoscopy shows colonic ulcers, strictures, "**cobble-stoning**," fissures, and normal areas of colon between involved segments
  - **Treatment**:
    - Aminosalicylates are the first line therapy for the disease
    - Antibiotics are frequently administered to prevent infection via the perianal disease
    - Corticosteroids and immunomodulators are used in resistant disease
    - Surgical resection of strictures, fissures, and fistulas may be required
  - **Outcomes**:
    - Exacerbations are common over the life of the disease
    - Complications include the extraintestinal manifestations, abscess formation, fistula and fissure formation, and toxic megacolon
    - The increased risk of colon cancer is similar to that for ulcerative colitis in patients who have **colonic involvement**
  - **Why eliminated from differential**: the presence of a bloody diarrhea, the continuous involvement of the colon seen on colonoscopy, and the histologic inflammation limited to the mucosa are more suggestive of UC as the diagnosis
- **Gastroenteritis (bacterial or parasitic)**
  - More thorough discussion in prior case
  - **Why eliminated from differential**: the chronic nature of the condition and colonoscopy findings rule out these diagnoses
- **Celiac sprue**
  - More thorough discussion in prior case
  - **Why eliminated from differential**: the bloody diarrhea, normal D-xylose test, and colonic involvement (as opposed to just small bowel) seen on colonoscopy rule out this diagnosis
- **Lactose intolerance**
  - More thorough discussion in prior case
  - **Why eliminated from differential**: the negative lactose breath and tolerance tests help to rule out this diagnosis
- **Irritable bowel disease**
  - More thorough discussion in prior case
  - **Why eliminated from differential**: the bloody diarrhea, labs suggesting an inflammatory process, and colonoscopy findings rule out this diagnosis
- **Whipple disease**
  - More thorough discussion in prior case
  - **Why eliminated from differential**: the lack of CNS, pulmonary, and cardiac symptoms make this diagnosis unlikely; colonic involvement would not be expected for this diagnosis

- **Carcinoid tumor**
  - Intestinal neoplasm that arises from neuroectodermal cells that function as amine-precursor-uptake and decarboxylation (APUD) cells
    - Most commonly occurs in the **appendix**, ileum, rectum, and stomach
  - History:
    - May be asymptomatic, but common symptoms include abdominal pain, fatigue, weight loss, and possible painless rectal bleeding
    - **Carcinoid syndrome** is seen in 10% of cases
      - **Diarrhea**, **flushing**, asthmatic symptoms (e.g., bronchoconstriction), heart murmurs (from tricuspid or pulmonary valve disease)
      - Results from serotonin secretion by the tumor
  - **Physical examination**: abdominal distension and tenderness are possible findings, but patients with carcinoid syndrome are notable for flushing, facial telangiectasias, wheezing, systolic heart murmurs, hepatomegaly, and lower extremity edema
  - Tests:
    - Increased serum serotonin
    - Increased urine 5-HIAA (5-hydroxyindoleacetic acid)
    - CT or **indium-labeled octreotide scintigraphy** may be used to localize the tumor
  - **Treatment**:
    - Tumors <2 cm are excised locally or via appendectomy
    - Tumors >2 cm require a wide resection because of a high risk of metastases
    - Metastatic disease is treated with chemotherapy, α-interferon (α-IFN), octreotide, or embolization
  - **Outcomes**: full resection carries an excellent prognosis; the 5-year survival for metastatic disease is 67%
  - **Why eliminated from differential**: the presence of diarrhea and the absence of the other findings seen in carcinoid syndrome make this diagnosis less likely; the colonoscopy results confirm that IBD is the cause of the patient's symptoms

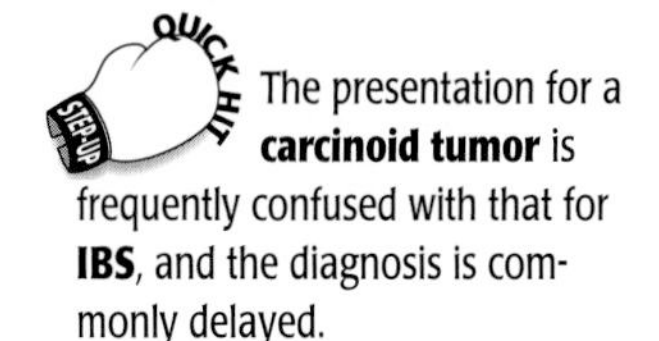

The presentation for a **carcinoid tumor** is frequently confused with that for **IBS**, and the diagnosis is commonly delayed.

CASE 3-7 "My belly hurts and I keep throwing up"

A 36-year-old woman presents to the emergency department with a week-long history of abdominal pain and bilious vomiting. She said that she has had intermittent crampy abdominal pain over the past week that has gradually increased in frequency and intensity. She has had multiple episodes of bilious vomiting over the past few days. She is having difficulty eating because of the vomiting. She has begun to feel fatigued due to poor food consumption. She denies hematemesis, melena, hematochezia, back pain, urinary symptoms, or pelvic pain. She noted that she has not had a bowel movement for 4 days. Her last menstrual period ended 1 week ago. She reports a history of Crohn disease that has been well controlled on a regimen of sulfasalazine and mercaptopurine. She takes no other medications. She notes a history of two prior partial bowel resections related to her Crohn disease, the most recent of which was performed 1 year ago. She denies substance use. She uses condoms as contraception. On examination, she is thin, pale, and looks fatigued. She has no palpable lymphadenopathy. Auscultation of her heart and lungs detects no extra sounds and mild tachycardia. She has diffuse moderate abdominal tenderness that is more pronounced in the central portion of her abdomen. Her bowel sounds are high-pitched and difficult to hear. She has some voluntary guarding but no rebound tenderness. No organomegaly is detected. A rectal examination detects no occult blood. A pelvic examination detects no abnormal fluid, no pelvic masses, and no cervical motion tenderness. The following vital signs are measured:

T: 99.5°F, HR: 110 bpm, BP: 105/70 mm Hg, RR: 18 breaths/min

Differential Diagnosis

- Small bowel obstruction, large bowel obstruction, ileus, appendicitis, volvulus, intussusception, cholecystitis, diverticulitis, gastroenteritis, mesenteric ischemia, pancreatitis, endometriosis, pregnancy, ectopic pregnancy, pelvic inflammatory disease

GASTROENTEROLOGY

Laboratory Data and Other Study Results

- CBC: WBC: 11.5, Hgb: 13.1, Plt: 200
- Chem10: Na: 144 mEq/L, K: 4.1 mEq/L, Cl: 105 mEq/L, CO_2: 24 mEq/L, BUN: 25 mg/dL, Cr: 1.2 mg/dL, Glu: 80 mg/dL, Mg: 2.1 mg/dL, Ca: 10.1 mg/dL, Phos: 4.1 mg/dL
- LFTs: AlkPhos: 96 U/L, ALT: 25 U/L, AST: 21 U/L, TBili: 1.1 mg/dL, DBili: 0.3 mg/dL
- Lactate: 2.2 mEq/L
- Amylase: 54 U/L
- Lipase: 120 U/L
- ESR: 28 mm/hr
- CRP: 1.1 mg/dL
- UA: straw-colored, pH: 5.0, specific gravity: 1.010, no glucose/ketones/nitrites/leukocyte esterase/hematuria/proteinuria
- Urine pregnancy test: negative
- Fecal occult blood test (rectal): positive
- *Neisseria gonorrhoeae* and *Chlamydia trachomatis* testing of vaginal fluid: pending
- AXR: multiple dilated loops of small bowel with air-fluid levels; no free air
- Abdominal CT: dilation of proximal jejunum to >4 cm with a collapsed middle and distal jejunum; mild proximal jejunal bowel wall thickening; mesenteric fat fibrosis with stranding; no masses, abscesses, biliary tree abnormalities, appendoliths, appendiceal thickening, or hernias

Diagnosis

- Small bowel obstruction

Treatment Administered

- A nasogastric tube was inserted, immediate intravenous (IV) fluids were initiated, and the patient was kept NPO (nulla per orem [nothing by mouth])
- The patient had continued intermittent abdominal pain and was taken to surgery the following morning for a lysis of adhesions obstructing a section of the jejunum

Follow-up

- The patient recovered following surgery with resolution of her symptoms and an improvement in her vital signs
- The patient was able to eat food normally after resolution of a postoperative ileus
- The patient continued to be followed for her Crohn disease
- *N. gonorrhoeae* and *C. trachomatis* testing was negative

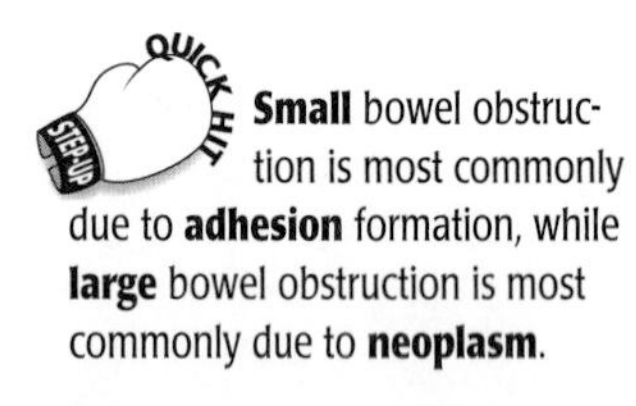

Small bowel obstruction is most commonly due to **adhesion** formation, while **large** bowel obstruction is most commonly due to **neoplasm**.

MNEMONIC

Some causes of the acute abdomen may be remembered by the mnemonic **SAUCED HIPPO**: **S**trangulation of bowel, **A**ppendicitis, **U**lcer (peptic), **C**holangitis, **E**ctopic pregnancy, **D**iverticulitis, **H**emorrhage (GI), **I**schemia (e.g., mesenteric, splenic, cardiac), **P**ancreatitis, **P**ID (pelvic inflammatory disease), **O**bstruction.

Steps to the Diagnosis

- **Small bowel obstruction** (SBO)
  - Mechanical or inflammatory obstruction of the bowel preventing the passage of food and leading to progressive local bowel ischemia
    - Common causes include **adhesions**, incarcerated hernias, neoplasm, intussusception, volvulus, Crohn disease, and congenital strictures
    - Progressive obstruction can present as an **acute abdomen** (i.e., severe abdominal pain and rigidity requiring **emergent intervention**) (Table 3-7)
  - **History**: colicky abdominal pain, nausea, vomiting, **constipation**, possible history of previous abdominal surgery or intra-abdominal neoplasm
  - **Physical examination**: abdominal tenderness, abdominal distention, visible peristaltic waves, **high-pitched or absent bowel sounds**, fever
  - **Tests:**
    - Increased BUN and Cr suggest dehydration due to obstruction; lactate is increased with strangulation or bowel ischemia

TABLE 3-7 Causes of an Acute Abdomen

Condition	H/P	Diagnosis	Treatment
Obstruction/strangulation (due to adhesions, hernias, tumors)	**Previous surgery**, abdominal distention, crampy pain, nausea, vomiting, high-pitched bowel sounds	CT or AXR shows distended loops of bowel and air-fluid levels; barium studies may locate site of obstruction	**Surgical lysis of adhesions**, hernia repair, surgical excision of tumors
Diverticulitis	**Left lower quadrant** pain (may progress over several days), blood in stool	CT or AXR may show free air from perforation; increased WBC	Surgical repair
Massive GI hemorrhage (e.g., perforation)	Sudden severe pain, **hematemesis**, **hematochezia**, hypotension	Colonoscopy or EGD visualizes lesion; technetium scan may detect smaller bleeding sources	Octreotide, **angiography with embolization**, surgical repair of detectable site of bleeding
Appendicitis	**Right lower quadrant** and **periumbilical** pain, psoas sign, rectal examination tenderness	Increased WBC; thickened appendix or fecalith on CT if unruptured; free air on CT or AXR if perforated	**Appendectomy**
Mesenteric ischemia	Severe abdominal pain **out of proportion to examination**, bloody diarrhea	Bowel wall thickening and air within bowel wall on CT; increased WBC and serum lactate	NPO, antibiotics, resection of necrotic bowel
Pancreatitis	**Upper abdominal and back pain**, nausea, vomiting, history of gallstones or alcoholism	CT shows inflamed pancreas; increased amylase and lipase	Nasogastric tube, NPO, analgesics
Ruptured ectopic pregnancy	**Amenorrhea**, lower abdominal pain, possible vaginal bleeding, or palpable pelvic mass	US **unable** to locate intrauterine pregnancy in presence of **positive urine pregnancy test**	Surgical excision
Pelvic inflammatory disease	Lower abdominal pain, vaginal discharge, cervical motion pain	Increased WBC; positive serology for *Chlamydia* or *Neisseria gonorrhoeae*	Antibiotics, treat sexual partners

AXR, abdominal x-ray; CT, computed tomography; EGD, esophagogastroduodenoscopy; GI, gastrointestinal; H/P, history and physical; NPO, nothing by mouth; US, ultrasound; WBC, white blood cell count.

- AXR will show **multiple ladderlike dilated loops of bowel** with **air-fluid levels**; the use of barium increases the sensitivity of the study (Figures 3-12)
- Abdominal CT can detect the location of an obstruction based on the presence of dilated bowel proximal to the obstruction and collapsed bowel distal to it; CT is also useful for detecting masses, abscesses, or herniations related to the obstruction

- **Treatment:**
  - Keep patient **NPO** and administer IV fluids
  - **Nasogastric suction** may decompress the bowel and relieve the obstruction in some simple cases
  - **Surgical correction** of the obstruction (e.g., lysis of adhesions, hernia repair) is required if the obstruction is unable to be decompressed
- **Outcomes:**
  - Prompt treatment is associated with a good prognosis
  - SBOs treated nonsurgically have a higher recurrence rate than those treated surgically
  - Complications include mesenteric ischemia, abscess formation, sepsis, and short-bowel syndrome following surgery
- **Clues to the diagnosis:**
  - History: abdominal pain, bilious vomiting, constipation, history of Crohn disease with previous abdominal surgeries
  - Physical: abdominal tenderness, high-pitched bowel sounds
  - Tests: mildly increased BUN and Cr, high normal lactate, appearance of the AXR and abdominal CT (consistent with Crohn disease)

FIGURE 3-11 **Barium enema in a patient with Crohn disease. Appreciable disease of variable severity is seen throughout the colon and distal ileum. Significant strictures are seen in the distal ileum and descending colon.**

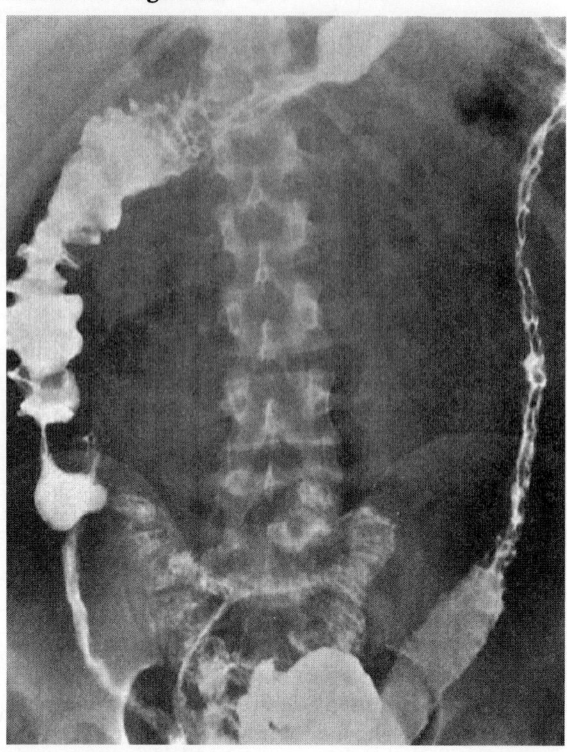

(Taken from Eisenberg RL. *Gastrointestinal radiology: a pattern approach.* 4th ed. Philadelphia: Lippincott Williams & Wilkins, 2003. Fig. 48-17. Used with permission of Lippincott Williams & Wilkins.)

FIGURE 3-12 **Abdominal radiograph in a patient with a small bowel obstruction. Note the multiple loops of dilated bowel with a ladderlike appearance.**

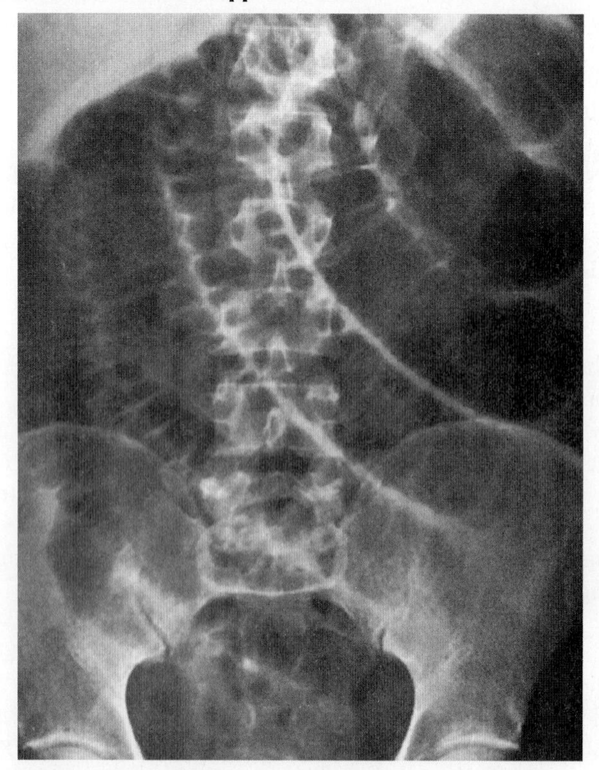

(Taken from Eisenberg RL. *Gastrointestinal radiology: a pattern approach.* 3rd ed. Philadelphia: Lippincott-Raven Publishers, 1996. Used with permission of Lippincott Williams & Wilkins.)

- **Large bowel obstruction** (LBO)
  - Mechanical obstruction of the colon leading to constipation and possible bowel ischemia
    - Common causes are **neoplasm**, diverticulitis, volvulus, and congenital strictures
  - **History**: abdominal pain, **obstipation**, nausea, feculent vomiting (progressed stages)
  - **Physical examination**: abdominal tenderness and distention, palpable abdominal mass, high-pitched or absent bowel sounds, hyperresonance to percussion
  - **Tests**:
    - Increased BUN and Cr suggest dehydration due to obstruction; lactate is increased with strangulation or bowel ischemia
    - AXR shows significant colonic distention; barium enema may detect distal obstructions (Figure 3-13)
    - Abdominal CT may show a mass causing the obstruction or a thickened bowel wall
  - **Treatment**:
    - Keep patient **NPO** and administer IV fluids
    - **Colonoscopy** may be used to reduce a LBO due to volvulus
    - Surgical resection of the obstructed segment is frequently required
  - **Outcomes**:
    - Prognosis is good with early treatment
    - When obstruction is due to neoplasm, the prognosis is dependent on the stage of the cancer
    - Complications include abscess formation and perforation
  - **Why eliminated from differential**: bilious vomiting is more suggestive of SBO; the abdominal CT demonstrates jejunal wall thickening and no obstructive masses

FIGURE 3-13 **Abdominal radiograph in patient with large bowel obstruction due to sigmoid volvulus. Note the significantly dilated bowel lumen. Of further note is the dense line marking where the walls of two dilated loops of bowel are pressed against each other (*open arrow*) and the dense marking where a dilated loop of bowel is compressed against the cecum (*solid arrow*).**

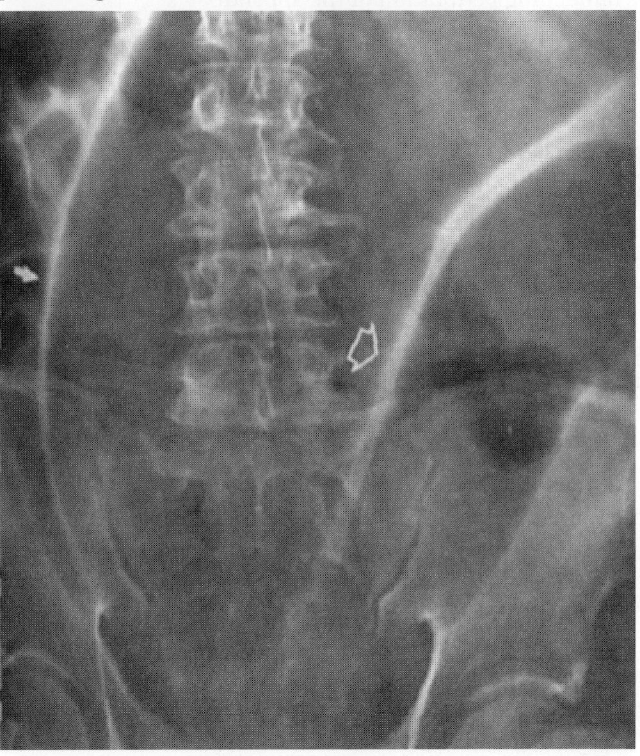

(Taken from Eisenberg RL. *Gastrointestinal radiology: a pattern approach.* 4th ed. Philadelphia: Lippincott Williams & Wilkins, 2003. Used with permission of Lippincott Williams & Wilkins.)

- **Ileus**
  - Paralytic obstruction of the bowel as a sequelae of decreased peristalsis
    - Common causes are **recent surgery**, infection, ischemia, DM, and **opioid use**
  - **History:** vague abdominal pain, nausea, vomiting, bloating, constipation, intolerance of food
  - **Physical examination:** abdominal distention, decreased bowel sounds, no guarding or rebound tenderness
  - **Tests:** AXR will show dilated bowel with possible air-fluid levels; barium enema can confirm the absence of a distal obstruction
  - **Treatment:**
    - Stop opioids and keep patient NPO
    - Prokinetic agents and ambulation may speed recovery of bowel function
    - Cases will **self-resolve**
  - **Outcomes:** prognosis is excellent with uncomplicated self-resolution considered the norm
  - **Why eliminated from differential:** the length of symptoms, severity of signs, and the radiographic findings suggest an actual obstruction and not just impaired peristalsis

QUICK HIT: Postoperative ileus typically lasts <**5 days.** Small bowel recovers in 24 hours, the stomach recovers in 48 to 72 hours, and large bowel recovers in 3 to 5 days.

MNEMONIC

Possible causes of right lower quadrant pain may be remembered by the mnemonic **APPENDICITIS**: **A**ppendicitis, **P**elvic issues (e.g., **P**ID, ectopic pregnancy, menstruation, ovarian cyst), **P**ancreatitis, **E**ndometriosis, **N**eoplasm, **D**iverticulitis (rare), **I**ntussusception, **C**rohn disease, **I**BD, **T**orsion (e.g., ovary, testicle), **I**BS, **S**tones (e.g., kidney, gallbladder).

- **Appendicitis**
  - Inflammation of the appendix with an increased risk of perforation
    - Due to lymphoid hyperplasia (common in children), fecalith impaction (adults), or fibroid bands (adults)
    - Obstruction of the appendiceal lumen leads to **infection** and progressive **inflammation**
  - **History:** dull periumbilical pain followed later by nausea, vomiting, anorexia, and migration of pain to the right lower quadrant
  - **Physical examination: tenderness at McBurney point** (i.e., one third of the distance from the right anterior superior iliac spine to the umbilicus), rebound tenderness, **psoas sign** (i.e., psoas pain on hip extension), fever, **Rovsing sign** (i.e., right lower quadrant pain with left lower quadrant palpation); signs of an **acute abdomen** (e.g., severe pain, distention, rebound tenderness, and involuntary guarding) suggest perforation or impending perforation of the appendix
  - **Tests:**
    - Increased WBC, ESR, and CRP
    - Ultrasound (US) may be useful to detect an enlarged, inflamed appendix
    - Abdominal CT with oral contrast can detect impaired appendiceal filling, wall thickening, an obstructing fecalith, abscess formation, free abdominal fluid, or fat stranding
  - **Treatment: appendectomy** is the standard of care; antibiotics are generally administered including coverage of anaerobic and Gram-negative organisms
  - **Outcomes:** prognosis is excellent with no mortality associated with an unruptured appendix and <1% mortality in cases of rupture (5% in elderly patients); complications include abscess formation and perforation without timely treatment
  - **Why eliminated from differential:** the classic signs of appendicitis are missing from the physical examination in this case, and the CT does not detect abnormalities of the appendix

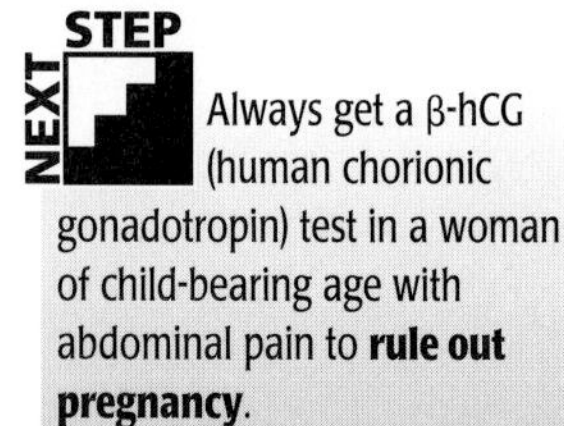

NEXT STEP: Always get a β-hCG (human chorionic gonadotropin) test in a woman of child-bearing age with abdominal pain to **rule out pregnancy**.

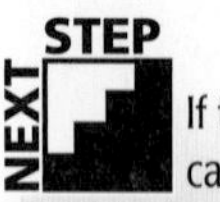

NEXT STEP: If there is a high clinical suspicion of appendicitis, go right to surgery and do not wait for radiologic examinations.

- **Volvulus**
  - **Rotation** of the bowel upon itself, resulting in obstruction and possible ischemia
    - The **cecum** and **sigmoid colon** are the most common sites in the adult
    - Elderly patients and infants are the most common age groups affected
  - **History:** abdominal pain, vomiting, obstipation
  - **Physical examination:** abdominal distention and tenderness, possible palpable mass
  - **Tests:** AXR may show a "**double bubble**" of air proximal and distal to the site of involvement; barium enema may show a distal "bird's beak" sign
  - **Treatment:**
    - May be self-limited with automatic derotation
    - Colonoscopic decompression may be performed for a sigmoid volvulus

- Surgical reduction is frequently required for a cecal volvulus or following failed colonoscopic detorsion
- **Outcomes:** reducible volvuli have a good prognosis but may recur; bowel ischemia is the most significant complication
- **Why eliminated from differential:** findings consistent with this diagnosis are not seen on the AXR and abdominal CT in the case

- **Intussusception**
  - **Telescoping** of one segment of bowel into another, leading to obstruction
    - Occurs most commonly proximal to the ileocecal valve
  - **Risk factors:** Meckel diverticulum, Henoch-Schonlein purpura, adenovirus infection, cystic fibrosis, young age (i.e., more common in children)
  - **History:** paroxysmal abdominal pain lasting <1 minute, pallor, diaphoresis, vomiting, bloody mucus in stool (i.e., currant-jelly stool)
  - **Physical examination:** abdominal tenderness, **palpable sausagelike abdominal mass**
  - **Tests:** barium enema will demonstrate the obstruction; US or CT may be able to detect the abnormal section of bowel
  - **Treatment:** barium enema may reduce the obstruction, but resistant cases require surgical reduction
  - **Outcomes:** prognosis is excellent; bowel ischemia may occur in cases with delayed presentation
  - **Why eliminated from differential:** the chronology of the abdominal pain and other symptoms and appearance of the CT make this diagnosis unlikely
- **Cholecystitis**
  - More thorough discussion in later case
  - **Why eliminated from differential:** the presence of bilious vomiting and the normal LFTs rule out this diagnosis, but an abdominal US could be performed if concern for this diagnosis further existed
- **Diverticulitis**
  - More thorough discussion in later case
  - **Why eliminated from differential:** the minimally elevated WBCs and the absence of free air or abscess formation on imaging help to rule out this diagnosis
- **Gastroenteritis**
  - More thorough discussion in prior case
  - **Why eliminated from differential:** the bilious nature of the emesis, length of symptoms, significance of the abdominal examination, and absence of diarrhea help to rule out this diagnosis
- **Mesenteric ischemia**
  - Ischemia and necrosis of a section of bowel due to vascular compromise
    - Due to embolization of mesenteric vessels, bowel obstruction, inadequate cardiac output (i.e., impaired systemic perfusion), or iatrogenic vascular compromise (e.g., medication, surgery)
    - Although the left side of the colon is the most common site of involvement, the rectum is typically spared because of collateral circulation
  - **Risk factors:** DM, atherosclerosis, congestive heart failure (CHF), systemic lupus erythematosus (SLE), peripheral vascular disease
  - **History:** acute severe abdominal pain, bloody diarrhea, vomiting
  - **Physical examination:** mild abdominal tenderness, tachycardia, tachypnea, fever, hypotension
  - **Tests:**
    - WBC and **lactate** are increased
    - Barium enema will demonstrate mucosal changes in the affected region
    - CT will demonstrate **bowel wall thickening** and **air within the bowel wall**
    - Sigmoidoscopy may show a bloody and edematous mucosa
  - **Treatment:**
    - Patients should be made NPO and given IV hydration
    - Antibiotics are administered to prevent bacteremia of GI flora
    - **Surgical resection** of necrotic bowel is required

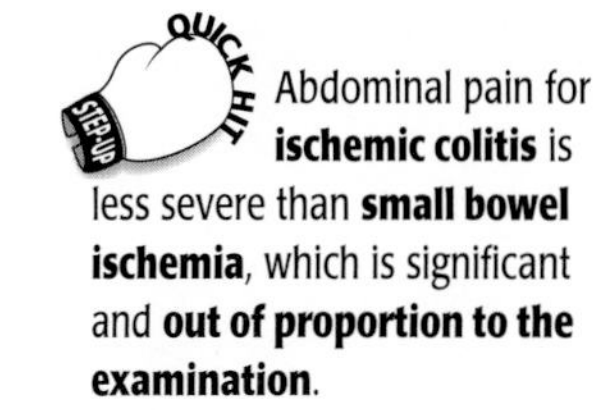

Abdominal pain for **ischemic colitis** is less severe than **small bowel ischemia**, which is significant and **out of proportion to the examination**.

- **Outcomes:** mortality is 50% for prompt treatment and 90% for missed diagnoses
- **Why eliminated from differential:** the absence of a high lactate, bloody diarrhea, and air within the bowel wall make this diagnosis unlikely

- **Pancreatitis**
  - More thorough discussion in later case
  - **Why eliminated from differential:** the normal amylase and lipase levels and the CT findings rule out this diagnosis
- **Pregnancy/ectopic pregnancy**
  - More thorough discussion in Chapter 12
  - **Why eliminated from differential:** the negative pregnancy test helps to rule out these diagnoses
- **Pelvic inflammatory disease**
  - More thorough discussion in Chapter 11
  - **Why eliminated from differential:** the normal findings on pelvic examination make this diagnosis unlikely
- **Endometriosis**
  - More thorough discussion to follow in Chapter 11
  - **Why eliminated from differential:** the absence of pelvic signs and symptoms make this diagnosis unlikely

The following additional Gastroenterology cases may be found online:

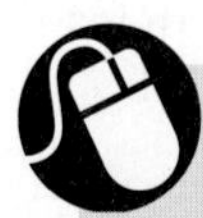

CASE 3-8 "I'm bleeding when I go to the bathroom"

CASE 3-9 "Just 'gimme' a drink to make my stomach feel okay"

CASE 3-10 "My right side hurts really bad"

CASE 3-11 "I just feel terrible"

CASE 3-12 "My little boy keeps throwing up"

CASE 3-13 "My baby is yellow"

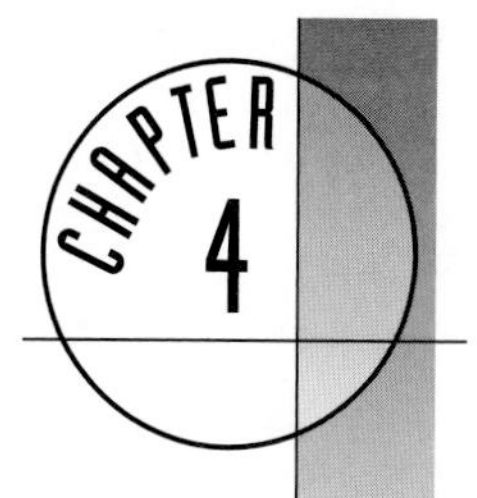

Nephrology and Urology

BASIC CLINICAL PRIMER

RENAL PHYSIOLOGY

- The key functions of the kidneys are to filter plasma (20% of all plasma flow), regulate intravascular fluid volume and electrolyte composition, aid in the maintenance of homeostasis between intravascular and extravascular fluids, and secrete several hormones that are important to systemic hemodynamics (Figure 4-1, Table 4-1)

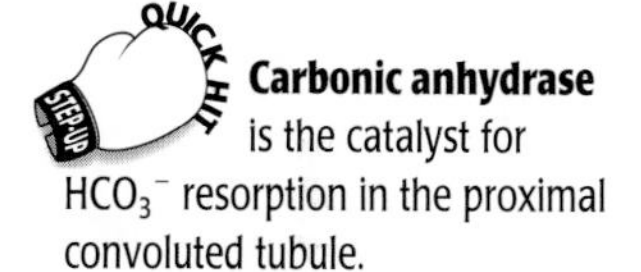

Carbonic anhydrase is the catalyst for HCO_3^- resorption in the proximal convoluted tubule.

DIURETICS

- Medications that affect the resorption of electrolytes and fluids function at distinct locations along the renal tubular system to modulate the composition and volume of body fluids (Table 4-2)

DIALYSIS

- Therapeutic filtering of intravascular serum through either artificial or induced means
  - Indicated for severe hyperkalemia or metabolic acidosis, intravascular fluid overload, uremic syndrome, or chronic kidney disease with a creatinine >12 mg/dL and a blood urea nitrogen >100 mg/Dl
- **Hemodialysis**
  - The creation of an arteriovenous fistula or the placement of a synthetic graft is performed to allow consistent vascular access
  - Blood is filtered by a machine and returned to the systemic circulation via the selected conduit
- **Peritoneal dialysis**
  - Dialysis fluid is temporarily pumped into the peritoneal cavity via an access catheter
  - The osmotic gradient drives the diffusion of substances from the intravascular serum to the peritoneum with the peritoneal membrane serving as a filter
  - Following dialysis, the fluid is pumped out of the peritoneal cavity

ACID-BASE PHYSIOLOGY

- In healthy individuals, serum pH is regulated by the reabsorption of **bicarbonate** (**HCO_3^-**) and the partial pressure of carbon dioxide (**pCO_2**) of blood
  - pH, partial pressure of oxygen (pO_2), and pCO_2 are measured directly by an arterial blood gas, and bicarbonate may be measured by the Henderson-Hasselbach equation:

$$pH = pKa + \log\left(\frac{[HCO_3]}{0.03 \times P_{CO2}}\right)$$

FIGURE 4-1 **Anatomy of the nephron and major sites of ion, water, and molecule exchange. Ca, calcium; Cl, chloride; H, hydrogen; H_2O, water; HCO^3, ; K, potassium; Mg, magnesium; Na, sodium.**

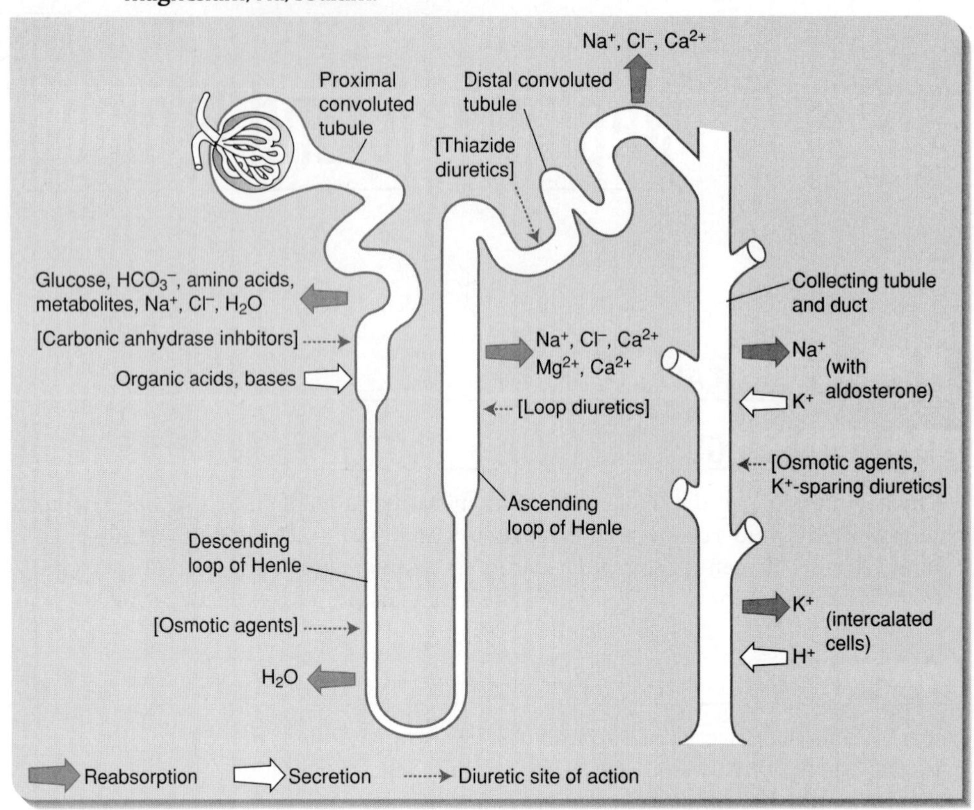

MNEMONIC

Causes of high-anion gap metabolic acidosis can be remembered by the mnemonic **MUD PILES**: **M**ethanol, **U**remia, **D**iabetic ketoacidosis, **P**araldehyde, **I**soniazid (INH), **L**actic acidosis, **E**thanol, **S**alicylates.

- Disturbances due to HCO_3^- abnormalities are **metabolic**; disturbances due to pCO_2 levels are **respiratory**
- Compensatory mechanisms attempt to keep the serum pH normalized (Table 4-3)

- Anion gap
  - Difference between the sodium positive ion concentration and chloride and bicarbonate negative ion concentrations

    Anion gap = $[Na] - [Cl] - [HCO_3^-]$ (normal = 8–12)

TABLE 4-1 Functions of Regions of the Nephron

Region	Location	Absorption	Secretions	Notes
Proximal convoluted tubule	Cortex	Glucose, bicarbonate, amino acids, metabolites, Na; Cl and water (passively)	Organic acids and bases	—
Descending loop of Henle	Medulla	Water (due to increasing interstitial osmotic gradient)	—	Descending limb is permeable to water
Ascending loop of Henle	Medulla	Na, Cl, K (Na/K/Cl cotransporter); Mg, Ca, K (paracellular diffusion)	—	—
Distal convoluted tubule	Cortex	Na and Cl (Na/Cl transporter); Ca (PTH activity)	—	Cells impermeable to water
Collecting tubule and duct	Cortex, medulla	Na (aldosterone activity on principal cells); water (ADH activity); K (intercalated cells)	K (aldosterone activity); H^+ (intercalated cells)	—

ADH, antidiuretic hormone; Ca, calcium; Cl, chloride; H^+, hydrogen ions; K, potassium; Mg, magnesium; Na, sodium; PTH, parathyroid hormone

NEPHROLOGY AND UROLOGY

TABLE 4-2 Common Diuretics and Their Effects Within the Nephron

Diuretic	Site of Action	Mechanism of Action	Indications	Adverse Effects
Carbonic anhydrase inhibitors (e.g, acetazolamide)	Proximal convoluted tubule	Inhibition of carbonic anhydrase causes mild diuresis and prevents HCO_3^- reabsorption	Glaucoma, epilepsy, altitude sickness, metabolic alkalosis	Mild metabolic acidosis, hypokalemia, nephrolithiasis
Osmotic agents (e.g., mannitol, urea)	Proximal convoluted tubule, loop of Henle, collecting tubule	Increased tubular osmotic gradient increases H_2O excretion	Increased intracranial pressure, acute renal failure (due to shock or drug toxicity)	No effect on Na excretion, relative hypernatremia
Loop diuretics (e.g., furosemide)	Ascending loop of Henle	Inhibit Na/Cl/K cotransporter to decrease reabsorption and indirectly inhibit Ca reabsorption	CHF, pulmonary edema, hypercalcemia; rapid onset useful in emergent situations	Ototoxicity, hyperuricemia, hypokalemia, hypocalcemia
Thiazides (e.g., hydrochlorothiazide)	Distal convoluted tubule	Inhibit Na/Cl cotransporter to decrease reabsorption and indirectly increase K excretion and increase Ca reabsorption	HTN, CHF, hypercalciuria, diabetes insipidus	Hypokalemia, hyperuricemia, hypercalcemia
K-sparing (e.g., spironolactone)	Collecting tubules	Aldosterone antagonist that inhibits Na-K exchange	Secondary hyperaldosteronism, CHF, K-preserving diuresis	Gynecomastia, menstrual irregularity, hyperkalemia

Ca, calcium; CHF, congestive heart failure; HCO_3, bicarbonate; H_2O, water; HTN, hypertension; K, potassium; Na, sodium.

    - Metabolic acidosis with a **normal** anion gap suggests **bicarbonate loss**
    - Metabolic acidosis with an **increased** anion gap suggests **hydrogen ion excess**
  - **Mixed** acid-base disturbances
    - Apparent if the corrected bicarbonate is different than the measured value:

      Corrected HCO_3^- = measured anion gap − normal anion gap + measured HCO_3^-
    - The normal anion gap is considered to be **12**
    - A normal corrected bicarbonate suggests a high anion gap acidosis alone
    - An increased corrected bicarbonate suggests a metabolic alkalosis with a high anion gap acidosis
    - A decreased corrected bicarbonate suggests a normal anion gap acidosis and a high anion gap acidosis through separate mechanisms

PREOPERATIVE RENAL RISK ASSESSMENT

- Electrolyte abnormalities, anemia, and impaired immune function are more common in patients with renal insufficiency
- **Preoperative dialysis** is frequently indicated in patients with renal insufficiency to decrease the risk of complications due to serum composition
- **Acetylcysteine** may be used as a preoperative renal protectant in patients with renal insufficiency who are scheduled to receive intravascular contrast during surgery

KIDNEY TRANSPLANTATION

- Indicated for end-stage renal disease requiring dialysis for survival
- Contraindicated in patients with significant comorbidities that carry a poor prognosis
- Living donor transplants are associated with a 20% risk of acute rejection and a 5-year survival of 91%
- Allografts carry a 40% acute rejection rate and a 5-year survival rate of 85%

TABLE 4-3 Acid-Base Disturbances and Compensatory Mechanisms

Disorder	Common Causes	pH	[H+]	$[HCO_3^-]$	pCO_2	Compensatory Mechanism	Compensation Formulas
Metabolic acidosis	Diarrhea, diabetic ketoacidosis, lactic acidosis, renal tubular acidosis	↓	↑	↓↓	↓	Hyperventilation	**Expected pCO_2 = 1.5 $[HCO_3^-]$ + (8±2)** If pCO_2 less than expected, then additional respiratory alkalosis If pCO_2 greater than expected, then additional respiratory acidosis
Metabolic alkalosis	Vomiting, diuretics, Cushing syndrome, hyperaldosteronism, adrenal hyperplasia	↑	↓	↑↑	↑	Hypoventilation	If $pCO_2 > 50$, then additional respiratory acidosis If $pCO_2 < 40$, then additional respiratory alkalosis
Respiratory acidosis	COPD, respiratory depression, neuromuscular diseases	↓	↑	↑	↑↑	Increased HCO_3^- reabsorption	Acute: Expected pH decrease = $\frac{1}{10} \times 0.08 \times (pCO_2 - 40)$ Chronic: Expected pH decrease = $\frac{1}{10} \times 0.03 \times (pCO_2 - 40)$
Respiratory alkalosis	Hyperventilation, high altitude, asthma, aspirin toxicity, pulmonary empolism	↑	↓	↓	↓↓	Decreased HCO_3^- reabsorption	Acute: Expected pH increase = $\frac{1}{10} \times 0.08 \times (pCO_2 - 40)$ Chronic: Expected pH increase = $\frac{1}{10} \times 0.03 \times (pCO_2 - 40)$

COPD, chronic obstructive pulmonary disease; H, hydrogen; HCO_3, bicarbonate; pCO_2, partial pressure of oxygen; ↑, high; ↓, low; ↑↑, very high ↓↓, very low.

CASE 4-1 "It hurts when I go to the bathroom"

A 26-year-old woman presents to her primary care physician (PCP) with complaints of multiple urinary symptoms and back pain that have not responded to therapy. She was seen in the same clinic 2 weeks prior to the current presentation with pain during urination, increased urinary frequency, and urgency prior to urination. She was given a 3-day prescription for trimethoprim-sulfamethoxazole at that visit. The patient did not fill the prescription until 2 days ago because of her busy schedule, although she was continuing to have symptoms. Today she reports nausea, vomiting, chills, and flank pain in addition to continued dysuria, urgency, and urinary frequency. She denies diarrhea, abdominal pain, hematochezia, dyspareunia, or dizziness. She denies any past medical history and uses oral contraceptive pills. She is in a monogamous relationship, and her last menstrual period was 1 week ago. She drinks alcohol socially but denies any other substance use. On examination, she is an uncomfortable-appearing thin woman. She has no palpable lymphadenopathy. Auscultation finds no abnormal sounds of her heart, lungs, or bowels.

She does not have any abdominal masses but has mild suprapubic tenderness. She is tender to palpation along the posterior aspects of her lower ribs. Pelvic examination reveals no tenderness, vaginal discharge, or masses. Neurologic examination is normal. The following vital signs are measured:

Temperature (T): 102.7°F, heart rate (HR): 96 beats per minute (bpm), blood pressure (BP): 115/80 mm Hg, respiration rate (RR): 16 breaths/min

Differential Diagnosis

- Urinary tract infection, pyelonephritis, nephrolithiasis, appendicitis, cervicitis, endometriosis, ectopic pregnancy, gastroenteritis

Laboratory Data and Other Study Results

- Complete blood cell count (CBC): white blood cells (WBC): 20.1, hemoglobin (Hgb): 14.9, platelets (Plt): 320
- Urinalysis (UA): cloudy, pH: 7.5, specific gravity: 1.030, positive nitrites and leukocyte esterase; no glucose/ketones/hematuria/proteinuria; 2 RBC/hpf (red blood cells/high-power field), 35 WBC/hpf
- Urine culture: Gram stain shows multiple Gram-negative rods and leukocyte casts; culture pending
- Blood culture: Gram stain and culture pending
- Vaginal fluid microscopy (saline): no mobile organisms or clue cells
- Vaginal fluid microscopy potassium hydroxide (KOH): no hyphae or pseudohyphae
- Vaginal fluid culture: culture pending
- Abdominal CT with contrast: no bowel or vascular abnormalities; no renal masses or stones
- Urine pregnancy test: negative

Diagnosis

- Pyelonephritis

Treatment Administered

- The patient was admitted to the hospital for intravenous (IV) antibiotics because of her prior noncompliance with prescribed treatment and concern over her ability to take oral medication (she had reported new episodes of emesis)
- The patient was started on empiric levofloxacin while awaiting the culture results

Follow-up

- The urine culture grew >10,000 colonies of *Escherichia coli*
- The patient was continued on IV levofloxacin for 2 additional days until her symptoms improved
- The patient was discharged to home to complete a 14-day course of oral levofloxacin
- The patient had full resolution of her symptoms and completed the full antibiotic course

Steps to the Diagnosis

- **Acute pyelonephritis**
  - Infection of the renal parenchyma
    - *E. coli*, *Staphylococcus saprophyticus*, *Klebsiella pneumoniae*, *Proteus mirabilis*, and *Candida albicans* are the most common causes
    - Most commonly occurs as a sequela of an **ascending urinary tract infection (UTI)**

    - **Risk factors:** urinary obstruction, immunocompromised, previous pyelonephritis, diabetes mellitus (DM), frequent sexual intercourse (more than 3 times per week), spermicide use, and intercourse with a new partner
    - **History: flank pain**, chills, nausea, vomiting, urinary frequency, dysuria, urinary urgency
    - **Physical examination:** fever, **costovertebral tenderness**, suprapubic tenderness
    - **Tests:**
        - Increased WBCs, erythrocyte sedimentation rate (ESR), and C-reactive protein (CRP)
        - **UA** will be positive for nitrites, leukocyte esterase, and WBCs
        - Urine Gram stain will show **white cell casts**, and **culture** will grow more than 10,000 bacteria/mL of urine
    - **Treatment:**
        - **IV fluoroquinolones**, aminoglycosides, or third-generation cephalosporins are given empirically until an organism is identified
        - Patient may be changed to oral medications after a few days and may be allowed to complete a 14-day course as an outpatient
        - Severe cases may require up to 14 days of IV antibiotics
        - Reliable patients who are hemodynamically stable, lack other medical comorbidities, and are capable of taking oral medications may be amenable to oral antibiotics alone in an outpatient setting

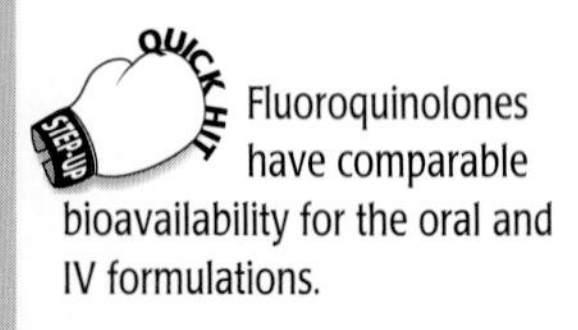
Fluoroquinolones have comparable bioavailability for the oral and IV formulations.

    - **Outcomes:** complications include renal abscess formation, acute renal failure, chronic kidney disease, and increased risks for preterm labor and low neonatal birth weight in pregnant females; the prognosis for uncomplicated cases is good
    - **Clues to the diagnosis:**
        - History: multiple urinary symptoms, flank pain, noncompliance with treatment for a diagnosis of UTI
        - Physical: fever, flank tenderness
        - Tests: UA and urine Gram stain suggestive of infection
- **Urinary tract infection**
    - Ascending infection of the urethra, bladder, and ureters
        - Most commonly due to direct inoculation of the lower urinary tract; rarely caused by hematogenous spread
        - *E. coli*, *S. saprophyticus*, *K. pneumoniae*, *P. mirabilis*, or *Enterobacter faecalis* are the most common causes
    - **Risk factors: obstruction, catheterization**, vesicoureteral reflux, pregnancy, DM, sexual intercourse, immunocompromise, female gender
    - **History: urinary frequency and urgency, dysuria**, suprapubic pain
    - **Physical examination:** suprapubic tenderness
    - **Tests:** UA will show nitrites, leukocyte esterase, and WBCs; urine culture will show more than 10,000 colony-forming units/mL
    - **Treatment:** oral amoxicillin, trimethoprim-sulfamethoxazole (TMP-SMX), or fluoroquinolones for 3 days; the treatment time increases to 14 days for relapsing infecting
    - **Outcomes:** complications include abscess formation and pyelonephritis; prognosis is excellent unless patient is elderly, immunocompromised, or has underlying kidney disease
    - **Why eliminated from differential:** the patient likely initially had a UTI that ascended and progressed to pyelonephritis, but the worsening of her symptoms and the onset of fever and back pain are more suggestive of a diagnosis of pyelonephritis

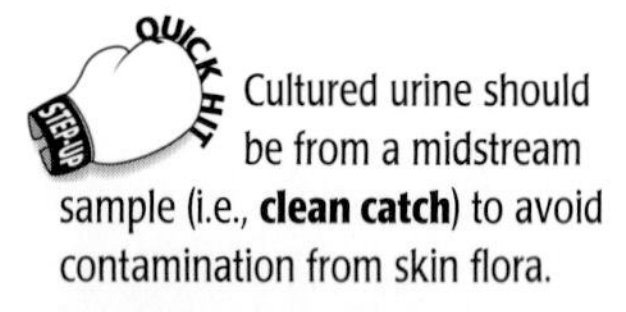
Cultured urine should be from a midstream sample (i.e., **clean catch**) to avoid contamination from skin flora.

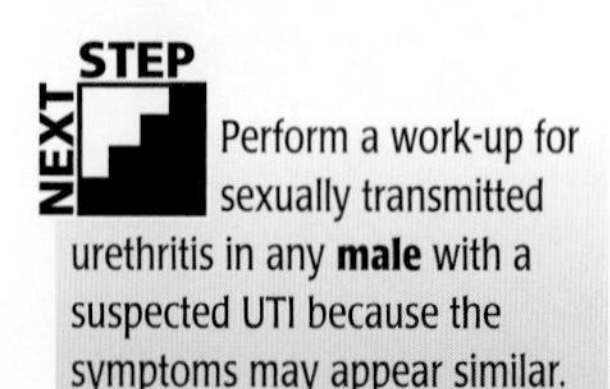
Perform a work-up for sexually transmitted urethritis in any **male** with a suspected UTI because the symptoms may appear similar.

- **Nephrolithiasis**
    - Formation of concentrated masses of minerals (i.e., kidney stones) in the ductal system of the urinary tract (Table 4-4)
    - **Risk factors: hypercalcemia, hyperparathyroidism**, prior nephrolithiasis, family history, low fluid intake, frequent UTIs, hypertension (HTN), DM, gout, renal tubular acidosis, allopurinol, acetazolamide, loop diuretics, and male gender
    - **History:** stones remain asymptomatic until **obstruction** of the urinary outflow tract occurs and then **acute severe colicky flank pain**, nausea, vomiting, and dysuria occur

TABLE 4-4 Types of Nephrolithiasis (Renal Stones)

Type	Frequency (%)	Cause	Radiology	Notes
Calcium oxalate	72	**Idiopathic hypercalciuria**, small bowel diseases	Radiopaque	Most patients have no identifiable cause
Struvite (Mg-NH_4-PO_4)	12	**Urinary tract infection**	Radiopaque	More common in **women**; may form staghorn calculi
Calcium phosphate	8	**Hyperparathyroidism**, renal tubular acidosis	Radiopaque	—
Uric acid	7	Chronic acidic/concentrated urine, chemotherapeutic drugs, gout	**Radiolucent**	Treat by alkalinizing urine
Cystine	1	Cystinuria, amino acid transport defects	Radiopaque	May form staghorn calculi

- **Physical examination:** acute costovertebral tenderness
- **Tests:**
  - UA will show **hematuria** in most cases (Table 4-5)
  - Serum electrolytes (including calcium and phosphorus), uric acid level, and parathyroid hormone level are useful for determining the etiology of stones
  - Twenty-four-hour urine collection is useful for determining the composition of stones and their etiology
  - Abdominal x-ray (AXR), computed tomography (CT), or ultrasound (US) will detect the majority of stones
  - **Intravenous pyelogram** (IVP) is the gold standard for detecting stones and measuring their size but is performed uncommonly because of the time requirements and contrast dye load (Figure 4-2)
    - Water-soluble dye is injected intravenously and excreted by the kidneys
    - Appropriate timing of postinjection imaging will demonstrate filling defects associated with impacted stones and hydronephrosis (i.e., dilation) of the renal calyces

QUICK HIT: Patients with **impacted stones** will be in pain and will **shift position frequently** in unsuccessful attempts to find a comfortable position; patients with **peritonitis** will remain **rigid**.

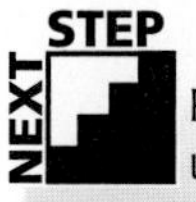

Rule out bladder or urethral obstruction in an anuric patient by attempting bladder catheterization.

MNEMONIC

The differential diagnosis for adult hematuria can be remembered by mnemonic **INEPT GUN**: **I**diopathic, **N**eoplasm (e.g., bladder, kidney, prostate), **E**xercise, **P**olycystic kidney disease, **T**rauma, **G**lomerular disease (nephritic, nephrotic), **U**TI, **N**ephrolithiasis.

TABLE 4-5 Common Causes of Hematuria

Age	Temporary Hematuria	Persistent Hematuria
Below 20 years old	Idiopathic UTI Exercise Trauma Endometriosis (women)	Glomerular disease
20–50 years old	Idiopathic UTI Nephrolithiasis Exercise Trauma Endometriosis (women)	Adult polycystic kidney disease Neoplasm (e.g., bladder, kidney, prostate) Glomerular disease
Beyond 50 years old	Idiopathic UTI Nephrolithiasis Trauma	Adult polycystic kidney disease BPH (men) Neoplasm (e.g., bladder, kidney, prostate) Glomerular disease

BPH, benign prostatic hyperplasia; UTI, urinary tract infection.

FIGURE 4-2 **Intravenous pyelogram demonstrating hydronephrosis in the right kidney (*asterisk*). Renal pelvis dilation is evident as is a radiopaque stone in the right ureter (*arrow*). The left kidney appears normal.**

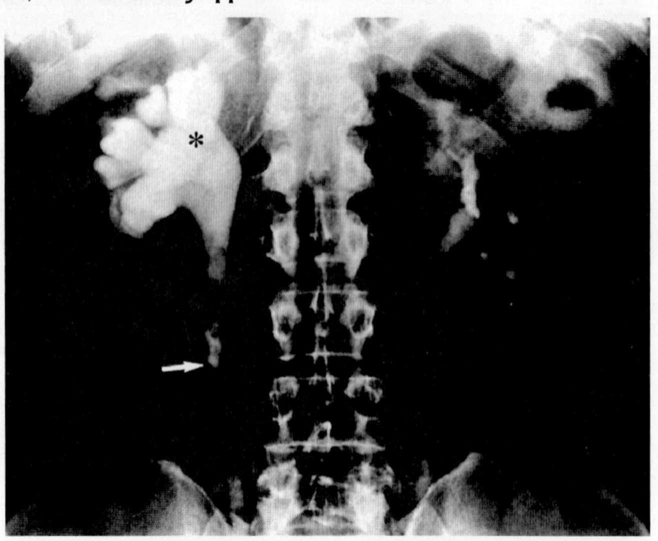

(Taken from Daffner RH. *Clinical radiology: the essentials.* 2nd ed. Philadelphia: Lippincott Williams & Wilkins, 1999. Used with permission of Lippincott Williams & Wilkins.)

- **Treatment:**
  - Hydration and **analgesics** for pain control
  - Shockwave lithotripsy may be useful to break up stones <3 cm and allow them to pass through the ureters
  - Surgical removal is indicated for large impacted stones
  - Chronic cases with the development of hydronephrosis may require drainage with a **nephrostomy tube** and placement of a double-J stent to allow continued urine flow
- **Outcomes:** potential complications include hydronephrosis, renal failure, recurrent stones, fistula formation, and ureteral stricture formation; recurrences occur in 50% of cases within 5 years of the first episode
- **Why eliminated from differential:** the absence of stones seen on the CT and the multiple signs suggestive of an infectious process (e.g., fever, WBCs) make this diagnosis unlikely

- **Appendicitis**
  - More thorough discussion in Chapter 3
  - **Why eliminated from differential:** the appearance of the CT makes this diagnosis less likely; although nausea and abdominal pain may be seen in each diagnosis, the presence of flank pain and urinary symptoms are more suggestive of pyelonephritis
- **Cervicitis**
  - More thorough discussion in Chapter 11
  - **Why eliminated from differential:** the normal pelvic examination rules out this diagnosis
- **Endometriosis**
  - More thorough discussion in Chapter 11
  - **Why eliminated from differential:** the normal pelvic examination makes this diagnosis unlikely; likewise, urinary frequency and urgency are not typically seen in this diagnosis
- **Ectopic pregnancy**
  - More thorough discussion in Chapter 12
  - **Why eliminated from differential:** the negative pregnancy test rules out this diagnosis
- **Gastroenteritis**
  - More thorough discussion in Chapter 3
  - **Why eliminated from differential:** the absence of epigastric pain and diarrhea makes this diagnosis less likely

CASE 4-2 "My sides are lumpy"

A 35-year-old man presents to his PCP with flank pain and palpable flank masses. He says that a few weeks prior to his appointment he began to experience mild pain in his right flank. When he went to rub the area that was sore, he realized that he had a palpable lumpy mass in that location. He also detected a smaller lumpy mass on the left flank that was painless. He does not recall noticing these lumps prior to this episode of back pain. He denies any weight loss, weakness, nausea, vomiting, diarrhea, hematemesis, hematochezia, constipation, dysuria, or urinary frequency. He does admit to occasional headaches and infrequent episodes of brown urine upon questioning. He denies any past medical history but has not seen a physician for 5 years. He drinks alcohol socially and denies other substance use. On examination, he is a healthy appearing man in no distress. Head and neck, lung, and heart examinations are normal. Auscultation of his abdomen detects normal bowel sounds. He has no abdominal tenderness or hepatosplenomegaly. He has palpable irregular masses on both posterior flanks that are mildly tender to palpation. The masses feel deep. There is no overlying erythema or swelling. Neurologic examination is normal. The following vital signs are measured:

T: 98.5°F, HR: 74 bpm, BP: 142/88 mm Hg, RR: 16 breaths/min

Differential Diagnosis

- Renal cell carcinoma, polycystic kidney disease, Wilms tumor, neuroblastoma, nephrolithiasis, pyelonephritis

Laboratory Data and Other Study Results

- CBC: WBC: 7.5, Hgb: 16.7, Plt: 279
- 10-electrolyte chemistry panel (Chem10): sodium (Na): 141 mEq/L, potassium (K): 4.2 mEq/L, chloride (Cl): 106 mEq/L, carbon dioxide (CO_2): 27 mEq/L, blood urea nitrogen (BUN): 33 mg/dL, creatinine (Cr): 1.6 mg/dL, glucose (Glu): 87 mg/dL, magnesium (Mg): 1.9 mg/dL, calcium (Ca): 8.1 mg/dL, phosphorus (Phos): 3.2 mg/dL
- UA: light brown colored, pH: 6.0, specific gravity: 1.030, 1+ proteinuria, 1+ hematuria, no glucose/ketones/nitrites/leukocyte esterase
- Urine culture: Gram stain negative; culture pending
- Renal US: significantly enlarged multicystic kidneys bilaterally; no renal stones

Diagnosis

- Adult polycystic kidney disease

Treatment Administered

- The patient was started on enalapril to control his HTN
- The patient was given acetaminophen for pain control

Follow-up

- The patient continued to be followed closely to trace any worsening of his renal function
- The patient was able to maintain sufficient renal function for another 15 years before reaching end-stage renal disease and requiring dialysis
- The patient eventually received a renal transplant

Steps to the Diagnosis

- **Polycystic kidney disease (adult)**
  - Hereditary syndrome characterized by the formation of multiple cysts in the kidneys and possibly the liver or spleen (Color Figure 4-1)

NEPHROLOGY AND UROLOGY

- Multiple cysts cause impaired renal function and eventual renal failure
- Types:
  - **Autosomal dominant: most common form** and is diagnosed in adults; characterized by large multicystic kidneys with impaired function
  - **Autosomal recessive**: rare form that is diagnosed in **children**; fatal in the initial years of life without a renal transplant
- **History**: typically asymptomatic until adulthood and then characterized by flank pain, possible chronic UTIs, and gross hematuria
- **Physical examination**: palpable kidneys, HTN, flank tenderness that becomes worse with cyst rupture
- **Tests:**
  - Increased creatinine and BUN; increased Hgb (due to increased erythropoietin activity)
  - UA will show proteinuria and hematuria
  - Renal US or CT will show **large multicystic kidneys**
- **Treatment:**
  - **Controlling HTN** (angiotensin receptor blockers [ARBs] or angiotensin-converting enzyme inhibitors [ACE-Is]) and **treating UTIs** will help to preserve renal function
  - Vasopressin receptor antagonists or amiloride may help prevent the accumulation of fluid in cysts
  - Therapeutic drainage of large cysts may improve pain
  - Dialysis or renal transplant is required when renal function deteriorates
- **Outcomes:**
  - End-stage renal disease will occur in 50% of patients before 60 years of age, and renal transplant is a common need in these patients
  - Hepatic and splenic cysts compromise the function of those respective organs
  - **Intracranial aneurysm** may occur in up to 10% of patients
  - Other complications include subarachnoid hemorrhage, mitral valve prolapse, diverticulosis, and nephrolithiasis
- **Clues to the diagnosis:**
  - History: flank pain, palpable flank masses, hematuria
  - Physical: palpable flank masses, HTN
  - Tests: increased creatinine and BUN, hematuria and proteinuria on UA, renal US findings

- **Renal cell carcinoma**
  - Most common **primary** malignant neoplasm of the renal parenchyma
  - **Risk factors: tobacco use**, cadmium or asbestos exposure
  - **History**: weight loss, flank pain, hematuria, malaise
  - **Physical examination**: palpable abdominal or flank mass, HTN, fever
  - **Tests:**
    - Increased Hgb
    - UA shows hematuria
    - US, magnetic resonance imaging (MRI), or CT with contrast may show a renal mass (cystic or solid)
    - Biopsy provides a histologic diagnosis but is rarely performed because the diagnosis is frequently made with imaging alone
  - **Treatment**: nephrectomy or a renal-sparing resection with lymph node dissection is routinely performed for localized disease; immunotherapy, radiation therapy, or chemotherapy are utilized in unresectable disease
  - **Outcomes**: localized tumors have at least an 88% 5-year survival rate with timely resection; regional disease and disease with metastases carry 5-year survival rates of 59% and 20%, respectively
  - **Why eliminated from differential**: although renal cell carcinoma may be cystic, a multicystic kidney is more characteristic of polycystic kidney disease

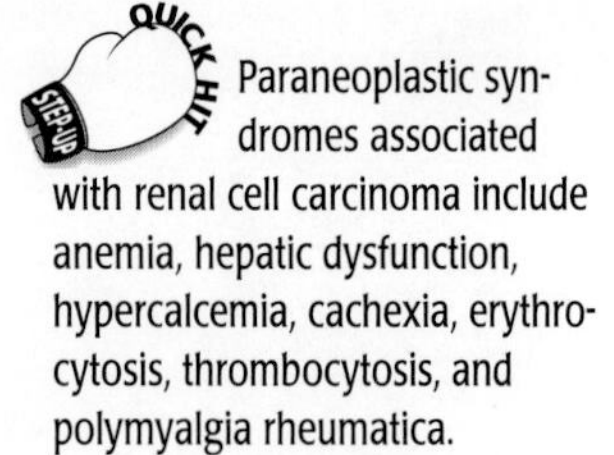

Paraneoplastic syndromes associated with renal cell carcinoma include anemia, hepatic dysfunction, hypercalcemia, cachexia, erythrocytosis, thrombocytosis, and polymyalgia rheumatica.

- **Wilms tumor**
  - A malignant renal tumor that is most commonly diagnosed in young children (average age is 4 years old)

- **Risk factors:** family history, neurofibromatosis, congenital genitourinary abnormalities
- **History:** weight loss, nausea, vomiting, dysuria, urinary frequency
- **Physical examination:** palpable abdominal or flank mass, HTN, fever
- **Tests:**
  - Increased creatinine and BUN
  - A renal mass will be apparent on CT, MRI, or US
  - Biopsy of the tumor will demonstrate a combination of epithelial cells, blast cells, and stromal cells
- **Treatment:** surgical resection or nephrectomy, chemotherapy, and radiation therapy
- **Outcomes:** survivorship is 90% in cases without regional or metastatic spread
- **Why eliminated from differential:** the age of the patient in this case is greater than the typical age for this cancer

- **Neuroblastoma**
  - Tumors of a neural crest cell origin that may arise in the adrenal glands or sympathetic ganglia
    - The majority of patients are younger than 2 years old
  - **Risk factors:** neurofibromatosis, tuberous sclerosis, pheochromocytoma, Beckwith-Wiedemann syndrome, Turner syndrome, low maternal folate consumption
  - **History:** abdominal or flank distention and pain, weight loss, malaise, bone pain, diarrhea
  - **Physical examination:** fever, palpable abdominal or flank mass, HTN, possible Horner syndrome, proptosis, movement disorders, hepatomegaly, periorbital bruising
  - **Tests:** possible increased vanillylmandelic and homovanillic acids in a 24-hour urine collection; CT may detect an adrenal or ganglion tumor
  - **Treatment:** surgical resection of tumors followed by postoperative chemotherapy and radiation therapy
  - **Outcomes:** poor prognosis if presenting after one year of age with metastases to the bone and brain
  - **Why eliminated from differential:** the patient's age makes this an unlikely diagnosis
- **Nephrolithiasis**
  - More thorough discussion in prior case
  - **Why eliminated from differential:** the presence of the flank masses makes this diagnosis unlikely, and the US helps to rule it out
- **Pyelonephritis**
  - More thorough discussion in prior case
  - **Why eliminated from differential:** the absence of findings suggesting an infectious process makes this diagnosis unlikely

CASE 4-3 "I just don't want to eat anything"

A 75-year-old man is brought to the emergency department by his wife because of worsening fatigue and anorexia over the past week. His wife says that he had gastroenteritis 2 weeks ago and was having frequent diarrhea for several days before the condition self-resolved. He says that he never got his appetite back after the illness and has eaten little over the past week. He says that he has felt progressively worse over this time. He also reports headaches and nausea over this same time. He has had difficulty moving his bowels and has urinated only a couple of times in the past week. He denies chest or abdominal pain, dyspnea, chills, current vomiting or diarrhea, hematemesis or hematochezia, paresthesias, or chronic weight loss. He notes a history of HTN, coronary artery disease (CAD), and type II DM and takes aspirin (ASA), hydrochlorothiazide (HCTZ), atenolol, and metformin. He says that his blood pressure and blood sugar levels have been well controlled on this regimen. He denies substance use. On examination, he is a tired-appearing man in no significant distress. He has dry mucous membranes and decreased skin turgor. Auscultation of his heart and lungs finds clear breathing sounds, tachycardia, and a mild friction rub. Examination of his abdomen finds no abdominal tenderness or masses, mild flank tenderness, and decreased bowel sounds. Rectal examination detects no gross blood or masses. Neurologic examination is normal. The following vital signs are measured:

T: 100.1°F, HR: 117 bpm, BP: 90/75 mm Hg, RR: 16 breaths/min

Differential Diagnosis

- Acute renal failure, interstitial nephropathy, chronic kidney disease, diabetic ketoacidosis, pyelonephritis, congestive heart failure (CHF)

Laboratory Data and Other Study Results

- CBC: WBC: 7.2, Hgb: 15.7, Plt: 278
- Chem10: Na: 146 mEq/L, K: 5.1 mEq/L, Cl: 108 mEq/L, CO_2: 23 mEq/L, BUN: 93 mg/dL, Cr: 3.9 mg/dL, Glu: 96 mg/dL, Mg: 2.1 mg/dL, Ca: 8.7 mg/dL, Phos: 4.1 mg/dL
- BNP: 34 pg/mL
- UA: dark yellow colored, pH: 6.0, specific gravity: 1.041, no glucose/ketones/nitrites/leukocyte esterase/hematuria/proteinuria
- Urine culture: Gram stain negative; culture pending

Based on these results, the following tests are performed following admission to the hospital:

- Urine electrolytes: Na: 20 mEq/L, K: 18 mEq/L, Cr: 70 mg/dL
- Fractional excretion of sodium: 0.8
- Renal US: normal size kidneys; no hydronephrosis; no detectable obstruction

Diagnosis

- Acute renal failure secondary to volume depletion

Treatment Administered

- HCTZ and metformin were held following his admission; insulin was used to regulate his glucose levels
- IV hydration was administered to gradually improve his volume depletion

Follow-up

- After 2 days of supportive care, the patient's BUN and creatinine began to trend downward
- Patient was discharged to home once his BUN and creatinine reached 35 mg/dL and 2.0 mg/dL, respectively
- The patient was kept on a low salt and low protein diet as an outpatient
- The patient had further improvement in his renal function but maintained a new baseline creatinine of 1.4 mg/dL

MNEMONIC

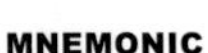

Causes of acute renal failure may be remembered by the mnemonic "Patients with ARF can't **VOID RIGHT**": **V**asculitis, **O**bstruction (e.g., calyces, bladder, or ureters), **I**nfection, **D**rugs (i.e., acute tubular necrosis [ATN]), **R**enal artery stenosis, **I**nterstitial nephropathy, **G**lomerular disease, **H**ypovolemia, **T**hromboembolism.

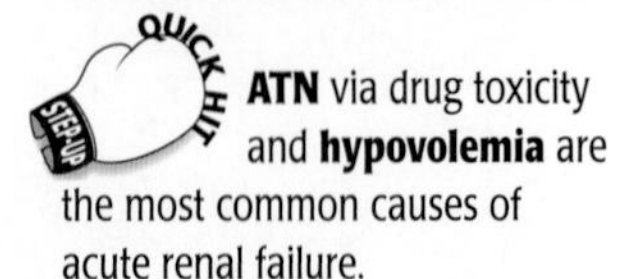

ATN via drug toxicity and **hypovolemia** are the most common causes of acute renal failure.

Steps to the Diagnosis

- **Acute renal failure** (ARF)
  - Acute worsening in renal function (e.g., impaired glomerular filtration, urine production, and chemical excretion) due to either a prerenal, intrarenal, or postrenal cause
    - **Prerenal** causes include **hypovolemia**, sepsis, and renal artery stenosis
    - **Intrarenal** causes include ATN (e.g., drugs, toxins), glomerular disease, and renal vascular disease
    - **Postrenal** disease is due to the **obstruction** (e.g., stones, tumor, adhesions) of the renal calyces, ureters, or the bladder
  - History:
    - Patients are **asymptomatic** until a significant degree of glomerular filtration (approximately 50%) is lost

- Early symptoms include fatigue, anorexia, nausea, **oliguria or anuria**, and flank pain
- Gross hematuria and mental status changes develop with progressive renal injury and the development of uremia
- **Physical examination:** possible pericardial friction rub, hypotension, fever, diffuse rash, or edema
- **Tests:**
  - **Increased BUN** and **creatinine**
  - **UA findings** vary with the etiology
    - Normal results may be seen with hypovolemia
    - Hematuria and red cell casts are seen in glomerular or vasculitic diseases
    - Granular casts are seen with ATN
    - Pyuria is seen in infection
    - Pyuria with waxy casts are seen in interstitial disease and in obstruction
  - **Fractional excretion of sodium (FENa)** is useful to differentiate hypovolemia from other causes
    - FENa <1% suggests hypovolemia, and FENa >1% is consistent with ATN:

$$\text{FENa} = \frac{(\text{UrineNa}/\text{SerumNa})}{(\text{UrineCr}/\text{SerumCr})}$$

    - Renal US, CT, IVP, or renal angiography may be used to detect hydronephrosis, obstruction, renal masses, abnormal blood flow, or vasculitis
    - Renal biopsy is frequently indicated to diagnose intrarenal pathology
- **Treatment:**
  - Intravascular volume should be carefully regulated with IV hydration and furosemide
  - Use of any potentially nephrotoxic substances should be stopped
  - Dietary salt and protein restriction helps reduce the risks of volume and protein overload
  - Dialysis is indicated for severe disease with hyperkalemia, metabolic acidosis, or uremia
- **Outcomes:**
  - Uremia and multiorgan dysfunction are possible complications
  - Negative prognostic factors include advanced age, oliguria, need for transfusions, recent surgery, hypotension, need for vasoactive medications, and multiorgan dysfunction
  - Mortality varies with the cause of the disease and may be as high as 70% in severe cases
- **Clues to the diagnosis:**
  - History: fatigue, anorexia, oliguria
  - Physical: dehydration, friction rub, flank pain
  - Tests: increased BUN and Cr, FENa <1%

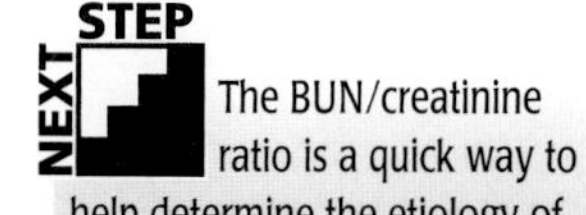

The BUN/creatinine ratio is a quick way to help determine the etiology of ARF (i.e., **ratio >20 if a prerenal cause**).

- **Chronic kidney disease (CKD)**
  - Progressive damage of the renal parenchyma taking place over multiple years
    - Greater than 90% of the renal parenchyma is sclerotic or necrotic at the time of diagnosis
    - Chronic **HTN** and **DM** are the most common causes
  - **History:** patients are initially asymptomatic and gradually develop fatigue, nausea, anorexia, vomiting or diarrhea, paresthesias, weakness, and hematochezia or melena
  - **Physical examination:** changes in mental status, hypertension, brownish discoloration of the skin
  - **Tests:**
    - Increased BUN, creatinine, potassium, and phosphate; decreased sodium and calcium
    - Metabolic acidosis is common
    - Anemia occurs due to impaired erythropoietin production
    - Urine osmolality will be similar to serum osmolality
    - Renal US will show hydronephrosis or small, sclerotic kidneys

- **Treatment:**
  - Dietary salt and protein restriction helps to prevent additional taxing of the residual kidney function
  - Any underlying conditions should be treated to prevent further secondary degeneration
  - Dialysis or renal transplantation are required for survival as kidney function deteriorates (i.e., end-stage renal disease)
- **Outcomes:** complications include uremia with encephalopathy, dangerous electrolyte imbalances, renal osteodystrophy, and severe anemia; survival is longer with renal transplantation than chronic dialysis
- **Why eliminated from differential:** the length of symptoms, pattern of electrolyte abnormalities, and findings on the renal US are more indicative of acute renal injury

- **Interstitial nephropathy/acute tubular necrosis**
  - Damage of renal tubules or parenchyma due to an acute toxic insult
    - **Drugs** are the most common cause, but industrial toxins (e.g., cadmium, lead, copper, mercury), infection, or autoimmune conditions (e.g., sarcoidosis, amyloidosis) may also be etiologies
      - The most common culprit drugs are β-lactam antibiotics, sulfonamides, **aminoglycosides, nonsteroidal anti-inflammatory drugs (NSAIDs)**, allopurinol, proton pump inhibitors (PPIs), and diuretics
  - **History:** fatigue, malaise, nausea, vomiting
  - **Physical examination:** fever, rash, pericardial friction rub
  - **Tests:**
    - Increased BUN and creatinine; eosinophilia
    - UA may show granular casts
    - Toxicology screens may be useful to detect a causative drug
    - Renal biopsy will demonstrate numerous inflammatory cells and renal tubular necrosis
  - **Treatment:**
    - **Stop the offending agent**
    - Supportive care with hydration and furosemide
    - Corticosteroids may be beneficial to recovery in refractory cases
  - **Outcomes:** complications include acute and chronic renal failure, renal papillary necrosis, uremia, electrolyte imbalances, and anemia; the mortality for full ATN with histologic evidence of renal necrosis is 50%
  - **Why eliminated from differential:** the UA results and FENa rule out this diagnosis in favor of ARF
- **Diabetic ketoacidosis (DKA)**
  - More thorough discussion in Chapter 5
  - **Why eliminated from differential:** the normal serum and urine glucose levels and the absence of urinary ketones rule out this diagnosis
- **Pyelonephritis**
  - More thorough discussion in prior case
  - **Why eliminated from differential:** the absence of urinary leukocytes and the normal WBC count make this diagnosis unlikely
- **Congestive heart failure**
  - More thorough discussion in Chapter 1
  - **Why eliminated from differential:** the benign lung examination and the normal brain natriuretic peptide (BNP) make this diagnosis unlikely

CASE 4-4 "My urine is brown"

A 12-year-old boy is brought to his pediatrician by his mother because he has had brown urine for the past 3 days. The boy says that he has had no pain or urgency during urination and that he first noticed the unusual color incidentally 3 days ago. He reports feeling tired and achy for the past 5 days. His mother says that he had a bad cold 3 weeks ago that resolved and that they initially attributed these constitutional symptoms to a recurrence of the illness. The boy denies brown urine during his recent illness. He denies flank pain, recent trauma, dyspnea, nausea, vomiting or diarrhea, and hematemesis or hematochezia. His mother says that he is a healthy boy with no previous medical problems and takes a children's vitamin on a daily basis. The patient denies using any illicit substances. He plays organized soccer but has had no sudden changes in his activity level or recent trauma. On examination, he is a healthy appearing boy in no distress. He has some mild puffy swelling of his facial characteristics. No lymphadenopathy is palpable. Tests of his hearing are normal. Auscultation of his heart and lungs finds no abnormalities. Abdominal examination detects no tenderness or masses. A genital examination detects no penile abnormalities and normally descended testes. Neurologic examination is normal. The following vital signs are measured:

T: 98.7°F, HR: 72 bpm, BP: 140/85 mm Hg, RR: 16 breaths/min

Differential Diagnosis

- Acute renal failure, polycystic kidney disease, poststreptococcal glomerulonephritis, immunoglobulin A (IgA) nephropathy, Goodpasture syndrome, Alport syndrome, nephrotic syndrome, cold-antibody hemolytic anemia, rhabdomyolysis

Laboratory Data and Other Study Results

- CBC: WBC: 6.5, Hgb: 15.5, Plt: 345
- Chem7: Na: 141 mEq/L, K: 3.9 mEq/L, Cl: 105 mEq/L, CO_2: 27 mEq/L, BUN: 32 mg/dL, Cr: 1.9 mg/dL, Glu: 79 mg/dL
- UA: brown colored, pH: 6.3, specific gravity: 1.020, multiple red cell casts, 3+ hematuria, 1+ proteinuria, no glucose/ketones/nitrites/leukocyte esterase
- Twenty-four-hour urine protein: 1,025 mg/d
- Antistreptolysin O titer: positive
- Antibasement membrane IgG antibodies: negative
- Renal US: normal-sized kidneys; no hydronephrosis or obstruction

Diagnosis

- Poststreptococcal glomerulonephritis

Treatment Administered

- The patient was put on a temporary salt-restricted diet with no excessive water consumption
- The patient and his mother were reassured that the disease would likely be self-limited

Follow-up

- The patient had symptomatic improvement over the following few days
- His hypertension was normalized 1 week later on a follow-up visit
- Proteinuria and hematuria resolved over the following 2 months

Steps to the Diagnosis

- **Poststreptococcal glomerulonephritis**
  - Acute glomerulonephritis that occurs as a sequela of recent **streptococcal infection** (Table 4-6)
    - Most common in children between 1 and 12 years of age
  - **History: recent streptococcal infection (1 to 2 weeks prior** to symptoms), **hematuria**, malaise, possible oliguria
  - **Physical examination**: periorbital edema, hypertension

MNEMONIC

The list of nephritic glomerular diseases may be remembered by the mnemonic **PIG WAIL**: **P**ostinfectious glomerulonephritis, **I**gA nephropathy, **G**oodpasture syndrome, **W**egener granulomatosis, **A**lport syndrome, **I**diopathic crescentic glomerulonephritis, **L**upus nephritis.

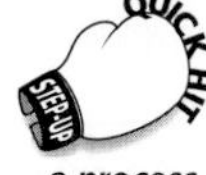

All nephritic syndromes involve a process of **glomerular inflammation**.

TABLE 4-6 Nephritic Syndromes

Type	Pathology	H/P	Tests	Treatment	Prognosis
Poststreptococcal glomerulonephritis	Sequela of **streptococcal** infection	Recent infection (**1–2 weeks prior** to onset of symptoms), oliguria, edema, brown urine, hypertension; more common in **children** (1 to 12 years old)	• UA shows hematuria and proteinuria • High antistreptolysin O titer • **Bumpy deposits** of IgG and C3 on renal basement membrane on electron microscopy	• Self-limited • Supportive treatment (decrease edema and hypertension) • Antihypertensives for refractory HTN	Excellent in children; 25% mortality in adults if CHF develops
IgA nephropathy (i.e., Berger disease)	Unclear relation to infection or autoimmune process; deposition of IgA antibodies in mesangial cells	Intermittent hematuria, flank pain, low-grade fever; rare HTN and edema; symptoms **coincide** with the onset of infection	• **Increased serum IgA** • Mesangial cell proliferation on electron microscopy • Histology is indistinguishable from that for Henoch-Schonlein purpura renal disease	• Occasionally self-limited • ACE-Is and statins are given for persistent proteinuria • Give corticosteroids if nephrotic syndrome develops	Disease course is highly variable, but the prognosis is generally good (especially in children)
Goodpasture syndrome	Rare progressive autoimmune disease of the lungs and kidneys characterized by deposition of antiglomerular and anti-alveolar **basement membrane antibodies**	**Dyspnea**, chest pain, **hemoptysis**, recurrent respiratory infections, arthralgias, hematuria, chills, nausea, vomiting, fever, tachypnea, rales	• Anemia • Pulmonary infiltrates on CXR • Restrictive disease on PFTs • **Serum IgG antiglomerular basement membrane antibodies** • **Linear pattern of IgG antibody deposition** on fluorescence microscopy of glomeruli	• Corticosteroids or immunosuppressive agents may ease symptoms • Plasmapheresis may be required to remove autoantibodies	Prognosis generally poor without aggressive treatment
Alport syndrome	Hereditary defect in collagen IV in basement membrane	Hematuria, symptoms of renal failure, **high-frequency hearing loss**	• UA shows red cell casts, hematuria, proteinuria, and pyuria • Renal biopsy shows **glomerular basement membrane inconsistency** on electron microscopy	• ACE-Is may reduce proteinuria • Renal transplant may be required in progressive disease	90% of cases will end in renal failure, although some cases may have a benign course
Idiopathic crescentic glomerulonephritis	**Rapidly progressive renal failure** due to idiopathic causes, other glomerular diseases, or systemic infection	Sudden renal failure, weakness, nausea, vomiting, weight loss, dyspnea, hemoptysis, myalgias, fever, oliguria	• Positive ANCA • Renal biopsy shows inflammatory cell deposition in Bowman capsule and **crescent formation** (i.e., basement membrane wrinkling) on electron microscopy	• Corticosteroids, plasmapheresis, and immunosuppressive agents may be helpful to slow progression • Renal transplant is frequently required	Poor prognosis with rapid progression to renal failure
Lupus nephritis (mesangial, membranous, focal proliferative, and diffuse proliferative types)	Sequela of systemic lupus erythematosus involving proliferation of endothelial and mesangial cells	Possibly asymptomatic, possible HTN, renal failure, or nephrotic syndrome	• **Positive ANA** and **anti-DNA antibodies** • Hematuria and possible proteinuria on UA	• Corticosteroids or immunosuppressive agents can delay renal failure • ACE-I and statins help reduce proteinuria	Prognosis and risk of renal failure correlates with severity of the systemic disease
Wegener granulomatosis (also see Chapter 2)	Systemic vasculitis characterized by granulomatous inflammation and necrosis of pulmonary and renal vessels	Dyspnea, chronic sinusitis, hemoptysis, myalgias, fever, hematuria, sensory neuropathy, arrhythmias, visual deficits	• Positive **c-ANCA** • Deposition of immune complexes in renal vessels seen on electron microscopy • Pulmonary and renal biopsies may detects areas of noncaseating necrosis	• Corticosteroids and cyclophosphamide may slow disease progression	Rapidly fatal if untreated; gradual multiorgan deterioration is typical with a 30% 5-year survival

ACE-Is, angiotensin converting enzyme inhibitors; ANA, antinuclear antibody; ANCA, antineutrophil cytoplasmic antibody; c-ANCA, cytoplasmic antineutrophil cytoplasmic antibody; CHF, congestive heart failure; CXR, chest x-ray; HTN, hypertension; H/P, history and physical; Ig, immunoglobulin; IV, intravenous; PFTs, pulmonary function tests; UA, urinalysis.

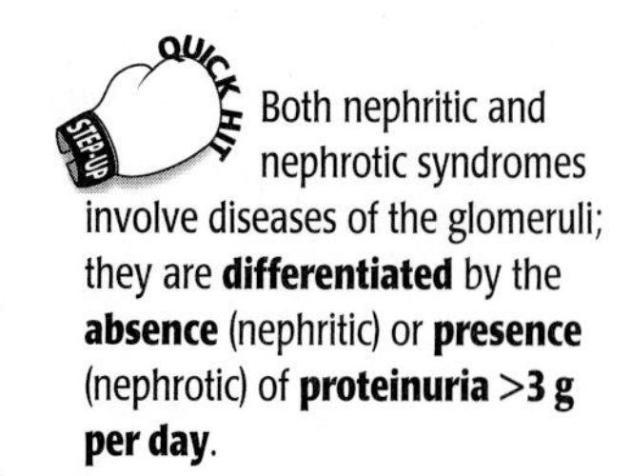

Both nephritic and nephrotic syndromes involve diseases of the glomeruli; they are **differentiated** by the **absence** (nephritic) or **presence** (nephrotic) of **proteinuria >3 g per day**.

- **Tests:**
  - UA will show hematuria, proteinuria, and red cell casts
  - Twenty-four-hour urine protein is <3 g
  - High antistreptolysin O titer
  - Renal biopsy will show **bumpy deposits** of IgG and C3 complement on the renal basement membrane when examined under electron microscopy (Figure 4-3)
- **Treatment:**
  - The condition is self-limited and generally requires only supportive care and a low salt diet with water restriction
  - Diuretics, calcium channel blockers, and ACE-Is may be used to treat significant HTN
  - Dialysis is very rarely required
- **Outcomes:**
  - Children have an excellent prognosis
  - Adults with the diagnosis may develop CHF and have mortality rates up to 25%
  - Complications include CHF, CKD, and nephrotic syndrome and are more common in adults
- **Clues to the diagnosis:**
  - History: hematuria, malaise, recent upper respiratory infection
  - Physical: periorbital edema
  - Tests: UA with hematuria, proteinuria, and red cell casts, positive antistreptolysin O titer

- **Immunoglobulin A nephropathy**
  - More thorough discussion in Table 4-6
  - **Why eliminated from differential:** symptoms of this diagnosis typically occur at the same time as the related infection, so this diagnosis is less likely than poststreptococcal glomerulonephritis
- **Goodpasture syndrome**
  - More thorough discussion in Chapter 2 and in Table 4-6 (Color Figure 4-2)
  - **Why eliminated from differential:** the absence of dyspnea in the history and the absence of antibasement membrane antibodies rule out this diagnosis
- **Alport syndrome**
  - More thorough discussion in Table 4-6
  - **Why eliminated from differential:** the absence of hearing loss makes this diagnosis less likely than the correct diagnosis
- **Nephrotic syndrome**
  - More thorough discussion in later case
  - **Why eliminated from differential:** the 24-hour urine protein level is indicative of a nephritic and not nephrotic condition
- **Acute renal failure**
  - More thorough discussion in prior case
  - **Why eliminated from differential:** some degree of mild ARF is apparent from the mildly increased BUN and creatinine, but the diagnosis of poststreptococcal glomerulonephritis is a better description of the actual etiology of the condition
- **Polycystic kidney disease**
  - More thorough discussion in prior case
  - **Why eliminated from differential:** the normal appearance of the kidneys on the renal US rules out this disease
- **Cold-antibody hemolytic anemia**
  - More thorough discussion in Chapter 6
  - **Why eliminated from differential:** the normal hemoglobin in the patient makes a hemolytic anemia unlikely
- **Rhabdomyolysis**
  - A syndrome following **skeletal muscle injury** in which the intracellular muscular components (e.g., myoglobin) enter the circulation and clog the renal filtration system
  - **History:** history of a precipitating factor (e.g., trauma, DKA, heat stroke, heavy drug use), weakness, myalgias, dark urine

FIGURE 4-3 **Electron microscopy of a renal biopsy from a patient with poststreptococcal glomerulonephritis. Bumpy deposits of immunoglobulin G and complement (*arrows*) are present on the basement membrane, and the capillary lumens (*Ls*) are compressed.**

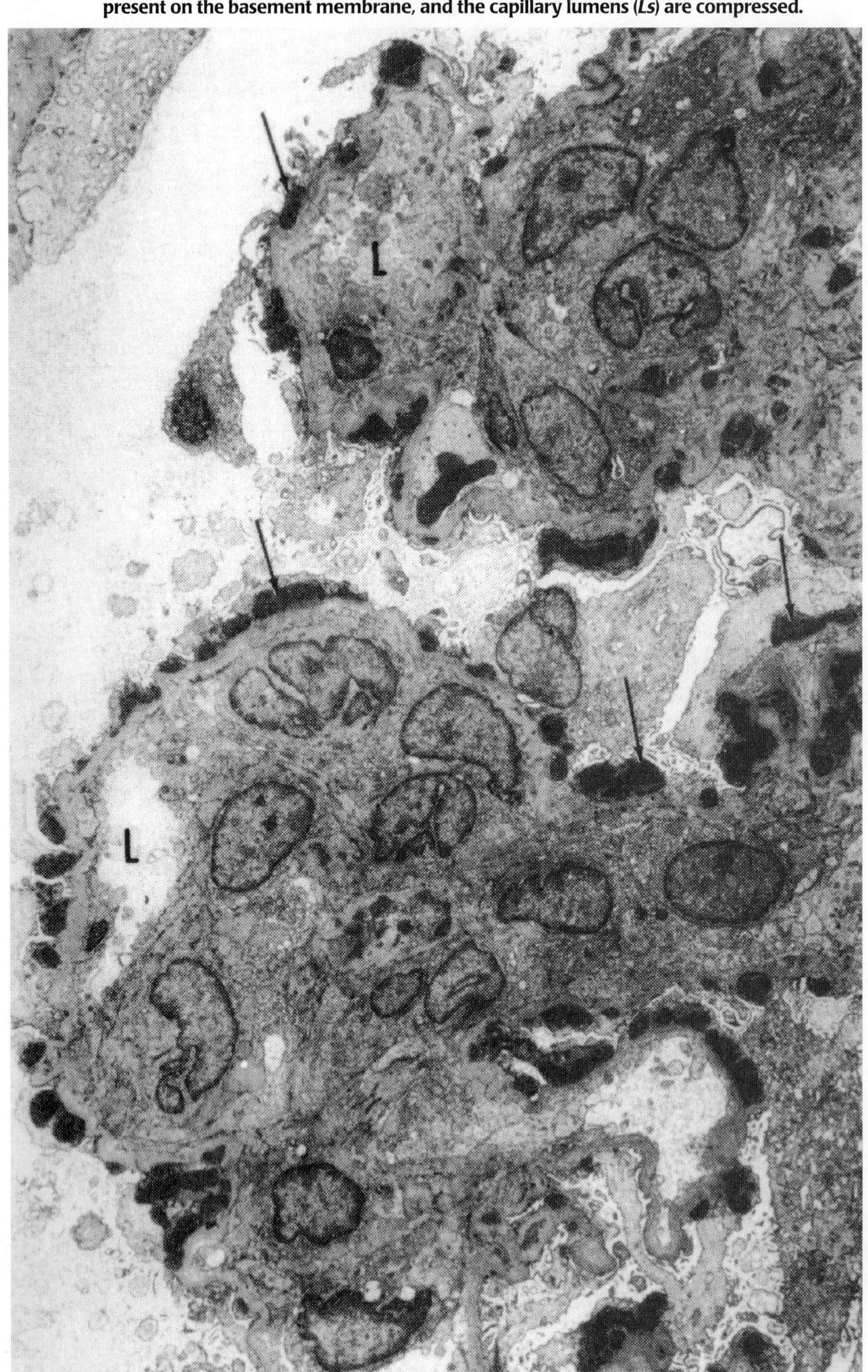

(Taken from Rubin E, Farber JL. *Pathology*. 3rd ed. Philadelphia: Lippincott Williams & Wilkins, 1999. Fig. 16-34. Used with permission of Lippincott Williams & Wilkins.)

- **Physical examination:** muscle tenderness, edema
- **Tests:** serum creatine kinase will be significantly increased; UA will indicate the presence of hematuria, but **no red cells will be seen**
- **Treatment:**
  - Use of a causative agent should be stopped
  - **IV hydration** helps to maintain glomerular filtration; simultaneous use of diuretics may also help to increase glomerular blood flow
  - Abnormal electrolyte levels should be corrected
  - Dialysis may be required in patients with severe renal failure
  - Strenuous activities and substance use should be avoided to prevent further muscle breakdown
- **Outcomes:** one third of cases will be complicated by renal failure; the outcome correlates with the rapidity of starting therapy
- **Why eliminated from differential:** the absence of a history of trauma and the presence of red cell casts on the UA make this diagnosis unlikely

CASE 4-5 "I'm having problems breathing, and my legs are swollen"

A 63-year-old man presents to his PCP with the complaint of progressive edema and dyspnea that have worsened over the past month. He was in his usual state of health until the onset of these symptoms and has never experienced them previously. He states that over this time he has also experienced fatigue, weakness, and a lack of appetite. He denies headache, dizziness, chest pain, abdominal pain, nausea, vomiting or diarrhea, hematemesis or hematochezia, urinary symptoms, hematuria, or paresthesias. He has a history of rheumatoid arthritis that has been controlled with celecoxib and methotrexate. He denies other medical conditions and medication use. He drinks alcohol infrequently and denies other substance use. On examination, he is a tired-appearing man who is mildly dyspneic. He has 4+ pitting edema in his legs and milder edema in his upper body. He has no palpable lymphadenopathy. Auscultation of his lungs detects mild coarse breath sounds but no areas of focal consolidation. Auscultation of his heart and bowels is normal. He has no abdominal masses. His proximal interphalangeal, metacarpophalangeal, and knee joints are mildly swollen and hypertrophic. The following vital signs are measured:

T: 98.8°F, HR: 87 bpm, BP: 128/81 mm Hg, RR: 22 breaths/min

Differential Diagnosis

- Rheumatoid arthritis, CHF, cirrhosis, nephrotic syndrome, pneumonia, acute renal failure, sarcoidosis

Laboratory Data and Other Study Results

- CBC: WBC: 10.1, Hgb: 13.7, Plt: 240
- Chem10: Na: 137 mEq/L, K: 5.3 mEq/L, Cl: 106 mEq/L, CO_2: 29 mEq/L, BUN: 43 mg/dL, Cr: 2.1 mg/dL, Glu: 79 mg/dL, Mg: 2.3 mg/dL, Ca: 9.7 mg/dL, Phos: 4.2 mg/dL
- BNP: 89 pg/mL
- Liver function tests (LFTs): alkaline phosphatase (AlkPhos): 56 U/L, alanine aminotransferase (ALT): 35 U/L, aspartate aminotransferase (AST) 21 U/L, total bilirubin (TBili): 1.0 mg/dL, direct bilirubin (DBili): 0.4 mg/dL
- UA: cloudy, pH: 5.5, specific gravity: 1.031, multiple fatty casts, 3+ proteinuria, no glucose/ketones/nitrites/leukocyte esterase/hematuria
- CXR: mild diffuse infiltrates; no focal consolidations; small pleural effusions at the costodiaphragmatic gutters

Based on these results, the following studies are ordered:

- Albumin: 2.3 g/dL
- Twenty-four-hour urine protein: 5,036 mg/day

- Renal US: normal-sized kidneys; no apparent hydronephrosis or obstruction
- Renal biopsy (US-guided): histology shows generalized thickening of glomerular capillaries with spiky endothelial deposits

Diagnosis

- Membranous glomerulonephritis (nephrotic syndrome)

Treatment Administered

- The patient was admitted to the hospital and placed on a low salt diet
- Enalapril, furosemide, and prednisone were initiated

MNEMONIC

The list of nephrotic glomerular diseases may be remembered by the mnemonic "**M**ost **D**ogs **F**ind **M**eat **M**esmerizing": **M**inimal change disease, **D**iabetic nephropathy, **F**ocal segmental glomerular sclerosis, **M**embranous glomerulonephritis, **M**embranoproliferative glomerulonephritis.

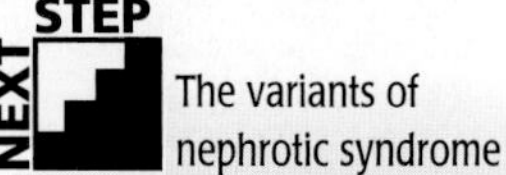

NEXT STEP

The variants of nephrotic syndrome are frequently difficult to differentiate, and a **renal biopsy** is often indicated to provide a definitive diagnosis.

QUICK HIT

Minimal change disease is more common in children, while focal segmental glomerular sclerosis is more common in adults.

Follow-up

- The patient had a gradual improvement in his edema following the initiation of therapy
- During his inpatient stay, the patient developed a deep vein thrombosis (DVT) of the left femoral vein and was anticoagulated with heparin and transitioned to warfarin
- The patient was discharged to home when his edema had decreased enough to significantly improve his symptoms
- Due to lingering edema and proteinuria, the patient was eventually started on cyclophosphamide as an outpatient
- Over the course of the subsequent year, the patient experienced progressive renal failure that required the eventual initiation of dialysis

Steps to the Diagnosis

- **Membranous glomerulonephritis**
  - More thorough discussion in Table 4-7 (Color Figure 4-3)
  - **Clues to the diagnosis:**
    - History: anorexia, fatigue, weakness, progressive edema and dyspnea
    - Physical: anasarca
    - Tests: significant proteinuria, hypoalbuminemia, renal biopsy findings
- **Minimal change disease**
  - More thorough discussion in Table 4-7
  - **Why eliminated from differential:** the edema in the case is more severe than that expected for this diagnosis, and the renal biopsy appearance is more consistent with membranous glomerulonephritis
- **Focal segmental glomerular sclerosis**
  - More thorough discussion in Table 4-7
  - **Why eliminated from differential:** the renal biopsy is more consistent with membranous glomerulonephritis
- **Membranoproliferative glomerulonephritis**
  - More thorough discussion in Table 4-7 (Color Figure 4-4)
  - **Why eliminated from differential:** the renal biopsy is more consistent with membranous glomerulonephritis
- **Rheumatoid arthritis**
  - More thorough discussion in Chapter 9
  - **Why eliminated from differential:** although the patient does have an existing diagnosis of rheumatoid arthritis, severe edema is not a characteristic of this disease, and an alternative explanation must be provided
- **Congestive heart failure**
  - More thorough discussion in Chapter 1
  - **Why eliminated from differential:** the normal range BNP makes this diagnosis less likely, and the edema seen in severe CHF is not associated with significant proteinuria

TABLE 4-7 Nephrotic Syndromes

Type	Pathology	H/P	Tests	Treatment	Prognosis
Minimal change disease	Autoimmune injury of foot processes on basement membrane leading to protein leaking	**Edema**, malaise, weight gain, possible HTN or increased frequency of infections	• Hyperlipidemia • Hypoalbuminemia • Proteinuria on UA • Renal biopsy shows flattening of basement membrane foot processes on electron microscopy	• Corticosteroids • Cyclophosphamide may be used in refractory cases	Relapse is possible, but most patients have a very good prognosis with eventual cessation of relapses and a low rate of renal failure
Focal segmental glomerular sclerosis	Segmental sclerosis of the glomeruli that is either idiopathic or associated with drug use or HIV	Edema, HTN, possible rapid renal deterioration	• Hyperlipidemia • Hypoalbuminemia • Hematuria and high proteinuria on UA • Renal US may show shrunken kidneys • Renal biopsy shows solidification of some glomeruli due to sclerosis on electron microscopy	• Salt restriction and diuretics help improve edema • ACE-Is decrease proteinuria and HTN • Corticosteroids with/without cyclophosphamide are used to induce disease remission	Disease course is variable, but most patients require dialysis within 10 years
Membranous glomerulonephritis	Deposition of immune complexes in the glomeruli basement membrane	Edema, dyspnea; history of infection or medication use may lead to diagnosis	• Hyperlipidemia • Hypoalbuminemia; proteinuria on UA • **"Spike and dome" basement membrane thickening** on electron microscopy	• Low salt diet and diuretics to improve edema • ACE-Is to improve proteinuria and HTN • Corticosteroids with/without cyclophosphamide are used to induce disease remission • Anticoagulants if DVT occurs	Risk of end-stage renal disease increases with the degree of proteinuria and renal failure at the time of diagnosis; increased risk of DVT
Membranoproliferative glomerulonephritis	Chronic proliferation of mesangial cells with interposition into the capillary walls due to an idiopathic, infectious, or autoimmune process	Edema, HTN, history of systemic infection or autoimmune condition, hematuria, oliguria, fatigue, retinal lesions	• Hyperlipidemia • Hypoalbuminemia; possible hypocomplementemia • Proteinuria and hematuria on UA • Renal biopsy shows IgG deposits on the basement membrane on fluorescence microscopy and **basement membrane thickening** with **a double-layer "train track"** appearance on electron microscopy	• Treat underlying infectious or rheumatic conditions • Corticosteroids may be beneficial in children • ASA or dipyridamole is useful in adults	Gradual progression to end-stage renal disease occurs over >10 years
Diabetic nephropathy (e.g., diffuse, nodular)	Basement membrane and mesangial thickening related to diabetic vascular changes	History of DM, HTN, edema, foamy urine	• Hyperlipidemia • Hypoalbuminemia; proteinuria on UA • Basement membrane thickening on electron microscopy seen in both types • Round nodules **(Kimmelstiel-Wilson nodules)** are seen within glomeruli in the nodular type	• Treat underlying DM • Dietary protein restriction • ACE-I for proteinuria and HTN	End-stage renal disease occurs in 50% of patients with DM type I and in 10% of patient with DM type II within 10 years of the diagnosis of nephropathy

ACE-Is, angiotensin converting enzyme inhibitors; ASA, aspirin; DM, diabetes mellitus; DVT, deep vain thrombosis; HIV, human immunodeficiency virus; HTN, hypertension; H/P, history and physical; Ig, immunoglobulin; UA, urinalysis; US, ultrasound.

- **Cirrhosis**
  - More thorough discussion in Chapter 3
  - **Why eliminated from differential:** the normal LFTs rule out a primary hepatic pathology
- **Pneumonia**
  - More thorough discussion in Chapter 2
  - **Why eliminated from differential:** the normal WBC count, lack of a fever, and unimpressive chest x-ray (CXR) rule out this diagnosis
- **Acute renal failure**
  - More thorough discussion in prior case
  - **Why eliminated from differential:** although some of the clinical signs and lab abnormalities are consistent with renal failure (e.g., edema, increased BUN and creatinine), the significant proteinuria requires a more definitive explanation for the patient's condition
- **Sarcoidosis**
  - More thorough discussion in Chapter 2
  - **Why eliminated from differential:** the absence of hilar adenopathy on the CXR and the normal calcium, alkaline phosphatase, and WBC lab values make this diagnosis less likely

CASE 4-6 "I am always so thirsty"

A 36-year-old woman presents to a trauma surgeon for a follow-up appointment 2 months after a motor vehicle accident. She was a restrained passenger in a car without airbags that was hit on the side by another car. Her trauma work-up was significant for a minor splenic laceration and small subarachnoid hemorrhage, both of which were able to be treated non-operatively. She was able to be discharged to home 10 days after her admission to the hospital and denies any current neurologic deficits. She reports some gradually resolving left abdominal and flank pain. Her main complaint, however, is significant thirst that has been present since she returned home. She reports urinating frequently, but feeling the need to drink constantly because of a feeling of being "dry." She denies headaches, nausea, vomiting or diarrhea, dysuria, paresthesias, or weakness. Prior to her trauma, she was healthy with no medical problems. She takes no medications. She drinks alcohol socially. On examination, she is a healthy appearing woman in no distress. She has a large bottle of water with her in the office. Her mucus membranes are mildly dry, and she has slightly decreased skin turgor. She has no palpable lymphadenopathy. Auscultation of her heart and lungs is normal. She has minimal abdominal tenderness in her left upper quadrant. She has no hepatosplenomegaly, but a distended bladder is palpable in the suprapubic region. Neurologic examination is normal. The following vital signs are measured:

T: 98.5°F, HR: 88 bpm, BP: 110/78 mm Hg, RR: 24 breaths/min

Differential Diagnosis

- Diabetes mellitus, chronic kidney disease, diabetes insipidus, psychogenic polydipsia

Laboratory Data and Other Study Results

- Chem7: Na: 157 mEq/L, K: 3.6 mEq/L, Cl: 108 mEq/L, CO_2: 25 mEq/L, BUN: 14 mg/dL, Cr: 0.5 mg/dL, Glu: 83 mg/dL
- UA: light straw colored, pH: 6.0, specific gravity: 1.003, no glucose/ketones/nitrites/leukocyte esterase/hematuria/proteinuria
- Urine electrolytes: Na: 4 mEq/L, K: 2 mEq/L
- Urine osmolality: 68 mOsm/kg
- Plasma osmolality: 298 mOsm/kg
- Brain MRI: continued resolution of small subarachnoid hemorrhage in the pituitary region when compared to imaging performed 2 months prior

After receipt of these results, the following test is ordered:

- Water deprivation test: urine osmolality increased from 70 mOsm/kg to 125 mOsm/kg following administration of vasopressin

Diagnosis

- Central diabetes insipidus secondary to cerebral trauma

Treatment Administered

- Intranasal desmopressin was prescribed on an outpatient basis
- The patient was encouraged to drink enough water to avoid dehydration

Follow-up

- Following the initiation of therapy, the patient's urine and serum osmolalities normalized, and she was able to reduce her water intake

Steps to the Diagnosis

- **Diabetes insipidus (DI)**
  - A disorder of antidiuretic hormone (ADH)-directed water reabsorption leading to dehydration and hypernatremia
    - **Types:**
      - **Central:** failure of the posterior pituitary to secrete ADH due to idiopathic causes, cerebral trauma, pituitary tumors, hypoxic encephalopathy, or anorexia nervosa
      - **Nephrogenic:** failure of the kidneys to respond to ADH due to congenital kidney disease, lithium toxicity, hypercalcemia, or hypokalemia
  - **Hypernatremia**
    - Serum sodium **>155 mEq/L**
      - Causes include dehydration, cutaneous water loss (e.g., burns, wounds), gastrointestinal (GI) fluid losses (e.g., vomiting, diarrhea), diabetes insipidus, and excess aldosterone secretion (Figure 4-4)
    - Symptoms and signs include oliguria, polydipsia, weakness, mental status changes, and seizures

MNEMONIC

Causes of hypernatremia may be remembered by the six **D**s: **D**iuretics, **D**ehydration, **D**iabetes insipidus, **D**ocs (iatrogenic), **D**iarrhea (and vomiting), **D**isease of kidney (hyperaldosteronism).

FIGURE 4-4 **Algorithm for the evaluation of hypernatremia. Na, sodium.**

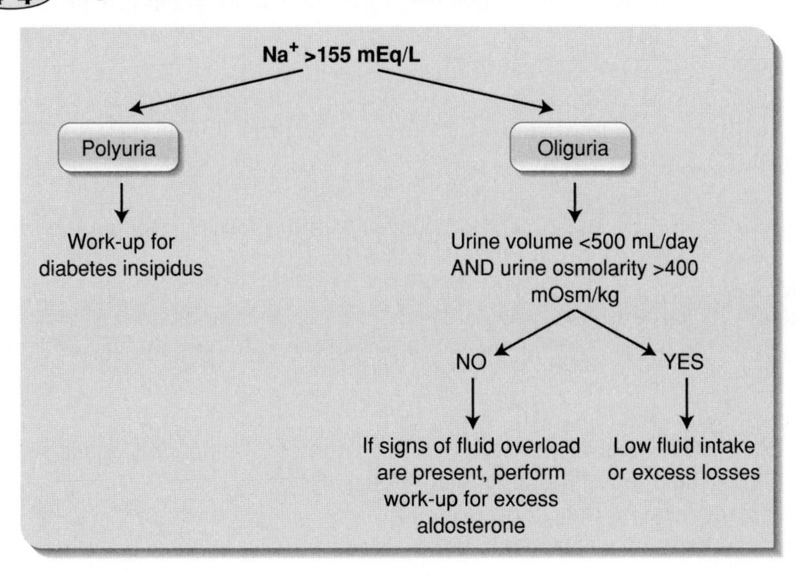

- **Fluid correction**
  - Gradual hydration with hypotonic saline for an inadequate fluid intake or excess fluid loss at a maximum rate of **12 mEq Na per day**
  - **Calculation of the water deficit** is used to determine the approximate required correction in a patient with fluid loss as a cause for the hypernatremia:

$$\text{Water Deficit} = \text{Total body water} \times \left(\frac{[\text{Na}]}{140} - 1\right)$$
$$= 0.60 \times (\text{mass in kg}) \times \left(\frac{[\text{Na}]}{140} - 1\right)$$

  - Half of the deficit is given in 24 hours in addition to maintenance fluids, and the remainder is given over the following 24 to 48 hours
  - Sodium levels are closely monitored to avoid overcorrection
  - The calculated water deficit may be artificially high because the normal total body water content will be slightly greater than the patient's body water content in the presence of hypernatremia
- **History**: polydipsia, polyuria
- **Physical examination**: signs of dehydration may be present, or the examination may be normal
- **Tests**:
  - **Hypernatremia**
  - **Low urine osmolality** in the presence of a large urine volume
  - **Water deprivation test**
    - The patient is deprived of water for 2 to 3 hours followed by administration of vasopressin
    - Normal patients will show normal or mildly increased urine osmolality before vasopressin administration with little change afterward
    - Patients with central DI will show low urine osmolality before vasopressin administration and normal osmolality afterward
    - Patients with nephrogenic DI will have low urine osmolality before and after vasopressin administration
- **Treatment**:
  - Any underlying causes are treated
  - Daily intranasal **desmopressin** is given in central DI
  - Salt restriction and high water consumption are required in patients with nephrogenic DI; thiazide diuretics may reduce net fluid loses by inducing distal convoluted tubule water secretion to cause a reflexive increase in proximal tubule water reabsorption
- **Outcomes**: complications include dehydration, seizures, and iatrogenic cerebral edema from excessive rehydration; treatable cases have an excellent prognosis
- **Clues to the diagnosis**:
  - History: polydipsia, polyuria, recent head trauma
  - Physical: signs of dehydration
  - Tests: hypernatremia, low urine osmolality, water deprivation test results

- **Diabetes mellitus**
  - More thorough discussion in Chapter 5
  - **Why eliminated from differential**: the normal serum glucose level and absence of glucosuria or urinary ketones on the UA rule out this diagnosis
- **Chronic kidney disease**
  - More thorough discussion in prior case
  - **Why eliminated from differential**: the normal BUN and creatinine levels rule out this diagnosis
- **Psychogenic polydipsia**
  - Excess water consumption related to a psychiatric cause and possibly associated with dysfunction of the cerebral thirst regulation system
  - **History**: polydipsia, polyuria, confusion
  - **Physical examination**: edema, mental status changes

- **Tests:** hyponatremia
- **Treatment:** treat underlying psychiatric conditions; water restriction
- **Outcomes:** success in correcting the electrolyte abnormality is tied to the success in treating the underlying disease
- **Why eliminated from differential:** the presence of hypernatremia rules out this diagnosis

The following additional Nephrology and Urology cases may be found online:

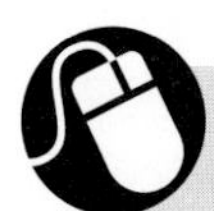

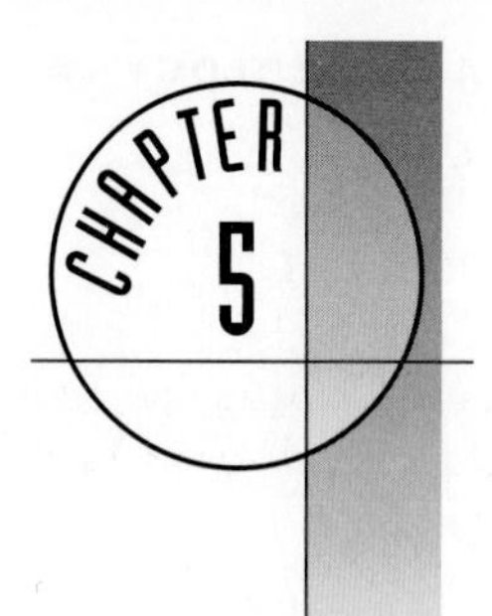

Endocrinology

BASIC CLINICAL PRIMER

NORMAL GLUCOSE METABOLISM

- **Postprandial period**
  - Feeding results in an increase in the blood concentration of **glucose**
  - **Insulin** is secreted by pancreatic **β-islet** cells in response to the increased serum glucose concentration (also induced to a lesser extent by other protein and neural input)
  - Insulin drives glucose anabolism
    - Glucose is converted into glycogen, fatty acids, and pyruvate (Figure 5-1)
    - Glycogen is stored in the liver and in skeletal muscle; fatty acids (i.e., triglycerides) are stored in adipose cells
    - Pyruvate and fatty acids are also incorporated into amino acid production
    - Lipolysis of adipose tissue is inhibited by insulin secretion
- **Fasting period**
  - Fasting results in a decrease in the blood glucose concentration
  - **Glucagon** is secreted by pancreatic **α-islet** cells in response to the dropping glucose level
  - Glucagon drives catabolism of glycogen and fatty acids

PRESURGICAL ASSESSMENT OF DIABETIC PATIENTS

- Diabetic patients have greater surgical risks of postoperative infection, complicated wound healing, adverse cardiac events, and postoperative mortality
- Tight glycemic control should be achieved postoperatively via frequent serum glucose checks and the administration of insulin as needed
- Insulin needs of the patient frequently **increase** from the baseline level postoperatively due to an augmented body stress response

THYROID FUNCTION

QUICK HIT: If TBG levels increase (e.g., pregnancy, oral contraceptive use), total T_4 increases but free T_4 remains normal.

QUICK HIT: Nephrotic syndrome and androgen use decrease TBG levels, leading to a decreased total T_4 but a normal free T_4.

- Thyroid hormones (i.e., thyroxine, or T_4, and triiodothyronine, or T_3) are important for determining the body's basal metabolic rate, promoting bone growth, increasing cardiac output in times of stress, and driving the maturation of the central nervous system (CNS) during fetal growth
- The hypothalamus secretes thyrotropin-releasing hormone (TRH) to induce the secretion of thyroid stimulating hormone (TSH) from the anterior pituitary (Figure 5-2)
- Free T_4 and T_3 determine the degree of metabolic activity; nonfree thyroid hormones are bound to thyroid-binding globulin (TBG) in the circulation
- The serum T_4 level is responsible for the feedback inhibition of TSH secretion
- Calcitonin is secreted by the parafollicular cells of the thyroid and plays a minor role in serum calcium regulation

FIGURE 5-1 **Glucose metabolism and its dependence on feeding states. (A) During the postprandial stage, insulin induces the anabolism of glucose to form glycogen and fatty acids, which are stored in the liver and skeletal muscle and in adipocytes, respectively. (B) During fasting, glucagon induces the breakdown of glycogen and fatty acids to increase the blood glucose level.**

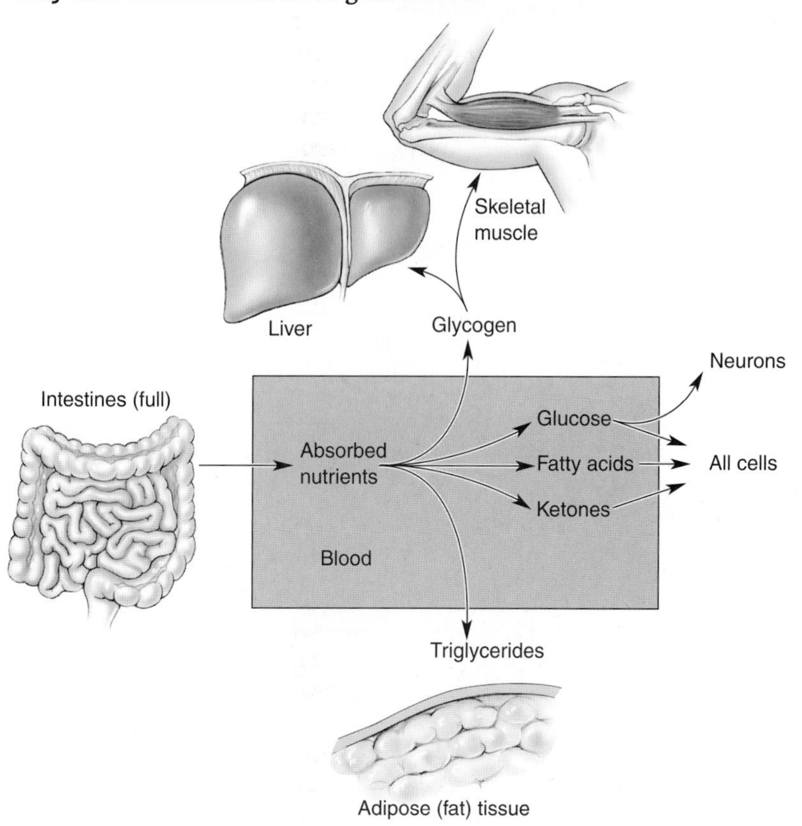

A Anabolism during the postprandial state

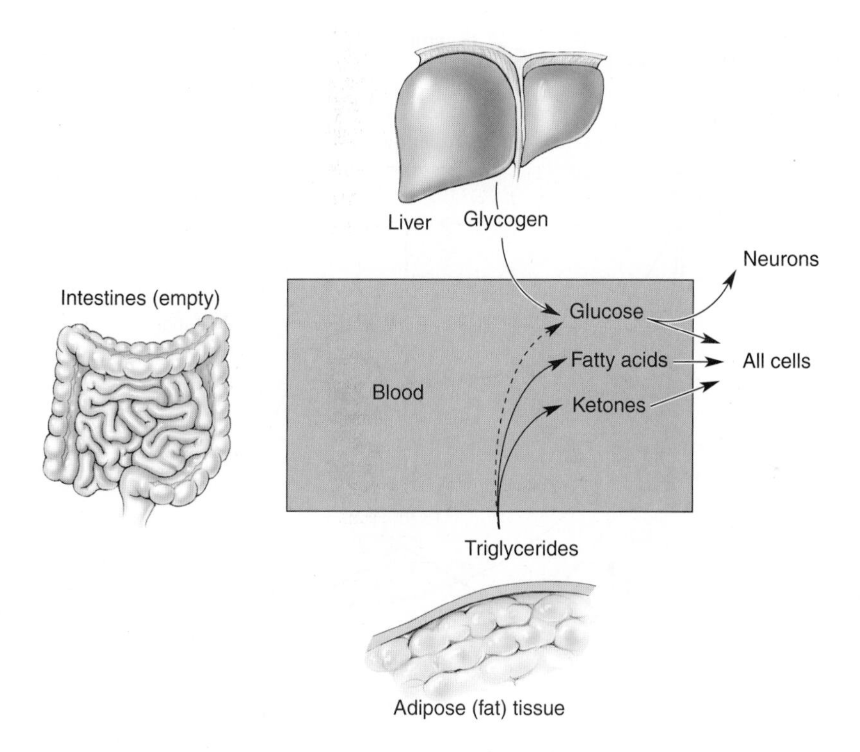

B Catabolism during the postabsorptive state

(Taken from Bear MF, Conners BW, Parasido MA. *Neuroscience–exploring the brain*. 2nd ed. Philadelphia: Lippincott Williams & Wilkins, 2001. Fig. 16.1. Used with permission of Lippincott Williams & Wilkins.)

FIGURE 5-2 Normal thyroid hormone secretion within the hypothalamic-pituitary axis. I^-, iodine; T_3, triiodothyronine; T_4, thyroxine; TRH, thyroid-releasing hormone; TSH, thyroid-stimulating hormone.

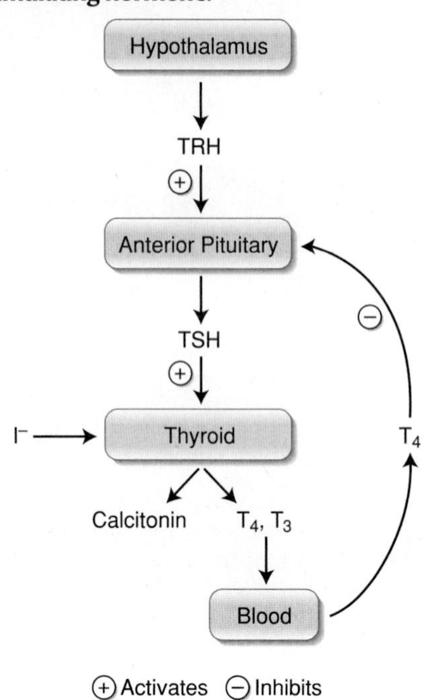

FIGURE 5-3 Regulation of serum calcium levels. Ca, calcium; PTH, parathyroid hormone.

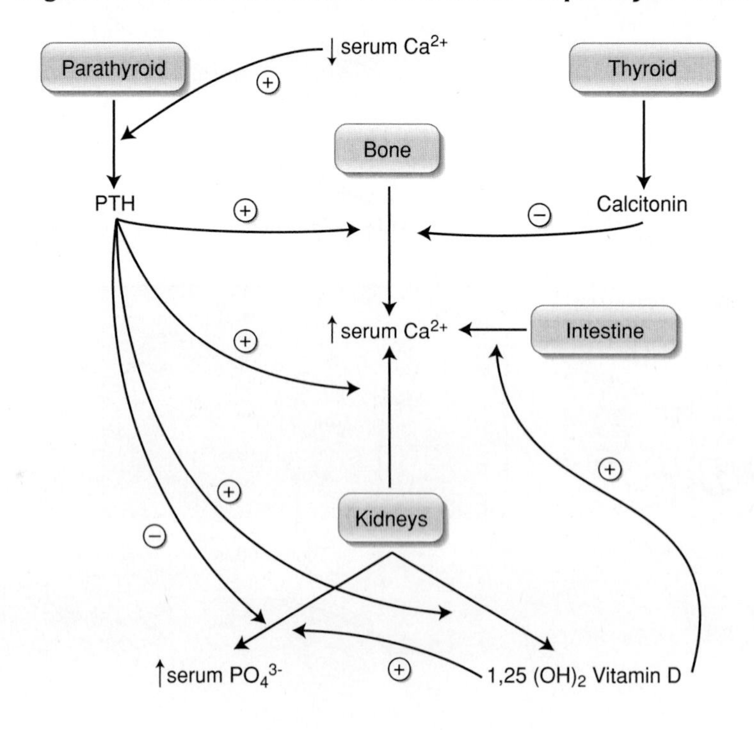

PARATHYROID FUNCTION

- The parathyroid glands secrete **parathyroid hormone (PTH)**, the chief hormone behind maintaining serum calcium concentrations (Figure 5-3)
  - Secretion of PTH increases with low serum calcium levels
  - PTH induces osteoclasts to reabsorb bone and subsequently increase serum calcium levels
  - PTH induces the conversion of 25-(OH) vitamin D to **1,25-$(OH)_2$ vitamin D**, induces distal tubule calcium reabsorption, and **inhibits** phosphate reabsorption in the kidneys
    - 1,25-$(OH)_2$ vitamin D increases the intestinal absorption of calcium and **increases** proximal tubule reabsorption of phosphate in the kidney to balance the activity of PTH

HYPOTHALAMIC-PITUITARY AXIS

- The hypothalamus is responsible for the modulation of pituitary gland activity (Figure 5-4)

FIGURE 5-4 Modulation of pituitary activity by the hypothalamus. ACTH, adrenocorticotropic hormone; ADH, antidiuretic hormone; CRH, corticotrophin-releasing hormone; FSH follicle-stimulating hormone; GH, growth hormone; GHRH, growth hormone-releasing hormone; GnRH, gonadotropin-releasing hormone; H_2O, water; LH, luteinizing hormone; PRH, prolactin-releasing hormone; T_3, triiodothyronine; T_4, thyroxine; TRH, thyrotropin-releasing hormone; TSH, thyroid-stimulating hormone.

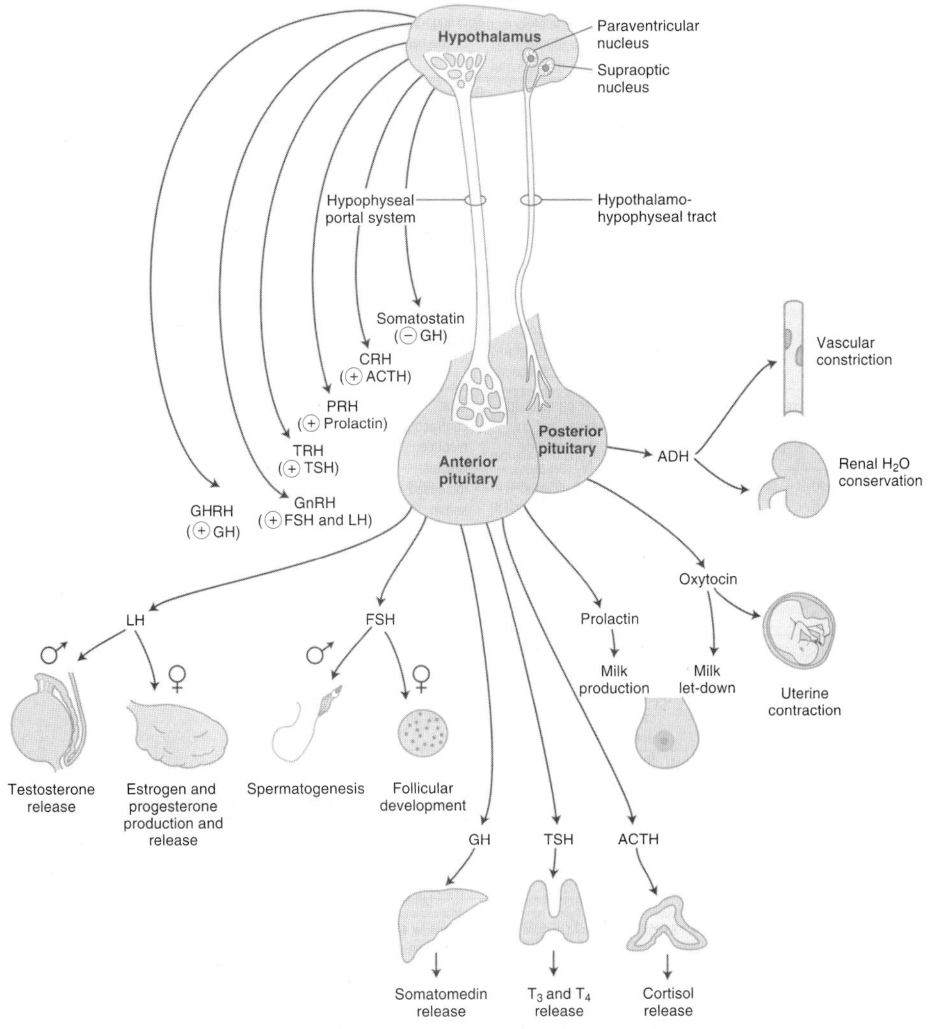

(From Mehta S, Milder EA, Mirachi AJ, Milder E. *Step-up: a high-yield, systems-based review for the USMLE step 1.* 2nd ed. Philadelphia: Lippincott Williams & Wilkins, 2003. Used with permission of Lippincott Williams & Wilkins.)

MNEMONIC

The hormones produced by the pituitary gland may be remembered by the mnemonic **GOAT FLAP**: **G**H (growth hormone), **O**xytocin (posterior), **A**DH (posterior; antidiuretic hormone), **T**SH, **F**SH (follicle-stimulating hormone), **L**H (luteinizing hormone), **A**CTH (adrenocorticotropic hormone), **P**rolactin.

- The **anterior pituitary** is regulated by the release of hormones from the hypothalamus into the hypophyseal portal system and by the feedback mechanisms of pituitary hormones
  - The anterior pituitary is responsible for the secretion of prolactin, ACTH, TSH, GH, FSH, and LH
- The **posterior pituitary** is regulated by neural impulses sent from the hypothalamus through the hypothalamo-hypophyseal tract
  - The posterior pituitary is responsible for the secretion of ADH and oxytocin

ADRENAL FUNCTION

MNEMONIC

The layers and activities of the adrenal cortex may be remembered by the mnemonic "**G**reat **A**ttire **A**nd **F**ast **C**ars **A**re **R**eally **S**exy **A**ttributes": **G**ranulosa secretes **A**ldosterone after **A**ngiotensin II stimulation, **F**asciculata secretes **C**ortisol after **A**CTH stimulation, **R**eticularis secretes **S**ex hormones after **A**CTH stimulation.

- The adrenal glands are divided into layers that differ in their enzyme products and function
- **Zona glomerulosa**
  - Outer layer of the cortex
  - Activity is stimulated by the renin-angiotensin system
  - Aldosterone is the main product, which serves to maintain body sodium and fluid volume
- **Zona fasciculata**
  - Middle layer of the cortex
  - Activity is stimulated by ACTH
  - Cortisol is the main product, which maintains glucose production from proteins, aids in fat metabolism, aids in vascular regulation, influences immune function, and aids in neural regulation
- **Zona reticularis**
  - Deep layer of the cortex
  - Activity is stimulated by ACTH
  - Androgens are the main products, which drive the development of secondary sexual characteristics, increase bone and muscle mass, and promote male sexual differentiation and sperm production
- **Medulla**
  - Activity is stimulated by preganglionic sympathetic neurons
  - Norepinephrine and epinephrine are the main products, which function as postsynaptic neurotransmitters in the sympathetic autonomic nervous system

CASE 5-1 "My son drinks too much"

A 10-year-old boy is brought to his pediatrician by his mother, who is concerned that he drinks large amounts of water frequently. She says that he is constantly thirsty and drinking water and that he needs to go to the bathroom many times every day. She is not sure how long this has been occurring, but it has been noticeable at least over the past month. The boy says that he feels thirsty very frequently and guesses that he needs to urinate at least five times per day. He wakes up in the middle of the night needing to urinate on most nights. He also reports being hungry during most of the day. He occasionally feels very tired and not well and usually eats something during these episodes. He denies any areas of pain, dizziness, numbness, dysuria, vomiting or diarrhea, or hematochezia. His mother says that he is a generally healthy boy but has had several colds in the past year. He takes children's vitamins but no other medications. There are no particular conditions that are common in the family. On examination, he is a thin boy in no distress. Auscultation of his heart, lungs, and bowels is normal. He has no pain in his flanks or abdomen and no palpable masses. His neurologic examination is normal. His mucous membranes are mildly dry. He appears to have no abnormalities of his penis or genitals. The following vital signs are measured:

Temperature (T): 98.8°F, heart rate (HR): 85 beats per minute (bpm), blood pressure (BP): 110/70 mm Hg, respiratory rate (RR): 16 breaths/min

Differential Diagnosis

- Diabetes insipidus, hyperthyroidism, diabetes mellitus (types 1 and 2), psychogenic polydipsia, acute renal failure

Laboratory Data and Other Study Results

- Complete blood cell count (CBC): white blood cells (WBC): 7.1, hemoglobin (Hgb): 15.8, platelets (Plt): 239
- 7-electrolyte chemistry panel (Chem7): sodium (Na): 133 mEq/L, potassium (K): 4.2 mEq/L, chloride (Cl): 101 mEq/L, carbon dioxide (CO_2): 25 mEq/L, blood urea nitrogen (BUN): 14 mg/dL, creatinine (Cr): 0.5 mg/dL, glucose (Glu): 265 mg/dL
- Urinalysis (UA): straw colored, pH: 5.7, specific gravity: 1.010, 3+ glucose, 1+ ketones, no nitrites/leukocyte esterase/hematuria/proteinuria
- Thyroid panel: TSH 1.2 μU/mL, T_4: 5.7 μg/dL, free T_4: index 6.3, T_3: 1.0 ng/mL, T_3 reuptake: 0.87

Based on these results, the following tests are performed on a different day:

- Chem7: Na: 132 mEq/L, K: 4.1 mEq/L, Cl: 101 mEq/L, CO_2: 25 mEq/L, BUN: 15 mg/dL, Cr: 0.5 mg/dL, Glu: 267 mg/dL
- Hemoglobin A1c (HbA1c): 9.8%
- Serum osmolality: 310 mOsm/kg

Diagnosis

- Diabetes mellitus type 1

Treatment Administered

- The patient was started on a insulin regimen of regular insulin at breakfast and dinner and NPH (neutral protamine Hagedorn) insulin at breakfast and bedtime
- The patient and his family were trained in home glucose measurements and a self-measurement program was initiated
- The patient was referred to a nutritionist for dietary counseling
- The patient was referred to an endocrinologist and ophthalmologist to be evaluated for any renal or retinal deficits

Follow-up

- The patient and his family were able to comply with the recommended therapeutic regimen
- The patient's follow-up HbA1c levels were able to be maintained near 7%
- The patient's symptoms improved following the successful control of his glucose levels

Steps to the Diagnosis

- **Diabetes mellitus type 1 (DM type 1)**
  - Impairment or loss of pancreatic insulin production due to an **autoimmune destruction of β-islet cells**
    - Strong association with human leukocyte antigen (HLA) DR3, DR4, and DQ genotypes
    - Most frequently diagnosed before puberty
  - **History:** polyuria, polydipsia, polyphagia, weight loss, rapid onset of symptoms
  - **Physical examination:** signs of mild dehydration
  - **Tests:**
    - **Increased serum glucose**; decreased insulin (Table 5-1)
    - HbA1c is increased and is a more accurate assessment of glucose levels over the most recent 3 months than individual random serum glucose levels
    - UA will demonstrate glycosuria and possible urinary ketones

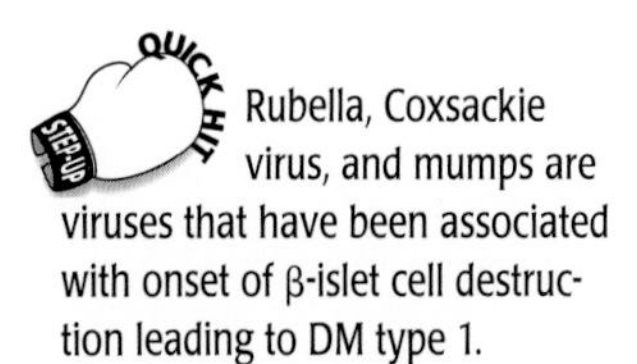

Rubella, Coxsackie virus, and mumps are viruses that have been associated with onset of β-islet cell destruction leading to DM type 1.

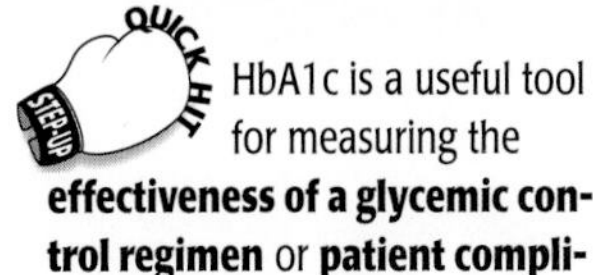

HbA1c is a useful tool for measuring the **effectiveness of a glycemic control regimen** or **patient compliance** because it indicates the trends of serum glucose levels over an extended period of time.

TABLE 5-1 Plasma Glucose Diagnostic Criteria for Diabetes Mellitus[1]

Plasma Glucose Test	Level (mg/dL)	And...
Random plasma glucose	>200	With symptoms of DM
Fasting plasma glucose	>126	On two separate occasions
Plasma glucose	>200	Two hours after 75 g oral glucose load[2]

DM, diabetes mellitus.

[1]Diagnosis is based on the occurrence of at least one of the following findings.

[2]This is a positive oral glucose tolerance test.

- Treatment:
  - An insulin regimen of scheduled injections or a continuous infusion pump is the keystone to glycemic control (Figure 5-5, Table 5-2)
  - A healthy diet is important to controlling glucose levels, and referral to a nutritionist may be appropriate

FIGURE 5-5 **Examples of insulin regimens in diabetes mellitus. (A) Injection of regular and NPH (neutral protamine Hagedorn) insulin (in 2:1 ratio) together at breakfast followed by a second regular insulin dose at dinner and a second NPH dose at bedtime. In some cases the second dose of NPH may be given concomitantly with the second regular insulin dose at dinner. (B) Adjustment in regimen (A) to achieve tighter, shorter time control by adding an additional dose of regular insulin at lunch and only administering NPH at bedtime. In patients with overnight hypoglycemia, insulin detemir may be substituted for NPH. (C) Tight control regimen using very-rapid-acting insulin at meals and a bedtime dose of insulin glargine.**

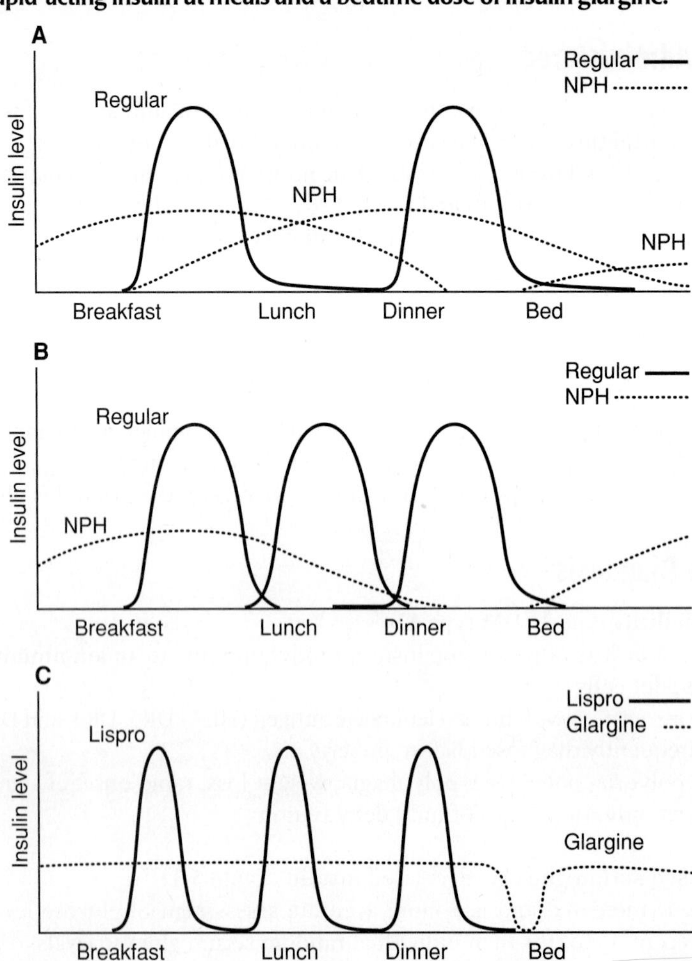

(Modified from Feibusch KC, Breaden RS, Bader CD, Gomperts SN. *Prescription for the boards: USMLE step 2.* 3rd ed. Philadelphia: Lippincott Williams & Wilkins, 2002. Used with permission of Lippincott Williams & Wilkins.)

TABLE 5-2 Formulations of Injected Insulin

Type of Insulin	Time of Onset of Action	Peak Effect	Duration of Action
Very-rapid-acting[1] (e.g., lispro, aspart, glulisine)	10 min	1 hr	2–4 hr
Regular	30 min	2–4 hr	5–8 hr
NPH	2 hr	6–10 hr	18–24 hr
Insulin glargine	2 hr	No peak	24+ hr
Insulin detemir	2 hr	No peak	~24 hr

[1]Appropriate for use in continuous infusion pump.

  - Self-monitoring of serum glucose levels is important to guide insulin dosing
  - Inclusion of a multidisciplinary team (e.g., diabetes specialists, ophthalmologists) is helpful to maintain adequate glycemic control and to avoid the onset of complications
- **Outcomes:**
  - **Diabetic ketoacidosis** may result from acute glycemic instability and poor control
  - Complications from chronic poor glycemic control include retinopathy, nephropathy, neuropathy, impaired wound healing, vascular insufficiency, and atherosclerosis
  - Although the life expectancy for type 1 diabetics is somewhat less than for unaffected individuals, patients should be able to avoid significant complications with tight glycemic control
- **Clues to the diagnosis:**
  - History: polyuria, polydipsia, polyphagia
  - Physical: mild dehydration
  - Tests: increased serum glucose, increased HbA1c, glycosuria and urinary ketones

- **Diabetes mellitus type 2 (DM type 2)**
  - Development of **tissue resistance to insulin** leading to hyperglycemia and an eventual decrease in the β-islet cells' ability to produce insulin
    - Although chronic hyperglycemia has similar deleterious effects for both type 1 and type 2 DM, their pathologies and presentations are different (Table 5-3)
    - Type II DM constitutes almost all cases of DM **diagnosed in adults** (especially in those >40 years old), but may be detected during childhood at similar ages to DM type 1

TABLE 5-3 Comparisons of Diabetes Mellitus Types 1 and 2

	DM Type 1	DM Type 2
Cause	Likely autoimmune destruction of β-islet cells	Development of insulin resistance in tissues
Inheritance/genetics	HLA-linked	Strong family history
Age of onset	Usually <13 years old	Frequently >40 years old
Onset of symptoms	Rapid	Gradual
Pancreatic effects	β-islet cell depletion	Gradual decrease in β-islet cells
Serum insulin	Low	Increased or normal; low in later disease
Body type	Thin	Obese
Acute complications	DKA	HHNC
Treatment	Insulin	Oral hypoglycemic agents, possibly insulin

DKA, diabetic ketoacidosis; DM, diabetes mellitus; HHNC, hyperosmolar hyperglycemic nonketotic coma; HLA, human leukocyte antigen.

TABLE 5-4 Oral Hypoglycemic Drugs Used in Treatment of Diabetes Mellitus Type 2

Drug	Mechanism	Role	Adverse Effects
Biguanides (e.g., metformin)	**Decreases hepatic gluconeogenesis, increases insulin activity**, reduces hyperlipidemia	Frequently first-line drug	GI disturbance, rare lactic acidosis, possible decreased vitamin B_{12} absorption; contraindicated in patients with hepatic and renal insufficiency
Sulfonylureas (e.g., tolbutamide, glyburide, glipizide)	**Stimulates insulin release** from β-islet cells, reduces serum glucagon, increases binding of insulin to tissue receptors	Frequently used after metformin or as first-line drug	**Hypoglycemia**; contraindicated in patients with hepatic or renal insufficiency (greater risk of hypoglycemia)
Thiazolidinediones ("glitazones")	Decreases hepatic gluconeogenesis, increases tissue uptake of glucose	Adjunct to other drugs	Weight gain, increase serum LDL, rare liver toxicity in some drugs
α-Glucosidase inhibitors (e.g., acarbose)	**Decreases GI absorption** of starch and disaccharides	Monotherapy in patients with good dietary control of DM; adjunct to other drugs; may be used in patients with DM type 1	Diarrhea, flatulence, GI disturbance
Meglitinides (e.g., repaglinide, nateglinide)	**Stimulates insulin release** from β-islet cells	Used as secondary drug with metformin or rarely as initial drug	**Hypoglycemia**; significantly more expensive than sulfonylureas with no therapeutic advantage

DM, diabetes mellitus; GI, gastrointestinal; LDL, low-density lipoprotein.

- **Risk factors:** family history, obesity, lack of exercise
- **History:** generally asymptomatic in the early stages and associated with a gradual onset of symptoms including polyuria, polydipsia, polyphagia, and symptoms associated with complications
- **Physical examination:** frequent obesity, signs associated with complications
- **Tests:**
  - **Increased serum glucose** and **HbA1c** (Table 5-1)
  - Serum insulin levels are not a reliable indicator of the condition
  - UA will show glycosuria and urinary ketones
- **Treatment:**
  - Initial therapy focuses on nutrition (e.g., reduced calorie intake, carbohydrate control, and consistency), exercise, and weight loss
  - Metformin is typically the first oral agent prescribed in patients who are unable to control their glycemic level with lifestyle modification alone (Table 5-4)
  - A sulfonylurea or thiazolidinedione is added to the regimen if the HbA1c is >7% after 3 months of therapy
  - An insulin regimen is initiated if the HbA1c is consistently >8.5% or if the patient demonstrates consistent low insulin levels
  - Self-monitoring of blood glucose levels is important to guide therapy
- **Outcomes:**
  - **Hyperosmolar hyperglycemic nonketotic coma (HHNC)** may result from acute glycemic instability and poor control
  - Complications include retinopathy, nephropathy, neuropathy, impaired wound healing, vascular insufficiency, and atherosclerosis (Figure 5-6, Table 5-5)
  - Prognosis is directly linked to the ability to control glucose levels and avoid the development of complications
- **Why eliminated from differential:** the patient's age, body habitus, and rapid onset of symptoms make type 1 DM the most likely form of the disease

QUICK HIT: **Background retinopathy** involves **no neovascularization** and constitutes the majority of cases; **proliferative diabetic retinopathy** consists of **neovascularization** and carries a much higher risk of **retinal hemorrhage**.

QUICK HIT: Diabetic patients are at an increased risk of **silent myocardial infarction (MI)** because of impaired pain sensation.

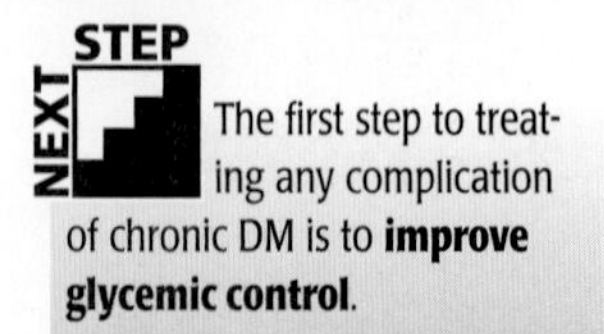

NEXT STEP: The first step to treating any complication of chronic DM is to **improve glycemic control**.

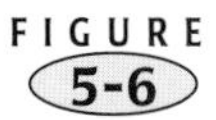

FIGURE 5-6 **Anteroposterior x-ray of the right shoulder in a patient with Charcot arthropathy. There is complete destruction of the right proximal humerus following a prior fracture. Due to peripheral neuropathy, these patients may be unaware of the severe destructive process in their joints.**

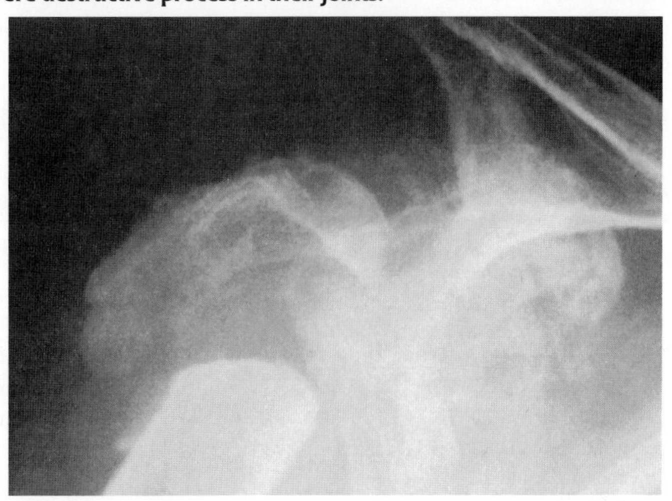

(Taken from Bucholz RW, Heckman JD. *Rockwood and Green's fractures in adults.* 5th ed. Philadelphia: Lippincott, Williams & Wilkins, 2001. Fig. 25-33. Used with permission of Lippincott Williams & Wilkins.)

- **Diabetes insipidus**
  - More thorough discussion in Chapter 4
  - **Why eliminated from differential:** hypernatremia would be expected for this diagnosis instead of the hyponatremia seen in this case
- **Hyperthyroidism**
  - More thorough discussion in later case
  - **Why eliminated from differential:** the normal thyroid panel rules out this diagnosis
- **Psychogenic polydipsia**
  - More thorough discussion in Chapter 4
  - **Why eliminated from differential:** low serum osmolality would be expected for this diagnosis and not the elevated serum osmolality seen in this case
- **Acute renal failure**
  - More thorough discussion in Chapter 4
  - **Why eliminated from differential:** the normal BUN and creatinine seen in this case rule out this diagnosis

CASE 5-2 "My ankle looks funny"

A 58-year-old woman presents to her primary care provider (PCP) because she feels that her ankle has a strange appearance. She says that she broke her right ankle in a car collision 1 year ago and required open reduction and internal fixation to repair the fractures. She followed up two times with the orthopedic surgeon after her surgery but neglected to follow-up after she felt comfortable walking again. She continues to walk on her right leg without pain but feels that her ankle is unstable. In addition, she feels that her ankle looks swollen and misshapen. She denies having seen this appearance several months prior to the current presentation. She denies any additional episodes of trauma. She feels that her extremities are strong and denies paresthesias. She denies fevers, wounds over her ankle, or drainage from the ankle. She says that she does not have this problem in any of her other joints. She recalls being told by the orthopedic surgeon to follow-up with a PCP because of elevated blood sugar, but she never followed his recommendation. She has not seen an internist for several years because her last PCP told her to stop eating sweets and fried food and to start

TABLE 5-5 Complications of Chronic Diabetes Mellitus

Condition	Pathology	Diagnosis	Treatment	Prognosis
Retinopathy	Vascular occlusion of retinal vessels with possible neovascularization, leading to microaneurysms, hemorrhage, infarcts, and macular edema	Progressive vision loss, premature cataracts, retinal changes (e.g., arteriovenous nicking, hemorrhages, edema, infarcts)	Anti-HTN therapy, routine ophthalmologic follow-up, laser photocoagulation of neovascularization, reduction of macular edema with intervitreal corticosteroid injections	Progressive vision loss without control of HTN and DM; other complications include retinal detachment, cataracts, and glaucoma
Nephropathy	Progressive intercapillary glomerulosclerosis, mesangial expansion, and basement membrane degeneration leading to **renal insufficiency** and eventual **nephrotic syndrome**	Chronic DM, HTN, **proteinuria**, hypoalbuminemia, **increased BUN and Cr**, basement membrane thickening and Kimmelstiel-Wilson nodules on electron microscopy of renal biopsies	ACE-I or ARBs are used to control HTN, low-protein diet, dialysis in late stages	End-stage renal disease occurs in 50% of patients with DM type 1 and in 10% of patients with DM type 2 within 10 years of the diagnosis of nephropathy
Neuropathy	Progressive neural damage and conduction abnormalities due to metabolic and vascular insufficiency leading to **sensory**, **autonomic**, and **motor** dysfunction	Sensory abnormalities include stocking-glove paresthesias, neural pain, and **decreased vibratory and pain sensation**; autonomic abnormalities include hypotension, impotence, incontinence, and delayed gastric emptying; motor abnormalities include weakness and a loss of coordination	Neural pain may be treated with tricyclic antidepressants, phenytoin, carbamazepine, gabapentin, or analgesics; patients should be instructed in **regular foot examinations** to detect skin breakdown	Chronic sensory impairment leads to **Charcot joints** and **foot ulcers** that may eventually require amputations
Atherosclerosis	Microvascular insufficiency leading to CAD, PVD, and impaired wound healing	Increased incidence of MI, extremity ischemia, and ulcer formation	Control of HTN and hyperlipidemia, daily ASA	Complications include MI, PVD necessitating amputations, and poor wound healing; cardiac issues are the greatest cause of death in diabetics

ACE-I, angiotensin converting enzyme inhibitor; ARB, angiotensin receptor blocker; ASA, aspirin; BUN, blood urea nitrogen; CAD, coronary artery disease; Cr, creatinine; DM, diabetes mellitus; HTN, hypertension; MI, myocardial infarction; PVD, peripheral vascular disease

eating healthier. She is only seeing a PCP today because her insurance policy requires a new referral for her to see an orthopedic surgeon. She is unsure of her past medical history and denies taking any medications currently. Her previous doctor wanted her to start "some drugs," but she forgets what he wanted to prescribe for her. She denies any substance use. On examination, she is an obese woman in no acute distress. Auscultation of her heart, lungs, and bowels is normal. She has no pain on palpation of her chest or abdomen. She has no lymphadenopathy. She is able to perform coordinated movements well. She has a slight limp due to some instability with weight on her right leg. She has minimally decreased motor strength in her lower extremities (5–/5) compared to her upper extremities. Testing of her sensation reveals significant sensory deficits in both lower extremities below the midcalf level in regards to two-point discrimination. She demonstrates some impaired lower extremity proprioception deficits with her eyes closed. Her right ankle appears to be mildly swollen and erythematous. Raising her right leg causes the erythema to resolve after a minute of elevation. The following vital signs are measured:

T: 98.5°F, HR: 79 bpm, BP: 145/90 mm Hg, RR: 16 breaths/min

Differential Diagnosis

- Diabetic neuropathy, Charcot-Marie-Tooth disease, rheumatoid arthritis, osteoarthritis, Lyme disease, osteomyelitis, septic arthritis

Laboratory Data and Other Study Results

- Right ankle x-ray: significant destruction of the ankle joint with near eradication of the distal tibia and fibula and proximal talus; no focal lesions outside of the remaining joint region
- CBC: WBC: 6.5, Hgb: 14.5, Plt: 431
- 10-electrolyte chemistry panel (Chem10): Na: 142 mEq/L, K: 4.4 mEq/L, Cl: 109 mEq/L, CO_2: 24 mEq/L, BUN: 19 mg/dL, Cr: 1.2 mg/dL, Glu: 223 mg/dL, magnesium (Mg): 2.3 mg/dL, calcium (Ca): 10.2 mg/dL, phosphorus (Phos): 4.2 mg/dL
- Erythrocyte sedimentation rate (ESR): 11 mm/hr
- C-reactive protein (CRP): 0.5 mg/dL
- Rheumatoid factor (RF): negative
- Lyme antibody enzyme-linked immunosorbent assay (ELISA): negative
- Electromyography (EMG): significantly decreased bilateral lower extremity sensory action potentials; low normal conduction velocities; mild decrease in motor action potentials

Diagnosis

- Diabetic neuropathy (DM type 2) with associated Charcot arthropathy

Treatment Administered

- The patient was started on metformin to control her hyperglycemia
- The patient was provided education on foot examinations, healthy life choices, and diabetic diets
- The patient was referred to a nutritionist to improve her eating habits and an orthopedic surgeon for immobilization of her ankle and possible fusion

Follow-up

- The patient was able to achieve control of her blood glucose levels with metformin
- She required close follow-up for the detection of additional diabetic complications
- A tibial-talar fusion was performed on her right ankle because of her severe degree of joint destruction

Steps to the Diagnosis

- **Diabetic neuropathy, DM type 2**
  - More thorough discussion in prior case
  - **Clues to the diagnosis:**
    - History: prior fracture, prior concerns regarding diet and blood sugar
    - Physical: swollen and erythematous joint, impaired sensation, impaired proprioception
    - Tests: increased glucose, x-ray appearance, EMG findings

- **Charcot-Marie-Tooth disease**
  - More thorough discussion in Chapter 7
  - **Why eliminated from differential:** the patient's hyperglycemia makes this diagnosis less likely, and the lack of conduction velocity delays on the EMG helps to rule this diagnosis out
- **Rheumatoid arthritis**
  - More thorough discussion in Chapter 9
  - **Why eliminated from differential:** this degree of joint destruction is not common in rheumatoid arthritis, and the negative rheumatoid factor helps to rule this diagnosis out
- **Osteoarthritis**
  - More thorough discussion in Chapter 9
  - **Why eliminated from differential:** this degree of joint destruction is rare for this diagnosis
- **Lyme disease**
  - More thorough discussion in Chapter 9
  - **Why eliminated from differential:** the negative antibody test for Lyme infection and the normal ESR and CRP rule this diagnosis out
- **Osteomyelitis/septic arthritis**
  - More thorough discussion in Chapter 9
  - **Why eliminated from differential:** the normal WBC count, ESR, and CRP rule out this diagnosis

CASE 5-3 "I found my roommate passed out"

A 19-year-old man is brought into the emergency department by his college roommate after the latter found him poorly responsive in their dorm room. He said that when he came home from dinner he found the patient lying on the floor passed out. When he tried to arouse him, the patient opened his eyes and tried to speak but otherwise was barely interactive. The roommate says that the patient had been "cramming" for upcoming final exams and had been getting very little sleep over the prior week. He notes that the patient said he had not been feeling well for a few days because of nausea and abdominal pain and had been going to the bathroom often. He has never seen his roommate in this condition prior to tonight. The roommate says that the patient is diabetic and uses insulin, but he does not know of any other medical history. He says that the patient drinks socially, but he does not think that the patient has been drinking while he has been studying. On examination, the patient is a thin male who is minimally responsive to questioning. His mucous membranes appear very dry, and he has decreased skin turgor. His breath smells very fruity. Auscultation of his heart and lungs detects slow deep breathing in all lung fields and tachycardia. His abdomen has no detectable masses and has normal bowel sounds. He withdraws to painful stimuli but does not follow commands. The following vital signs are measured:

T: 98.4°F, HR: 110 bpm, BP: 100/65 mm Hg, RR: 10 breaths/min

Differential Diagnosis

- Diabetic ketoacidosis, hyperosmolar hyperglycemic nonketotic coma, intoxication, hypoglycemia, MI

Laboratory Data and Other Study Results

- CBC: WBC: 13.7, Hgb: 16.5, Plt: 340
- Chem10: Na: 131 mEq/L, K: 4.4 mEq/L, Cl: 93 mEq/L, CO_2: 17 mEq/L, BUN: 45 mg/dL, Cr: 0.9 mg/dL, Glu: 589 mg/dL, Mg: 1.8 mg/dL, Ca: 9.7 mg/dL, Phos: 2.1 mg/dL
- Arterial blood gas (ABG; room air): pH: 7.18, partial pressure of oxygen (pO_2): 96 mm Hg, partial pressure of carbon dioxide (pCO_2): 20 mm Hg, bicarbonate (Bicarb): 18 mEq/L, oxygen saturation (O_2 sat): 99%

- Serum osmolality: 317 mOsm/kg
- UA: dark yellow colored, pH: 5.2, specific gravity: 1.411, 4+ glucose, 4+ ketones, no nitrites/leukocyte esterase/hematuria/proteinuria
- Urine toxicology screen: negative for alcohol or any illicit substances
- Blood cultures: Gram stain and culture pending
- Urine culture: Gram stain and cultures pending
- Electrocardiogram (ECG): sinus tachycardia; no abnormal wave morphology

Diagnosis

- Diabetic ketoacidosis

Treatment Administered

- The patient was promptly given intravenous (IV) hydration and placed on an IV insulin infusion
- The patient was admitted to the intensive care unit (ICU) for close observation, correction of his calculated fluid deficit, and the titration of his serum glucose levels with IV insulin
- He was started on empiric vancomycin and gentamicin while cultures remained pending

Follow-up

- The patient's mental status progressively improved with the normalization of his serum glucose level and the correction of his fluid deficit
- All culture results were negative, and all antibiotics were stopped
- The patient's insulin schedule was adjusted to maintain control of his glucose levels
- Prior to discharge, the patient was educated regarding risk factors and precautions for diabetic ketoacidosis (DKA) and how to avoid future episodes

Steps to the Diagnosis

- **Diabetic ketoacidosis**
  - A complication of DM due to **extremely low insulin** levels and an excess of glucagon
    - Significant degradation of glycogen into glucose and triglycerides into fatty acids occurs
    - Significant hyperglycemia occurs, and metabolism of the fatty acids produces **ketones and ketoacids**
    - Most commonly occurs in patients with DM type 2 who are noncompliant with their insulin regimens or who have infections, significant stress, recent MI, or significant alcohol use
  - **History**: weakness, polyuria, polydipsia, abdominal pain, vomiting
  - **Physical examination: signs of dehydration** (e.g., dry mucous membranes, decreased skin turgor), **fruity breath odor**, tachypnea or Kussmaul respirations (i.e., slow and deep breathing), mental status changes
  - **Tests:**
    - **Serum glucose 300 to 800 mg/dL**; increased serum ketones
    - Decreased sodium and phosphate; normal or increased potassium and BUN
    - Increased serum osmolality
    - High anion gap metabolic acidosis
    - UA will show **glycosuria and urine ketones**
  - **Treatment:**
    - IV rehydration with replacement of the fluid deficit over 24 to 48 hours
    - IV insulin titrated to achieve a consistent normal serum glucose
    - Any underlying pathology should be treated
    - The patient's insulin regimen should be adjusted to avoid relapses

MNEMONIC

Inciting factors for DKA and HHNC may be remembered by the mnemonic **PHAT MINDS**: **P**ancreatitis, **H**ot weather, **A**lcohol, **T**rauma, **MI**, **I**nsufficient water intake, **N**oncompliance with therapy, **D**rugs, **S**troke.

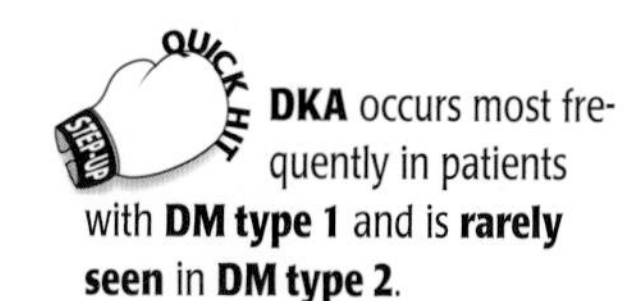

DKA occurs most frequently in patients with **DM type 1** and is **rarely seen** in **DM type 2**.

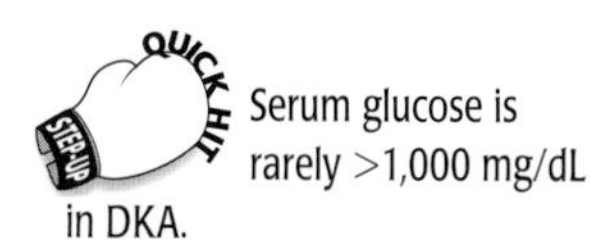

Serum glucose is rarely >1,000 mg/dL in DKA.

- **Outcomes:** prognosis is generally excellent with prompt treatment, but comatose patients carry a poor prognosis
- **Clues to the diagnosis:**
  - History: history of DM and insulin use, stressful environment, abdominal pain
  - Physical: dehydration, fruity breath, Kussmaul respirations
  - Tests: increased glucose, glycosuria and urine ketones, metabolic acidosis

- **Hyperosmolar hyperglycemic nonketotic coma**
  - Significant dehydration in diabetic patients due to hyperglycemia and significant osmotic diuresis
    - Occurs in patients with **DM type 2** who are able to maintain a **sufficient insulin production to prevent DKA**
    - Often associated with lengthy infections, stress, or other illnesses
  - **History:** polyuria, polydipsia
  - **Physical examination:** signs of dehydration, mental status changes, tachypnea
  - **Tests:**
    - Serum glucose is frequently **>800 mg/dL**
    - Decrease sodium and potassium; increased BUN
    - **No metabolic acidosis**
    - UA shows glycosuria and possible urine ketones
  - **Treatment:**
    - IV hydration with gradual correction of the fluid deficit
    - IV insulin is used to control the serum glucose level
    - Patient education is needed to prevent recurrences
  - **Outcomes:** complications include multisystem organ dysfunction and MI; mortality is up to 20%
  - **Why eliminated from differential:** the patient's serum glucose level is lower than that expected for HHNC, the patient has significant urine ketones and a metabolic acidosis, and the patient's history is suggestive of an existing diagnosis of DM type 1
- **Hypoglycemia**
  - Abnormally low serum glucose that diffusely impairs normal tissue function
    - May occur due to several processes related to insulin excess or an insufficient glucose supply (Table 5-6)
  - **History:** weakness, diaphoresis, dizziness, palpitations, headache
  - **Physical examination:** mental status changes, impaired consciousness
  - **Tests:**
    - Decreased serum glucose with or without increased insulin
    - Computed tomography (CT) or magnetic resonance imaging (MRI) may be useful for detecting tumors
    - Low cortisol and either increased or decreased ACTH is indicative of a pituitary or adrenal cause
  - **Treatment:**
    - Prompt administration of glucose
    - Guidance for proper eating habits and titration of insulin use can help avoid recurrences in some patients
    - Patients with insulin-secreting tumors will frequently require surgical resection
    - Patients with pituitary or adrenal pathology will require cortisol replacement
  - **Outcomes:** easily treatable conditions have an excellent prognosis, but the prognosis for untreatable diseases is poor; untreated hypoglycemia leads to tissue death and mortality
  - **Why eliminated from differential:** although hypoglycemia is a complication of insulin use, this diagnosis is ruled out by the patient's elevated glucose level
- **Intoxication**
  - More thorough discussion in Chapter 13
  - **Why eliminated from differential:** the negative toxicology screen rules out this diagnosis
- **Myocardial infarction**
  - More thorough discussion in Chapter 1
  - **Why eliminated from differential:** the relatively normal ECG in a young patient rules out this diagnosis

TABLE 5-6 Causes of Hypoglycemia

Cause	Pathology	Diagnosis	Treatment
Reactive	Decrease in serum glucose **after eating** (e.g., post-surgical, idiopathic)	Hypoglycemia and symptoms improve with carbohydrate meal	**Frequent small meals**
Iatrogenic (e.g., excess insulin)	**Excess insulin** administration or an adverse effect of **sulfonylurea** or meglitinide use	**Increased insulin in the presence of hypoglycemia,** adjustment of drug regimen improves symptoms	Adjust insulin regimen, consider a different oral hypoglycemic drug
Insulinoma[1]	**β-islet cell tumor** producing excess insulin	Increased insulin in presence of hypoglycemia, may be detected on CT or MRI	Surgical resection if able to locate
Fasting	**Underproduction of glucose** due to hormone deficiencies, malnutrition, or liver disease	Lab abnormalities and history associated with particular etiology	Proper nutrition, enzyme replacement
Alcohol-induced	Glycogen depletion and **gluconeogenesis inhibition** by high concentrations of alcohol	History of alcohol use, serum ethanol >45 mg/dL	Proper nutrition, stopping high quantity alcohol use
Pituitary/adrenal insufficiency	Decreased cortisol production leads to insufficient hepatic gluconeogenesis in response to hypoglycemia	Low serum cortisol; site of defect determined by ACTH activity tests; possible other comorbid endocrine abnormalities	Cortisol replacement

ACTH, adrenocorticotropic hormone ; CT, computed tomography; MRI, magnetic resonance imaging.

[1]A similar presentation would be expected for tumors with paraneoplastic production of insulin or insulinlike substance.

CASE 5-4 "I can't stand the heat"

A 38-year-old woman presents to her PCP because of restlessness and heat intolerance that has developed over the past 3 months. She says that she does not remember a specific start to these symptoms and that they have developed insidiously. The symptoms are present most of the day. She says that whenever she is in a warm room she becomes very uncomfortable and feels the need to cool down as quickly as possible. She describes herself as being frequently on edge but tired at the same time. She works as an insurance adjuster and feels that her performance at work has deteriorated recently because she has a difficult time sitting still and focusing on her work. She finds that she has been irritable toward her coworkers when she has unproductive days. She has had difficulty sleeping at night recently. She notices that she is also losing weight despite eating large meals but attributes this to the fact that she tends to move her bowels soon after eating. She denies any headaches, paresthesias, or any episodes of anxiety or depression previous to 3 months ago. She denies any past medical history and currently takes a daily vitamin and oral contraceptive pill. She drinks socially and denies illicit substance use. On examination, she is a thin woman who appears agitated. Her eyes appear to protrude slightly from her orbits, and her eyelids are retracted. Her skin is warm and slightly sweaty. She has no palpable lymphadenopathy, but a nontender mass is palpable on the front of her throat. Auscultation of her heart and lungs detects tachycardia and mild tachypnea but no abnormal sounds. Her abdomen is nontender with no palpable masses, and she has normal bowel sounds. The anterior surfaces of her shins have very dry skin and are swollen. She has hyperactive reflexes but no weakness or paresthesias. The following vital signs are measured:

T: 99.3°F, HR: 105 bpm, BP: 130/86 mm Hg, RR: 22 breaths/min

Differential Diagnosis

- Graves disease, toxic multinodular goiter, subacute thyroiditis, silent thyroiditis, Hashimoto thyroiditis, thyroid cancer, pheochromocytoma, anxiety disorder, cocaine intoxication, heat exhaustion

Laboratory Data and Other Study Results

- CBC: WBC: 7.9, Hgb: 15.4, Plt: 298
- Chem10: Na: 141 mEq/L, K: 4.1 mEq/L, Cl: 103 mEq/L, CO_2: 27 mEq/L, BUN: 12 mg/dL, Cr: 0.6 mg/dL, Glu: 89 mg/dL, Mg: 1.9 mg/dL, Ca: 10.1 mg/dL, Phos: 4.6 mg/dL
- Thyroid panel: TSH: 0.2 μU/mL, T_4: 15.7 μg/dL, free T_4 index: 18.3, T_3: 4.0 ng/mL, T_3 reuptake: 2.35
- Thyroid scan: diffusely increased uptake in the region of the thyroid gland
- UA: straw colored, pH: 6.2, specific gravity: 1.010, no glucose/ketones/nitrites/leukocyte esterase/hematuria/proteinuria
- Urine toxicology screen: negative for alcohol or any illicit substances

Based on these results, the following test is ordered:

- Thyroid-stimulating immunoglobulins (TSIs): positive

Diagnosis

- Graves disease

Treatment Administered

- The patient was started on propylthiouracil (PTU) until iodine therapy could be performed
- Prednisone and artificial tears were prescribed for the ophthalmologic abnormalities
- Radioactive iodine therapy was administered to the patient on an outpatient basis
- PTU was discontinued following the completion of iodine therapy

Follow-up

- The patient had resolution of her symptoms over the following 3 months
- The ophthalmologic symptoms resolved, and prednisone was discontinued
- The patient developed hypothyroidism and required thyroid hormone replacement therapy

Steps to the Diagnosis

- **Graves disease**
  - Autoimmune condition in which TSIs bind to TSH receptors in the thyroid and stimulate excessive thyroid hormone production
  - **History: heat intolerance, anxiety**, restlessness, irritability, diaphoresis, palpitations, increased bowel activity, weight loss, fatigue, vision abnormalities, dyspnea
  - **Physical examination: exophthalmos**, lid lag, **pretibial myxedema**, tachycardia, tremor, warm skim, hyperreflexia, **painless goiter**, thyroid bruit, proximal muscle weakness (Color Figure 5-1)
  - **Tests:**
    - **Decreased TSH; increased T_4, free T_4, T_3, and T_3 resin uptake**
    - **Diffusely increased uptake** of tracer on thyroid nuclear imaging (i.e., thyroid scan)
    - Presence of **TSIs** in serum
    - Biopsy of thyroid tissue demonstrates lymphocytic infiltrates and hypertrophy of the follicles with minimal colloid material

MNEMONIC

Causes of hyperthyroidism and how they are differentiated with a thyroid scan may be remembered by the mnemonic "**L**ots (of) **T**hyroid **N**ever **F**ails **I**n **G**iving **A**nxiety": **L**ow thyroid scan uptake–**T**hyroiditis; **N**ormal thyroid scan uptake–**F**actitious hyperthyroidism; **I**ncreased thyroid scan uptake–**G**raves disease, **A**denomas.

- **Treatment:**
  - Thionamides (e.g., PTU, methimazole) may be used to control the concentration of thyroid hormones, but they are usually a bridge to more definitive therapy
  - β-blockers may be used to control the cardiac effects of excess thyroid hormones until definitive therapy can be administered
  - **Radioactive iodine therapy** is used to gradually ablate the gland and is frequently the primary definitive therapy
  - **Thyroidectomy** is performed in patients who do not respond to other therapies
  - Corticosteroids and eye lubricants are prescribed to avoid visual complications until the resolution of eye symptoms
- **Outcomes:**
  - Most patients respond well to therapy with a resolution of their hyperthyroidism
  - Patients will typically require thyroid hormone replacement therapy following thyroid ablation or resection
  - **Thyroid storm**
    - Acute severe hyperthyroidism resulting from a significant release of thyroid hormones
    - May be caused by stressful events (e.g., illness, pregnancy) or may be a rare reaction to changes in therapy
    - Symptoms, signs, and lab findings are similar to typical hyperthyroidism but are more severe
    - Treated with an aggressive combination of β-blockers, corticosteroids, thionamides, IV iodide, and appropriate definitive therapy
    - Mortality is up to 50%
- **Clues to the diagnosis:**
  - History: anxiety, restlessness, heat intolerance, insomnia, irritability, weight loss
  - Physical: exophthalmos, lid retraction, diaphoresis, warm skin, tachycardia, painless goiter, tachypnea, pretibial myxedema, hyperreflexia
  - Tests: increased thyroid hormones, decreased TSH, presence of TSIs, thyroid scan appearance

- **Toxic multinodular goiter/toxic adenoma (a.k.a. Plummer disease)**
  - Presence of one or more thyroid nodules that are responsible for the production of excess thyroid hormones
  - **History:** symptoms similar to those for Graves disease
  - **Physical examination:** one or more **palpable thyroid nodules**, tachycardia, tremor, warm skim, hyperreflexia, **painless goiter**, thyroid bruit, proximal muscle weakness
  - **Tests:**
    - Thyroid panel will be similar to that for Graves disease
    - **Increased uptake** of tracer on a thyroid scan at the site of the nodules
    - Ultrasound (US) may be useful to localize nodules
  - **Treatment:**
    - **Radioactive iodine** is considered the primary therapy
    - Thionamides and β-blockers may be used as temporary therapy until definitive treatment is performed
    - Surgical resection is performed for patients with large nodules causing compression of nearby structures
  - **Outcomes:** prognosis is good with definitive treatment; hypothyroidism occurs at a lower rate than for Graves disease following radioactive iodine therapy
  - **Why eliminated from differential:** the appearance of the thyroid scan in this case (diffuse uptake) is more consistent with Graves disease than this diagnosis
- **Subacute thyroiditis (a.k.a. de Quervain thyroiditis)**
  - Self-limited hyperthyroidism due to a **viral** cause
    - Diffuse enlargement of the thyroid gland occurs in response to the precipitating infection
  - **History:** neck pain, similar symptoms as toxic multinodular goiter but typically **milder** in nature
  - **Physical examination: painful goiter**, fever, tachycardia, tremor, warm skin, hyperreflexia, thyroid bruit, proximal muscle weakness

- Tests:
  - **Increased T_4, free T_4, T_3, T_3 resin uptake**; TSH is typically extremely low
  - Thyroid scan will show **decreased uptake** of tracer
  - ESR and CRP are frequently increased
  - Biopsies will show a significant infiltration of lymphocytes
- **Treatment:**
  - The condition is **self-limited**
  - **Supportive care** with hydration, nonsteroidal anti-inflamatory drugs (NSAIDs), and β-blockers are used to treat the symptoms
  - Thyroid hormone replacement may be required if hypothyroidism occurs during recovery
- **Outcomes:** almost all patients recover fully and have an excellent prognosis; <5% of patients will continue to have some degree of thyroid dysfunction following recovery
- **Why eliminated from differential:** the thyroid scan appearance and painless goiter seen in this case rule out this diagnosis

- **Silent thyroiditis**
  - Temporary hyperthyroidism that has an autoimmune etiology
    - Incitation of the condition may be related to pregnancy or certain medications (e.g., amiodarone, lithium)
  - **History:** similar symptoms to toxic multinodular goiter but milder in nature
  - **Physical examination:** painless goiter, tachycardia, tremor, warm skin, hyperreflexia, thyroid bruit, proximal muscle weakness
  - **Tests:**
    - **Decreased TSH; increased T_4, free T_4, T_3, T_3 resin uptake**
    - Thyroid scan shows **low uptake**
    - Biopsies will show an infiltration of lymphocytes
  - **Treatment:** self-limited; NSAIDs and β-blockers are used to treat symptoms
  - **Outcomes:** pregnancy-related cases tend to have relapses following future pregnancies and carry a higher risk of long-term thyroid dysfunction; otherwise, cases typically have an excellent prognosis
  - **Why eliminated from differential:** the thyroid scan appearance (increased uptake) rules out this diagnosis
- **Hashimoto thyroiditis**
  - More thorough discussion in later case
  - **Why eliminated from differential:** the decreased TSH, increased thyroid hormones, and increased uptake on the thyroid scan rule out this diagnosis
- **Thyroid cancer**
  - Malignant nodules of the thyroid that may arise from columnar epithelial, follicular, or parafollicular cells (Table 5-7)
    - The majority of thyroid nodules are not malignant in nature and become more common with increasing age
  - **Risk factors:** female gender, aged 20 to 60 years, history of neck irradiation, poor iodine uptake on a thyroid scan, solid nodules
  - **History:** asymptomatic or possible dysphagia and hoarseness
  - **Physical examination: solitary nontender** anterior neck mass, cervical lymphadenopathy
  - **Tests:**
    - Thyroid hormones may be increased or decreased and are not a reliable indicator of the diagnosis
    - Malignant nodules are more likely to show **decreased tracer uptake** (i.e., cold nodules) than increased tracer uptake (i.e., hot nodules) (Figure 5-7)
    - US may be used to localize nodules and guide biopsies
    - Biopsy via fine needle aspiration will demonstrate malignant transformation of cells
  - **Treatment:**
    - Benign nodules may be observed for any changes, and those associated with hyperthyroidism or hypothyroidism are treated accordingly

TABLE 5-7 Types of Thyroid Carcinoma

Type	Cells Affected	Frequency	Characteristics	Prognosis
Papillary	Columnar cells of gland	**Most common form** (80% cases); more common in **younger** patients	Begins as slow-growing nodule; eventually metastasizes to local cervical lymph nodes	**Good**; few recurrences
Follicular	Cuboid cells in follicles	10% of thyroid cancers; more common in **older** patients	May function like normal thyroid tissue; metastasizes to liver, lung, bone, and brain	Worse than papillary cancer; 50% 10-year survival
Medullary	Parafollicular C cells	4% of thyroid cancers	**Produces calcitonin;** may present with other endocrine tumors (e.g., MEN2a and MEN2b)	Worse in older patients; metastases common at diagnosis
Anaplastic	Poorly differentiated neoplasm	1% of thyroid cancers	**Very aggressive**; local extension causes hoarseness, dysphagia	Poor

MEN, multiple endocrine neoplasia.

- **Lobectomy** is performed for nonanaplastic tumors that are <1.0 cm; **total thyroidectomy** is performed for larger tumors
- Radioactive iodine therapy frequently accompanies surgical resection
- Radiation therapy is used for tumors with local extension
- Chemotherapy is used for metastatic tumors
- Thyroid hormone replacement may be required following resection
- **Outcomes:** prognosis depends on the type of tumor encountered but is best in papillary cancers
- **Why eliminated from differential:** the diffuse nature of the disease in the case (per examination and the thyroid scan) makes this diagnosis unlikely

QUICK HIT: A complication of thyroid surgery is hoarseness due to damage of the recurrent laryngeal nerve.

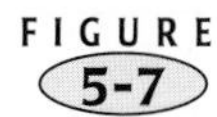

FIGURE 5-7 Thyroid scan in a patient with suspected thyroid carcinoma. Note that in the patient's right lobe (on the left side of the figure) there is a region of decreased uptake, suggesting a "cold nodule."

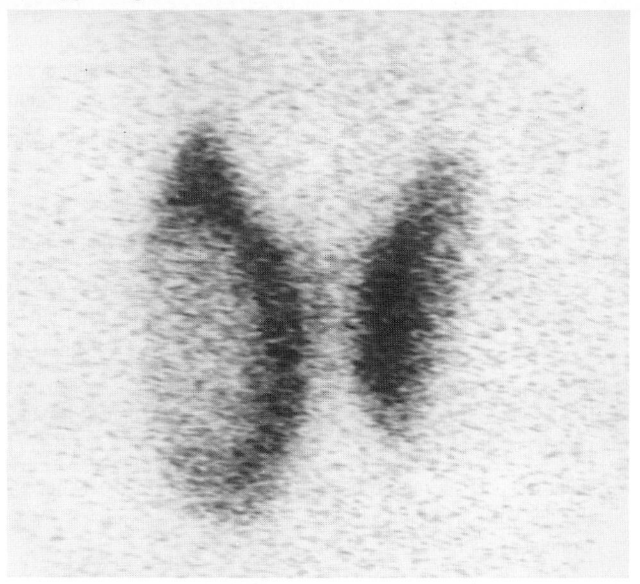

(Taken from Daffner RH. *Clinical radiology: the essentials*. 3rd ed. Philadelphia: Lippincott Williams & Wilkins, 2007. Fig. 1-28, p. 24. Used with permission of Lippincott Williams & Wilkins.)

- **Pheochromocytoma**
  - More thorough discussion in Chapter 1
  - **Why eliminated from differential:** the continuous nature of the patients symptoms and the multiple tests suggesting a thyroid pathology make this diagnosis very unlikely
- **Anxiety disorder**
  - More thorough discussion in Chapter 13
  - **Why eliminated from differential:** the multiple findings suggesting a thyroid pathology make this diagnosis unlikely; if the patient's symptoms of anxiety were to continue following treatment for Graves disease, a psychiatric work-up would be appropriate
- **Cocaine intoxication**
  - More thorough discussion in Chapter 13
  - **Why eliminated from differential:** the negative toxicology screen rules out this diagnosis
- **Heat exhaustion**
  - Acute dysfunction of the body's thermoregulatory system, leading to the onset of dehydration and electrolyte abnormalities (Table 5-8)
    - It occurs when the body's attempts to maintain a normal body temperature become **inadequate** to prevent hyperthermia (e.g, extremely hot environment, prolonged strenuous activity)
  - **History:** fatigue, weakness, headache, nausea, vomiting, irritability, **significant diaphoresis**
  - **Physical examination:** increased body temperature (**below 106°F**), tachycardia
  - **Tests:** typically noncontributory
  - **Treatment: rehydration**, removal from a hot environment, and rest are the primary therapies
  - **Outcomes:** the prognosis is excellent with the proper treatment; progression to heat stroke is associated with worse outcomes
  - **Why eliminated from differential:** although several of the symptoms for this diagnosis are present in this case, the chronology of the patient's complaints and the presence of findings suggestive of a thyroid pathology make this diagnosis unlikely

TABLE 5-8 Types of Heat Emergencies

	Heat Exhaustion	Heat Stroke	Malignant Hyperthermia
Cause	Thermoregulatory dysfunction	Thermoregulatory dysfunction	Genetic condition in which exposure to inhaled anesthetics causes uncontrolled muscle oxidative metabolism
Symptoms/signs	Fatigue, weakness, headache, nausea, vomiting, irritability, diaphoresis, tachycardia	Similar to heat exhaustion plus mental status changes, hallucinations, and late onset of anhydrosis	Muscular rigidity, tachycardia, cyanosis
Body temperature	Mildly elevated, <106°F	Frequently above 106°F	>104°F and may increase by 4°F per hour
Tests	Noncontributory	Increased LFTs, signs of DIC, increased creatine kinase, hematuria, proteinuria	A muscle biopsy will contract *in vitro* following exposure to caffeine or halothane in affected individuals
Treatment	Rehydration, rest, cooling	ABCs, aggressive cooling measures (e.g., evaporative cooling, ice baths, cooled fluids)	Aggressive cooling measures, dantrolene, immediate cessation of the offending agent
Complications	Progression to heat stroke	Cardiac ischemia, pulmonary edema, rhabdomyolysis, ARF, DIC, cerebral vascular accident	Similar to heat stroke

ABCs, airway, breathing, circulation; ARF, acute renal failure; DIC, disseminated intravascular coagulopathy; LFTs, liver function tests.

CASE 5-5 "What is this lump on my neck?"

A 38-year-old woman presents to an endocrinologist for the work-up of a painless anterior neck mass. She says that she first noticed the mass a few weeks ago and is unsure how long it has been present. She denies any neck pain, anxiety, restlessness, heat intolerance, palpitations, or weight loss. When asked about these symptoms, she says that she feels quite the opposite. She frequently feels tired, has little energy, cannot seem to lose any weight, generally feels down, and needs to wear several layers of clothing because she is always cold. She previously saw this endocrinologist because of a brief episode of hyperthyroidism that resolved by itself and was ruled to be a case of silent thyroiditis. She has a history of depression, constipation, and menstrual irregularity for which she takes fluoxetine, docusate sodium, and an oral contraceptive pill. She denies any substance use. On examination, she is an overweight woman who appears to be in no distress. She has generally dry skin and thinning of her cranial hair. There is mild swelling of her face. She has no lymphadenopathy. Fundoscopic examination is normal. She has a mass on her anterior neck in the region of the thyroid gland with several indistinct nodules. There is no audible bruit over this mass. Auscultation of her heart and lungs detects clear lung sounds and bradycardia. Her abdomen is nontender with no detectable masses. Her motor function is slightly weakened diffusely (4+/5), but her sensation is normal. Her reflexes are slow and difficult to elicit. The following vital signs are measured:

T: 98.3°F, HR: 54 bpm, BP: 118/87 mm Hg, RR: 13 breaths/min

Differential Diagnosis

- Hypothyroidism, toxic multinodular goiter, subacute thyroiditis, silent thyroiditis, Graves disease, hypopituitarism, acute renal failure, nephrotic syndrome, depression

Laboratory Data and Other Study Results

- CBC: WBC: 5.3, Hgb: 12.1, Plt: 328
- Chem7: Na: 133 mEq/L, K: 3.9 mEq/L, Cl: 102 mEq/L, CO_2: 28 mEq/L, BUN: 11 mg/dL, Cr: 0.6 mg/dL, Glu: 96 mg/dL
- Thyroid panel: TSH: 8.4 μU/mL, T_4: 2.1 μg/dL, free T_4 index: 1.9, T_3: 1.1 ng/mL, T_3 reuptake: 0.95
- Thyroid scan: heterogenous decreased uptake of tracer in the thyroid
- UA: straw colored, pH: 7.1, specific gravity: 1.010, no glucose/ketones/nitrites/leukocyte esterase/hematuria/proteinuria

Based on these results, the following tests are performed:

- US-guided thyroid biopsy: diffuse lymphocytic infiltration, follicular hyperplasia, parenchymal atrophy
- Antithyroglobulin antibodies: positive
- Antithyroid peroxidase antibodies: positive

Diagnosis

- Hashimoto thyroiditis with associated hypothyroidism

Treatment Administered

- The patient was started on levothyroxine for thyroid hormone replacement therapy

Follow-up

- The patient had improvement in her physical and mood symptoms following the start of treatment

- Subsequent measurements of the patient's thyroid panel demonstrated normalization of her thyroid hormones and TSH
- The patient was able to be weaned off of fluoxetine and docusate sodium following an improvement of her symptoms

Steps to the Diagnosis

QUICK HIT: **Hashimoto thyroiditis** is the most common cause of hypothyroidism in the United States, but **iodine deficiency** is the most common cause worldwide.

QUICK HIT: Symptoms of hyperthyroidism may be seen in early Hashimoto thyroiditis.

- **Hashimoto thyroiditis**
  - Chronic thyroiditis due to autoimmune destruction of the gland that results in hypothyroidism
    - Thyroid surgery, radioactive iodine ablation, pituitary dysfunction, and medications (e.g., lithium) are other potential causes of hypothyroidism
  - **History:** fatigue, weakness, **cold intolerance**, **weight gain**, constipation, menstrual irregularity, **depression**, hoarseness, memory loss, hair loss, somnolence
  - **Physical examination: bradycardia**, hyporeflexia, dry skin, facial and extremity edema, **painless goiter**, brittle nails
  - **Tests:**
    - **Increased TSH**; decreased T_4 and free T_4; T_3 and T_3 uptake tend to remain normal
    - Antithyroglobulin and antithyroid peroxidase antibodies are typically detected
    - Thyroid scan shows decreased tracer uptake
    - Thyroid biopsy will show lymphocytic infiltration, follicular hyperplasia, parenchymal atrophy, and damage to the basement membrane of the follicles
  - **Treatment:** lifelong thyroid hormone replacement is required
  - **Outcomes:** complications include osteoporosis, cardiomyopathy, and myxedema coma from significantly low thyroid hormone levels; the prognosis is excellent in patients who are correctly diagnosed and are placed on thyroid replacement therapy
  - **Clues to the diagnosis:**
    - History: fatigue, weakness, depression, cold intolerance, constipation, menstrual irregularity
    - Physical: painless goiter, dry skin, facial edema, bradycardia, hyporeflexia
    - Tests: increased TSH, decreased T_4 and free T_4, thyroid scan results, biopsy results, positive antibody screens
- **Graves disease, toxic multinodular goiter**
  - More thorough discussion in prior case
  - **Why eliminated from differential:** the thyroid panel results and thyroid scan appearance are opposite to what would be expected for these conditions, so they are ruled out
- **Subacute and silent thyroiditis**
  - More thorough discussion in prior case
  - **Why eliminated from differential:** these conditions do feature decreased uptake on thyroid scans, but since their thyroid panels would show hyperthyroidism and not hypothyroidism, they are ruled out
- **Hypopituitarism**
  - More thorough discussion in later case
  - **Why eliminated from differential:** hypothyroidism does occur in this condition, but the increased TSH level shows that the pituitary is functioning and rules out this diagnosis

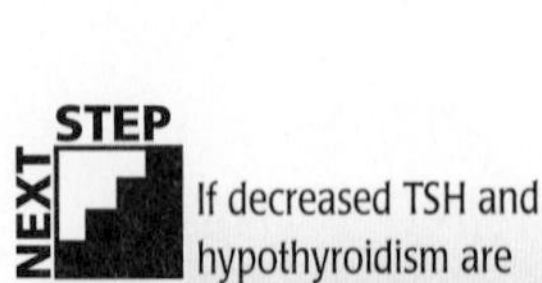

If decreased TSH and hypothyroidism are seen, suspect a pituitary or hypothalamic etiology.

- **Acute renal failure (ARF), nephrotic syndrome**
  - More thorough discussion in Chapter 4
  - **Why eliminated from differential:** the normal BUN, creatinine, and UA rule out these diagnoses
- **Depression**
  - More thorough discussion in Chapter 13
  - **Why eliminated from differential:** this condition may still exist in this patient, but given the evidence of hypothyroidism, a psychiatric evaluation should only be considered if the patient's mood symptoms do not improve after the start of thyroid replacement

The following additional Endocrinology cases may be found online:

CASE 5-6 "My lips and fingers keep tingling"

CASE 5-7 "My periods never came back"

CASE 5-8 "I'm starting to look like a hunchback"

CASE 5-9 "My diabetes is cured, but I feel awful"

CASE 5-10 "My baby isn't growing"

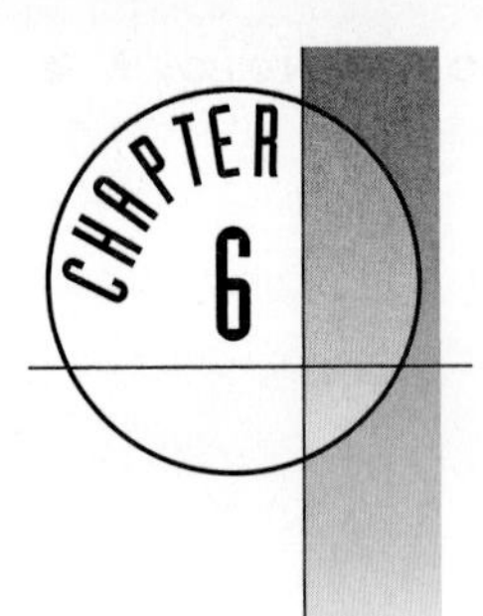

Hematology and Oncology

BASIC CLINICAL PRIMER

RED BLOOD CELL (RBC) PHYSIOLOGY

- RBCs function to transport oxygen (O_2) from alveoli to tissues and to transport carbon dioxide (CO_2) from tissues to the lungs using hemoglobin (Hgb) as the binding protein for both gases
- Binding of O_2 by Hgb A follows the **Hgb-O_2 dissociation curve** (Figure 6-1)
  - Changes in the inhaled air composition and pressure, Hgb subtype, body temperature, and activity level will cause the curve to shift
- Circulating RBCs, myeloid cells, and lymphoid cells originate from the same pluripotent stem cells in bone marrow (Figure 6-2)
  - As RBCs mature in bone marrow, they become **enucleated** and depend on glycolysis for survival

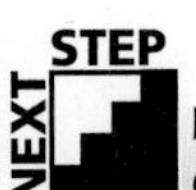

Monitor **heparin** anticoagulation with **PTT**.

CLOTTING FUNCTION

- **Platelets**
  - Circulate in plasma as the **primary** controllers of bleeding
  - Cause localized **vasoconstriction** and form a **platelet plug** at the site of vascular injury in response to adenosine diphosphate (ADP) that is secreted by the injured cells
  - Platelet response may be quantified by measuring the bleeding time (poorly reproducible)
- **Coagulation factors**
  - Responsible for the formation of **fibrin clot** at the site of vascular injury (Figure 6-3)
    - The **intrinsic** pathway is induced by exposure of vascular tissue to negatively charged foreign substances and is measured by the **partial thromboplastin time (PTT)**
    - The **extrinsic** pathway is induced by tissue factor exposed at the site of injury and is measured by **prothrombin time (PT)**

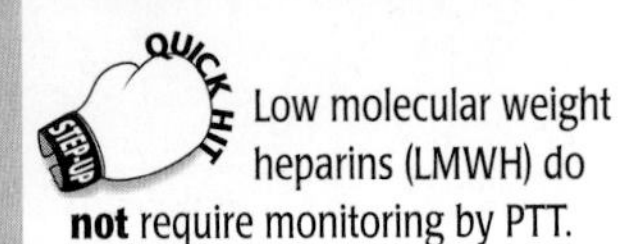

Low molecular weight heparins (LMWH) do **not** require monitoring by PTT.

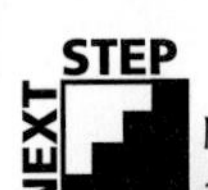

Monitor **warfarin** anticoagulation with a normalized PT (i.e., **international normalized ratio [INR]**) to track its relative effect on the extrinsic pathway.

ANTITHROMBOTIC MEDICATIONS

- Medications used to reduce the risk of pathologic clot formation (e.g., deep vein thrombosis [DVT], thromboembolic stroke, mural thrombus, pulmonary embolism [PE], postsurgical or traumatic thrombus)
- May affect platelet function and intrinsic or extrinsic pathway function (Table 6-1)

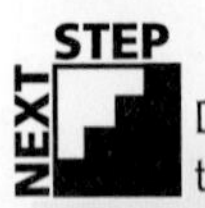

Do not start warfarin therapy for a thrombus until after starting LMWH or until the PTT is therapeutic on unfractionated heparin because warfarin inhibits proteins C and S to cause a short period of **hypercoagulability** immediately after therapy is initiated.

PRESURGICAL ASSESSMENT OF COAGULATION

- A history of **abnormal bleeding** or **easy bruising** should raise the concern for a coagulopathy

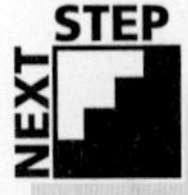

Treat a warfarin overdose with **vitamin K**.

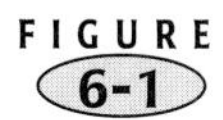

FIGURE 6-1 **The hemoglobin-oxygen dissociation curve. O_2, oxygen; pO_2, partial pressure of oxygen.**

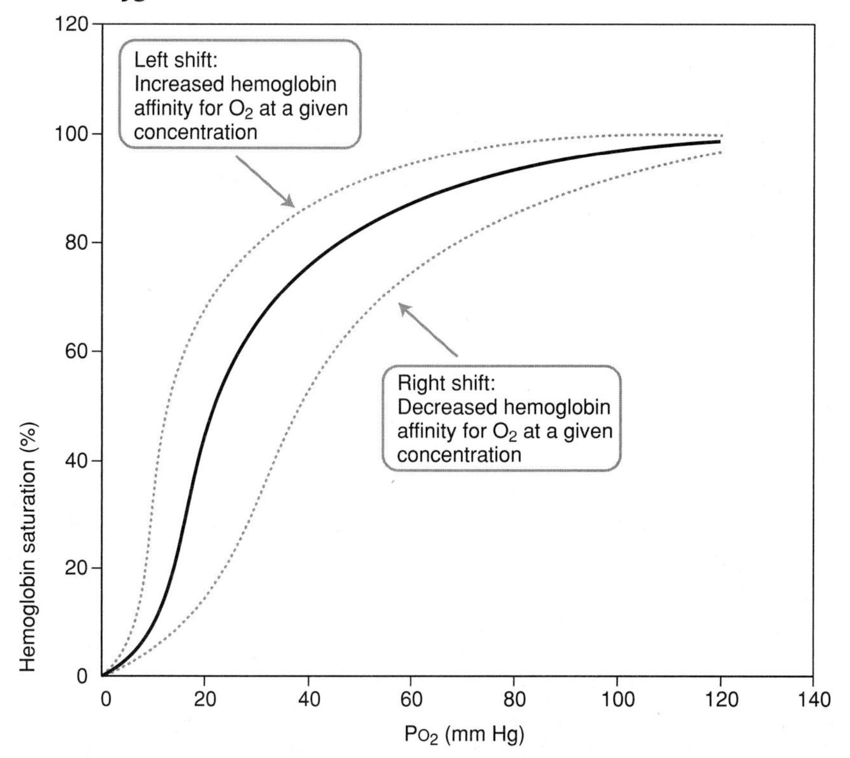

Left shift: metabolic alkalosis, decreased body temperature, increased Hgb F concentration
Right shift: metabolic acidosis, increased body temperature, high altitude, exercise

- Patients taking **warfarin** should stop this medication 3 to 4 days before surgery with a goal INR of <1.5
- **Fresh frozen plasma (FFP)** and **vitamin K** may be used for rapid warfarin reversal
- Patients with a recent thromboembolism should be anticoagulated with heparin or LMWH after stopping warfarin until the time of surgery and then restarted on warfarin postoperatively; heparin or LMWH should be restarted 12 hours postoperatively and continued until an INR >2.0 is achieved
- In general, warfarin, heparin, and LMWH are associated with a **lower risk** of postoperative **thromboembolism** than aspirin or antiplatelet medications but carry a **greater risk** of **postoperative bleeding complications**

QUICK HIT: LMWH should not be restarted for at least 2 hours after the removal of an epidural catheter to avoid formation of an epidural hematoma.

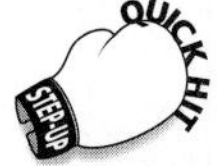

QUICK HIT: AB+ patients are **"universal recipients"**; they can **receive any** donor blood type because they have no antibodies to blood antigens in their plasma but can **only donate** to other **AB+** patients.

TRANSFUSIONS

- Use of an infusion of blood products to treat an insufficient supply of that component, improve oxygen-carrying capacity, or reverse coagulopathy (Table 6-2)
- **ABO blood groups**
  - Blood is defined by **A** and **B** antigens and their respective antibodies
  - Blood with **one** antigen only will have antibodies for the other antigen (i.e., A or B types)
  - Blood with **both** antigens will not have either form of antibody (i.e., AB type)
  - Blood with **neither** antigen will have antibodies to both antigens (i.e., O type)
- **Rh blood groups**
  - Blood with either carry the Rh antigen (i.e., Rh+) or will not (i.e., Rh−)
  - Rh− blood carries antibodies to the Rh antigen

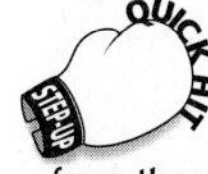

QUICK HIT: O− patients are **"universal donors."** RBCs from these patients will not induce antibody reactions in other patients, but they can **only receive** blood from other **O−** donors.

FIGURE 6-2 **Differentiation of hematopoietic stem cells in bone marrow.**

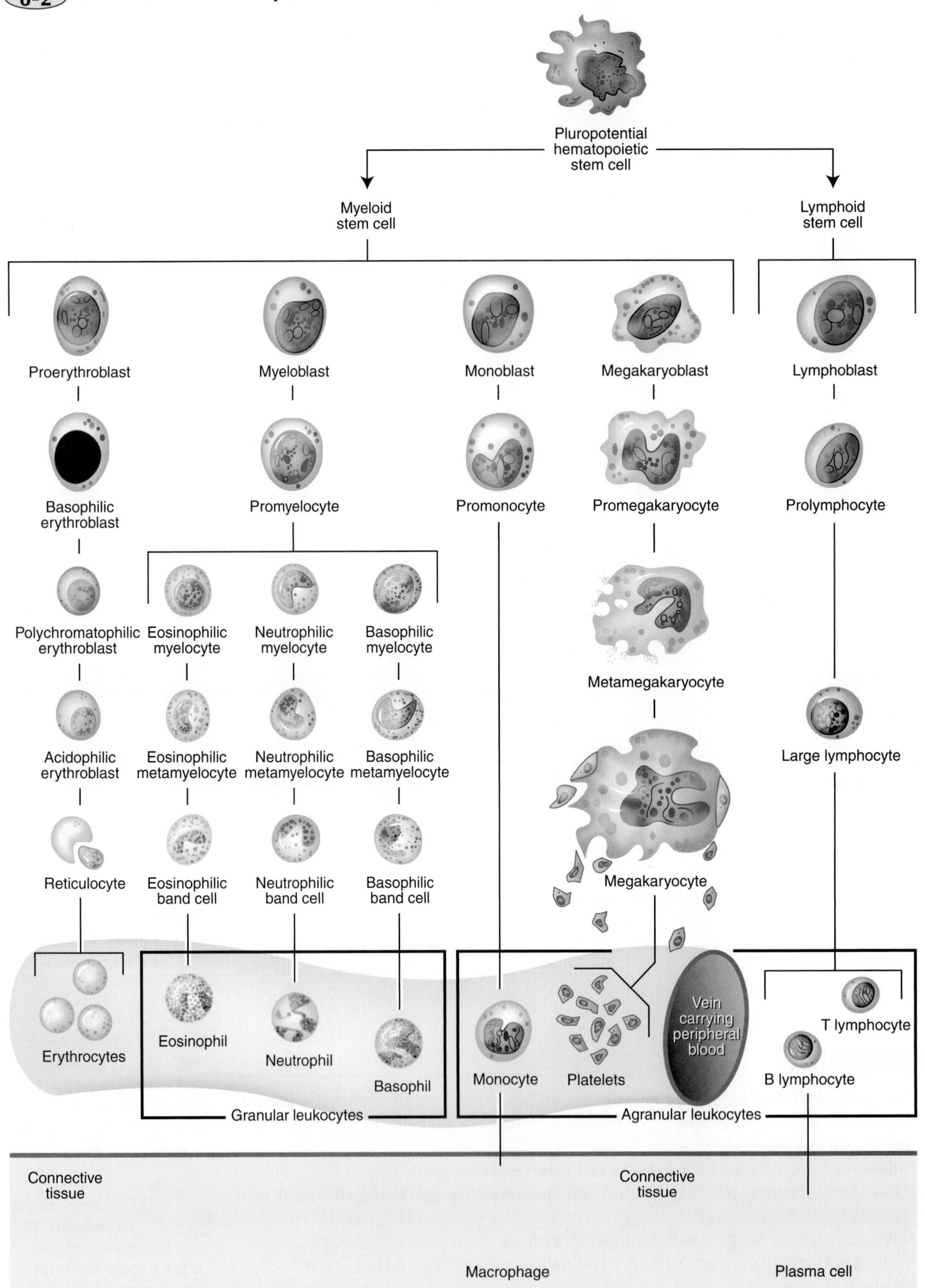

(Taken from Eroschenko VP. *DiFiore's atlas of histology with functional correlations*. 11th ed. Baltimore: Lippincott Williams & Wilkins, 2008. Used with permission of Lippincott Williams & Wilkins.)

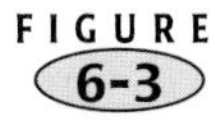

FIGURE 6-3 **The coagulation cascade. INR, international normalization ratio; PT, prothrombin time; PTT, partial thromboplastin time.**

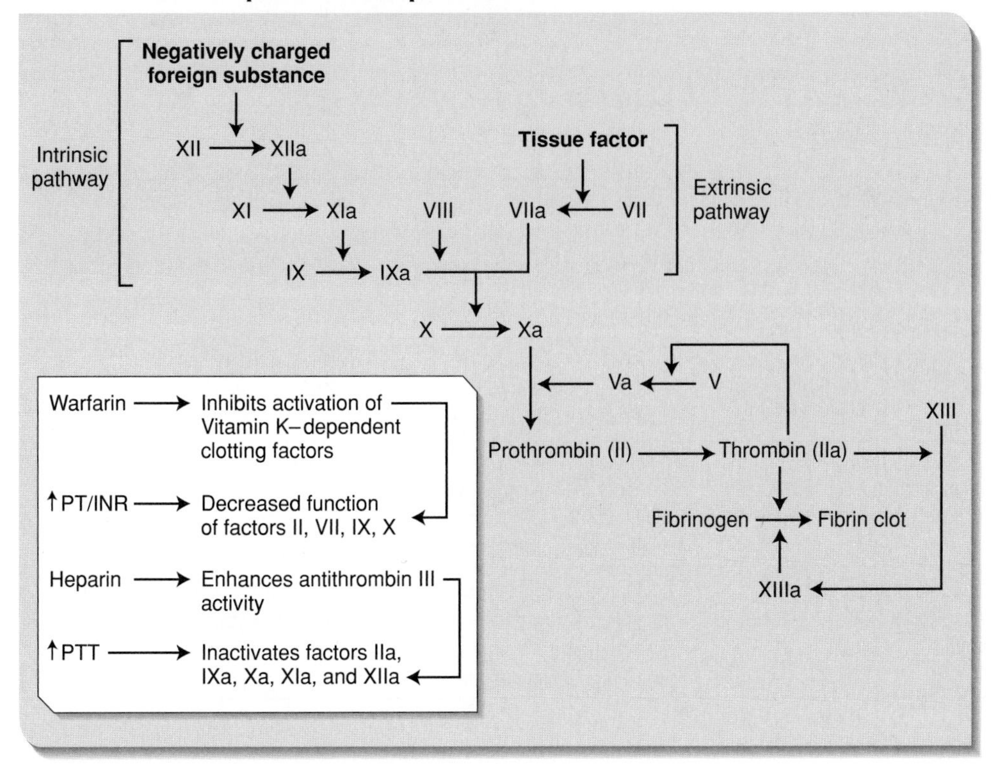

- Transfusions must be matched for the particular ABO and Rh blood types to avoid transfusion reactions (Table 6-3)

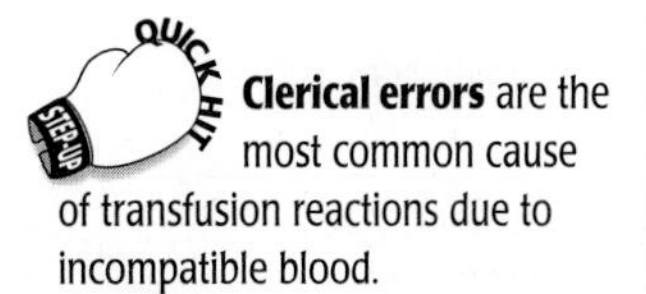

Clerical errors are the most common cause of transfusion reactions due to incompatible blood.

ORGAN TRANSPLANTATION

- Donors are selected based on **ABO blood type compatibility**, **cross-match compatibility** (i.e., presence of antidonor antibodies on recipient T cells), and **human leukocyte antigen (HLA) matching**
- Transplant rejection may be hyperacute, acute, or chronic (Table 6-4)
- All transplant recipients require immunosuppressive agents to reduce the risk of rejection (Table 6-5)
- Transplant patients have greater risks of **infection** (secondary to immunosuppression), **cancer** (e.g., skin, B cell lymphoma, oral squamous cell, cervical, vaginal), and **infertility**
- HLA mismatching may cause **graft versus host disease**, in which immune cells transplanted along with the donor tissue attack the immunocompromised host and cause hepatic, gastric, pulmonary, and dermatologic inflammation

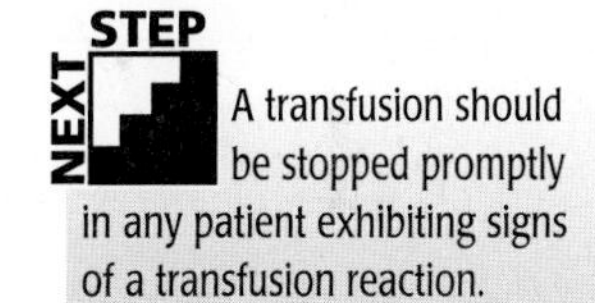

A transfusion should be stopped promptly in any patient exhibiting signs of a transfusion reaction.

ONCOLOGIC THERAPY

- The ultimate goal of therapy is the **eradication** of neoplastic cells
- Secondary goals are to **delay disease progression** or to serve as **palliative therapy**
- **Surgery**
  - Performed to **reduce the mass** of solid tumors or to **remove** well-contained tumors
  - Tissue surrounding a lesion is frequently removed to increase the likelihood of resecting microscopic extensions of the tumor
  - Many procedures are associated with significant morbidity

TABLE 6-1 Common Anticoagulant Drugs

Drug	Mechanism	Role	Adverse Effects
ASA	Inhibits platelet aggregation by inhibiting cyclooxygenase activity to suppress thromboxane A_2 synthesis	Decreases thrombus risk in CAD and post-MI, decreases postoperative thrombus risk	Increased risk of hemorrhagic stroke and **GI bleeding**
Thienopyridines (e.g., clopidogrel, ticlopidine)	Block ADP receptors to suppress fibrinogen binding and platelet adhesion to injury sites	Decreases risk of repeat MI or stroke in patients with prior MI, stroke, or PVD; decreases thrombus risk in postvascular intervention patients	Increased risk of hemorrhage and **GI bleeding**
GP IIb/IIIa inhibitors (e.g., abciximab)	Inhibit platelet aggregation by binding to platelet GP IIb/IIIa receptors	Reduce risk of thrombus in unstable angina or following coronary vessel intervention	Increased risk of hemorrhage, nausea, back pain, and hypotension
Adenosine reuptake inhibitors (e.g., dipyridamole)	Inhibit activity of adenosine deaminase and phosphodiesterase to inhibit platelet aggregation	Used in combination with ASA in patients with recent stroke or with warfarin following artificial heart valve replacement	Dizziness, headache, and nausea
Heparin	Binds to **antithrombin III** to increase activity and prevent clot formation	Postoperative prophylaxis for DVT and PE, dialysis, decreases post-MI thrombus risk, safer than warfarin during pregnancy	Hemorrhage, hypersensitivity, and **thrombocytopenia**; narrow therapeutic window
Low molecular weight heparin (e.g., enoxaparin, dalteparin)	Binds to **factor Xa** to prevent clot formation	Postoperative prophylaxis for DVT and PE, safest option during pregnancy	Hemorrhage, fever, and rare thrombocytopenia
Direct thrombin inhibitors (e.g., lepirudin, argatroban)	Highly selective inhibitors of thrombin to suppress activity of factors V, IX, and XIII and platelet aggregation	Alternative anticoagulation in patients with history of HIT	Hemorrhage and hypotension
Direct factor Xa inhibitors (e.g., fondaparinux)	Highly selective inhibition of factor Xa without activity against thrombin	DVT prophylaxis, anticoagulation following acute DVT or PE	Hemorrhage, fever, anemia, edema, rash, constipation
Warfarin	Antagonizes vitamin K–dependent carboxylation of factors II, VII, IX, and X	**Long-term** anticoagulation postthrombotic event or in cases of increased thrombus risk (postsurgery, Afib, artificial valves)	Hemorrhage, numerous **drug interactions**, and **teratogenicity**

Afib, atrial fibrillation; ASA, aspirin; CAD, coronary artery disease; DVT, deep vein thrombosis; GI, gastrointestinal; HIT, heparin-induced thrombocytopenia; MI, myocardial infarction; PE, pulmonary embolism; PVD, peripheral vascular disease.

- **Radiation therapy**
  - Performed to **necrose** tumor cells and to **decrease tumor size**
  - Adverse effects include impaired surgical wound healing, fibrosis of tissue, skin irritation, esophagitis, gastritis, pneumonitis, neurologic deficits, bone marrow suppression, and **radiation-induced malignancies** (e.g., thyroid, chronic myelogenous leukemia [CML], sarcomas)
- **Chemotherapy**
  - Aims to eradicate smaller populations of neoplastic cells and destroy cells not removed through surgery or radiation (Table 6-6)
  - May sensitize neoplastic cells to radiation therapy (i.e., radiosensitizers)
  - May be the primary treatment modality in certain cancers particularly receptive to pharmacological therapy

TABLE 6-2 Types of Blood Products Used in Transfusions

Blood Product	Definition	Indications
Whole blood	Donor blood not separated into components (full volume blood)	Rarely used except for massive transfusions for severe blood loss
Packed RBCs	RBCs separated from other donor blood components (two-thirds volume of transfusion unit is RBCs)	Product of choice for treatment of low Hct due to blood loss or anemia
Autologous blood	Blood donated by a patient prior to elective surgery or other treatments; blood is frozen until needed by patient	Elective surgery or chemotherapy
FFP	Plasma from which RBCs have been separated	Warfarin overdose, clotting factor deficiency, DIC, or TTP
Cryoprecipitate	Clotting factor and vWF-rich precipitate collected during thawing of FFP	Same indications as FFP; preferable to FFP in cases where a large transfusion volume is unwanted
Platelets	Platelets separated from other plasma components	Thrombocytopenia not due to rapid platelet destruction
Clotting factors	Concentrations of a specific clotting factor pooled from multiple donors	Specific clotting factor deficiencies (e.g., hemophilia)

DIC, disseminated intravascular coagulation; FFP, fresh frozen plasma; Hct, hematocrit; RBCs, red blood cells; TTP, thrombotic thrombocytopenic purpura; vWf, von Willebrand factor.

TABLE 6-3 Types of Transfusion Reactions

Type	Cause	Characteristics	Treatment
Febrile nonhemolytic	HLA antibodies in matched blood	Fevers during transfusion	Acetaminophen
Acute hemolytic	ABO incompatibility	Severe destruction of host RBCs	Aggressive supportive care
Delayed hemolytic	Kidd or Rh antibodies	Mild delayed hemolysis	Supportive care
Anaphylactic	Anti-IgA IgG antibodies transfused to patient with IgA deficiency	Rapid onset of shock and hypotension	Epinephrine, volume maintenance, and airway management
Urticarial	Donor plasma not filtered from blood	Urticarial rash forms on recipient	Diphenhydramine

HLA, human leukocyte antigen; Ig, immunoglobulin; RBCs, red blood cells.

TABLE 6-4 Forms of Transplant Rejection

Type	When Seen	Cause	Treatment
Hyperacute	**Initial 24 hours** after transplantation	Antidonor antibodies in recipient	**Untreatable**; should be avoided by proper cross-matching
Acute	**6 days to 1 year** after transplantation	Antidonor T cell proliferation in recipient	**Frequently reversible** through immunosuppressive agents
Chronic	**More than 1 year** after transplantation	Development of multiple cellular and humoral immune reactions to donor tissue	Usually untreatable; immunosuppression may serve some role

TABLE 6-5 Immunosuppressive Drugs to Prevent Transplant Rejection

Drug	Indication	Mechanism	Adverse Effects
Cyclosporine	Rejection prevention	**Helper** T cell inhibition	**Nephrotoxicity**, androgenic effects, HTN
Azathioprine	Rejection prevention	Inhibits T cell proliferation	**Leukopenia**
Tacrolimus	Rejection prevention and reversal	Inhibitor of T cell function	**Nephrotoxicity**, neurotoxicity
Corticosteroids	Rejection prevention and reversal	Inhibits **all leukocyte** activity	Cushing syndrome, weight gain, AVN of bone
Muromonab-D3 (OKT3)	Rejection reversal and **early** rejection maintenance	Inhibitor of T cell function and depletes T cell population	Induces **one-time cytokine release** (fever, bronchospasm), leukopenia; limited to **short-term therapy**
Rapamycin	Rejection prevention	Helper T cell inhibition	Thrombocytopenia, hyperlipidemia
Mycophenolic acid	Rejection prevention	Inhibits T cell proliferation	**Leukopenia**, GI toxicity
Antithymocyte globulin	Rejection reversal and **early** rejection maintenance	Depletes T cell population	Limited to **short-term therapy**, serum sickness
Hydroxychloroquine	Chronic graft vs. host disease	Inhibits antigen processing	Visual disturbances
Thalidomide	Chronic graft vs. host disease	Inhibits T cell function and migration	Sedation, constipation

AVN, avascular necrosis; HTN, hypertension.

- **Multiple drugs** with different cell cycle–specific targets are frequently combined to increase neoplastic cell death while minimizing the toxicity to normal tissues, to have an effect against a broader range of cells, and to slow the development of resistance
- Adverse effects include bone marrow suppression, alopecia, gastrointestinal (GI) upset, infertility, neurotoxicity, hepatotoxicity, skin changes, pulmonary fibrosis, cardiomyopathy, and renal toxicity

TABLE 6-6 Mechanisms and Classes of Chemotherapeutic Drugs

Mechanism	Drug Class	Examples
Free radical production causing cytotoxic alkylation of DNA and RNA	Nitrogen mustard alkylating agents	Cyclophosphamide, chlorambucil, ifosfamide, mechlorethamine
	Nitrosourea alkylating agents	Carmustine, streptozocin
	Alkyl sulfonate alkylating agents	Busulfan
	Ethylenimine/methylmelamine alkylating agents	Thiotepa, hexamethylmelamine
	Triazine alkylating agents	Dacarbazine
Inhibition of spindle proteins to stop mitosis or to cause cytotoxic polymerization	Vinca alkaloids Taxanes	Etoposide, vinblastine, vincristine Paclitaxel, docetaxel
Inhibition of DNA and RNA synthesis	Antibiotics	Bleomycin, dactinomycin, daunorubicin, doxorubicin, mitomycin
	Monoamine oxidase inhibitors	Procarbazine
Interference with enzyme regulation or DNA and RNA activity	Antimetabolites	Cytarabine, 5-flurouracil, methotrexate, mercaptopurine
	Platinum analogues	Carboplatin, cisplatin
Modulation of hormones to cause tumor remission	Steroid hormones and antagonists	Prednisone, tamoxifen, estrogens, leuprolide

CASE 6-1 "My father's anemia is keeping him from walking"

A 62-year-old man is seen in referral by a hematologist for microcytic anemia. The patient had initially seen his primary care provider (PCP) for symptoms of significant weakness, memory impairment, and impaired coordination, which developed over the past year, and the referral is directed toward finding a relationship between anemia that was detected during his initial work-up and his multiple symptoms. The PCP was unable to explain the patient's symptoms and feels that the elucidation of the cause of his anemia is the key to his work-up. He is accompanied to the office by his daughter. She says that she has noticed a gradual deterioration in her father's mobility and function over the past year. She says that her father was a very active man in the past, but he has gradually become less active. He has also been unsteady on his feet while walking and has fallen from standing five times over the past few months. The patient says that he feels tired all of the time. His daughter notes that once he awakens in the morning, he sits in his favorite chair and watches television all day. It is extremely difficult to get him to do any activities because he complains about not having "enough energy." He has stopped leaving the house to shop, visit family, or go to church because of his lethargy. She says that he also has had difficulty remembering simple instructions and quickly forgets things that have been told to him. The patient says that he is uncertain when his symptoms started. He notes frequent headaches and abdominal pain. He feels that his balance is impaired by constant aching in his knees and ankles. He is frustrated by his problems with short-term memory and his constant tiredness. He was working as a contractor for the military, and his primary assignment was the restoration of retired warships. He was removing old paint from these ships and cleaning them out, but has been unable to work for the past 6 months because of his impaired balance. He denies nausea, vomiting, diarrhea, hematemesis, or hematochezia. He has a past medical history of hypertension (HTN) and hyperlipidemia for which he takes enalapril and simvastatin. He drinks five alcoholic beverages per week and denies smoking. On examination, he appears well-nourished in no acute distress. His skin is mildly pale. He has mild papilledema on fundoscopic examination. He has grayish streaks in his gums at the bases of his teeth. He has no lymphadenopathy. Auscultation of his heart and lungs detects normal breath and heart sounds. His abdomen is soft and nontender with normal bowel sounds. A rectal examination detects no gross blood. Neurologic examination detects mild impairments of coordinated movement and normal sensation. He has a mildly unsteady gait when his walking is observed. The following vital signs are measured:

Temperature (T): 98.6°F, heart rate (HR): 89 beats per minute (bpm), blood pressure (BP): 132/91 mm Hg, respiratory rate (RR): 17 breaths/min

Differential Diagnosis

- Acute renal failure, hemolytic anemia, iron deficiency anemia, lead poisoning, sideroblastic anemia, acute intermittent porphyria, thalassemia, anemia of chronic disease, mononucleosis, Lyme disease, vitamin B_{12} deficiency, cerebral vascular accident, alcoholism

Laboratory Data and Other Study Results

The following studies were ordered by the patient's PCP:

- Complete blood cell count (CBC): white blood cells (WBC): 7.9, Hgb: 10.2, platelets (Plt): 301, mean corpuscular volume (MCV): 69 fL
- Blood smear: microcytic RBCs with basophilic stippling, no other RBC abnormalities
- 10-electrolyte chemistry panel (Chem10): sodium (Na): 139 mEq/L, potassium (K): 4.1 mEq/L, chloride (Cl): 109 mEq/L, carbon dioxide (CO_2): 27 mEq/L, blood urea nitrogen (BUN): 27 mg/dL, creatinine (Cr): 1.5 mg/dL, glucose (Glu): 102 mg/dL, magnesium (Mg): 2.2 mg/dL, calcium (Ca): 10.9 mg/dL, phosphorous (Phos): 3.3 mg/dL

- Liver function tests (LFTs): alkaline phosphatase (AlkPhos): 67 U/L, alanine aminotransferase (ALT): 68 U/L, aspartate aminotransferase (AST): 51 U/L, total bilirubin (TBili): 0.9 mg/dL, direct bilirubin (DBili): 0.5 mg/dL
- Head computed tomography (CT): no evidence of hemorrhage, ischemia, or volume loss

The following additional tests are ordered by the hematologist:

- Whole blood lead level: 63 μg/dL
- Free erythrocyte protoporphyrin: 42 μg/dL
- Reticulocyte count: 4%
- Nutrition panel: albumin: 4.6 g/dL, iron (Fe) 102 μg/dL, transferrin: 320 mg/dL, ferritin: 65 ng/mL
- Hemoglobin A_2: 2.0%
- Hemoglobin F: 0%
- Lyme antibody enzyme-linked immunosorbent assay (ELISA): negative
- Vitamin B_{12} level: 526 pg/mL
- Twenty-four-hour urine porphobilinogen level: 0.9 mg

Diagnosis

- Chronic lead poisoning

Treatment Administered

- The patient's employer was notified of the potential risk of lead exposure in the patient's job
- The patient was started on oral 2,3-dimercaptosuccinic acid (DMSA) with a tapering dose over 3 weeks

Follow-up

- Follow-up whole blood lead levels detected a decrease to 31 μg/dL after the 3 weeks of chelation therapy
- The patient's symptoms resolved over the following 4 months, and his lead levels were found to continue to decrease
- The patient was allowed to return to work after his symptoms improved, and he was reassigned to a job that was less likely to be at risk for lead exposure

Steps to the Diagnosis

- **Lead-poisoning anemia**
  - Anemia that results from the inhibition of heme synthesis following lead exposure (e.g., ingestion, inhalation)
    - More common in **children**, especially those in urban environments
    - Chronic alcoholism and isoniazid (INH) use may cause similar symptoms
  - **History:** fatigue, weakness, abdominal pain, arthralgias, headaches, impaired short-term memory
  - **Physical examination:** pallor, **gingival lead lines**, **peripheral motor neuropathy**, developmental delays in children
  - **Tests:**
    - **Decreased Hgb and MCV**; increased reticulocyte count (Table 6-7)
    - Increased erythrocyte protoporphyrin
    - Increased whole blood lead level
    - Mild increases in BUN and creatinine and liver transaminases
    - Blood smear will show **microcytic RBCs** with **basophilic stippling** and possible ringed sideroblasts (Color Figure 6-1)
  - **Treatment:** elimination of the lead source or removal of the patient from the site of exposure is frequently sufficient to prompt gradual reduction in blood lead levels; patients with a whole blood lead level >80 μg/dL or symptomatic patients with levels

MNEMONIC

The list of common microcytic anemias may be remembered by the mnemonic "**L**ook **F**or **T**hose **S**mall **C**ells": **L**ead-poisoning, **Fe** (iron) deficiency, **T**halassemia, **S**ideroblastic, **C**hronic disease.

TABLE 6-7 Classification of Anemias by Mean Corpuscular Volume and Common Etiologies

Microcytic (MCV <80 μL)	Normocytic (MCV 80–100 μL)	Macrocytic (MCV >100 μL)
Iron deficiency	Hemolytic	Folate deficiency
Lead poisoning	Chronic disease	Vitamin B_{12} deficiency
Chronic disease	Hypovolemia	Liver disease
Sideroblastic		
Thalassemias		

MCV, mean corpuscular volume.

>60 μg/dL may be treated with ethylenediamine tetraacetic acid (EDTA) or DMSA as chelation therapy
- **Outcomes:** complications include renal, hepatic, cardiac, and neurologic damage; patients who develop encephalopathy are at greater risk for chronic symptoms
- **Clues to the diagnosis:**
  - History: fatigue, short-term memory impairments, abdominal pain, headaches, possible work-related exposure
  - Physical: loss of coordination, gingival lead lines, pallor
  - Tests: increased lead level, microcytic anemia, increased erythrocyte protoporphyrin, increased reticulocyte count, blood smear appearance

- **Acute renal failure**
  - More thorough discussion in Chapter 4
  - **Why eliminated from differential:** the patient has mild increases in his BUN and creatinine, but these levels would not explain his constellation of symptoms or explain his multiple hematologic lab abnormalities
- **Hemolytic anemia**
  - Anemia that results from a combination of an abnormally shortened RBC lifespan (normally 120 days) and insufficient marrow replacement of RBCs
    - Common causes include RBC membrane defects, RBC enzyme defects, hemoglobinopathies, drug effects, or mechanical damage (Table 6-8, Color Figure 6-2)
  - **History:** weakness, fatigue, dyspnea on exertion, other symptoms depending on the particular etiology (Table 6-8)
  - **Physical examination: pallor**, tachycardia, tachypnea, palpitations, increased pulse pressure, **jaundice**, **hepatosplenomegaly**, **brownish discoloration of urine**, mental status changes, other signs per particular etiology (Table 6-8)
  - **Tests:**
    - Decreased Hgb, **increased reticulocyte count, normal MCV**
    - **Increased indirect bilirubin**, lactate dehydrogenase (LDH), and serum haptoglobin
    - **Coombs test** may help differentiate causes
      - In a direct test, Coombs reagent is mixed with the patient RBCs, and agglutination indicates the presence of immunoglobulin IgG and complement on the RBC membranes (e.g., warm and cold agglutinin diseases)
      - In an indirect test, the patient's RBC are mixed with type O RBCs, which are then mixed with Coombs reagent, and agglutination indicates the presence of anti-RBC antibodies in the serum (e.g., Rh alloimmunization)
    - Blood smear will show **schistocytes** (i.e., fragments of RBCs), spherocytes, and burr cells (Color Figure 6-3)
  - **Treatment:** treatments vary with each etiology and include avoidance of the underlying stimulus, corticosteroids, and splenectomy (Table 6-8)
  - **Outcomes:** prognosis varies with each etiology of anemia, but generally, patients will do better if they are able to be separated from the cause of hemolysis

TABLE 6-8 Types of Hemolytic Anemias

Type	Pathology	Blood Smear	Coombs Test	Other Diagnostic Aids	Treatment
Drug-induced	Substances bind to RBC membranes and cause oxidative destruction, induce production of **anti-drug antibodies,** form **immune complexes** that fix, complement, or induce **anti-Rh antibodies**	Burr cells, schistocytes	**Direct** + (unless due to oxidative destruction)	Recent penicillin, L-dopa, quinidine, other drug use	Stop offending agent
Immune	**Anti-RBC antibodies,** autoimmune disease, possibly drug-induced	Spherocytes (warm agglutinins), RBC agglutination (cold agglutinins)	**Direct** +	**Warm-reacting antibodies** (IgG) or **cold-reacting antibodies** (IgM)	Corticosteroids, **avoid cold exposure** (with cold-reacting antibodies), stop offending agent; splenectomy may be needed in persistent cases
Mechanical	RBCs broken by force or **turbulent flow**	**Schistocytes**	Negative	**Prosthetic heart valve**, HTN, coagulation disorder	Treat underlying cause
Hereditary spherocytosis	Genetic **defect of RBC membranes** resulting in spherical RBCs	**Spherocytes**	Negative	**Hepatosplenomegaly**	Splenectomy
G6PD deficiency	Deficiency of G6PD (i.e., enzyme required to repair oxidative damage to RBCs); ingestion of oxidant (e.g., fava beans, ASA, sulfa drugs) causes excessive RBC hemolysis	RBCs with **"bites"** taken out of them, **Heinz bodies** (i.e., small densities of Hgb in RBC)	Negative	**Low G6PD** (by indirect measurement); dizziness and fatigue begins within days of ingesting the oxidant; mild form in African Americans and more severe form in people of Mediterranean decent	Avoid oxidants; transfusion may be needed in severe cases

ASA, aspirin; G6PD, glucose 6-phosphate dehydrogenase; Hgb, hemoglobin; HTN, hypertension; Ig, immunoglobulin; RBC, red blood cell.

- **Why eliminated from differential:** the absence of the characteristic blood smear findings and the decreased MCV rule out this collection of disorders
- **Iron-deficiency anemia**
  - Anemia that results from an insufficient supply of iron, leading to an insufficient production of heme
    - Common causes include **hemorrhage**, poor dietary iron intake, poor GI absorption of iron, pregnancy, and menstruation
  - **History**: fatigue, weakness, dyspnea on exertion, **pica** (i.e., cravings to eat ice, dirt, etc.)
  - **Physical examination**: pallor, tachycardia, tachypnea, increased pulse pressure, **angular celitis** (i.e., irritation of the lips and the corners of the mouth), **spooning** of fingernails
  - **Tests:**
    - Decreased Hgb and MCV; decreased or normal reticulocyte count
    - **Decreased ferritin and iron**; increased transferrin (Table 6-9)
    - Blood smear shows hypochromic microcytic RBCs (Color Figure 6-4)
  - **Treatment:** the cause of iron loss must be determined to rule out malignancies; long-term iron supplementation is required to replete body stores

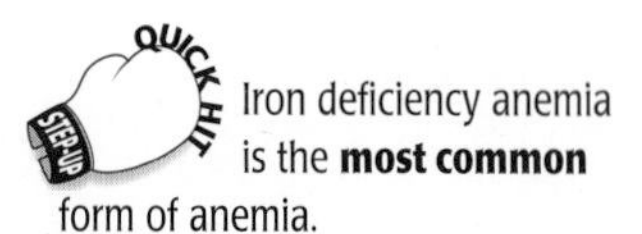

Iron deficiency anemia is the **most common** form of anemia.

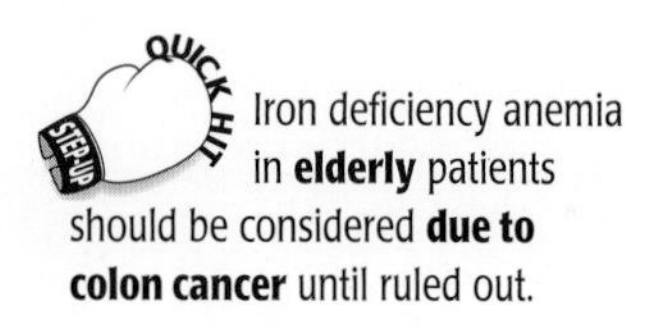

Iron deficiency anemia in **elderly** patients should be considered **due to colon cancer** until ruled out.

TABLE 6-9 Laboratory Distinction of Microcytic Anemias

Type	Serum Iron	Ferritin	TIBC (transferrin)	Mentzer Index[1]	Blood Smear
Iron deficiency	↓	↓	↑	>13	Hypochromic, microcytic RBCs
Lead poisoning	Normal or ↑	Normal	Normal	>13	Stippled, microcytic RBCs
Chronic disease	↓	Normal or ↑	↓	>13	Hypochromic, normocytic or microcytic RBCs
Sideroblastic	↑	↑	↓	>13	Ringed sideroblasts
Thalassemia	Normal or ↑	Normal	Normal	<13	Microcytic RBCs, target cells (α), basophilic stippling (β)

MCV, mean corpuscular volume; RBC, red blood cells; TIBC, total iron-binding capacity; ↑, increased; ↓, decreased.

[1]Mentzer index = MCV ÷ RBC count

- **Outcomes:** the prognosis is excellent with iron supplementation, but neoplasm as a cause must be ruled out
- **Why eliminated from differential:** the increased reticulocyte count and normal nutrition panel rule out this condition

- **Sideroblastic anemia**
  - Anemia resulting from a **defect in heme synthesis** that causes a decrease in Hgb levels in RBCs
    - May be due to genetic factors or induced by alcohol or INH use
  - **History:** fatigue, weakness, dyspnea on exertion, angina
  - **Physical examination:** pallor, tachycardia, tachypnea, increased pulse pressure, hepatosplenomegaly
  - **Tests:**
    - Decreased Hgb and possible decreased MCV
    - Increased ferritin and iron and decreased transferrin
    - Blood smear shows a significant variability in the size of RBCs and **ringed sideroblasts** (Color Figure 6-5)
  - **Treatment:**
    - Hereditary cases may respond to supplemental vitamin B_6
    - Supplemental erythropoietin (EPO) may be used in acquired cases
    - Therapeutic phlebotomy or iron chelation with deferoxamine may be required in cases of iron overload (occurs because the obstacle to heme synthesis causes a buildup of iron stores)
  - **Outcomes:** adverse reactions to vitamin B_6 therapy may occur; acute leukemia develops in 10% of patients
  - **Why eliminated from differential:** the normal nutrition panel and the consistency of microcytic RBCs on the blood smear rule out this diagnosis
- **Acute intermittent porphyria**
  - Defect in the metabolism of heme, leading to an accumulation of porphobilinogen and amino-levulinic acid
    - May be caused by a genetic defect or may be drug related
  - **History: severe prolonged abdominal pain**, nausea, vomiting, constipation, depression, **psychotic behavior**
  - **Physical examination:** tachycardia, HTN, areflexia, **motor dysfunction**

- **Tests:** increased urine porphyrins (particularly porphobilinogen); decreased serum sodium
- **Treatment:** hematin and high-dose glucose are used to stop exacerbations; precipitating factors should be avoided
- **Outcomes:** exacerbations rarely recur if the underlying causes are avoided
- **Why eliminated from differential:** the normal urinary porphobilinogen level rules out this diagnosis

- **Thalassemia**
  - Defects in Hgb resulting from an abnormal production of heme α-globin and β-globin subunits
    - The disease state arises from the **unbalanced production ratio** of subunits and not from the subunits themselves
    - Normally Hgb is composed of two α-subunits, whose synthesis is controlled by four genes, and two β-subunits, whose synthesis is controlled by two genes (Table 6-10)
      - **α-thalassemia** may feature defects in one to four of the genes and is more common in people of African or Asian descent
      - **β-thalassemia** may feature defects in one or both genes and is more common in people of Mediterranean descent

TABLE 6-10 Variants of α- and β-Thalassemias

Thalassemia Type	Variant	Number of Abnormal Genes	Characteristics
α	Hydrops fetalis	4	• No α-globin production • **Fetal death** occurs
	Hemoglobin H disease	3	• Minimal α-globin production • **Chronic hemolytic anemia**, pallor, splenomegaly • **Hemoglobin Barts** in serum • Microcytic RBCs on blood smear • Decreased patient lifespan
	α-thalassemia minor	2	• Reduced α-globin production • **Mild anemia** • Microcytic RBCs and target cells on blood smear
	α-thalassemia minima	1	• Generally **asymptomatic** • Children of carriers are at an increased risk for thalassemia pending the genotype of the other parent
β	β-thalassemia major	2	• No β-globin production • Asymptomatic until decline of fetal hemoglobin • Growth retardation, developmental delays, bony abnormalities, hepatosplenomegaly, anemia • Increase in hemoglobin A2 and F • Microcytic RBCs on blood smear • Patients die in childhood without transfusions
	β-thalassemia minor	1	• Reduced β-globin production • Mild anemia • Patients can lead normal lives • Transfusions may be needed during periods of stress

RBC, red blood cell.

- **History:** patients with only one defective gene are frequently asymptomatic, while patients with more severe forms of the conditions may experience fatigue and activity intolerance
- **Physical examination:** pallor, facial bony abnormalities, hepatosplenomegaly, jaundice, growth retardation
- **Tests:**
  - Decreased Hgb and MCV; increased reticulocyte count
  - Increased Hgb variants (e.g., Barts, F, A_2)
  - Blood smear will show abnormally shaped microcytic RBCs and target cells in α-thalassemia and RBCs with a variable size and shape and basophilic stippling in β-thalassemia (Color Figure 6-6)
- **Treatment:**
  - α-thalassemia with one or two defective genes and β-thalassemia with only one defective gene are frequently treated symptomatically only during periods of stress
  - Folate supplementation may help relive symptoms in all variants
  - Transfusions may be required for severe variants and for milder variants during symptomatic exacerbations; chronic transfusions may require iron chelation
  - Bone marrow transplant may benefit young children with an early diagnosis
- **Outcomes:** patients with more severe variants of the disease have a high mortality rate due to cardiac and hepatic failure; chronic iron overload from frequent transfusions may cause cardiac and hepatic complications
- **Why eliminated from differential:** the absence of increased RBC variability makes this diagnosis unlikely

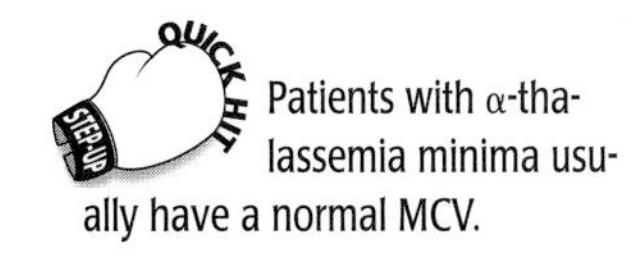
Patients with α-thalassemia minima usually have a normal MCV.

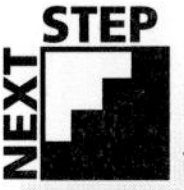
Differentiate between the causes of microcytic anemia using the ratio of MCV to RBC count (i.e., Mentzer index): MCV:RBC count >13 suggests iron deficiency; MCV:RBC count <13 suggests thalassemia.

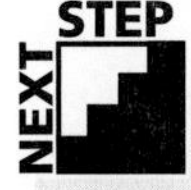
If microcytic anemia is found on blood smear, rule out thalassemia before administering supplemental iron to prevent iron overload.

- **Anemia of chronic disease**
  - Anemia common in patients with neoplasms, diabetes mellitus (DM), autoimmune disorders, or chronic infections
    - Frequently associated with the trapping of iron in macrophages, decreased erythropoietin production, and increased hepcidin levels (i.e., inhibitor of iron absorption and mobilization)
  - **History:** fatigue, weakness, dyspnea on exertion
  - **Physical examination:** pallor, tachycardia
  - **Tests:**
    - Mildly decreased Hgb and MCV
    - Decreased iron and transferrin; normal or increased ferritin
    - Blood smear shows mildly microcytic RBCs
  - **Treatment:** treat the underlying disorder; supplemental EPO may help increase Hgb
  - **Outcomes:** prognosis is more dependent on the underlying condition than the anemia itself
  - **Why eliminated from differential:** the lack of a causative medical diagnosis and the normal nutrition panel make this diagnosis unlikely
- **Mononucleosis**
  - More thorough discussion in later case
  - **Why eliminated from differential:** the normal WBC and the absence of atypical WBCs on the blood smear rule out this diagnosis
- **Lyme disease**
  - More thorough discussion in Chapter 9
  - **Why eliminated from differential:** the negative antibody assay makes this diagnosis unlikely
- **Vitamin B_{12} deficiency**
  - Anemia that results from an inadequate supply of vitamin B_{12}
    - **Pernicious anemia** is an autoimmune deficit of **intrinsic factor**, leading to the impaired GI absorption of vitamin B_{12}
    - Acquired causes include poor dietary intake, ileal resection, GI bacterial overgrowth, or a *Diphyllobothrium latum* parasitic infection
  - **History:** fatigue, weakness, dyspnea on exertion, memory loss
  - **Physical examination:** pallor, tachycardia, tachypnea, increased pulse pressure, **symmetric paresthesias**, **ataxia**, possible psychosis

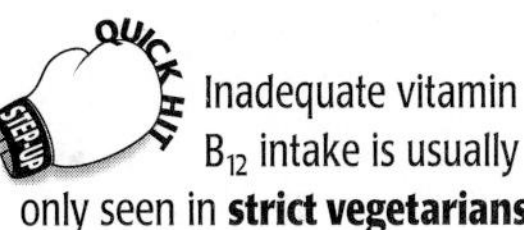
Inadequate vitamin B_{12} intake is usually only seen in **strict vegetarians** (e.g., vegans).

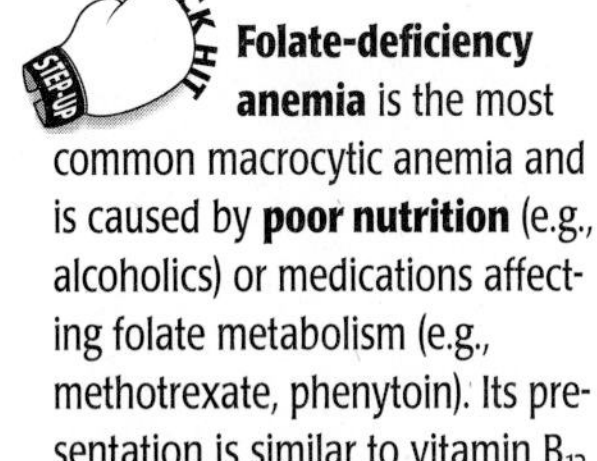
Folate-deficiency anemia is the most common macrocytic anemia and is caused by **poor nutrition** (e.g., alcoholics) or medications affecting folate metabolism (e.g., methotrexate, phenytoin). Its presentation is similar to vitamin B_{12} deficiency except it has **no neurologic symptoms**, a normal vitamin B_{12} level, and a decreased serum folate level. It is treated with **folate supplementation**.

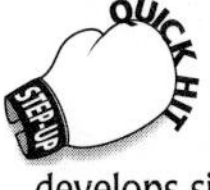
In cases of poor nutrition, folate deficiency develops significantly more quickly than vitamin B_{12} deficiency.

FIGURE 6-4 Testing protocol for the Schilling test. vit., vitamin.

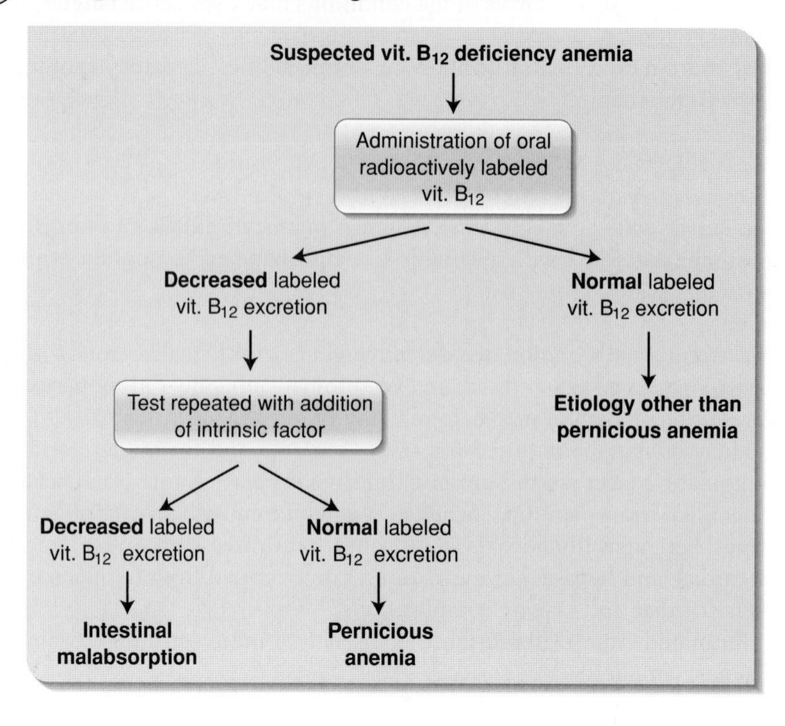

- **Tests:**
  - Decreased Hgb; increased MCV
  - Decreased serum vitamin B_{12} levels
  - The **Schilling test** is useful to determine the etiology of the condition (Figure 6-4)
  - Blood smear will show **macrocytic RBCs** and **hypersegmented neutrophils** (Color Figure 6-7)
- **Treatment:** periodic intramuscular injections (for pernicious anemia) or dietary supplementation of vitamin B_{12}
- **Outcomes:** the prognosis is more favorable in acquired forms of the disease; chronic neurologic abnormalities may not improve following therapy
- **Why eliminated from differential:** the MCV measured in the case and the appearance of the blood smear rule out this diagnosis

- **Cerebral vascular accident**
  - More thorough discussion in Chapter 7
  - **Why eliminated from differential:** the normal head CT makes this diagnosis unlikely
- **Alcohol-related liver disease**
  - More thorough discussion in Chapter 3
  - **Why eliminated from differential:** the minimally elevated transaminases and normal other LFTs make this diagnosis unlikely

CASE 6-2 "My daughter's hands and feet hurt"

A 4-year-old girl is brought by her parents to her pediatrician because of pain in her arms and legs. The patient's mother says that she and the patient's father first noticed that the child would periodically favor one of her arms or legs about 1 year ago. These episodes would last a couple of days and then resolve. In the past 6 months, the child has periodically complained that her feet or hands hurt. These episodes seem to occur randomly and self-resolve within a week. The parents estimate that such episodes have occurred three times in the past 6 months. When they took her to a local emergency department during one such episode, a radiographic work-up was negative for any bony pathology. They are also concerned because the patient refrains from normal activities when she has these symptoms. They deny any trauma to the patient, nausea, vomiting, seizures, or impaired coordination. She is notable for a case of streptococcal pneumonia when she was 3 years old that required an inpatient admission and treatment with intravenous (IV) antibiotics. The parents deny any other past medical history. She was the product of an uncomplicated full-term vaginal birth. The family is of African descent and is notable for HTN, hyperlipidemia, and breast cancer in the patient's grandparents. The parents deny smoking and say that they live in a relatively new house without any risks for lead paint or carbon monoxide. On examination, the girl is thin but well nourished and in no acute distress. Her sclera are mildly icteric. She has no lymphadenopathy. Her lungs are clear to auscultation without any abnormal breathing sounds. Auscultation of her heart detects a soft, blowing systolic murmur. Her abdomen is soft and nontender, and her spleen is moderately enlarged and palpable. Her extremities are nontender on palpation but she says that her hands hurt. Her joints have a normal range of motion. She is able to walk normally. Her neurologic examination is normal. The following vital signs are measured:

T: 99.0°F, HR: 86 bpm, BP: 105/80 mm Hg, RR: 18 breaths/min

Differential Diagnosis

- Thalassemia, mononucleosis, leukemia, sickle cell disease, rickets, cystic fibrosis, endocarditis, osteomyelitis

Laboratory Data and Other Study Results

- Height and weight: 38″ (14th percentile), 30 lb (10th percentile)
- CBC: WBC: 11.9, Hgb: 8.2, Plt: 203, MCV: 85 fL
- Chem10: Na: 139 mEq/L, K: 4.3 mEq/L, Cl: 100 mEq/L, CO_2: 23 mEq/L, BUN: 10 mg/dL, Cr: 0.4 mg/dL, Glu: 99 mg/dL, Mg: 1.9 mg/dL, Ca: 10.0 mg/dL, Phos: 3.4 mg/dL
- LFTs: AlkPhos: 80 U/L, ALT: 36 U/L, AST: 21 U/L, TBili: 1.4 mg/dL, DBili: 0.4 mg/dL, indirect bilirubin (IBili): 1.0 mg/dL
- Erythrocyte sedimentation rate (ESR): 2 mm/hr
- C-reactive protein (CRP): 0.3 mg/dL
- Sweat test: Cl: 26 mEq/L, Na: 32 mEq/L
- Blood smear: few sickled red cells and target cells; no abnormal leukocytes
- Chest x-ray (CXR): normal lung fields; no infiltrations or lymphadenopathy
- Echocardiogram: slight mitral and tricuspid regurgitation; no wall defects; normal wall motion, vasculature, and estimated chamber pressures

After these results are received, the additional studies are ordered:

- Reticulocyte count: 10%
- Serum haptoglobin: 39 mg/dL
- Hemoglobin A: 0%
- Hemoglobin A_2: 1.3%
- Hemoglobin F: 8.4%
- Hemoglobin S: 90.3%
- Transcranial Doppler ultrasound (US): normal carotid and cerebral blood flow

Diagnosis

- Sickle cell disease

Treatment Administered

- The family was referred to a sickle cell support group to discuss coping with recurrent pain, disease complications, and the expected outcomes
- The patient was provided the pneumococcal vaccine, and all other vaccinations were updated as indicated by the recommended vaccination calendar

- Prophylactic penicillin was initiated and scheduled as a daily dose until 5 years of age
- Folate supplementation was initiated

Follow-up

- Annual transcranial Doppler studies detected no changes in cerebral perfusion over the following several years
- The patient experienced sickle cell crises one to two times per year after the age of 8 years that required narcotic pain control and transfusion therapy
- Through midadolescence, the patient had developed no significant cerebral, musculoskeletal, or vascular complications

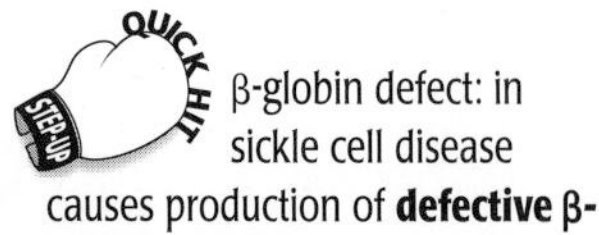

β-globin defect: in sickle cell disease causes production of **defective β-chains**; in β-thalassemia causes **decreased production** of **normal β-chains**.

Heterozygous **carriers** of the sickle cell defect (i.e., sickle cell trait) are **asymptomatic** and carry an **improved resistance to malaria**.

Steps to the Diagnosis

- **Sickle cell disease**
  - Autosomal recessive disease in which a defect in the β-globin chain of Hgb leads to the production of **Hgb S**, a form of Hgb that is poorly soluble when deoxygenated
    - Acidosis, hypoxia, and dehydration cause the polymerization of Hgb S, which leads to the distortion of RBCs into a **sickle shape** that is **susceptible to hemolysis** and **vascular clumping**
  - **Risk factors: African** or Latin American heritage
  - **History:**
    - Patients may be asymptomatic between crises or may note bone pain
    - Stressful events (e.g., infection, illness, trauma) incite **sickle cell crises** characterized by **severe bone pain**, chest pain, pain and swelling of the hands and feet, dyspnea, and priapism
  - **Physical examination:** decreased growth velocity, jaundice or pallor, **splenomegaly**, fever, possible leg ulcers
  - **Tests:**
    - Decreased Hgb and increased reticulocyte count; WBCs may be increased
    - Decreased serum haptoglobin
    - **No Hgb A**, increased Hgb F, and **presence of Hgb S** (normally not present) on electrophoresis
    - Increased indirect bilirubin
    - Solubility tests (e.g., SICKLEDEX, Streck, Omaha, Nebraska) can detect Hgb abnormalities but cannot differentiate between the carrier trait and homozygous disease states
    - Blood smear shows target cells, **sickle cells**, and nucleated RBCs; deoxygenation of blood significantly increases the number of sickled cells (Color Figure 6-8)
    - X-rays may show "fish-mouth" vertebrae and avascular necrosis of bony regions with a tenuous blood supply (e.g., femoral head)
    - Transcranial Doppler US is useful to measure the carotid and cerebral blood flow and determine the stroke risk
  - **Treatment:**
    - Referral of the patient to a sickle cell specialty group is beneficial to coordinate treatment and to counsel the patient on chronic pain issues and disease outcomes
    - Sickle cell crises are treated with **hydration**, **supplemental oxygen**, and **narcotic** pain control
    - **Transfusions**, exchange transfusions, and hydroxyurea are frequently useful to shorten crises or to decrease the number of crises in patients with frequent recurrences
    - All children should be kept current on their **vaccinations** (particularly pneumococcal vaccine) to reduce the risk of infection
    - **Bone marrow transplantation** has demonstrated success as a curative therapy, but due to the appreciable mortality and morbidity rates it is currently reserved for patients with severe disease and multiple complications

- **Outcomes:**
  - Complications include chronic anemia, pulmonary HTN, heart failure due to cardiac stresses, vascular insufficiency, renal failure, and infections
  - An **aplastic crisis** may follow infection (typically parvovirus B19) and is notable for severe anemia requiring aggressive transfusion therapy
  - **Acute chest syndrome** is severe chest pain due to pneumonia, embolization, or pulmonary infarction and requires pain control and respiratory support
  - Autosplenectomy, stroke, osteonecrosis of the femoral or humeral head, and multiorgan ischemia may result from **vascular occlusion**
  - Increased risk of infection by **encapsulated organisms** (e.g., *Streptococcus pneumoniae, Haemophilus influenzae, Neisseria meningitides, Klebsiella*)
  - Despite the multiple potential complications, survival at 18 years of age is 86%
- **Clues to the diagnosis:**
  - History: hand and foot pain, childhood pneumonia, African descent
  - Physical: lower than median height and weight for age, scleral icterus, splenomegaly, systolic murmur
  - Tests: normocytic anemia, increased reticulocyte count, decreased serum haptoglobin, blood smear appearance, Hgb electrophoresis results

MNEMONIC

Complications of sickle cell disease may be remembered by the mnemonic **SHARP MALICE**: **S**troke, **H**emolytic anemia, **A**utosplenectomy, **R**enal necrosis, **P**riapism, **M**yocardial infarction, **A**cute chest syndrome, **L**ung infarctions, **I**nfections, **C**rises (painful or aplastic), **E**ye disease (retinopathy).

QUICK HIT: Patients with sickle cell disease are particularly susceptible to ***Salmonella osteomyelitis*** (although *Staphylococcus aureus* is still the most common etiology) and **sepsis** by **encapsulated organisms**.

- Thalassemia
  - More thorough discussion in prior case
  - **Why eliminated from differential:** the normal MCV makes this diagnosis unlikely, and the Hgb electrophoresis results and the presence of sickle cells on the blood smear rule it out
- Mononucleosis
  - Infection by **Epstein-Barr virus (EBV)** affecting B leukocytes and oropharyngeal epithelium
    - Most common transmission is through **intimate contact** or exposure to saliva
  - **History: significant fatigue**, sore throat, malaise
  - **Physical examination: lymphadenopathy**, fever, splenomegaly, tonsillar exudates
  - **Tests:**
    - Increased WBCs
    - Positive heterophile antibodies and EBV serology
    - Blood smear shows an increased number of lymphocytes with some degree of atypia
  - **Treatment:** because the condition is self-limited, only supportive care is typically necessary; patients should refrain from contact sports during splenomegaly to reduce the risk of splenic rupture (at least 1 month)
  - **Outcomes:** prognosis is excellent; rare complications include splenic rupture and airway obstruction due to tonsillar hypertrophy
  - **Why eliminated from differential:** the minimally elevated WBC count and the appearance of the blood smear make this diagnosis unlikely

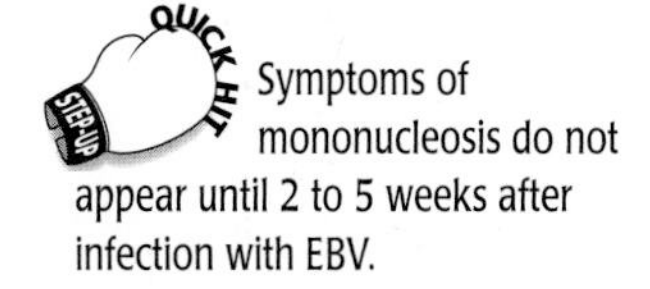

QUICK HIT: Symptoms of mononucleosis do not appear until 2 to 5 weeks after infection with EBV.

- Leukemia
  - More thorough discussion in later case
  - **Why eliminated from differential:** the minimally elevated WBC count and appearance of the blood smear make this diagnosis unlikely
- Rickets
  - More thorough discussion in Chapter 9
  - **Why eliminated from differential:** the history of normal-appearing x-rays, normal alkaline phosphatase, and normal calcium and phosphorus levels rule out this diagnosis
- Cystic fibrosis
  - More thorough discussion in Chapter 2
  - **Why eliminated from differential:** the normal results of the sweat test rule out this diagnosis
- Endocarditis
  - More thorough discussion in Chapter 1
  - **Why eliminated from differential:** the minimally elevated WBC count and the absence of vegetations on the echocardiogram make this diagnosis unlikely

CASE 6-3 "My baby is sick all of the time"

A 13-month-old infant boy is seen by a pediatric immunologist in referral because of frequent infections that are unexplained by his pediatrician. The child's parents say that he has had three cases of *S. pneumoniae* since birth that have required hospitalization. The first of these cases occurred at 6 months of age. His parents say that he has also had recurrent otitis media that has been treated with antibiotics. He is notable for a chronic cough that never seems to completely resolve. More recently he has had bouts of diarrhea that last for several days and then gradually resolve over a week. His parents deny vomiting, poor feeding, or significant developmental delays. Besides his recurrent respiratory infections, they deny a history of cutaneous, cerebral, or urinary infections. His mother is concerned because her brother and a male cousin exhibited a similar history when they were infants, and both died from pneumonia before the age of 5 years. His parents say that he has not been diagnosed with any medical conditions up to this time. He has not received medications other than antibiotics and has no history of radiation exposure. He has not yet received his 12-month vaccinations but is otherwise current. He was a product of an uncomplicated full-term vaginal birth. There is no significant family history besides that described above. No one in the household is a smoker. The patient is the couple's first child. On examination, the infant appears well nourished and is in no acute distress. He intermittently coughs during the office visit. No anatomic abnormalities of the face are detectable. No tonsils are visible on inspection of his oropharynx. His eardrums appear mildly inflamed. He has no palpable lymphadenopathy. Auscultation of his lungs detects rhonchi and mild wheezing. There is variation in the volume of his breath sounds across his lung fields. Auscultation of his heart detects no abnormal sounds. His abdomen is soft and nontender with normal bowel sounds. He is actively moving all extremities and has normal reflexes. The following vital signs are measured:

T: 99.4°F, HR: 90 bpm, BP: 104/76 mm Hg, RR: 22 breaths/min

Differential Diagnosis

- Recurrent pneumonia, cystic fibrosis, human immunodeficiency virus (HIV), agammaglobulinemia, leukopenia without immune deficiency, common variable immunodeficiency, IgA deficiency, severe combined immunodeficiency, DiGeorge syndrome, hyper-IgM disease, Wiskott-Aldich syndrome, Fanconi anemia

Laboratory Data and Other Study Results

- Length, weight, and head circumference: 31″ (41th percentile), 24 lb (40th percentile), 18.5″ (41th percentile)
- CBC: WBC: 7.2, Hgb: 14.1, Plt: 402
- Lymphocyte flow cytometry: T cells: normal, B cells: significantly decreased
- Chem10: Na: 138 mEq/L, K: 4.0 mEq/L, Cl: 103 mEq/L, CO_2: 28 mEq/L, BUN: 14 mg/dL, Cr: 0.7 mg/dL, Glu: 81 mg/dL, Mg: 2.1 mg/dL, Ca: 10.1 mg/dL, Phos: 4.4 mg/dL
- HIV ELISA: negative
- Sweat test: Cl: 29 mEq/L, Na: 28 mEq/L
- CXR: mild patchy infiltrates in both lung bases; no areas of consolidation; no lymphadenopathy

The following additional tests are then performed:

- IgA: 0 mg/dL
- IgG: 79 mg/dL
- IgM: 0 mg/dL
- IgE: 0.002 mg/dL

Diagnosis

- Agammaglobulinemia (X-linked)

Treatment Administered

- Regular infusions of IV immunoglobulin were initiated
- Bronchodilators and inhaled corticosteroids were prescribed for an as needed basis
- The measles, mumps, rubella (MMR) vaccine and varicella zoster vaccine (VZV) were withheld, but all other vaccines were administered on schedule

Follow-up

- Annual pulmonary function tests (PFTs) were started at the age of 5 years
- Aggressive antibiotic regimens were prescribed in cases of respiratory infection
- By consistently adhering to a regular IV immunoglobulin schedule, the patient was doing well into his adolescent years with no significant pulmonary complications at the time of most recent follow-up

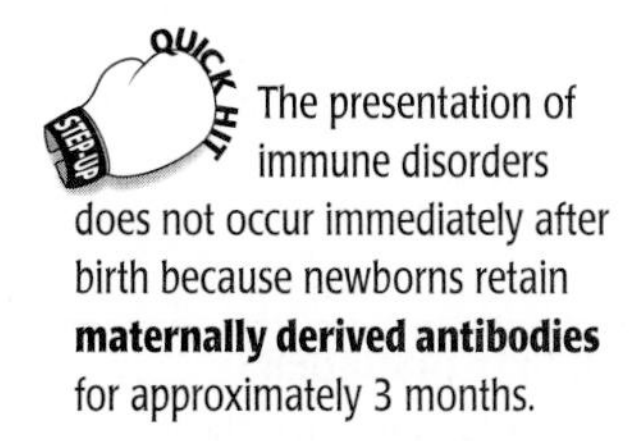

The presentation of immune disorders does not occur immediately after birth because newborns retain **maternally derived antibodies** for approximately 3 months.

Steps to the Diagnosis

- **X-linked agammaglobulinemia**
    - A defect in B lymphocyte differentiation leading to **low B cell and immunoglobulin** levels (Table 6-11)
        - Occurs as a X-linked disorder affecting only males, with females acting as carriers
    - **History: recurrent sinopulmonary bacterial infections** that become more common after 6 months of age, diarrhea that cannot be explained by antibiotic use, chronic cough, possible arthralgias, and symptoms of inflammatory bowel disease in adulthood
    - **Physical examination:** hypoplastic tonsils and lymph nodes, rhonchi, rales, wheezing
    - **Tests:**
        - Normal WBC count
        - Flow cytometry detects very low levels of B lymphocytes
        - **Low IgG levels; undetectable IgA and IgM levels**
    - **Treatment:**
        - **IV immunoglobulin (IVIG)** is able to maintain the humoral immune defenses and can provide a normal life if given on a regular basis
        - Aggressive and prolonged antibiotic therapy for bacterial infections
        - Bronchodilators and inhaled corticosteroids help improve symptoms during respiratory disease
        - Live vaccines (e.g., MMR, VZV) should be avoided because of the risk of inducing the respective infections
    - **Outcomes:** patients on IVIG frequently live into their fifth decade
    - **Clues to the diagnosis:**
        - History: recurrent pulmonary infections, diarrhea
        - Physical: undetectable tonsils, signs of pulmonary infection
        - Tests: decreased B cell numbers, low immunoglobulin levels
- **Recurrent pneumonia**
    - More thorough discussion in Chapter 2
    - **Why eliminated from differential:** three episodes of pneumonia in 15 months is unusual in a child without an underlying condition; the low B cell and immunoglobulin levels confirm that there is an immune disorder causing these infections
- **Cystic fibrosis**
    - More thorough discussion in Chapter 2
    - **Why eliminated from differential:** the negative sweat test rules out this diagnosis
- **Human immunodeficiency virus**
    - More thorough discussion in later case
    - **Why eliminated from differential:** the negative HIV ELISA test rules out this diagnosis
- **Leukopenia without immune deficiency**
    - Decreased **lymphocyte** or **neutrophil** (i.e., agranulocytosis) counts that are not attributable to an underlying immune disorder

TABLE 6-11 Types of Congenital Immunodeficiency Disorders

Disease	Description	Diagnosis	Treatment
T CELL DISORDERS			
DiGeorge syndrome	• Chromosomal deletion in 22q11 resulting in **thymic and parathyroid hypoplasia**, **congenital heart disease**, tetany, and abnormal facial structure • Recurrent viral and fungal infections occur because of insufficient T cells	• **Tetany** and **facial abnormalities** on examination • Decreased serum calcium • Evidence of congenital heart disease • CXR may show absence of thymic shadow • Genetic screening can detect chromosomal abnormality	• Calcium, vitamin D, thymic transplant, bone marrow transplant, surgical correction of heart abnormalities • IVIG or prophylactic antibiotics may be helpful to prevent infections
Chronic mucocutaneous candidiasis	• Persistent infection of skin, mucous membranes, and nails by ***Candida albicans*** due to T cell deficiency • Frequent associated adrenal pathology	• Poor reaction to cutaneous *C. albicans* anergy test • Possible decreased IgG	• Antifungal agents (e.g., fluconazole)
B CELL DISORDERS			
X-linked agammaglobulinemia	• Abnormal B cell differentiation resulting in low B cell and antibody levels • X-linked disorder with **boys** experiencing recurrent sinopulmonary infections after 6 months of age	• **No B cells in peripheral smear** • Low total immunoglobulin levels	• IVIG, appropriate antibiotics, supportive pulmonary care
IgA deficiency	• Specific IgA deficiency due to an abnormal immunoglobulin production by B cells • Patients have increased incidence of respiratory and gastrointestinal infections and food allergies	• **Decreased IgA** with **normal** levels of **other immune globulins**	• Prophylactic antibiotics • IVIG is infrequently used because of an increased risk of anaphylaxis
Hyper-IgM disease	• Defect in T cell CD40 ligand resulting in a poor interaction with B cells that leads to low IgG and excessive IgM • Infections by **encapsulated bacteria** (pulmonary and GI) are common	• Decreased IgG and IgA, **increased IgM** • Possible decreased Hgb, Hct, platelets, and neutrophils	• IVIG, prophylactic antibiotics • Bone marrow transplant
Common variable immunodeficiency	• Autosomal disorder of B cell differentiation into plasma cells leading to low immunoglobulin levels • Patients experience recurrent respiratory and GI infections beginning in second decade of life • Associated with increased risk of **malignant neoplasms** and **autoimmune disorders**	• Decreased but not absent immunoglobulin levels • Poor response to vaccines • Decreased CD4:CD8 T cell ratio • Family history shows **both men and women affected**	• IVIG, appropriate antibiotics
COMBINED B AND T CELL DISORDERS			
Severe combined immunodeficiency syndrome (SCID)	• Absence of T cells and frequently B cells resulting in **severe immune compromise** • Patients experience significant recurrent infections by all types of pathogens from an early age • **Frequently fatal at an early age**	• Significantly decreased WBCs, T cell counts are always low or absent, decreased immunoglobulins	• Isolation, antibiotics, **bone marrow transplant** • **No live or attenuated vaccines** should be administered

(*continued*)

TABLE 6-11 Types of Congenital Immunodeficiency Disorders (*Continued*)

Disease	Description	Diagnosis	Treatment
Wiskott-Aldrich syndrome	• X-linked disorder of actin polymerization in hematopoietic cells resulting in significant susceptibility to **encapsulated** bacteria and opportunistic pathogens • Associated with **eczema** and **thrombocytopenia**	• Recurrent infections in presence of **eczema** and **easy bleeding** • Decreased platelets, decreased IgM with normal or high other immune globulins • Genetic analysis detects abnormal *WASP* gene	• **Splenectomy**, antibiotic prophylaxis, IVIG, bone marrow transplant
Ataxia-telangiectasia	• Autosomal recessive disorder causing **cerebellar dysfunction**, **cutaneous telangiectasias**, increased risk of cancer, and impaired WBC and IgA development	• **Telangiectasia** and **ataxia** develop after third year of life • Recurrent pulmonary infections begin a few years later • Decreased WBCs and IgA	• IVIG and prophylactic antibiotics may be helpful, but treatment is usually unable to limit disease progression
PHAGOCYTIC CELL DISORDERS			
Chronic granulomatous disease	• Defect in neutrophils with **impaired phagocytosis** of bacteria, resulting in recurrent bacterial and fungal infections	• Cutaneous, pulmonary, and perirectal abscess formation • Chronic lymphadenopathy • Genetic analysis detects causative genetic mutations	• Prophylactic antibiotics, γ-interferon, corticosteroids, bone marrow transplant
Hyper-IgE disease	• Defect in neutrophil chemotaxis, T cell signaling, and overproduction of IgE that results in **chronic dermatitis**, **recurrent skin abscesses**, and pulmonary infections • Patients commonly have coarse facial features and retained primary teeth	• Increased IgE, increased eosinophils • Defective chemotactic response of neutrophils upon stimulation	• Prophylactic antibiotics • Skin hydration and emollient use
Chediak-Higashi syndrome	• Autosomal recessive dysfunction of intracellular protein transport in neutrophils and other cell resulting in recurrent *Staphylococcus aureus*, streptococcal, Gram-negative bacteria, and fungal infections • Associated with **abnormal platelets**, **albinism**, and **neurologic dysfunction**	• Large granules seen in granulocytes on peripheral smear	• Prophylactic antibiotics, bone marrow transplant
Leukocyte adhesion deficiency (types 1 and 2)	• Inability of neutrophils to leave circulation due to abnormal leukocyte integrins (type 1) or E-selectin (type 2) • Recurrent bacterial infections of upper respiratory tract and skin • Short stature, abnormal facies, and cognitive impairment seen in type 2 disease	• Increased serum neutrophils • Defective chemotactic response of neutrophils upon stimulation	• Prophylactic antibiotics • Bone marrow transplant needed in type 1 disease • Type 2 disease treated with fucose supplementation
COMPLEMENT DISORDERS			
Complement deficiencies	• Multiple inherited deficiencies of one or more complement components resulting in recurrent bacterial infections and **predisposition to autoimmune disorders (i.e., SLE)**	• Hemolytic complement tests are abnormal and indicate problem in pathway • Direct testing of components can detect exact deficiency	• Appropriate antibiotics • Treat autoimmune disorders as needed

CXR, chest x-ray; GI, gastrointestinal; Hct, hematocrit; Hgb, hemoglobin; Ig, immunoglobulin; IVIG, intravenous immune globulin; SLE, systemic lupus erythematosus; TMP-SMX, trimethoprim-sulfamethoxazole; WBC, white blood cell.

    - May be due to diseases associated with an increased cortisol level, medications (e.g., chemotherapeutics, antithyroid drugs, trimethoprim-sulfamethoxazole [TMP-SMX]), radiation, viral infection (e.g., hepatitis, EBV), or aplastic anemia
  - **History: recurrent infections**, weakness, chills, exposure to an appropriate causal factor
  - **Physical examination:** fever
  - **Tests:** decreased WBCs (either lymphocytes or neutrophils, depending on which cell line is affected)
  - **Treatment:**
    - Stop exposure to the offending agent
    - Bone marrow transplant, granulocyte colony-stimulating factor, or corticosteroids may be required to induce repletion of the deficient cell line
    - Antibiotic therapy should be used to treat any suspected infection
  - **Outcomes:** prognosis is dependent on the ability to eliminate the inciting factor and restore the depleted leukocytes
  - **Why eliminated from differential:** the absence of exposure to an obvious agent and the normal WBC count make this diagnosis less likely
- **Common variable immunodeficiency**
  - More thorough discussion in Table 6-11
  - **Why eliminated from differential:** this diagnosis tends to occur later in childhood or adolescence, and the immunoglobulin levels tend to be higher than those seen in agammaglobulinemia, so the latter is a more likely diagnosis
- **IgA deficiency**
  - More thorough discussion in Table 6-11
  - **Why eliminated from differential:** deficiencies in all of the immunoglobulins and not just IgA in this case rules out this diagnosis
- **Severe combined immunodeficiency syndrome (SCID)**
  - More thorough discussion in Table 6-11
  - **Why eliminated from differential:** the maintained presence of T lymphocytes rules out this diagnosis
- **DiGeorge syndrome**
  - More thorough discussion in Table 6-11
  - **Why eliminated from differential:** the normal facial appearance, normal reflexes, and normal T lymphocyte numbers help to rule out this diagnosis
- **Hyper-IgM disease**
  - More thorough discussion in Table 6-11
  - **Why eliminated from differential:** the undetectable IgM level in this case rules out this diagnosis
- **Wiskott-Aldrich syndrome**
  - More thorough discussion in Table 6-11
  - **Why eliminated from differential:** the low levels of all immunoglobulins and not only IgM in this case rules out this diagnosis
- **Fanconi anemia**
  - An autosomal recessive disorder associated with bone marrow failure, pancytopenia, and an increased risk of leukemia
  - **History:** fatigue, dyspnea, frequent infections,
  - **Physical examination: short stature, abnormal skin pigmentation**, thumb abnormalities, abnormal gonads, microcephaly, possible anatomical defects of any organ system
  - **Tests:**
    - Decreased Hgb, WBCs, and platelets
    - Increased serum α-fetoprotein
    - Chromosome analysis demonstrates multiple strand breakages
    - Bone marrow biopsy shows hypocellularity
  - **Treatment:**
    - Antibiotics are required for infections
    - Transfusions, bone marrow transplant, or hematopoietic growth factors may be required to induce hematopoietic cell production
    - Androgens or corticosteroids may improve bone marrow activity

- **Outcomes:** prognosis is poor with death frequently occurring in childhood due to bone marrow failure or leukemia; aggressive use of blood products and marrow stimulation can prolong survival
- **Why eliminated from differential:** the normal cell count on the CBC rules out this diagnosis

CASE 6-4 "He just started having problems breathing"

A 47-year-old man is brought intubated into the emergency department via ambulance after the acute onset of dyspnea. He is accompanied by his wife who is able to quickly describe the chain of events that led to this presentation. She says that she was having lunch with her husband during their respective lunch hours. While eating a salad, her husband began to complain of tightness in his chest and difficulty breathing and swallowing. He also began to break out in a red rash. The patient's wife says that this is the first time she has ever seen this happen. She denies that he mentioned any difficulty breathing, feeling ill, or chest pain prior to the onset of his symptoms. She thought that he was choking and tried to perform the Heimlich maneuver, which did not improve his symptoms. Emergency medical services was called because of his continued difficulty breathing, and he was immediately placed on oxygen via a face mask. During transport to the hospital, the emergency medical technicians (EMTs) were forced to intubate the patient because of further worsening in his ability to breathe. The EMTs note that this procedure was performed with minimal difficulty, but that the patient was notable for moderate tracheal and glottic swelling. The patient's wife says that he has a history of gastric reflux for which he takes ranitidine. She is unaware of any allergies that he has, but he avoids eating peanuts because his father experienced a bad reaction to them on one occasion. She says he drinks about six alcoholic beverages per week and does not use any other substances. On examination, the patient is sedated and intubated. He has a palpable red rash over his face and upper body. Auscultation of his heart and lungs detects no extra heart sounds and significant wheezing in all lung fields. His abdomen is soft with normal bowel sounds. The patient opens his eyes when addressed. The following vital signs are measured:

T: 98.7°F, HR: 96 bpm, BP: 102/74 mm Hg, RR: 18 breaths/min while intubated

Differential Diagnosis

- Anaphylaxis, aspirated foreign body, myocardial infarction (MI), pulmonary embolism

Laboratory Data and Other Study Results

- Electrocardiogram (ECG): regular rate and rhythm; no abnormal wave morphology
- Arterial blood gas (ABG) (40% O_2): pH: 7.38, partial pressure of oxygen (pO_2): 228 mm Hg, partial pressure of carbon dioxide (pCO_2): 43 mm Hg, bicarbonate (Bicarb): 24 mEq/L, oxygen saturation (O_2 sat): 97%

Diagnosis

- Anaphylaxis

Treatment Administered

- Epinephrine, methylprednisolone, and diphenhydramine were immediately administered intravenously
- Albuterol was administered via the endotracheal tube

Follow-up

- Following the administration of treatment, the patient's oxygen saturation improved to 100%, and the urticaria began to resolve
- The patient was able to be extubated in the emergency department and was able to be weaned from supplemental oxygen
- A follow-up CXR detected no infiltrates or unventilated areas
- The patient was admitted overnight for observation and was discharged to home the next day
- Follow-up allergy testing detected a strong reaction to peanuts; discussion with the restaurant revealed that they used peanut oil in their salad dressing
- The patient was provided a portable subcutaneous epinephrine injector and instructed to avoid any food containing peanuts or peanut oil

Steps to the Diagnosis

- **Anaphylaxis**
  - A severe type I hypersensitivity reaction following exposure to an allergen (e.g., penicillin, insect stings, latex, certain foods)
    - Hypersensitivity reactions are allergen-induced immune responses involving either cellular or humoral mechanisms (Table 6-12)
  - **History**: symptoms occur 5 to 60 minutes after exposure and include skin tingling, pruritis, cough, chest tightness, **difficulty swallowing and breathing** (secondary to angioedema), and syncope
  - **Physical examination**: tachycardia, **urticaria**, **hypotension**, arrhythmias
  - **Tests**:
    - Typically a clinical diagnosis in the acute setting
    - Skin allergen testing or radioallergosorbent testing (RAST) can confirm a specific allergic response
    - Increased histamine and tryptase levels are apparent immediately following exposure

MNEMONIC

The types of hypersensitivity reactions may be remembered by the mnemonic **ACID**: **A**naphylactic, **C**omplement-mediated, **I**mmune complex-mediated, **D**elayed.

TABLE 6-12 Types of Hypersensitivity Reactions

Type	Mediated By	Mechanism	Examples	Treatment
I	IgE antibodies attached to mast cells	Allergens react with antibodies to cause **mast cell degranulation** and histamine release	Allergic rhinitis, asthma, **anaphylaxis**	**Epinephrine**, **antihistamines**, leukotriene inhibitors, bronchodilators, or corticosteroids used during an acute reaction; **desensitization** is considered to avoid recurrent reactions
II	IgM and IgG antibodies	Allergens react with antibodies to initiate **complement cascade** and cell death	**Drug-induced or immune hemolytic anemia**, hemolytic disease of the newborn	Anti-inflammatories or immunosuppressive agents
III	IgM and IgG immune complexes	Antibodies form **immune complexes** with allergens which are then deposited in tissue and initiate complement cascade	Arthus reaction, serum sickness, glomerulonephritis	Anti-inflammatories
IV	T cells and macrophages	**T cells** present allergens to macrophages and secrete lymphokines that induce macrophages to destroy surrounding tissue	Transplant rejection, **allergic contact dermatitis**, PPD testing	Corticosteroids or other immunosuppressive agents

Ig, immunoglobulin; PPD, purified protein derivative.

- **Treatment:**
  - **Subcutaneous or IV epinephrine** is administered to maintain blood pressure and decrease angioedema by inducing vasoconstriction
  - **Intubation** must be considered if airway patency is at risk
  - **Antihistamines** and corticosteroids are important to reduce the acute inflammatory reaction to the allergen
  - Bronchodilators are used to decrease bronchoconstriction
  - Continued vasopressor use may be required for recalcitrant hypotension
  - Patient should be observed for at least 12 hours after the reaction because of the rare incidence of delayed rebound anaphylactic reactions in some patients
  - Avoidance of the particular allergen is the key to avoiding recurrence; subcutaneous epinephrine injectors should be carried at all times to avoid a reaction to future exposures
  - Desensitization therapy may be appropriate following recurrent episodes
  - It can only be performed for IgE-mediated type I hypersensitivity reactions
  - **Anaphylactoid** reactions (i.e., non-IgE-mediated mast cell degranulation) cannot be treated with desensitization
- **Outcomes:** mortality and morbidity correlates with delays in treatment and the inability to maintain a patent airway
- **Clues to the diagnosis:**
  - History: reaction while eating, acute difficulty swallowing and breathing
  - Physical: urticaria, wheezing, glottic edema
  - Tests: noncontributory in the acute setting (postevent allergy testing helps to confirm the diagnosis)

- **Aspirated foreign body**
  - More thorough discussion in Chapter 2
  - **Why eliminated from differential:** the lack of visualization of a foreign body during intubation and the presence of adequate oxygenation following the intubation make this diagnosis less likely
- **Myocardial infarction**
  - More thorough discussion in Chapter 1
  - **Why eliminated from differential:** the normal-appearing ECG makes this diagnosis less likely
- **Pulmonary embolism**
  - More thorough discussion in Chapter 2
  - **Why eliminated from differential:** the normal A-a gradient, adequate oxygen saturation following intubation, and normal ECG all make this diagnosis unlikely

The following additional Hematology and Oncology cases may be found online:

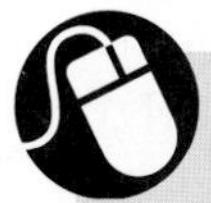

CASE 6-5 "My face is horribly bruised"

CASE 6-6 "My cousin is wasting away"

CASE 6-7 "All of my blood cells are low"

CASE 6-8 "My baby is going yellow"

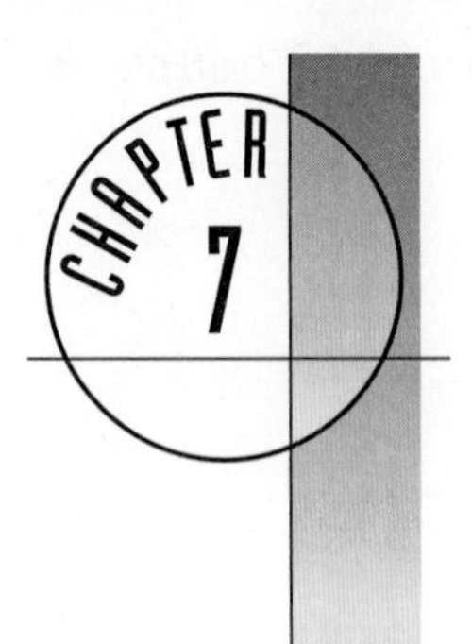

Neurology

MNEMONIC

The order of cranial nerves may be remembered by the mnemonic "**O**oh, **O**oh, **O**oh, **T**o **T**ouch **A**nd **F**eel **V**ery **G**reen **V**egetables, **A**h **H**eaven!": **O**lfactory, **O**ptic, **O**culomotor, **T**rochlear, **T**rigeminal, **A**bducens, **F**acial, **V**estibulocochlear, **G**lossopharyngeal, **V**agus, **A**ccessory, **H**ypoglossal.

MNEMONIC

The function (sensory, motor, or both) of the cranial nerves may be remembered by the mnemonic "**S**ome **S**ay **M**arry **M**oney, **B**ut **M**y **B**rother **S**ays **B**ig **B**rains **M**atter **M**ost": **S**ensory, **S**ensory, **M**otor, **M**otor, **B**oth, **M**otor, **B**oth, **S**ensory, **B**oth, **B**oth, **M**otor, **M**otor (in order of cranial nerves).

QUICK HIT: First-order neurons are **preganglionic**; second-order neurons are **postganglionic**.

QUICK HIT: Upper motor neuron conditions are those that originate in the brain or first-order neurons; lower motor neuron conditions are those caused by pathology in second-order neurons.

QUICK HIT: Rapid eye movements (REM) and dreams occur during REM sleep.

BASIC CLINICAL PRIMER

NEUROANATOMY

- **Vasculature**
  - The **circle of Willis** forms the backbone of the cerebral vasculature (Figure 7-1, Table 7-1)
- **Neurons**
  - Cranial nerves originate in cerebral nerve roots and function primarily in the head and neck (Table 7-2)
  - The spinal cord is organized into distinct tracts of sensory and motor neurons (Figure 7-2, Table 7-3)

SLEEP

- Sleep cycles are divided into several stages that describe the depth of sleep and the corresponding electroencephalogram (EEG) activity (Table 7-4)

CASE 7-1 "My neck feels really stiff"

A 19-year-old man presents to his college's student health office because of a constant headache and neck pain that has worsened over the past 3 days. The headache is diffuse but is worse posteriorly. He says that a few other people in his dorm have come down with similar symptoms, and he is concerned that they all have a similar illness. He denies having had these symptoms previously. He has been unable to eat for the past day because he feels nauseous. He did not go to class yesterday or today because he did not feel well. He denies any recent head or spine trauma or animal or insect bites. He denies any past medical history and does not take any medications regularly. He has been taking ibuprofen over the past few days and says that it has had little benefit. He drinks heavily on weekends (last use 4 days ago) and denies other substance use. On examination, he is an ill-appearing young adult. He asks that the examination room lights be dimmed because the bright lights worsen his headache. Fundoscopic examination is normal. He has no palpable lymphadenopathy. He has scattered red petechiae on his trunk. Flexion of his neck does not change his perceived neck pain. Auscultation of his heart and lungs is normal. His abdomen is nontender with no masses, but palpation worsens his nausea. His sensory and motor function is normal, but he is slow to move because of his neck pain. The following vital signs are measured:

Temperature (T): 102.3°F, heart rate (HR): 96 beats per minute (bpm), blood pressure (BP): 110/80 mm Hg, respiratory rate (RR): 20 breaths/min

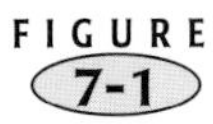

(A) Arteries of the brain, including the circle of Willis, and their anatomical relationship to selected cranial nerves. (B) Arterial blood supply to the cortex. CN, cranial nerve.

A. Arteries of the base of the brain and brainstem

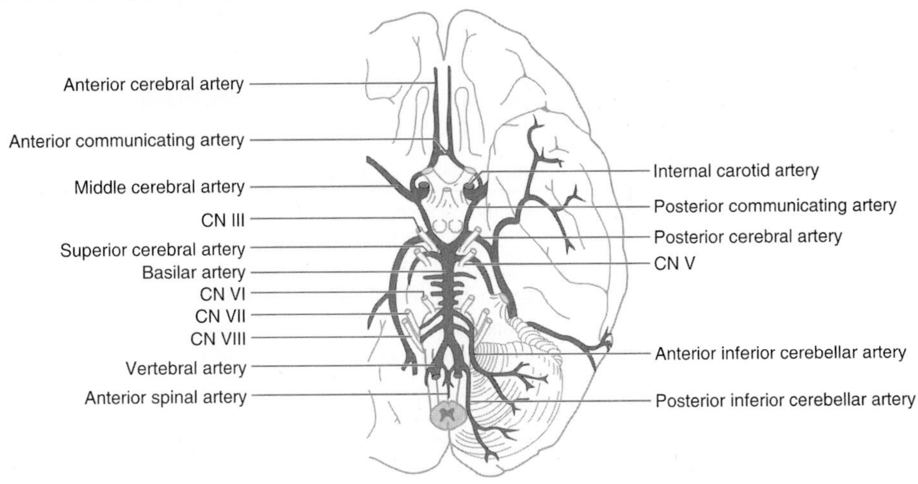

B. Arterial blood supply to the cortex

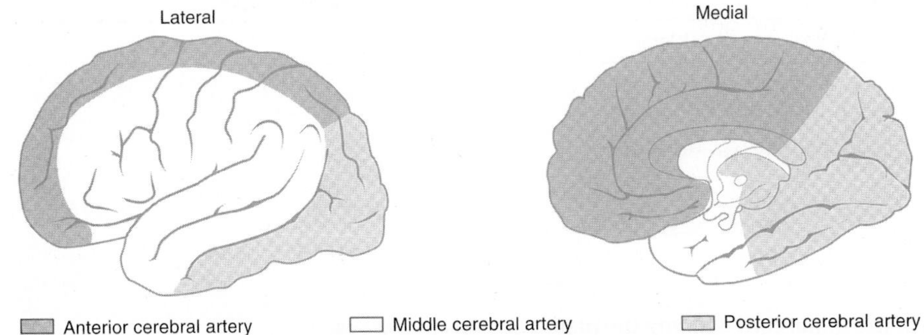

(Taken from Mehta S, Milder EA, Mirachi AJ, Milder E. *Step-up: a high-yield, systems-based review for the USMLE step 1.* 2nd ed. Philadelphia: Lippincott Williams & Wilkins, 2003. Used with permission of Lippincott Williams & Wilkins.)

Differential Diagnosis

- Bacterial meningitis, viral meningitis, alcohol intoxication/withdrawal, migraine headache, cluster headache, tension headache, mononucleosis, cerebrovascular accident, subarachnoid hemorrhage, brain abscess, viral encephalitis, rabies, cervical spine injury

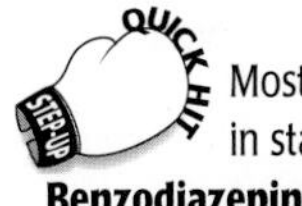

Most of sleep is spent in stage 2. **Benzodiazepines** increase stage 2 sleep and decrease stages 3 and 4, and do not reproduce the normal sleep architecture.

TABLE 7-1 Regions of the Brain Supplied by Vessels in the Circle of Willis

Artery	Region of Brain Supplied
Anterior cerebral artery	Medial and superior surfaces and frontal lobes
Middle cerebral artery	Lateral surfaces and temporal lobes
Posterior cerebral artery	Inferior surfaces and occipital lobes
Basilar artery	Midbrain, brainstem (pons)
Anterior inferior cerebellar artery	Brainstem (pons)
Posterior inferior cerebellar artery	Brainstem (medulla)

TABLE 7-2 Cranial Nerves and Their Functions

Nerve	Type	Function/Innervation
Olfactory (CN I)	Sensory	Smell
Optic (CN II)	Sensory	Sight
Oculomotor (CN III)	Motor	Medial/superior/inferior rectus muscles, inferior oblique muscle, ciliary muscle, sphincter muscle of eye
Trochlear (CN IV)	Motor	Superior oblique muscle of eye
Trigeminal (CN V)	Both	Sensation of face; muscles of mastication
Abducens (CN VI)	Motor	Lateral rectus muscle of eye
Facial (CN VII)	Both	Taste (anterior two thirds of tongue); muscles of facial expression, stapedius muscle, stylohyoid muscle, digastric muscle (posterior belly); lacrimal, submandibular, sublingual glands
Vestibulocochlear (CN VIII)	Sensory	Hearing, balance
Glossopharyngeal (CN IX)	Both	Taste (posterior one third of tongue), pharyngeal sensation; stylopharyngeus muscle; parotid gland
Vagus (CN X)	Both	Sensation of trachea, esophagus, viscera; laryngeal, pharyngeal muscles; visceral autonomics
Accessory (CN XI)	Motor	Sternocleidomastoid and trapezius muscles
Hypoglossal (CN XII)	Motor	Tongue

CN, cranial nerve.

FIGURE 7-2 **(Cross-sectional anatomy of the spinal cord defining the main neuronal pathways. Generally for each pathway, fibers closer to the center of the cord supply the upper body, and fibers closer to the periphery supply the lower half of the body.**

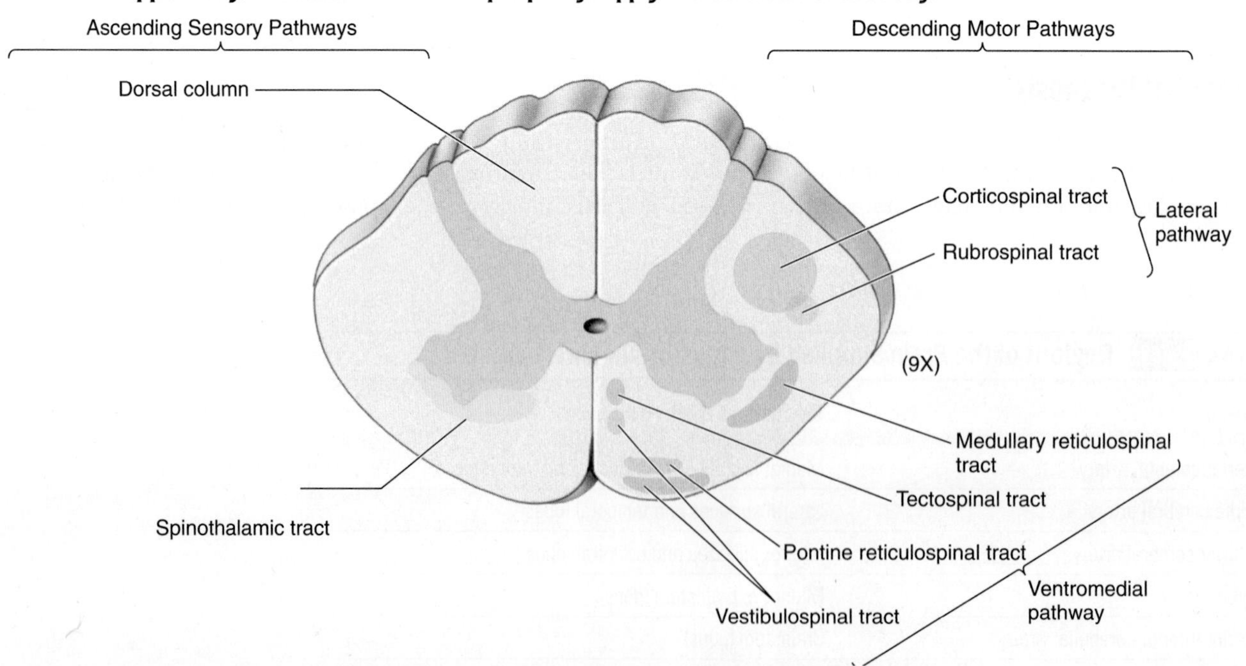

(Taken from Bear MF, Connors BW, Parasido MA. *Neuroscience–exploring the brain*. 2nd ed. Philadelphia: Lippincott Williams & Wilkins, 2001. Fig. 7A-35. Used with permission of Lippincott Williams & Wilkins.)

TABLE 7-3 Primary Sensory and Motor Tracts of the Spinal Cord

Pathway	Location	First-Order Neurons	Second-Order Neurons	Function
Dorsal columns	Posterior spinal cord	Enter at ipsilateral dorsal horn, ascend in fasciculus gracilis and cuneatus, synapse in nucleus gracilis and cuneatus	Decussate at medulla, ascend as medial lemniscus	**Two point discrimination**, sense vibration, sense **proprioception**
Spinothalamic tract	Anterior spinal cord	Originate in dorsal root ganglion, synapse in dorsolateral tract of Lissauer	Decussate in ventral white commissure, ascend in lateral spinothalamic tract	**Senses pain**, senses **temperature**
Corticospinal tract	Lateral spinal cord	Descend from internal capsule and midbrain, decussate in medullary pyramids, descend in corticospinal tract, synapse in ventral horn through interneurons	Exit cord through ventral horn	**Voluntary movement** of striated muscle

Laboratory Data and Other Study Results

The patient is immediately sent to the local emergency department where the following tests are performed:

- Complete blood cell count (CBC): white blood cells (WBC): 21.6, hemoglobin (Hgb): 14.1, platelets (Plt): 412
- 7-electrolyte chemistry panel (Chem7): sodium (Na): 141 mEq/L, potassium (K): 4.5 mEq/L, chloride (Cl): 102 mEq/L, carbon dioxide (CO_2): 27 mEq/L, blood urea nitrogen (BUN): 17 mg/dL, creatinine (Cr): 0.5 mg/dL, glucose (Glu): 89 mg/dL
- Liver function tests (LFTs): alkaline phosphatase (AlkPhos): 78 U/L, alanine aminotransferase (ALT): 34 U/L, aspartate aminotransferase (AST): 23 U/L, total bilirubin (TBili): 1.1 mg/dL, direct bilirubin (DBili): 0.3 mg/dL
- Ethyl alcohol (EtOH) level: 0 mg/dL
- Head and cervical spine computed tomography (CT): no hemorrhage; no cerebral atrophy; no focal lesions; no spinal fracture, dislocation, or malalignment

After receipt of these results, a lumbar puncture is performed with the following results:

- Appearance: cloudy
- Opening pressure: 230 mm Hg
- WBCs: 6,538/μL
- Glucose: 32 mg/dL
- Protein: 64 mg/dL

Diagnosis

- Bacterial meningitis

TABLE 7-4 Normal Stages of Sleep

Stage	Depth of Sleep	EEG
1	Light	Fast θ waves
2	Intermediate	Sleep spindles, k-complexes
3 and 4	Deep	δ waves
REM	Increased brain activity every 90–120 minutes of sleep	Low-voltage, high-frequency waves

EEG, electroencephalogram; REM, rapid eye movement.

Treatment Administered

- The patient was admitted to the hospital and immediately placed on dexamethasone and cefotaxime while cerebral spinal fluid (CSF) cultures were pending
- Cultures grew *Neisseria meningitides*, and the antibiotic was changed to ampicillin for a total of seven days of treatment

Follow-up

- Two other students in the same dorm room were diagnosed with *N. meningitides* and were treated in a similar fashion
- All close contacts of the infected students were administered prophylactic rifampin
- The patient was able to recover without any significant neurologic sequelae but continued to have intermittent headaches that gradually improved over 3 months

Steps to the Diagnosis

- **Bacterial meningitis**
  - Infection of the meningeal tissue surrounding the brain and spinal cord by a bacterial pathogen
    - The most common agents of infection vary by age group (Table 7-5)
    - Infection may be caused by close contact with infected individuals, hematogenous spread, local extension, or exposure of CSF to bacteria (e.g., neurosurgical procedures, skull fracture)
  - **Risk factors:** ear infection, sinusitis, immunocompromise, neurosurgery, maternal group β streptococcus infection during birth
  - **History:** headache, **neck pain**, photophobia, malaise, nausea, vomiting, confusion
  - **Physical examination:** fever, **Brudzinski sign** (i.e., neck flexion in a supine patient prompts reflexive hip flexion), **Kernig sign** (i.e., painful knee extension occurs with hip flexion in a supine patient), petechiae (especially *N. meningitides* infection), change in mental status, impaired consciousness, seizures
  - **Tests:**
    - Increased serum WBCs
    - Possible positive blood cultures
    - **Lumbar puncture** is the best diagnostic test and may be used to differentiate the causes of meningitis (Table 7-6)
      - CSF appearance, WBC count, protein level, glucose level, and culture are important analyses for CSF collected from a lumbar puncture
    - Imaging is rarely helpful for making the diagnosis
  - **Treatment:**
    - Empiric antibiotic therapy is started initially and usually consists of a **third-generation cephalosporin**
    - Intravenous (IV) corticosteroids have been shown to improve outcomes in some cases but are not helpful for all types of infection

NEUROLOGY

QUICK HIT: While considered "classic" signs of meningitis, **Kernig** and **Brudzinski** signs are **not reliable signs** for diagnosis and are particularly unreliable in **children**.

NEXT STEP: Neurologic examination must be performed before lumbar puncture. If there are signs of **increased intracranial pressure** (e.g., papilledema, focal neurologic deficits, pupil asymmetry), do **not** perform a lumbar puncture because of the increased risk of **uncal herniation**.

TABLE 7-5 Common Causes of Meningitis by Age Group

Age	Most Common Agent	Other Common Agents
Newborn	Group β streptococci	*Escherichia coli, Listeria, Haemophilus influenzae*
1 month–2 years old	*Streptococcus pneumoniae, Neisseria meningitidis*	Group β streptococci, *Listeria, H. influenzae*
2–18 years old	*N. meningitidis*	*S. pneumoniae, Listeria*
18–60 years old	*S. pneumoniae*	*N. meningitidis, Listeria*
60+ years old	*S. pneumoniae*	*Listeria*, Gram-negative rods

TABLE 7-6 Cerebral Spinal Fluid Findings for Different Causes of Meningitis

Status	WBCs	Pressure	Glucose	Protein
Healthy patient	<5	50–180 mm H_2O	40–70 mg/dL	20–45 mg/dL
Bacterial infection	↑↑ (PMNs)	↑↑	↓	↑
Viral infection	↑ (lymphocytes)	↑	Normal	Normal
Fungal infection or tuberculosis	↑ (lymphocytes)	↑↑	↓	↑

H_2O, water; PMNs, polymorphonuclear cells; WBCs, white blood cells; ↑, mild increase; ↑↑, significant increase.

- Specific antibiotic therapy is based on the CSF cultures
- Prophylactic **rifampin** may be given to close contacts of an infected patient
- **Outcomes:**
  - One third of patients will develop neurologic sequelae, including cranial nerve palsies, cerebral infarcts, and brain abscesses
  - Prognosis is best in healthy patients treated promptly with antibiotics
  - Immunocompromised patients and the very young and old have worse outcomes
- **Clues to the diagnosis:**
  - History: headache, neck pain, close contacts with similar symptoms, photophobia
  - Physical: fever, petechiae
  - Tests: increased serum WBCs, lumbar puncture results

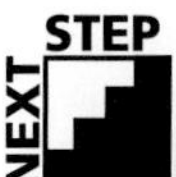

Treat fungal meningitis with amphotericin B, and treat tuberculosis meningitis with the combination of isoniazid, ethambutol, pyrazinamide, and rifampin.

- **Viral meningitis (a.k.a. aseptic meningitis)**
  - Meningitis due to infection by an enterovirus, echovirus, herpes simplex virus, lymphocytic choriomeningitis virus, or mumps virus
  - **History**: headache, neck pain, nausea, vomiting, photophobia, malaise
  - **Physical examination**: fever, viral rash
  - **Tests**: lumbar puncture is useful for differentiating this cause of meningitis from a bacterial cause (Table 7-6); viral culture provides a more definitive diagnosis
  - **Treatment**: empiric antibiotics are typically started while the results of a lumbar puncture are pending but may be stopped once a viral cause is suspected; supportive care only is required once the diagnosis has been established
  - **Outcomes**: the prognosis is **better** than for bacterial meningitis, and most patients fully recover
  - **Why eliminated from differential**: the results of the lumbar puncture rule out this diagnosis

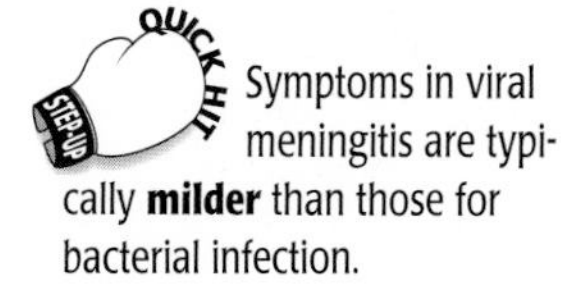

Symptoms in viral meningitis are typically **milder** than those for bacterial infection.

- **Migraine headache**
  - More thorough discussion in later case
  - **Why eliminated from differential**: the length of symptoms, diffuse nature of the headache, lack of an aura, and poor response to nonsteroidal anti-inflammatory drugs (NSAIDs) make this diagnosis unlikely
- **Cluster headache**
  - More thorough discussion in later case
  - **Why eliminated from differential**: the length of symptoms, diffuse nature of the headache, and lack of Horner syndrome make this diagnosis unlikely
- **Tension headache**
  - More thorough discussion in later case
  - **Why eliminated from differential**: this diagnosis would be considered until the further testing ruled it out (i.e., lumbar puncture, CBC), but the length of symptoms would make it less likely
- **Alcohol intoxication/withdrawal**
  - More thorough discussion in Chapter 13
  - **Why eliminated from differential**: given the patient's drinking history, this diagnosis should be considered, but the lab values rule it out as a diagnosis

- **Cerebrovascular accident/subarachnoid hemorrhage**
  - More thorough discussion in later case
  - **Why eliminated from differential:** the normal-appearing head CT rules out these diagnoses
- **Mononucleosis**
  - More thorough discussion in Chapter 6
  - **Why eliminated from differential:** this diagnosis should be seriously considered, but is less likely given the lack of lymphadenopathy; the lumbar puncture results further rule it out
- **Viral encephalitis**
  - Inflammation of brain parenchyma due to **viral** infection
    - Varicella zoster virus, herpes simplex virus, mumps virus, poliovirus, rhabdovirus, Coxsackie virus, arbovirus, flavivirus, and measles virus are all common pathogens
    - The condition may actually reflect an immunologic response to systemic viral infection
  - **History:** malaise, headache, vomiting, neck pain
  - **Physical examination:** decreased consciousness, **focal neurologic deficits** (e.g., hemiparesis, pathologic reflexes, palsies), fever, **change in mental status**, possible skin lesions (for herpes virus), possible parotid swelling (for mumps), possible flaccid paralysis with a maculopapular rash (for West Nile virus)
  - **Tests:**
    - Lumbar puncture shows increased WBCs and a normal glucose
    - CSF cultures frequently are negative and are not reliable
    - Serologic viral testing is useful to identify a pathogen
    - Brain biopsy may provide a definitive diagnosis but is generally impractical
    - CT and magnetic resonance imaging (MRI) may show cerebral inflammation with an associated effusion
  - **Treatment:** supportive care (e.g., maintenance of normal intracranial pressure, seizure prophylaxis); antivirals may demonstrate some usefulness to improving outcomes
  - **Outcomes:** neurologic sequelae happen in up to 40% of patients and include seizures and motor dysfunction; mortality varies significantly between causative viruses
  - **Why eliminated from differential:** the lack of neurologic deficits and the results of the lumbar puncture rule out this diagnosis

QUICK HIT: Common arboviruses include the St. Louis and California strains. Common flaviviruses include the **West Nile** and Japanese strains.

QUICK HIT: In young children encephalitis may be due to **Reye syndrome** (i.e., reaction in children with a viral infection who are given aspirin [ASA]).

- **Brain abscess**
  - A collection of purulent material in the brain parenchyma that results from extension of a local bacterial infection, head wound, or hematogenous spread of bacteria
  - **History: headache**, neck pain, malaise, vomiting
  - **Physical examination:** change in mental status, focal neurologic deficits, papilledema, seizures
  - **Tests:** MRI or CT is useful to detect the lesion; CT-guided biopsy may be used to culture the abscess fluid and determine the bacterial identity
  - **Treatment: surgical drainage** is required; empiric antibiotics and corticosteroids are administered until the culture results are finalized
  - **Outcomes:** the prognosis is poor with any delays to diagnosis or therapeutic intervention
  - **Why eliminated from differential:** the negative head CT and normal fundoscopic examination help to rule out this diagnosis
- **Rabies**
  - Rhabdovirus infection transmitted to humans via the **bite of an infected animal**
    - Infection causes a severe encephalitis with neuronal degeneration and cerebral inflammation
  - **History:** malaise, headache, restlessness, painful laryngospasms, **fear of water ingestion** (secondary to laryngospasm)
  - **Physical examination:** significant CNS excitability, **foaming at the mouth**, **alternating mania and stupor**
  - **Tests:**
    - A suspected animal should be caught and tested or observed for signs of rabies
    - Animals suspected of infection should be euthanized, and their brains should be tested for the presence of the virus and histologic **Negri bodies** (i.e., round eosinophilic inclusions within the neurons)

  - Viral testing of symptomatic patients (including CSF, skin, and serum) provides a confirmatory diagnosis
- **Treatment:** animal bites should be thoroughly cleaned and bandaged; rabies immunoglobulin and vaccine should be administered promptly to any patient bitten by an infected or suspicious animal
- **Outcomes:** once symptoms develop, mortality is nearly 100%
- **Why eliminated from differential:** the absence of a history of being bitten by any animals makes this diagnosis unlikely

- **Cervical spine injury**
  - More thorough discussion in later case and in Chapter 9
  - **Why eliminated from differential:** the normal-appearing cervical spine CT makes this diagnosis unlikely

CASE 7-2 "My head is killing me"

A 19-year-old man presents to his college's student health office with recurrent severe headaches. He says that his pain is located in the front of his head near his forehead and eye and on the right side only. He has no pain in his neck. The headaches have been intermittent in nature over the past 5 days and have occurred about three times each day. Each headache lasts approximately 1 hour before resolving. During these headaches the patient has nasal congestion on the right side but has no upper respiratory symptoms in between headaches. He denies any visual abnormalities prior to the headaches. He also denies any numbness or weakness in any of his extremities. He says that he had a similar experience 2 years ago. At that time he had several headaches over a 1-week period that self-resolved, and he has had no recurrences until the present time. A head CT performed during the previous episode was normal. He has a history of childhood asthma that has improved with age, and he no longer requires any medications other than antihistamines during peak seasonal allergy periods. He drinks socially and estimates that he consumes eight alcoholic beverages per week. He says that he used marijuana two times in his previous year at school but has not used this substance in over a year. On examination, he is a well-developed, tall young man who appears mildly uncomfortable. He has a mild lid sag in his right eye. His right eye conjunctiva is mildly injected, and his pupils are asymmetric (the right is smaller). Fundoscopic examination of both eyes is normal. There are no lesions visible on his face or body. He has no lymphadenopathy. Flexion of his neck while he is supine does not elicit any pain. Auscultation of his heart and lungs is normal. His abdomen is nontender with no masses, and he has regular bowel sounds. All of his extremities have normal and symmetric motor and sensory function, and his gait is normal. The following vital signs are measured:

T: 98.5°F, HR: 88 bpm, BP: 133/87 mm Hg, RR: 17 breaths/min

Differential Diagnosis

- Migraine headache, cluster headache, tension headache, sinusitis, cerebrovascular accident, viral meningitis, bacterial meningitis, subarachnoid hemorrhage, shingles, trigeminal neuralgia

Laboratory Data and Other Study Results

- CBC: WBC: 6.6, Hgb: 15.2, Plt: 285
- Head MRI: no masses within the brain or face; no areas of hemorrhage or ischemia

Diagnosis

- Cluster headaches

Treatment Administered

- The patient was placed on oral sumatriptan and low-dose verapamil
- Sumatriptan was stopped after 3 days with no additional headaches

Follow-up

- The patient continued to take low-dose verapamil for prophylaxis
- The patient experienced a single similar headache 9 months later after a night of high alcohol consumption; after restarting sumatriptan, he experienced no additional headaches during that episode
- The patient was able to remain headache free by remaining on verapamil and refraining from heavy drinking

Steps to the Diagnosis

- **Cluster headache**
  - A primary headache disorder affecting young men that is poorly understood and typified by recurrent (i.e., "**clustered**") severe headaches (Table 7-7)
    - Clusters may last for a week up to a year
    - **Alcohol** and vasodilators have been suggested as precipitating factors
  - **History:** severe unilateral headaches in the periorbital region that last 30 minutes to 3 hours, nasal congestion, lacrimation
  - **Physical examination:** possible Horner syndrome (i.e., ptosis, miosis, anhydrosis), conjunctival injection, diaphoresis
  - **Tests:** typically this is a clinical diagnosis, but head and neck imaging may be useful to rule out other diagnoses
  - **Treatment:** ergots, 100% oxygen, or sumatriptan are used to break acute headaches; tricyclic antidepressants, calcium channel blockers, β-blockers, and ergots may be used as prophylaxis

NEXT STEP
Any sudden onset of severe headache or focal neurologic deficits should be further examined using **CT without contrast** or MRI to rule out hemorrhage.

NEUROLOGY

TABLE 7-7 Primary Headache Disorders

Variable	Migraine	Cluster	Tension
Patients	10–30 years old, **female** more commonly than male	Young **men**	Female and male
Pathology	Incompletely understood but related to generalized dysfunctional cerebral activity	Poorly understood but likely an extracerebral cause	Poorly understood but related to muscular and psychogenic causes
Precipitating factors	Stress, oral contraceptives, **menstruation**, exertion, foods containing tyramine or nitrates (e.g., chocolate, cheese, processed meats)	Alcohol, vasodilators	Stress, fatigue, depression
Pain characteristics	Unilateral, throbbing	Severe, unilateral, **periorbital**, recurrent (i.e., "in clusters" over time)	**Bilateral**, head or scalp tightness, occipital or neck pain
Other symptoms	**Nausea**, **vomiting**, preceding aura (i.e., visual abnormalities), photophobia, temporary neurologic deficits	**Horner syndrome** (i.e., ptosis, myosis, anhidrosis), lacrimation, nasal congestion	Anxiety, insomnia, photophobia
Duration	4–72 hours	30 minutes–3 hours per headache; clusters last 1 week–1 year	30 minutes–1 week
Acute treatment	NSAIDs, ergots, sumatriptan, possible antiemetics	100% O_2, ergots, sumatriptan	NSAIDs, ergots, sumatriptan, relaxation exercises
Prophylactic treatment	Tricyclic antidepressants, β-blockers, calcium channel blockers, ergots	Tricyclic antidepressants, β-blockers, calcium channel blockers, ergots	Treating underlying depression and stress helps reduce frequency
Outcomes	Typically recurrent but responsive to abortive therapies	Typically recurrent but becomes a near-constant chronic disorder in 15% of cases	Correction of the underlying factors reduces frequency

O_2, oxygen; NSAIDs, nonsteroidal anti-inflammatory drugs.

- **Outcomes:** the disease course will be episodic in most patients, with a small subset developing near continuous clusters
- **Clues to the diagnosis:**
  - History: multiple headaches in a brief period of time, nature of headaches (e.g., unilateral, periorbital, severe), nasal congestion
  - Physical: Horner syndrome
  - Tests: noncontributory

- **Migraine headache**
  - More thorough discussion in Table 7-7
  - **Why eliminated from differential:** the absence of auras and recurrent nature of the headaches makes this diagnosis less likely
- **Tension headache**
  - More thorough discussion in Table 7-7
  - **Why eliminated from differential:** the nature of the headaches (e.g., location, frequency) makes this diagnosis unlikely
- **Sinusitis**
  - More thorough discussion in Chapter 2
  - **Why eliminated from differential:** the absence of continuous upper respiratory symptoms makes this diagnosis unlikely
- **Cerebrovascular accident/subarachnoid hemorrhage**
  - More thorough discussion in later case
  - **Why eliminated from differential:** the negative head MRI rules out these diagnoses
- **Bacterial/viral meningitis**
  - More thorough discussion in prior case
  - **Why eliminated from differential:** the absence of fever and neck pain and the normal serum WBC count rule out these diagnoses
- **Shingles**
  - More thorough discussion in Chapter 10
  - **Why eliminated from differential:** the absence of skin lesions rules out this diagnosis
- **Trigeminal neuralgia**
  - Significant head and **facial pain** due to compression or irritation of the trigeminal nerve root
  - **History:** sudden severe pain in the trigeminal nerve maxillary and mandibular distributions that lasts from a few seconds to a couple of minutes and recurs throughout the day
  - **Physical examination:** stimulation of "trigger points" in the affected nerve distribution may induce pain
  - **Tests:** MRI may identify lesions compressing the trigeminal nerve
  - **Treatment: carbamazepine**, baclofen, phenytoin, gabapentin, valproate, clonazepam, or other **anticonvulsants** are useful to eliminating the pain; surgical decompression may help to alleviate symptoms when deemed appropriate
  - **Outcomes:** typically becomes a chronic episodic disease unless nerve decompression is achieved
  - **Why eliminated from differential:** the location and length of the headaches make this diagnosis less likely

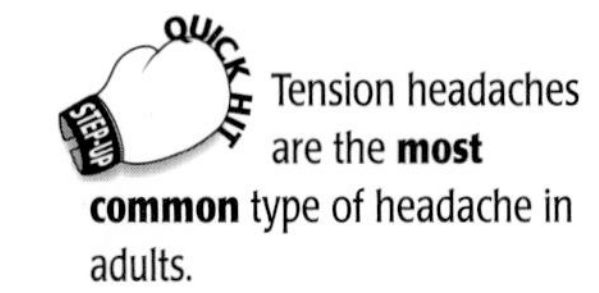

Tension headaches are the **most common** type of headache in adults.

CASE 7-3 "My father started talking funny, and he can't walk correctly"

A 78-year-old man is brought to an emergency department by his daughter after the acute onset 6 hours ago of right-sided weakness and slurred speech. The patient's daughter says that she was visiting her father for dinner. During the meal he developed progressive deterioration in the clarity of his voice and began to slur his words. The daughter later convinced him to go to the hospital, and when he tried to stand, he found that he had weakness in his right arm. He also noted slight weakness in his right leg. He denies any numbness in any of his extremities, headache, neck pain, or difficulty seeing objects. The patient and his daughter both deny that he has had any prior symptoms of this nature. The patient says that he has a history of hypertension (HTN), hypercholesterolemia, and stable angina. His medications are ASA, lisinopril, atenolol, simvastatin, and hydrochlorothiazide (HCTZ). He had an uncomplicated hip replacement at the age of 67 years. He drinks a glass of wine each day. He has a 80-pack-year smoking history but quit smoking 18 years ago. On examination, he is a well-nourished man in no acute distress. His speech is somewhat slurred during conversation, and he frequently has difficulty finding words. He has a subtle facial droop on the right side. Fundoscopic examination demonstrates arteriovenous nicking in both eyes. He has difficulty seeing objects to the left side of his face. He has no lymphadenopathy. Auscultation of his lungs and heart detects clear breathing sounds and an S_3 extra heart sound. His abdomen is nontender with no masses and normal bowel sounds. Neurologic examination detects 3/5 weakness in his right arm and 4/5 weakness in his right leg. He has a mildly impaired gait due to a slight drag in his right leg. His sensory examination is normal. His coordination is mildly impaired in his right arm. The following vital signs are measured:

T: 98.7°F, HR: 95 bpm, BP: 155/90 mm Hg, RR: 20 breaths/min

Differential Diagnosis

- Cerebrovascular accident, transient ischemic attack, migraine headache, seizure, multiple sclerosis, parenchymal hemorrhage, subdural hematoma, subarachnoid hemorrhage

Laboratory Data and Other Study Results

- CBC: WBC: 8.1, Hgb: 13.9, Plt: 421
- 10-electrolyte chemistry panel (Chem10): Na: 139 mEq/L, K: 3.9 mEq/L, Cl: 108 mEq/L, CO_2: 29 mEq/L, BUN: 17 mg/dL, Cr: 0.7 mg/dL, Glu: 90 mg/dL, magnesium (Mg): 2.1 mg/dL, calcium (Ca): 10.3 mg/dL, phosphorus (Phos): 4.1 mg/dL
- Coagulation panel (Coags): protime (PT): 11.1 sec, international normalized ratio (INR) 1.0, partial thromboplastin time (PTT): 28.5 sec
- Cardiac enzymes: creatine kinase (CK): 213 U/L, creatine kinase myocardial component (CK-MB): 1.0 ng/mL, troponin-I: 0.1 ng/mL
- Electrocardiogram (ECG): normal sinus rhythm; no abnormal wave morphology
- Head CT: no hemorrhage; abnormal signal seen in the superior region of the left hemisphere

The patient is admitted to the hospital, and his right-sided weakness increases slightly over the next 12 hours. Besides the treatments listed below, the following additional studies are performed:

- Head MRI angiogram: near complete occlusion of a branch off of the left middle cerebral artery (MCA), causing impaired perfusion of part of the superior left hemisphere; no hemorrhage; no white matter lesions
- Echocardiogram: mild-to-moderate systolic dysfunction; mild aortic stenosis; no intracardiac thrombus; mild left ventricular wall thickening; no wall anatomic abnormalities
- Carotid duplex ultrasound (US): 75% stenosis of the left common carotid artery; 10% stenosis of the right common carotid artery

Diagnosis

- Cerebrovascular accident, likely thrombotic or embolic in nature and related to carotid artery atherosclerosis

Treatment Administered

- The patient was deemed inappropriate for fibrinolytic therapy because of the time passed since the onset of his symptoms
- ASA was continued, and simvastatin was increased to the maximum dose
- Percutaneous transluminal angioplasty and stenting was performed on the left carotid artery
- Clopidogrel was started postoperatively

Follow-up

- The patient's weakness and speech defects stabilized within the first 24 hours after admission but did not resolve
- The patient was kept on ASA and clopidogrel as long-term antiplatelet therapy
- The patient was referred to speech therapy and physical therapy
- The patient's speech improved over time, and he regained most of his voice clarity
- The patient's right leg weakness improved to near normal
- His right arm weakness improved partially, and he was forced to use his left arm as his primary functioning arm

> **QUICK HIT** Atherosclerosis of the carotid, basilar, or vertebral arteries is the most common cause of **thrombotic** ischemic stroke.

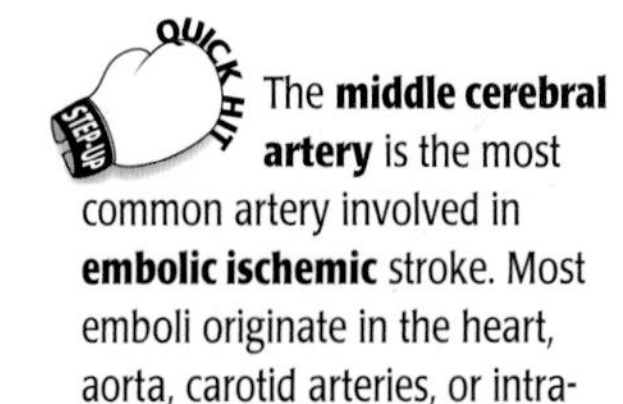

> **QUICK HIT** The **middle cerebral artery** is the most common artery involved in **embolic ischemic** stroke. Most emboli originate in the heart, aorta, carotid arteries, or intracranial arteries.

Steps to the Diagnosis

- **Cerebrovascular accident (CVA) (a.k.a. stroke)**
  - An acute focal neurologic deficit **lasting more than 24 hours** due to cerebral ischemia
    - Ischemia may be a product of **impaired perfusion** (i.e., ischemic stroke) or **hemorrhage** (i.e., hemorrhagic stroke)
      - Ischemic strokes may be **thrombotic** (i.e., obstruction via occlusive thrombus formation in a supplying artery) or **embolic** (i.e., embolization of a distant thrombus occludes a supplying artery)
  - **Risk factors:** increased age, family history, obesity, diabetes mellitus (DM), HTN, tobacco, atrial fibrillation (Afib)
  - **History:**
    - Acute development of focal neurologic deficits that last **more than 24 hours**
    - The characteristic neurologic deficits correspond to the arteries involved and their distribution (Figure 7-3, Table 7-8)

> **MNEMONIC** Risk factors for stroke may be remembered by the mnemonic **HEADACHES**: **H**TN, **E**lderly, **A**fib, **D**M, **A**therosclerosis, **C**ardiac defect (patent foramen ovale), **H**yperlipidemia, **E**xcess weight (obesity), **S**moking.

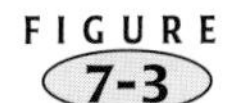

FIGURE 7-3 **Homunculus representing the sensory (A) and motor (B) cortex and its corresponding arterial supply.**

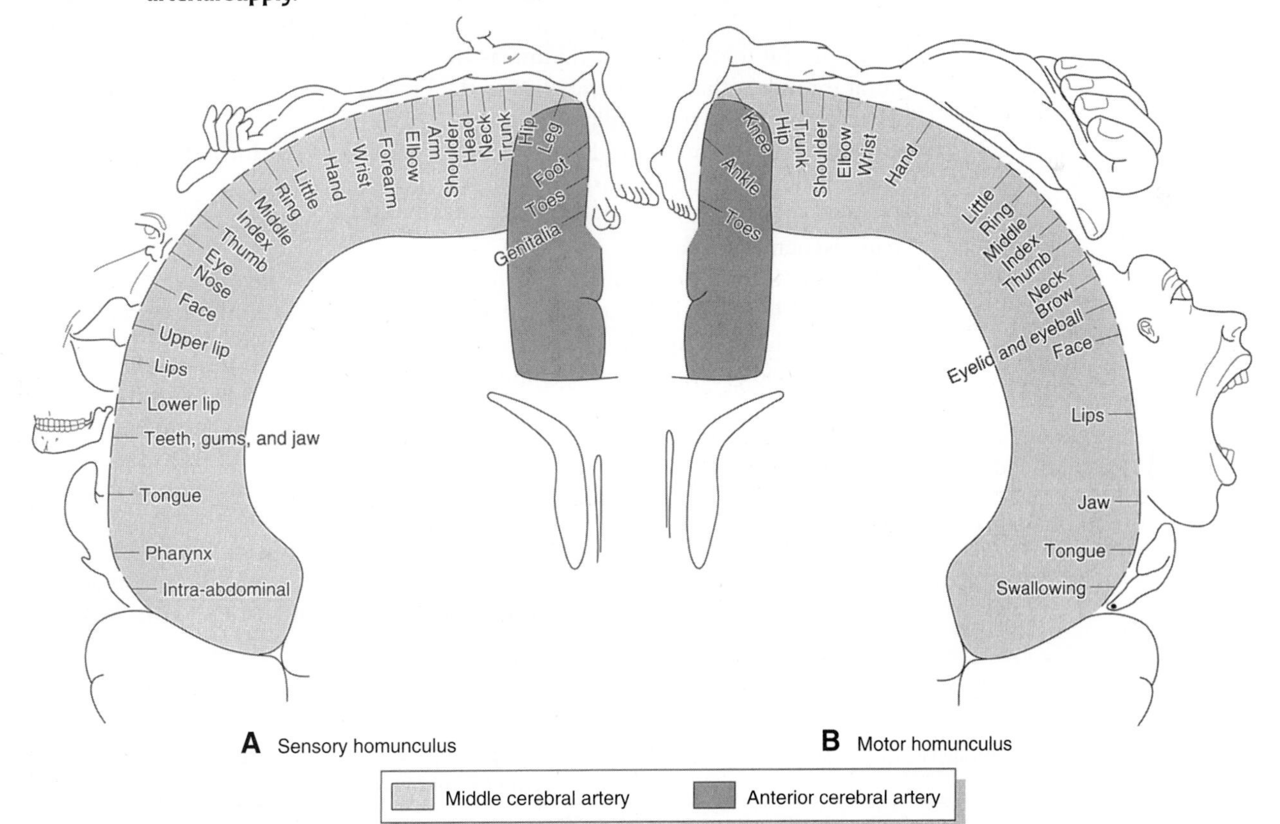

(Taken from Mehta S, Milder EA, Mirachi AJ, Milder E. *Step-up to the bedside: clinical case review for USMLE step 1.* Philadelphia: Lippincott Williams & Wilkins, 2002. Used with permission of Lippincott Williams & Wilkins.)

TABLE 7-8 Common Stroke Locations and Corresponding Signs and Symptoms

Location of Stroke	Signs and Symptoms
ACA	Contralateral lower extremity and trunk weakness
MCA	Contralateral face and upper extremity weakness and decreased sensation, bilateral visual abnormalities, aphasia (if dominant hemisphere), neglect and inability to perform learned actions (if nondominant hemisphere)
PCA	Contralateral visual abnormalities, blindness (if bilateral PCA involvement)
Lacunar arteries	Focal motor or sensory deficits, loss of coordination, difficulty speaking
Basilar artery	Cranial nerve abnormalities, contralateral full body weakness and decreased sensation, vertigo, loss of coordination, difficulty speaking, visual abnormalities, coma

ACA, anterior cerebral artery; MCA, middle cerebral artery; PCA, posterior cerebral artery.

MNEMONIC

Causes of stroke in young patients may be remembered by the **seven Cs**: **C**ocaine, **C**ancer, **C**ardiogenic emboli, **C**oagulation (excessive), **C**NS infection (septic emboli), **C**ongenital vascular lesion, **C**onsanguinity (genetic disease).

- **Aphasias** are communication disorders that may develop due to ischemia of distinct brain centers (Table 7-9)
- **Physical examination:**
  - Thorough serial neurovascular examinations are important to determining the region of involvement and stroke evolution
  - Consistent physical findings indicate a stabilized stroke
  - Progressive findings indicate an evolving stroke in which the full extent of the ischemic involvement has not been defined
- **Tests:**
  - **Head CT without contrast** is frequently the first radiographic tool used to differentiate ischemic from hemorrhagic strokes and to determine the extent of injured cerebrum
  - **MRI** is more sensitive than CT in defining an ischemic area, and MRI angiogram (CT angiogram to a slightly lesser extent) is useful for defining the site of vascular insult
  - ECG is useful to detect any arrhythmias that may contribute to the formation of a mural thrombus that might embolize to the brain; cardiac enzymes are helpful for detecting an underlying cardiac pathology
  - Echocardiogram and carotid artery duplex US are useful for detecting sites of thrombus and vascular stenosis in the heart and great vessels
- **Treatment:**
  - **Acute ischemic stroke**
    - **Thrombolytic therapy** may be administered for ischemic stroke if performed **within 3 hours** of onset and in the absence of any contraindications (e.g., evidence of hemorrhage on CT, recent surgery, anticoagulant use, recent hemorrhage, blood pressure >185/110 mm Hg) (Figure 7-4)

TABLE 7-9 Common Classifications of Aphasias

Type	Area Injured	Characteristics
Broca (i.e., expressive)	Inferior frontal gyrus, dorsolateral frontal cortex, anterior parietal cortex	Few words, difficulty producing words (i.e., **nonfluent**), **good comprehension**, face and arm hemiparesis, loss of oral coordination
Wernicke (i.e., receptive)	Posterior superior temporal gyrus, inferior parietal lobe	Word substitutions, meaningless words, meaningless phrases (i.e., **poor comprehension**, "word salad")
Conduction	Supramarginal gyrus, angular gyrus	**Fluent speech**, word substitutions, **frequent attempts to correct words**, word-finding pauses
Global	Large infarcts of left cerebral hemisphere	Difficulty producing words, **nonfluent speech**, **poor comprehension**, limb ataxia

Treatment algorithm for a suspected acute stroke. CT, computed tomography; ECG, electrocardiogram; IV, intravenous; LP, lumbar puncture; O_2, oxygen; t-PA, tissue plasminogen activator.

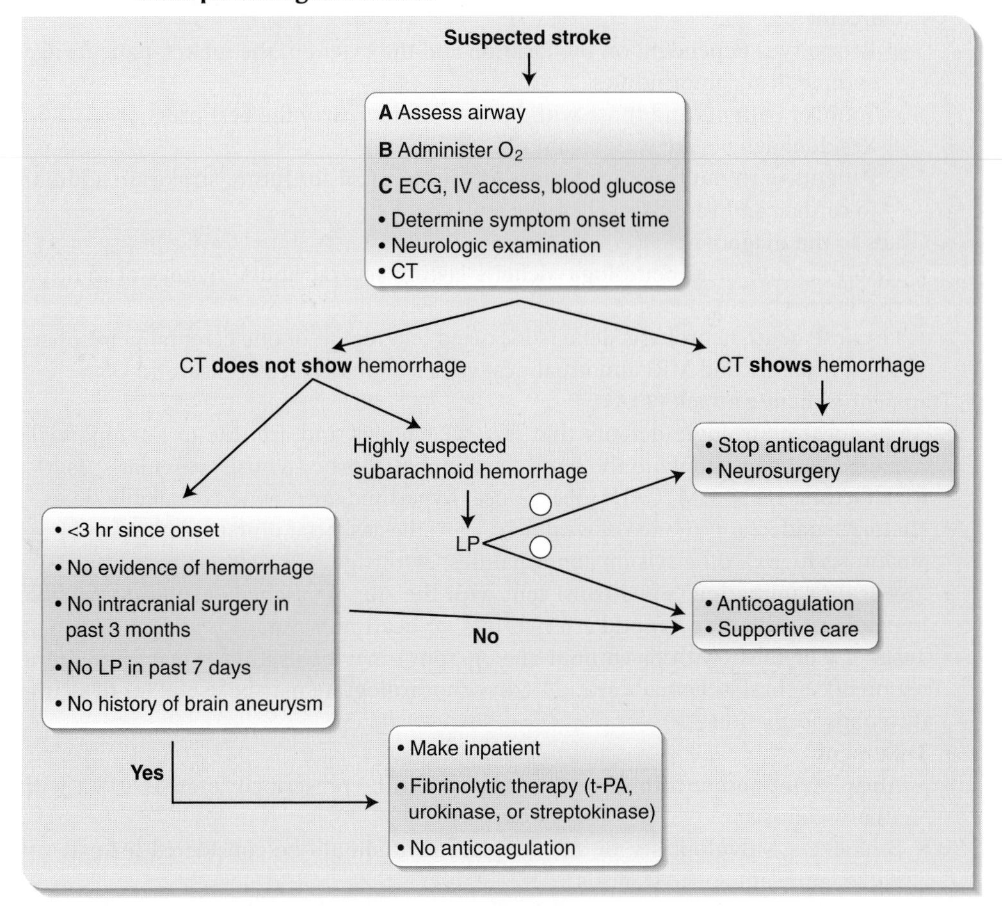

- **Antiplatelet therapy** (e.g., ASA, clopidogrel) should be started within 48 hours of the onset of symptoms to reduce the risk of additional vascular events
- Heparin and low molecular weight heparin have not been proven to be of benefit but should be considered in patients with an embolic stroke from a cardiac source
- Control of excessive HTN and the use of lipid-lowering medications are beneficial to preventing additional acute strokes

- **Acute hemorrhagic stroke**
  - Anticoagulation should be reversed
  - Tight control of blood pressure and intracranial pressure (e.g., mannitol, hyperventilation, anesthesia) are important to controlling evolving symptoms
  - Surgical decompression should be considered for bleeds causing a mass effect and impairing consciousness
  - Antiplatelet medications may be restarted 2 weeks after the stroke if the patient's deficits remain stable
- **Long-term care**
  - Patients will require multiple therapies to help treat neurologic deficits
  - Physical therapy is useful to optimizing functional disabilities
  - Speech therapy is useful for improving speaking clarity and may assist with treating aphasias
  - **Treatment of the underlying pathologies** (e.g., blood pressure control, lipid reduction, arrhythmia control) for stroke is vital to the **prevention** of future strokes
  - Long-term anticoagulation (e.g., warfarin) is indicated for patients with a cardiac mural thrombus

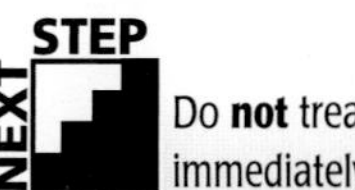

Do **not** treat HTN immediately following stroke unless it is extreme (>220/120) or if patient has coronary artery disease (CAD) in order to **maintain cerebral perfusion**.

- **Carotid endarterectomy or angioplasty with stenting** is performed for carotid narrowing >60% in asymptomatic men, >50% in symptomatic men, and >70% in symptomatic women
- **Outcomes:**
  - Recovery is dependent on the location and the extent of the infarct, patient's age, and medical comorbidities
  - Younger patients and those with limited infarcts carry the best prognosis
  - Residual deficits are very common
  - Patients with multiple risk factors are at high risk for future strokes in addition to cardiac and vascular ischemic events
- **Clues to the diagnosis:**
  - History: acute focal neurologic deficits lasting several hours, history of multiple risk factors
  - Physical: acute neurologic deficits localized to a region of one cerebral hemisphere
  - Tests: head CT and MRI abnormalities, vessel occlusion seen on carotid US

- **Transient ischemic attack (TIA)**
  - Acute focal neurologic deficits that last **<24 hours** and are due to a temporarily impaired vascular supply to the brain (e.g., emboli, aortic stenosis, vascular spasm)
  - **Risk factors:** HTN, DM, CAD, tobacco use, hyperlipidemia, hypercoagulable states
  - **History:** sudden appearance of weakness, paresthesias, brief unilateral blindness (i.e., amaurosis fugax), other vision abnormalities, or vertigo

Most TIAs last **<2 hours** and are **recurrent**.

  - **Physical examination:** signs consistent with the site of vascular insult and possible impaired coordination, carotid artery bruits, or heart murmurs
  - **Tests:** CT or MRI (with or without angiography) may be useful for determining the region of cerebral ischemia; carotid US or echocardiogram may be useful for detecting thrombus formation
  - **Treatment:**
    - **Antiplatelet** and **antilipid** medications should be prescribed to any patient with atherosclerosis
    - β-blockers, valvuloplasty, or valve replacement should be considered for patients with significant aortic stenosis
    - **Carotid endarterectomy** or **angioplasty** should be considered using the same guidelines as for stroke patients
    - Long-term anticoagulation is required for patients with arrhythmias
  - **Outcomes:**
    - TIAs tend to be recurrent
    - Patients have an increased risk of stroke, with 25% of patients having a stroke within 5 years of the initial TIA
    - Severe carotid artery disease significantly increases stroke risk
    - Long-term outcomes correlate with successful control of the underlying pathologies
  - **Why eliminated from differential:** although stroke and TIA may present identically, the persistent nature of this patient's deficits defines this process as a stroke
- **Migraine headache**
  - More thorough discussion in prior case
  - **Why eliminated from differential:** although focal neurologic deficits may be seen in some variants of migraines, the lack of a headache and persistent nature of the deficits rule out this diagnosis
- **Seizure**
  - More thorough discussion in later case
  - **Why eliminated from differential:** the absence of a witnessed seizure and persistent nature of the neurologic deficits make this diagnosis unlikely
- **Multiple sclerosis**
  - More thorough discussion in later case
  - **Why eliminated from differential:** the focal and acute onset of the neurologic deficits and the absence of any white matter lesions on the neuroimaging studies make this diagnosis less likely

- **Parenchymal hemorrhage**
  - Bleeding within the brain parenchyma due to excessive HTN (possibly related to stimulant use), arteriovenous malformation, or cerebral aneurysm
  - **History:** headache, nausea, vomiting, confusion, possible seizures
  - **Physical examination:** change in mental status, focal neurologic deficits
  - **Tests:** head CT without contrast is useful for detecting the region of hemorrhage; MRI or CT angiography is useful for localizing the site of bleeding
  - **Treatment:**
    - Supportive care is used to keep the patient hemodynamically stable
    - Intracranial pressure is managed to prevent dangerous increases
    - **Anticonvulsants** are administered for seizure prophylaxis
    - **Surgical decompression** may be required for large hemorrhages to reduce the risk of herniation
    - Surgical repair or embolization of bleeding aneurysms or arteriovenous malformations (AVMs) should be performed
  - **Outcomes:**
    - Prognosis is dependent on the size of hemorrhage
    - The early development of significant symptoms carries a worse prognosis
    - Complications include permanent neurologic deficits, seizures, spastic paralysis, and death
  - **Why eliminated from differential:** the absence of a hemorrhage on the CT and MRI rules out this diagnosis
- **Subdural hematoma/subarachnoid hemorrhage**
  - More thorough discussion in later case
  - **Why eliminated from differential:** the absence of an intracranial bleed on the CT and MRI rules out these diagnoses

CASE 7-4 "I was in a car crash"

A 27-year-old woman is brought to an emergency department by ambulance after being involved in a single-car collision. The patient says that her car slipped off a wet road and hit a telephone pole on the front left side of the car. She says that she was wearing her seat belt but that her car does not have any airbags. She does think that she lost consciousness. She says that she was able to get out of the car somehow and was able to walk around. She says that she has some mild neck and upper back soreness but denies any pain elsewhere in her body. She also denies any numbness or weakness in her extremities, nausea, vomiting, or loss of bowel control. The emergency medical technicians (EMTs) accompanying her say that it appeared that she may have hit her head on the driver's side window. She was found to have a 4 cm laceration on her scalp that was covered with a bandage. No significant amount of blood was visible at the scene, although she had bled an appreciable amount onto her shirt. She was fully alert and oriented at the scene of the event and was placed in a cervical collar and on a backboard for spinal precautions. The patient says that she has no past medical history and only takes birth control medication. She drinks socially but cannot remember if she drank any alcohol this evening. On examination, she is a healthy appearing woman in no acute distress. Her airway is confirmed to be intact by her speech, auscultation of her heart and lungs detects clear bilateral lung sounds and mild tachycardia. Her abdomen is nontender with no masses and has normal bowel sounds. She has a laceration on the left scalp that is bandaged and only bleeds slowly when the bandage is removed. When she is log-rolled she has some minor paraspinal tenderness in her thoracic and cervical spine but no deformities or palpable step-offs. A rectal examination shows normal tone and no gross blood. She has no gross deformities of any extremities and is fully intact on motor and sensory examinations. On her secondary survey, she is oriented to her name but not the date or location. She also perseverates on several of the questions surrounding the details of her collision and begins to complain of a severe headache. A repeat neurologic examination is normal. The following vital signs are measured:

T: 98.9°F, HR: 110 bpm, BP: 127/87 mm Hg, RR: 18 breaths/min

Differential Diagnosis

- Cerebrovascular accident, subarachnoid hemorrhage, subdural hematoma, epidural hematoma, intoxication, seizure, spinal cord injury

Laboratory Data and Other Study Results

- CBC: WBC: 5.9, Hgb: 14.2, Plt: 433
- Chem10: Na: 140 mEq/L, K: 3.8 mEq/L, Cl: 104 mEq/L, CO_2: 26 mEq/L, BUN: 15 mg/dL, Cr: 0.7 mg/dL, Glu: 91 mg/dL, Mg: 2.0 mg/dL, Ca: 10.1 mg/dL, Phos: 4.0 mg/dL
- Coags: PT: 11.3 sec, INR: 1.0, PTT: 27.8 sec
- EtOH level: 0 mg/dL
- Urine toxicology screen: negative
- Chest x-ray (CXR): clear lung fields; no rib fractures; no pneumothorax
- Head CT: nondisplaced cranial fracture on the left side of the skull; convex fluid collection under the cranium on the left side, causing a mass effect and midline shifting of the cerebrum; no interparenchymal or intraventricular hemorrhage
- Full spine CT: no fractures or dislocations; no impingement on the spinal cord
- Abdomen/pelvis CT: no hemorrhage; no masses; no free abdominal fluid or air; no visceral abnormalities

Diagnosis

- Epidural hematoma

Treatment Administered

- The patient was taken emergently to the operating room with neurosurgery for drainage of the hematoma and placement of an intracranial pressure (ICP) monitor
- The patient was admitted to the neurosurgical intensive care unit (ICU) following the procedure
- Initially following surgery, the patient was placed on anticonvulsants and kept sedated

Follow-up

- The ICP monitor was removed after the patient demonstrated consistent stabilization of her intracranial pressure
- Sedation was discontinued, and the patient was allowed to fully awaken
- The tertiary examination detected no neurologic deficits, and the patient was found to be fully awake and oriented
- The patient was able to be discharged to home in stable condition after a 1-week inpatient admission

Steps to the Diagnosis

- **Epidural hematoma**
  - Collection of blood between the dura mater and the skull due to arterial hemorrhage
    - The most common cause of arterial bleeding is an injury to the **middle meningeal artery** following blunt head trauma
  - **History**: initial "**lucid interval**" after trauma in which the patient demonstrates no neurologic signs of injury followed later by severe headache, confusion, nausea, and possible seizures
  - **Physical examination:** altered mental status, possible hemiparesis, hemiplegia, and pupil abnormalities (i.e., "blown pupil")
  - **Tests:** CT without contrast shows a **convex** hyperdensity compressing the brain at the site of injury and a possible adjacent skull fracture (Figure 7-5)
  - **Treatment: emergent** drainage of the hematoma either via burr hole or craniotomy; stabilization of the blood pressure and ICP is required to reduce the risk of herniation

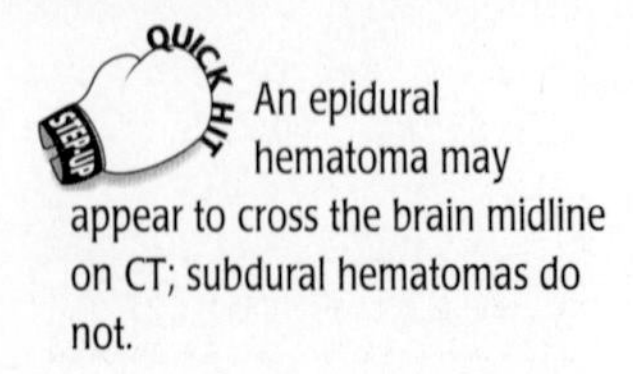

An epidural hematoma may appear to cross the brain midline on CT; subdural hematomas do not.

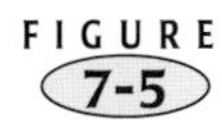

FIGURE 7-5 Head computed tomography without contrast, demonstrating an epidural hematoma with a convex hyperdensity due to blood accumulation above the dura (*arrowheads*).

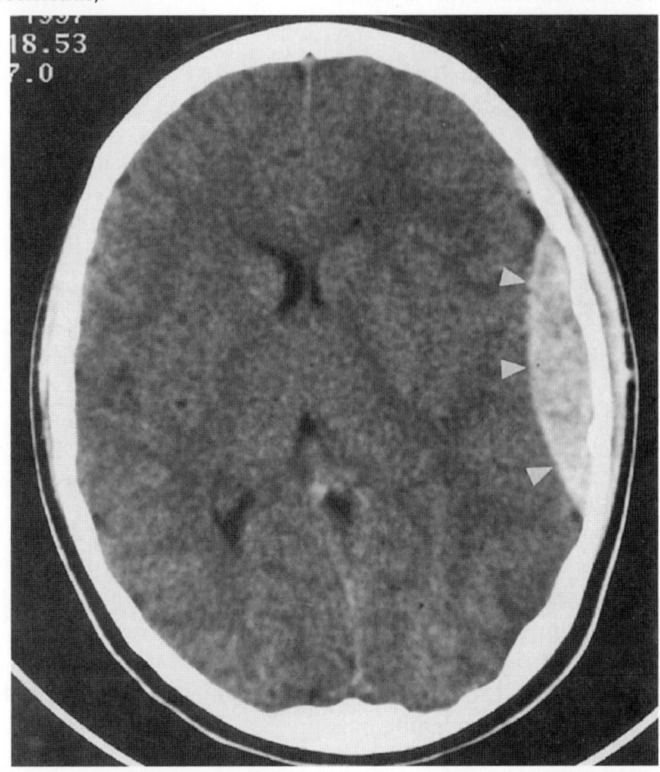

(Taken from Daffner RH. *Clinical radiology: the essentials.* 2nd ed. Philadelphia: Lippincott Williams & Wilkins, 1999. Used with permission of Lippincott Williams & Wilkins.)

- **Outcomes:** complications include seizures and neurologic deficits; the prognosis worsens with increasing age, additional intracranial injuries, decreasing Glasgow coma scale, and delays to intervention
- **Clues to the diagnosis:**
  - History: head trauma, initial normal mental function with delayed deterioration and amnesia
  - Physical: mental status changes
  - Tests: findings of head CT
- **Subdural hematoma**
  - Collection of blood between the dura and arachnoid meningeal layers due to rupture of the bridging veins
    - Frequently follows head trauma
  - **History: slowly progressive headache** (days to weeks), blunt head trauma
  - **Physical examination:** change in mental status, contralateral hemiparesis, increased deep tendon reflexes, papilledema, gait abnormalities, visual field defects
  - **Tests:** head CT shows a **concave** hyperdensity compressing the brain but not crossing the midline (Figure 7-6)
  - **Treatment:** supportive care is appropriate for small hematomas with minimal neurologic effects; surgical decompression is required for large hematomas or those with significant neurologic deficits
  - **Outcomes:** prognosis worsens with increasing age, decreasing Glasgow coma scale scores, and greater pupil asymmetry
  - **Why eliminated from differential:** the appearance of the bleed on the head CT is characteristic for an epidural hematoma
- **Subarachnoid hemorrhage**
  - Bleeding between the pia and arachnoid meningeal layers due to rupture of an **arterial aneurysm** (i.e., berry aneurysm) or AVM or due to head trauma

NEXT STEP

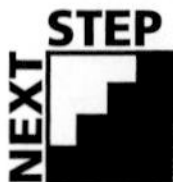

If you see mental status changes in an elderly patient with a history of **falls**, perform a work-up for a subdural hematoma.

NEXT STEP

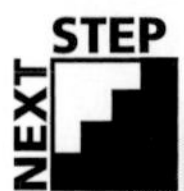

Do **not** perform a lumbar puncture in patients with a **subdural hematoma** because of the increased risk of herniation.

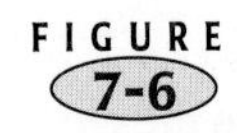

FIGURE 7-6 Head computed tomography without contrast, demonstrating a subdural hematoma with a concave hyperdensity due to blood accumulation between the dura and arachnoid layers (*arrows*).

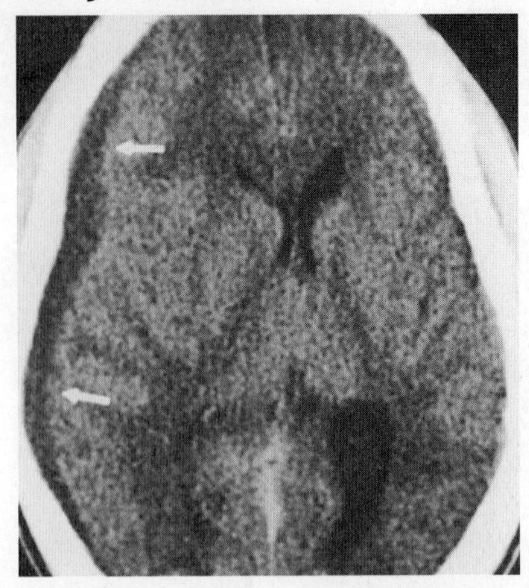

(Taken from Swischuk LE. *Emergency imaging of the acutely ill or injured child.* 3rd ed. Philadelphia: Lippincott Williams & Wilkins, 1994. Fig. 10.23. Used with permission of Lippincott Williams & Wilkins.)

QUICK HIT: **Berry aneurysms** are found more commonly in patients with **adult polycystic kidney disease**.

QUICK HIT: Patients may describe the headache in a subarachnoid hemorrhage as the "**worst headache of my life**."

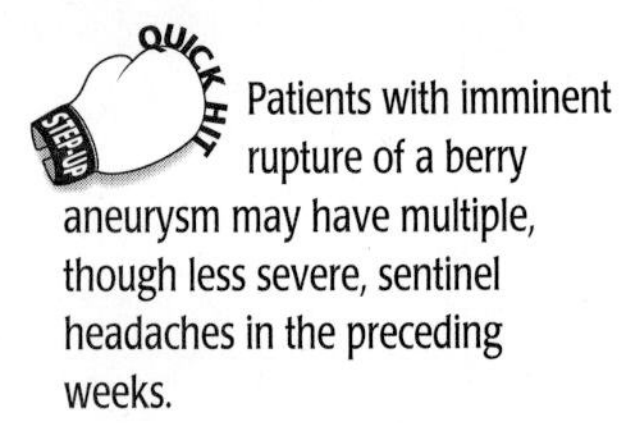

QUICK HIT: Patients with imminent rupture of a berry aneurysm may have multiple, though less severe, sentinel headaches in the preceding weeks.

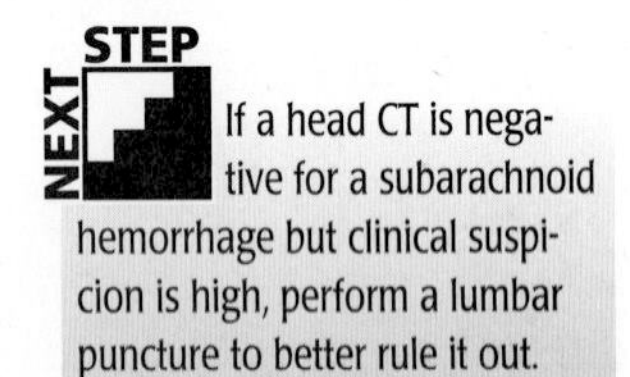

NEXT STEP: If a head CT is negative for a subarachnoid hemorrhage but clinical suspicion is high, perform a lumbar puncture to better rule it out.

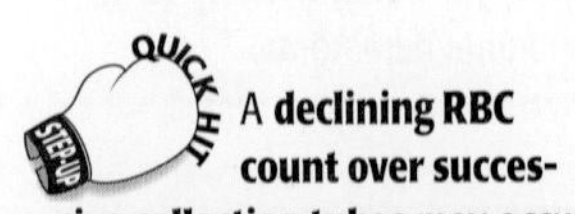

QUICK HIT: A **declining RBC count over successive collection tubes** may occur in a traumatic lumbar puncture and can help differentiate it from xanthochromia.

- **History:** sudden severe headache, neck pain, nausea, vomiting, possible seizure
- **Physical examination:** fever, mental status changes
- **Tests:**
  - Lumbar puncture will show RBCs, xanthochromia (i.e., yellowish discoloration of the CSF), and increased opening pressure
  - Head CT will show blood in the subarachnoid space (Figure 7-7)
  - MRI angiography or an angiogram can localize the site of bleeding
- **Treatment:**
  - **Control ICP** by elevating the head of the bed and administering mannitol
  - Control blood pressure to prevent HTN
  - Reverse any anticoagulation
  - Administer anticonvulsants for seizure prophylaxis
  - Perform interventional radiographic embolization of aneurysms or AVMs
- **Outcomes:**
  - Mortality ranges from 30% for asymptomatic cases to 90% for cases causing a coma
  - Some degree of cognitive impairment following hemorrhage is common
  - Long-term neurologic deficits are seen in 25% of cases
- **Why eliminated from differential:** the appearance of the bleed on the head CT is characteristic for an epidural hematoma

- **Cerebrovascular accident**
  - More thorough discussion in prior case
  - **Why eliminated from differential:** the relatively young age of the patient, lack of medical comorbidities, and relation to recent head trauma make this diagnosis less likely
- **Intoxication**
  - More thorough discussion in Chapter 13
  - **Why eliminated from differential:** the negative toxicology screening rules out this diagnosis
- **Seizure**
  - More thorough discussion in later case
  - **Why eliminated from differential:** the lack of a history of prior seizures and the recent head trauma make this diagnosis less likely
- **Spinal cord injury**
  - More thorough discussion in later case
  - **Why eliminated from differential:** the negative spinal CT and the patient's lack of neurologic deficits make this diagnosis unlikely

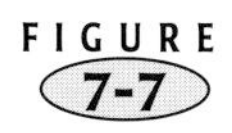
FIGURE 7-7 **Subarachnoid hemorrhage seen on computed tomography without contrast; blood is evident in the subarachnoid space (*arrows*).**

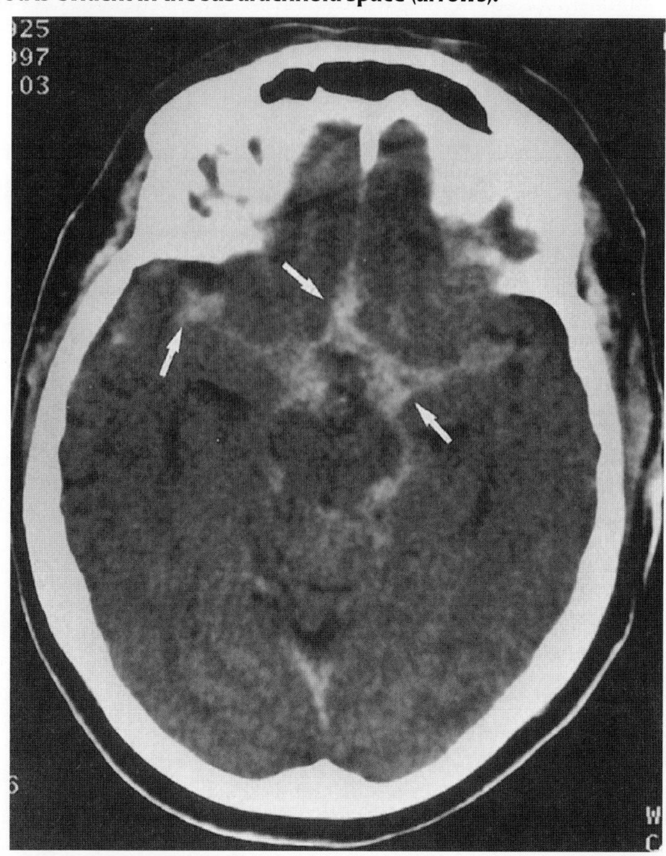

(Taken from Daffner RH. *Clinical radiology: the essentials.* 2nd ed. Philadelphia: Lippincott Williams & Wilkins, 1999. Used with permission of Lippincott Williams & Wilkins.)

CASE 7-5 "My daughter keeps having fits"

The 27-year-old patient from the previous case presents to a neurologist in follow-up for her epidural hematoma. She was seen 2 weeks after her discharge from the hospital to discuss the development of any abnormal neurologic symptoms, and at that time she reported no new issues. This is her second follow-up appointment and is occurring at 2 months after her discharge. The patient is accompanied by her mother, who reports the occurrence of multiple episodes of strange behavior. The patient's mother reports that on a half dozen occasions in the past month, her daughter will begin flapping her arms for approximately a minute. During these episodes she does not communicate with anyone around her. Following these episodes she is confused for <30 minutes and has no recollection of the arm flapping. The patient says that when these episodes have occurred, she will smell a strong sweet odor and will feel that air is blowing on her face. She is unable to remember what follows these experiences over the subsequent 20 to 30 minutes. All of these episodes have occurred at home. She has been staying with her parents since the car collision. She has not driven her car in the past 3 weeks because she is concerned that she will have an episode while driving, and she is currently on leave from work. She has occasional headaches and bouts of nausea that have been decreasing in frequency. She denies any new numbness or weakness. She has had no other medical issues since her car collision and takes no new medications. She denies any substance use. On examination, she is well appearing and in no acute distress. Her face appears symmetrical. Fundoscopic examination is normal. She has no lymphadenopathy. Auscultation of her heart, lungs, and abdomen is normal.

Her sensation is normal and symmetrical across her body. Her motor function is likewise normal including her coordination and gait. The following vital signs are measured:

T: 98.6°F, HR: 78 bpm, BP: 120/82 mm Hg, RR: 17 breaths/min

Differential Diagnosis

- Postconcussive syndrome, stroke, subarachnoid hemorrhage, subdural hematoma, epidural hemorrhage, seizure disorder, bacterial meningitis, viral meningitis

Laboratory Data and Other Study Results

- CBC: WBC: 5.9, Hgb: 13.9, Plt: 431
- Head MRI: no hemorrhage; increased signal in the left temporal lobe on T2-weighted images; normal cerebral volume

Following these tests, these additional studies are performed:

- Lumbar puncture: clear appearance, opening pressure 87 mm Hg, WBC: 3/μL, glucose: 52 mg/dL, protein: 34 mg/dL
- EEG: no abnormal activity

Diagnosis

- Seizure disorder, most likely complex partial seizures due to traumatic temporal lobe injury

Treatment Administered

- The patient was placed on phenytoin to prevent additional seizures
- The patient was instructed to refrain from driving until stable control of her seizures was achieved

Follow-up

- The patient experienced no additional seizures after starting phenytoin
- Attempted weaning of the patient from phenytoin was attempted after 6 months of therapy
- The patient experienced a similar complex partial seizure during medication weaning and was returned to her prescribed phenytoin dose; she had no new seizures after resumption of her anticonvulsant therapy

Steps to the Diagnosis

- **Seizure disorder (a.k.a. epilepsy)**
  - Recurrent sudden alterations in cortical neurologic activity due to the excessive synchronized discharge of cortical neurons in either a focal or generalized distribution of the brain
    - Causes vary with age (Table 7-10)
  - **History:**
    - The characteristics of a seizure vary with its subtype (Table 7-11)
    - Simple seizures have **no loss of consciousness**
    - Complex or generalized seizures are associated with an **altered state of consciousness**
    - Partial seizures may be associated with hallucinations or *déjà vu*
  - **Physical examination:**
    - **Partial** seizures involve a focal distribution of abnormal neurologic activity
    - **Generalized** seizures are characterized by a widespread abnormal neurologic activity
    - **Tonic-clonic** seizures feature a period of tonic muscle contraction followed by clonic contraction-relaxation movements

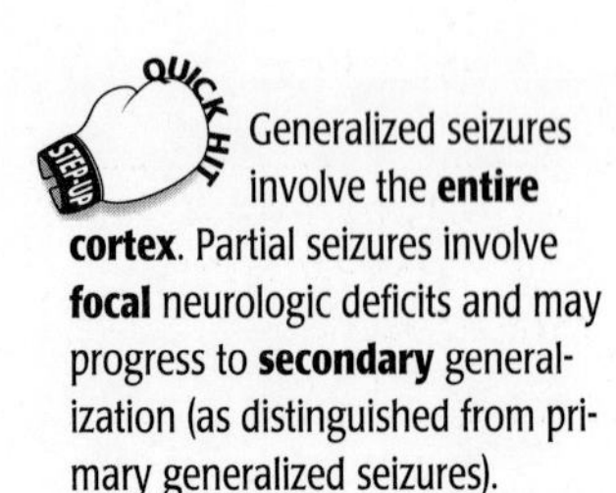

Generalized seizures involve the **entire cortex**. Partial seizures involve **focal** neurologic deficits and may progress to **secondary** generalization (as distinguished from primary generalized seizures).

TABLE 7-10 Common Causes of Seizures by Age Group

Age Group	Causes
Infant	Hypoxic injury Metabolic defects Genetic/congenital abnormality Infection
Children	Idiopathic Infection Fever
Adult	Trauma Idiopathic Metabolic defects Drugs/withdrawal Trauma Neoplasm Infection Cerebrovascular disease Psychogenic
Elderly	Stroke/cerebrovascular disease Metabolic defects Drugs/withdrawal Infection Trauma Neoplasm

TABLE 7-11 Types of Seizures

Type	Involvement	H/P	EEG
Simple partial	Focal cortical region of brain	**Focal** sensory (e.g., paresthesias, hallucinations) or motor (e.g., repetitive or purposeless movement) activity, **no loss of consciousness**	Distinct focal conductive abnormality in the causative region of the brain
Complex partial	Focal region of **temporal** lobe	**Hallucinations** (e.g., auditory, visual, olfactory), **automatisms** (i.e., repeated coordinated movement), déjà vu, impaired consciousness, postictal confusion	Focal abnormalities in temporal lobe
Generalized convulsive (e.g., tonic, clonic, tonic-clonic, myoclonic, atonic)	Bilateral cerebral cortex	Sustained contraction of extremities and back (**tonic**); repetitive muscle contraction and relaxation (**clonic**); brief contraction period followed by repetitive contraction-relaxation (**tonic-clonic**); brief repetitive contractions (**myoclonic**); loss of tone (**atonic**); loss of consciousness, incontinence, significant postictal confusion, possible focal neurologic deficits lasting several days after seizure (i.e., Todd paralysis) are common	**Generalized** electrical abnormalities
Absence	Bilateral cerebral cortex	**Brief** (few seconds) episodes of **impaired consciousness**, normal muscle tone, possible eye blinking, no postictal confusion; more common in **children**	Generalized three-cycle-per-second **spike and wave pattern** abnormalities

EEG, electroencephalogram; H/P, history and physical.

- Tests:
  - EEG is used to detect abnormal neurologic activity but is frequently normal between seizures
  - Patients may be admitted to an epilepsy observation unit to undergo constant EEG and video monitoring to try and record neurologic activity during a seizure
  - MRI is useful to detect intracranial lesions (e.g., tumors, abscesses, hemorrhage) and areas of brain contusion (increased signal on T2-weighted images)
- Treatment:
  - Anticonvulsant medications are the standardized first-line therapy (Table 7-12)
  - Only one medication is initially prescribed (e.g., phenytoin, carbamazepine, valproate), but a second-line drug may be added for incomplete control under monotherapy
  - Surgery may be considered for resectable foci of seizures but is complicated by the loss of nearby cerebral tissue
  - Vagal nerve stimulator implantation is an option for patients with refractory seizures not willing to undergo surgical resection

QUICK HIT: Anticonvulsant withdrawal is considered for patients after an extended seizure-free period of time but is frequently complicated by a recurrence of seizure activity.

TABLE 7-12 Anticonvulsant Medications Used in Epilepsy Treatment

Drug	Current Indications	Adverse Effects
Mechanism: Inhibition of voltage-dependent sodium channels		
Carbamazepine	Monotherapy for partial or generalized convulsive seizures	Nausea, vomiting, hyponatremia, Stevens-Johnson syndrome, drowsiness, vertigo, blurred vision, leukopenia
Phenytoin	Monotherapy for partial or generalized convulsive seizures, **status epilepticus**	Gingival hyperplasia, androgeny, lymphadenopathy, Stevens-Johnson syndrome, confusion, blurred vision
Lamotrigine	Partial seizures, second-line drug for tonic-clonic seizures	Rash, nausea, Stevens-Johnson syndrome, dizziness, sedation
Oxcarbazepine	Monotherapy for partial or generalized convulsive seizures	Hyponatremia, rash, nausea, sedation, dizziness, blurred vision
Zonisamide	Second-line drug for partial and generalized seizures	Somnolence, confusion, fatigue, dizziness
Mechanism: Inhibition of neuronal calcium channels		
Ethosuximide	**Absence** seizures	Nausea, vomiting, drowsiness, inattentiveness
Mechanism: Enhanced GABA activity		
Phenobarbital, pentobarbital	Nonresponsive status epilepticus	Drowsiness, general cognitive depression, vertigo, nausea, vomiting, rebound seizures
Benzodiazepines	**Status epilepticus**	Drowsiness, tolerance, rebound seizures
Tiagabine	Second-line drug for partial seizures	Dizziness, fatigue, nausea, inattentiveness, abdominal pain
Mechanism: Inhibition of sodium channels and enhanced GABA activity		
Valproate	Monotherapy or second drug for partial and generalized seizures	Hepatotoxicity, nausea, vomiting, drowsiness, tremor, weight gain, alopecia
Mechanism: Inhibition of NMDA-glutamate receptors and enhanced GABA activity		
Topiramate	Second-line drug for partial and generalized seizures	Weight loss, cognitive impairment, heat intolerance, dizziness, nausea, paresthesias, fatigue
Mechanism: Unknown		
Gabapentin	Monotherapy or second-line drug for partial seizures	Sedation
Levetiracetam	Monotherapy for partial seizures, second-line drug for partial or generalized seizures	Fatigue, somnolence, dizziness

GABA, γ-aminobutyric acid; NMDA, *N*-methyl-D-aspartate.

- **Outcomes:**
  - Partial seizures have a higher recurrence rate than generalized seizures
  - Mortality rates are twice as high in patients with partial seizures compared to the general population and considerably higher in patients with recurrent generalized seizures
  - Overall prognosis correlates with the success in controlling recurrences through medical or surgical means
  - **Status epilepticus**
    - **Repetitive, uncontrolled** seizures without any period of normal consciousness
    - Maintenance of a stable airway, breathing, and circulation is important to survival
    - **Intravenous benzodiazepines** and aggressive anticonvulsant therapy are required to break the seizure activity
    - Acute mortality is >20%
- **Clues to the diagnosis:**
  - History: recurrent abnormal neurologic activity, postictal confusion, preictal auras
  - Physical: automatisms (i.e., arm flapping)
  - Tests: MRI demonstrating a temporal lobe contusion at the site of the former epidural hematoma

- **Postconcussive syndrome**
  - A poorly understood constellation of symptoms that follow head trauma and lasts for several months after the initial injury
  - **History:** symptoms last for a few months and include headache, dizziness, vertigo, tinnitus, nausea, diplopia, anxiety, fatigue, irritability, sensitivity to noise and light, insomnia, or memory impairments
  - **Physical examination:** examination is frequently normal but may feature cognitive deficits on testing
  - **Tests:** there are no diagnostic tests but CT or MRI are useful to rule out other pathologies
  - **Treatment:** pain management and psychotherapy are beneficial during recovery
  - **Outcomes:** most patients recover within 3 months; up to 15% of patients will have chronic symptoms (more common in patients reporting dizziness)
  - **Why eliminated from differential:** this patient likely has some degree of postconcussive syndrome given her history of head trauma and her report of headaches and nausea; however, this diagnosis would not explain her unusual automatisms
- **Stroke**
  - More thorough discussion in prior case
- **Why eliminated from differential:** this diagnosis is unlikely because the patient has normal neurologic behavior in between her brief episodes
- **Subarachnoid hemorrhage/epidural hematoma/subdural hematoma**
  - More thorough discussion in prior case
  - **Why eliminated from differential:** these diagnoses are ruled out by the appearance of the brain MRI and by the normal lumbar puncture analysis
- **Bacterial/viral meningitis**
  - More thorough discussion in prior case
  - **Why eliminated from differential:** these diagnoses are ruled out by the normal serum WBC count and the normal lumbar puncture analysis

CASE 7-6 "My husband's shaking has gotten worse"

A 70-year-old man presents to a neurologist for the work-up of hand tremors. He is accompanied by his wife. He says that he is not sure why he is being seen and has to be reminded on several occasions by his wife that he is there to discuss his tremor. The patient's wife says that she first noticed the tremor in her husband's hands 6 months ago, but it has gradually worsened since that time. The tremor seems to be present both at rest and during activity. The tremor nearly resolves while he is sleeping. She is also concerned because he has become unstable on his feet and has fallen on a couple of occasions. He does not participate in the activities he previously enjoyed and seems to forget things easily. She says that she never saw any of these symptoms until the past year. The patient is able to contribute to the history, but relies on his wife to explain his symptoms. He says that he has a history of HTN and takes enalapril and a baby ASA daily. He formerly was a social drinker but has not consumed alcohol for over a year. On examination, he is a well-nourished man in no acute distress. He shows little emotion during the examination and history. Fundoscopic examination is normal. His face appears symmetric. He has no lymphadenopathy. Auscultation of his heart and lungs detects clear breath sounds and normal heart sounds. His abdomen is nontender with no masses. He has a resting tremor in both hands that consists of a regular beat of wrist and finger flexion. He has increased tone throughout his body, and it is difficult to passively range his extremities. His sensation is grossly intact. When his gait is observed, he has a difficult time initiating his first steps, walks in a shuffling pattern, and takes several extra steps when he tries to come to a stop. His deep tendon reflexes are moderately increased. The following vital signs are measured:

T: 98.4°F, HR: 67 bpm, BP: 130/90 mm Hg, RR: 16 breaths/min

Differential Diagnosis

- Essential tremor, Parkinson disease, normal pressure hydrocephalus, Alzheimer disease, stroke, subdural hematoma, Huntington disease

Laboratory Data and Other Study Results

- CBC: WBC: 8.8, Hgb: 13.9, Plt: 231
- Chem10: Na: 143 mEq/L, K: 3.7 mEq/L, Cl: 100 mEq/L, CO_2: 29 mEq/L, BUN: 19 mg/dL, Cr: 0.9 mg/dL, Glu: 85 mg/dL, Mg: 2.1 mg/dL, Ca: 9.9 mg/dL, Phos: 4.0 mg/dL
- Head MRI: no intracranial hemorrhage; normal ventricles; normal cortical volume; no focal lesions

Diagnosis

- Parkinson disease

Treatment Administered

- The patient was started on levodopa to improve his symptoms

Follow-up

- The patient experienced an improvement in his symptoms after starting levodopa
- Five years after initiating medical therapy, the patient began to experience further worsening of his neurologic function
- He was considered an appropriate candidate for implantation of a deep brain stimulator and underwent the procedure
- The patient experienced a further improvement in his symptoms after this surgery

Steps to the Diagnosis

- **Parkinson disease**
  - An idiopathic disease of dopamine depletion, loss of dopaminergic striated neurons in the substantia nigra, and Lewy body formation (i.e., eosinophilic cytoplasmic inclusions) in substantia nigra neurons, leading to an abnormally increased inhibition of the thalamic-cortical neural pathways
    - A similar syndrome may be seen following repeated blunt injuries to the head (e.g., boxers), MPTP (1-methyl-4-phenyl-1,2,3,6-tetrahydropyridine) intoxication (i.e., a side product of illicit opioid production), or exposure to certain industrial toxins
  - **History:** memory loss, sleep disturbances, depression, constipation

- **Physical examination: resting tremor** (i.e., "**pill-rolling**" in the hands), bradykinesia (i.e., decreased voluntary movement) with difficulty initiating movement, masklike face, **shuffling gait**, involuntary gait acceleration following initiation, "**cogwheel**" **rigidity** (i.e., increased tone of agonist and antagonist muscles), postural instability
- **Tests:** no lab tests or neuroimaging is reliable for the diagnosis; positron emission tomography (PET) scan is useful for detecting decreased dopamine uptake in the substantia nigra
- **Treatment:**
  - Dopaminergic agonists (e.g., levodopa, carbidopa, bromocriptine, amantadine), monoamine oxidase B inhibitors (MAOI; e.g., selegiline), anticholinergic agents (e.g., benztropine), and amantadine play a role in treatment (Table 7-13)
  - Initially a single dopaminergic agonist is prescribed; a second drug may be added if symptoms begin to worsen while on monotherapy
  - Deep brain stimulation is an approved option for disease that is refractory to medications or progressive in nature
- **Outcomes:** as the disease progresses, patients become susceptible to other medical comorbidities (e.g., pneumonia, dementia, falls) that increase their overall mortality rate
- **Clues to the diagnosis:**
  - History: memory loss, depression
  - Physical: pill-rolling tremor, gait disturbance, masklike face, cogwheel rigidity
  - Tests: noncontributory

MNEMONIC

Common signs of Parkinson's disease may be remembered by the mnemonic **SMART**: **S**huffling gait, **M**asklike face, **A**kinesia, **R**igidity ("cogwheel"), **T**remor (resting).

- **Essential tremor**
  - Development of a slowly progressive resting or activity-related tremor that is most common in the upper extremities
    - Involves abnormal neural activity in the thalamic-cortical-brainstem pathway
  - **History:** tremor worsens with stress and emotion, tremor resolves during sleep
  - **Physical examination:** fixed frequency tremor in either the head or upper extremities that occurs during activity
  - **Tests:** lab tests and imaging are nondiagnostic and typically are used to rule out other diagnoses
  - **Treatment:** primidone, propanolol, and anticonvulsants are used to reduce the degree of tremor; thalamotomy or implantation of a deep brain stimulator is considered for severe cases
  - **Outcomes:** the tremor is progressive and requires occasional adjustments in therapy

TABLE 7-13 Medications Used in Treatment of Parkinson Disease

Drug	Mechanism	Indications	Adverse Effects
Levodopa	Dopamine precursor	Initial therapy	Nausea, vomiting, anorexia, tachycardia, hallucinations, mood changes, dyskinesia with chronic use
Carbidopa	Dopamine decarboxylase inhibitor that reduces levodopa metabolism	Combined with levodopa to augment effects	Reduces adverse effects of levodopa by allowing smaller dosage
Bromocriptine	Dopamine receptor agonist	Increases response to levodopa in patients with declining response	Hallucinations, confusion, nausea, hypotension, cardiotoxicity
Selegiline	Monoamine oxidase type B inhibitor	Early disease; may help delay the need to start levodopa	Nausea, headache, confusion, insomnia
Amantadine	Increases synthesis, release, or reuptake of dopamine	More effective against rigidity and bradykinesia	Agitation, hallucinations
Antimuscarinic agents (e.g., benztropine)	Block cholinergic transmission	Adjuvant therapy	Mood changes, dry mouth, visual abnormalities, confusion, hallucinations, urinary retention

- **Why eliminated from differential:** the multiple additional symptoms seen in this case besides upper extremity tremor make this diagnosis unlikely
- **Normal pressure hydrocephalus**
  - The collection of excessive CSF in the cerebral ventricles and spinal thecal sac
    - May be a sequela of subarachnoid hemorrhage or chronic meningitis
  - **History:** cognitive impairments, incontinence
  - **Physical examination:** gait abnormalities
  - **Tests:** MRI will show enlarged cerebral ventricles, white matter lesions, and aqueduct atrophy
  - **Treatment:** ventriculoperitoneal shunting is performed to decompress the accumulation of CSF but improves symptoms in a minority of cases
  - **Outcomes:** the disease carries an unfavorable prognosis in which a minority of cases improve following shunting, and complications involving shunt occlusion are common
  - **Why eliminated from differential:** the normal appearance of the MRI rules out this diagnosis

MNEMONIC

The signs of normal pressure hydrocephalus may be remembered by the **three Ws**: **W**acky (cognitive impairment), **W**et (incontinence), **W**obbly (gait abnormalities).

- **Alzheimer disease**
  - Slowly progressive dementia due to the development of neurofibrillary tangles, neuritic plaques, amyloid deposition, and neuronal atrophy of cortical neurons
  - **Risk factors:** increased age, family history, Down syndrome, female gender
  - **History: progressive short-term memory loss**, depression, **confusion**, inability to complete complex movements or tasks, depression, possible personality changes or delusions
  - **Physical examination:** typically noncontributory, but spasticity may be seen
  - **Tests:** CT or MRI demonstrates cortical atrophy
  - **Treatment:**
    - Cholinesterase inhibitors (e.g., donepezil, rivastigmine, galantamine) and vitamin E may slow progression
    - Memantine may improve symptoms in moderate cases
    - Antidepressants are useful for treating comorbid depression
    - Occupational therapy is useful to prolong independence
  - **Outcomes:**
    - Dementia is progressive and associated with a worsening ability to perform daily activities and a greater susceptibility to other medical comorbidities
    - Mortality rates are based on the age at the time of diagnosis
      - Patients diagnosed at 65 may live 10 years
      - Patients diagnosed at 90 survive <5 years
  - **Why eliminated from differential:** the multiple physical findings detected in addition to the memory impairment make this diagnosis less likely

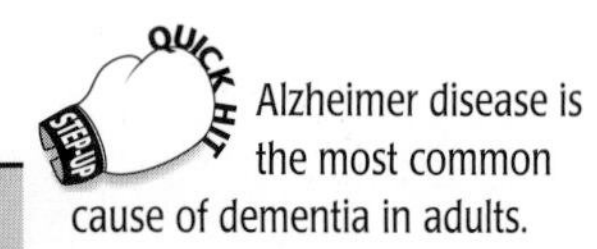
Alzheimer disease is the most common cause of dementia in adults.

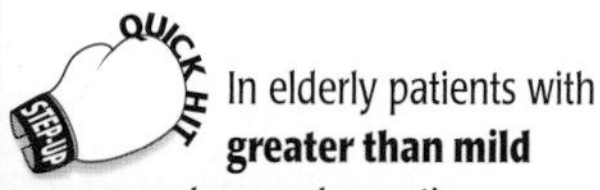
In elderly patients with **greater than mild** memory loss or dementia, Alzheimer disease is the most common explanation.

NEUROLOGY

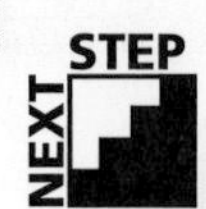
NEXT STEP

Distinguish dementia due to Alzheimer disease from that due to multiple cortical infarcts with MRI. Multiple small lesions or infarcts will be apparent on MRI when there is a **vascular** cause.

- **Stroke**
  - More thorough discussion in prior case
  - **Why eliminated from differential:** the normal-appearing MRI rules out this diagnosis
- **Subdural hematoma**
  - More thorough discussion in prior case
  - **Why eliminated from differential:** the normal-appearing MRI rules out this diagnosis
- **Huntington disease**
  - An autosomal dominant disease defined by the presence of multiple CAG repeats on chromosome 4
    - A higher number of CAG repeats correlates with an earlier development of the disease
  - **History:** symptoms develop in middle age and include dementia, irritability, antisocial behavior, and possible seizures
  - **Physical examination: chorea** of the extremities (i.e., rapid irregular involuntary movements)
  - **Tests:** genetic analysis can detect the chromosomal abnormality; CT or MRI will demonstrate atrophy of the caudate nucleus and putamen
  - **Treatment:** dopaminergic antagonists may improve choreatic movements; genetic screening may be useful for family members to help plan for future cases

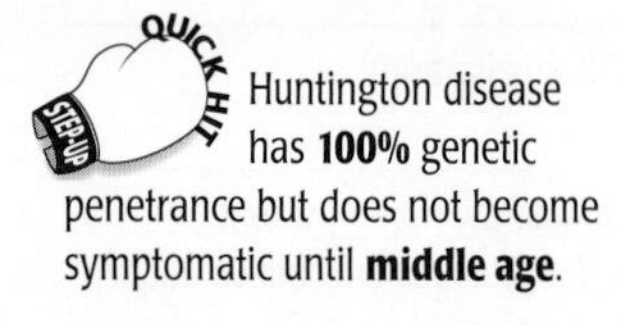
Huntington disease has **100%** genetic penetrance but does not become symptomatic until **middle age**.

- **Outcomes:** the prognosis is poor with mortality occurring <20 years from the time of diagnosis
- **Why eliminated from differential:** the movement abnormalities seen in this case are not choreatic in nature, and the patient is older than would be expected for the development of the characteristic symptoms

The following additional Neurology cases may be found online:

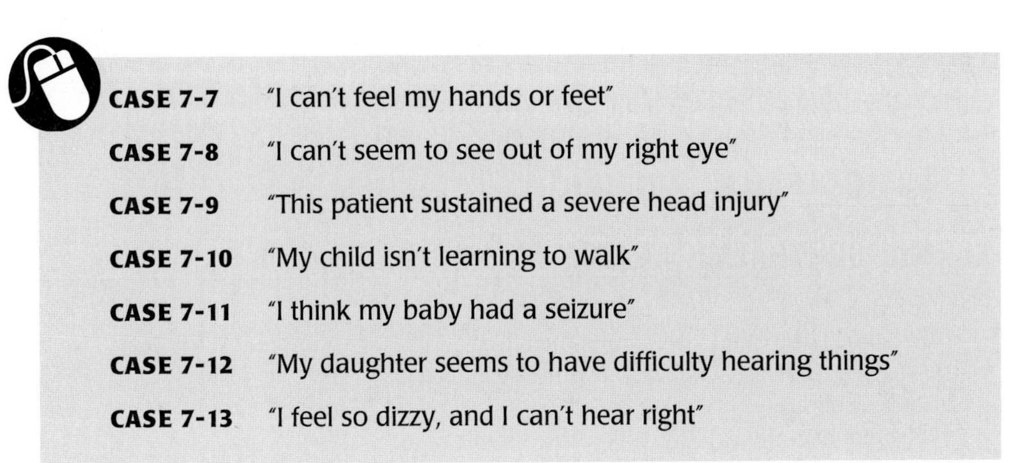

CASE 7-7	"I can't feel my hands or feet"
CASE 7-8	"I can't seem to see out of my right eye"
CASE 7-9	"This patient sustained a severe head injury"
CASE 7-10	"My child isn't learning to walk"
CASE 7-11	"I think my baby had a seizure"
CASE 7-12	"My daughter seems to have difficulty hearing things"
CASE 7-13	"I feel so dizzy, and I can't hear right"

Ophthalmology

BASIC CLINICAL PRIMER

NORMAL OPHTHALMIC ANATOMY

- **Vasculature**
  - The retinal artery and vein supply the retina
  - Vascular pathology is associated with visual defects
- **Neurologic supply**
  - The optic nerve (CN II) is responsible for vision
  - The trochlear nerve (CN IV) controls the superior oblique muscle (downward medial gaze, inward eye motion)
  - The abducens nerve (CN IV) controls the lateral rectus muscle
  - The oculomotor nerve (CN III) controls all of the other eye muscles
  - The medial longitudinal fasciculus (MLF) maintains conjugate gaze in one eye when the other eye abducts

COMMON VISUAL ABNORMALITIES

- **Pupil defects**
  - Typically occur due to an injury or defect along the neural signaling pathway for vision (Table 8-1)
- **Visual field or focal defects**
  - Typically occur because of eye shape or neural injury (Figure 8-1, Table 8-2)
  - May be correctable through **lenses**, visual training, or surgery

CASE 8-1 "I woke up, and my eye was all red"

A 19-year-old woman presents to her college's student health office after she woke up this morning with a red, painful left eye. She says that she had some mild itching in her left eye when she went to bed the previous night. She also reports that she has never had these symptoms previously. Her eye feels mildly painful, itchy, and teary. She denies any visual difficulties. She denies any problems in her right eye, fevers, headache, neck pain, sore throat, or ear pain. She denies any past medical history and takes no medications. She drinks alcohol socially on the weekends and works three afternoons per week in a children's day care center. On examination, she appears to be in no acute distress. The sclera and conjunctiva of her left eye are inflamed. No purulent discharge is notable, but the left eye is watery. Her right eye has slight inflammation of the conjunctiva. Her pupils are symmetrical, react equally to light, and track normally. Fundoscopic examination detects normal vascular markings in each eye. A slit lamp examination with fluorescein staining detects no corneal defects. Otoscopic examination detects mobile, pearly tympanic membranes. She has a mildly palpable preauricular lymph node on the left side. Her neck

TABLE 8-1 Common Pupil and Gaze Abnormalities

Abnormality	Presentation	Cause
Argyll-Robertson pupil	Normal accommodation to near objects, nonreactive to light	Syphilis, SLE, DM
Marcus Gunn pupil	Light in the affected pupil causes minimal bilateral constriction, light in the normal pupil causes normal bilateral constriction	Afferent nerve defect
Horner syndrome	Ptosis, miosis, anhidrosis	Sympathetic trunk lesion (e.g., Pancoast tumor)
Adie pupil	Minimally reactive dilated pupil	Abnormal innervation of the iris
MLF syndrome	With lateral gaze there is absent contralateral eye adduction	Intracranial lesion, MS

DM, diabetes mellitus; MLF, medial longitudinal fasciculus; MS, multiple sclerosis; SLE, systemic lupus erythematosus.

has no lymphadenopathy and is supple. Examination of her oropharynx is normal. The following vital signs are measured:

Temperature (T): 98.8°F, heart rate (HR): 70 beats per minute (bpm), blood pressure (BP): 115/80 mm Hg, respiratory rate (RR): 17 breaths/min

Differential Diagnosis

- Conjunctivitis, uveitis, closed-angle glaucoma, corneal abrasion

Laboratory Data and Other Study Results

- None performed

Diagnosis

- Viral conjunctivitis

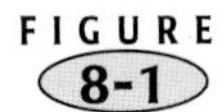

FIGURE 8-1 **Visual field defects resulting from neuronal injury.**

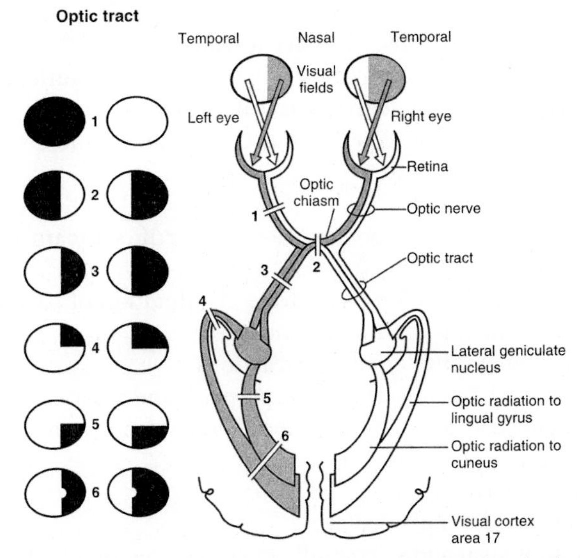

(Taken from Mehta S, Milder EA, Mirachi AJ, Milder E. *Step-up: a high-yield, systems-based review for the USMLE step 1.* 2nd ed. Philadelphia: Lippincott Williams & Wilkins, 2003. Used with permission of Lippincott Williams & Wilkins.)

TABLE 8-2 Common Vision Abnormalities

Disorder	Cause	H/P	Treatment
Myopia	Refracting power of the eye is too great, causing the image focal point to be anterior to the retina	Blurred vision, vision quality worsens as objects move farther away	Corrective lenses, laser correction
Hyperopia	Refracting power of the eye is insufficient, causing the image focal point to be posterior to the retina	Blurred vision, vision quality worsens as objects move closer	Corrective lenses, laser correction
Astigmatism	Asymmetrical cornea surface, causing an inconsistent refraction of light	Blurred vision	Corrective lenses
Strabismus	Deviation of an eye that is unable to be overcome by normal motor control	Gaze for each eye is in a different direction, double vision, progressive blindness	Vision training, surgery is frequently required to achieve bilateral alignment
Amblyopia (i.e., "lazy eye")	Developmental defect in the neural pathways of the eye	Poor visual acuity, spatial differentiation in the affected eye	Vision training, levodopa, carbidopa

H/P, history and physical.

Treatment Administered

- The patient was provided artificial tears and a 3-day course of ciprofloxacin drops

Follow-up

- The patient's symptoms resolved over the following 3 days

Steps to the Diagnosis

- Conjunctivitis
  - Inflammation of the eye mucosa that occurs as a result of viral infection, bacterial infection, or an allergic reaction
    - Typically **highly contagious** and spread by close contact or through towels and linens
    - Adenovirus is the most common cause
    - *Staphylococcus aureus* and *Streptococcus pneumoniae* are common bacterial causes
    - *Neisseria gonorrhoeae* and *Chlamydia trachomatis* may be transmitted by sexual contact or to a newborn by an infected mother
  - **History:** mild eye pain, pruritis, excessive tearing
  - **Physical examination: inflamed conjunctiva**, possible preauricular lymphadenopathy, possible purulent discharge (bacterial infections)
  - **Tests:** tests are typically not required, but Gram stain of the discharge is helpful to define a species in bacterial cases
  - **Treatment:**
    - Typically self-limited, so supportive care (e.g., **artificial tears**, cold compresses) is the mainstay of therapy
    - Broad-spectrum antibiotic drops decrease the duration of bacterial infections and serve a prophylactic role in viral infections
    - Antihistamines are useful for allergic reactions
    - **Prevention** through hand washing and proper laundry services is important
  - **Outcomes:** prognosis is good, but *N. gonorrhoeae* infections require aggressive therapy to prevent secondary meningitis
  - **Clues to the diagnosis:**
    - History: itchy, painful, inflamed eye
    - Physical: conjunctival and scleral inflammation, preauricular lymphadenopathy
    - Tests: noncontributory

- **Uveitis**
  - Inflammation of the iris, choroids, and ciliary bodies due to infectious (e.g., viral, syphilis), autoimmune (e.g., ankylosing spondylitis, **juvenile rheumatoid arthritis**), or inflammatory (e.g., ulcerative colitis, **Crohn** disease) conditions
    - May occur as an anterior or posterior eye process
  - **History:**
    - **Anterior uveitis:** eye pain, photophobia
    - **Posterior uveitis:** blurry vision
  - **Physical examination:**
    - **Anterior uveitis:** slit lamp examination shows eye inflammation and corneal keratin deposits
    - **Posterior uveitis:** slit lamp examination shows eye inflammation and retinal lesions
  - **Tests:** typically not required
  - **Treatment:**
    - Infectious cases should be treated with antibiotic drops
    - Noninfectious cases will benefit from topical or systemic corticosteroid use
    - Treatment of an underlying condition will help limit or prevent recurrences
  - **Outcomes:** the prognosis is good with treatment; an acute increase in the intraocular pressure is a rare complication and may cause permanent visual deficits
  - **Why eliminated from differential:** the normal slit lamp examination makes this diagnosis unlikely
- **Corneal abrasion**
  - Traumatic injury of the corneal epithelial surface
    - The injury may occur thorough mechanical means or due to chemical exposure
  - **History:** appropriate exposure to an irritant, eye pain, photophobia, **sensation of a foreign body in the eye**, excessive tearing
  - **Physical examination:** eye inflammation, slit lamp examination with fluorescein staining shows corneal defects
  - **Tests:** typically not required
  - **Treatment:** topical antibiotics are administered prophylactically; debridement may be performed for larger abrasions to reduce the risk of ulceration
  - **Outcomes:** the prognosis is good with most injuries healing in <2 days; inadequately treated abrasions that ulcerate may result in permanent vision deficits
  - **Why eliminated from differential:** the normal slit lamp examination rules out this diagnosis
- **Closed-angle-glaucoma**
  - More thorough discussion in later case
  - **Why eliminated from differential:** the normal symmetry and reactivity of the pupils and mild degree of eye pain make this diagnosis unlikely

CASE 8-2 "My eyesight is getting really bad"

An 84-year-old woman presents to an ophthalmologist with the complaint of progressive vision loss over several years. The patient says that she is unsure of when she first started to have difficulty seeing objects, but she knows that she cannot see things as well as she could 5 years ago. She was last seen by an ophthalmologist at that time for a vision examination and eyeglass prescription. She says that all objects look fuzzy. She especially has problems seeing in rooms with bright lights because of the glow surrounding the lights. She has not driven in the past year because she is afraid of hitting something. She feels that her vision is equally bad throughout her visual fields. She denies eye pain, pruritis, eye discharge, or any eye trauma. She notes a history of hypertension (HTN), hypercholesterolemia, and breast cancer treated with a lumpectomy 10 years ago. She takes losartan, hydrochlorothiazide (HCTZ), and simvastatin as medications. She denies any substance use. On examination, she appears to be in no distress. Her eyes both appear cloudy, with the right being worse than the left. Her pupils are equally reactive and track well. Fundoscopic examination is difficult but detects one example of arteriovenous nicking in each eye and no evidence of retinal hemorrhage or fragmentation. Visual acuity testing detects significant deficits in each eye, with the right worse than the left. Slit lamp examination detects no corneal lesions but does demonstrate opacity of both lenses. No lymphadenopathy is detected. The following vital signs are measured:

T: 98.5°F, HR: 80 bpm, BP: 120/82 mm Hg, RR: 18 breaths/min

Differential Diagnosis

- Cataracts, glaucoma, macular degeneration, retinal detachment, retinal vessel occlusion

Laboratory Data and Other Study Results

- Ocular tonometry: normal intraocular pressure in both eyes

Diagnosis

- Cataracts

Treatment Administered

- The patient was scheduled for lens replacement surgery of the right eye

Follow-up

- Following surgery, the patient reported a significant improvement in her right eye vision
- The patient elected to schedule lens replacement for her left eye following recovery from the first surgery

Steps to the Diagnosis

- Cataracts
  - Clouding of the lens of the eye, leading to progressive vision loss
    - May occur as an insidious process, following eye trauma, or as a congenital abnormality
  - **Risk factors:** trauma (e.g., caustic chemicals), diabetes mellitus (DM), corticosteroid use, advanced age, low education, alcohol use, tobacco use
  - **History: progressive hazy and blurred vision**, glare around lights, diplopia
  - **Physical examination: lens opacity**, decreased red reflex (Color Figure 8-1)
  - **Tests:** none required
  - **Treatment:** lens extraction and replacement is the definitive treatment for the condition
  - **Outcomes:**
    - The prognosis is good with lens replacement
    - Patients are at a risk for accidents due to impaired vision prior to treatment
    - Complications from lens replacement surgery may cause permanent visual deficits
  - **Clues to the diagnosis:**
    - History: progressive vision loss, hazy vision, glare from lights
    - Physical: lens opacity, impaired visual acuity
    - Tests: noncontributory
- Open-angle glaucoma
  - A gradual increase in intraocular pressure, leading to progressive vision loss
  - **Risk factors:** increased age, DM, myopia, family history, African heritage

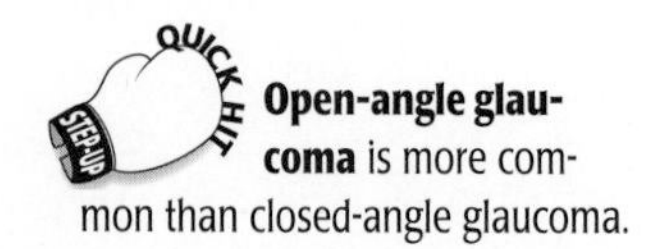

Open-angle glaucoma is more common than closed-angle glaucoma.

- **History**: gradual loss of visual fields (**peripheral to central**), halos seen around lights, headache, poor light adaptation
- **Physical examination:**
  - Fundoscopic examination shows cupping of the optic disc
  - Slit lamp examination shows corneal thickening with keratin deposits and iris atrophy
  - Visual field testing shows vision loss in the peripheral extent of the visual fields
- **Tests:** tonometry demonstrates increased intraocular pressure consistently for several tests performed at intervals over multiple weeks
- **Treatment:**
  - **Topical β-blockers** (e.g., timolol) and α-adrenergic agonists decrease the aqueous humor production to help reduce intraocular pressure
  - Prostaglandin analogues, α-adrenergic agonists, and cholinergic agonists (e.g., pilocarpine) increase aqueous humor removal
  - Laser surgery improves aqueous humor drainage in refractory cases
  - **Regular ophthalmologic examinations** are the key to prevention in at-risk groups
- **Outcomes:** prognosis correlates with the ability to normalize intraocular pressure; poor pressure control results in progressive vision loss and blindness
- **Why eliminated from differential:** the normal tonometry measurements rule out this diagnosis

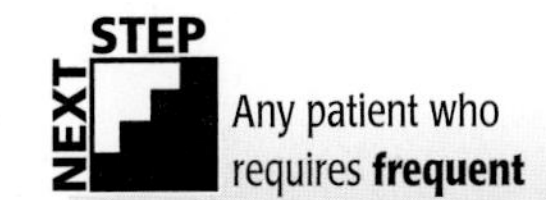

Any patient who requires **frequent changes of lens prescriptions** should be suspected for having glaucoma, and tonometry should be performed to rule out the condition.

- **Close-angle glaucoma**
  - An **acute** increase in intraocular pressure due to narrowing of the anterior chamber angle that causes obstructed drainage of aqueous humor from the eye
  - **Risk factors:** increased age, hyperopia, dilated pupils, Asian heritage
  - **History:** severe eye pain, blurry vision, halos seen around lights, nausea, vomiting
  - **Physical examination:** inflamed and **hard** eye, **dilated** and **nonreactive** pupil
  - **Tests:** tonometry demonstrates an increased intraocular pressure
  - **Treatment:**
    - Acetazolamide and β-blockers acutely decrease the intraocular pressure
    - Pilocarpine is administered after pressure reduction to reduce the degree of obstruction to aqueous humor drainage
    - Laser iridotomy should be performed to prevent recurrences and may be performed prophylactically on the unaffected eye
  - **Outcomes:** permanent vision loss will result without prompt treatment
  - **Why eliminated from differential:** the mild degree of eye pain, normal reactivity of the eye, and normal intraocular pressure rule out this diagnosis

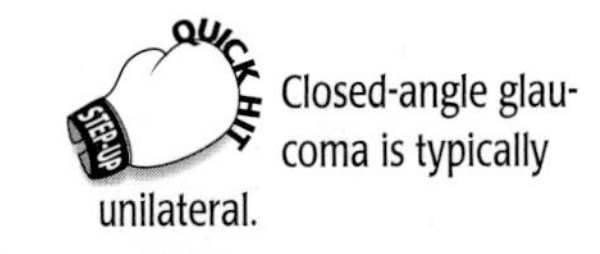

Closed-angle glaucoma is typically unilateral.

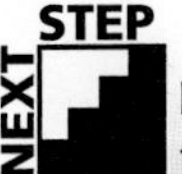

Never induce additional pupil dilation during an examination of the patient with suspected closed-angle glaucoma because it will acutely worsen the condition.

- **Macular degeneration**
  - Atrophic (slow) or exudative (rapid) degeneration of the retina leading to **retinal fibrosis** and **permanent vision loss**
  - **Risk factors:** tobacco use, family history, white race, increased age, prolonged sun exposure, HTN, female gender
  - **History:** painless gradual vision loss (**central to peripheral**) for all distances
  - **Physical examination:** fundoscopic examination shows either increased retinal pigmentation (atrophic type) or retinal hemorrhage (exudative type) in the macula and possible retinal detachment
  - **Tests:** fluorescein angiography may demonstrate neovascularization of the retina and membrane formation
  - **Treatment:**
    - Intravitreal ranibizumab may help treat exudative lesions near the fovea
    - Laser photocoagulation of discrete lesions may delay progression
  - **Outcomes:** prognosis is poor for the exudative type with a gradual loss of vision; the atrophic type is associated with a slower progression of vision loss
  - **Why eliminated from differential:** the findings of the fundoscopic examination make this diagnosis unlikely
- **Retinal detachment**
  - Separation of the retina from the adjacent epithelium leading to an acute loss of vision
  - **Risk factors:** trauma, cataract surgery, myopia, family history

- **History:** painless acute loss of vision, numerous "floaters" or the feeling of a "**window shade pulled over the eye**"
- **Physical examination:** fundoscopic examination shows retinal fragmentation or a gray retina floating in the vitreous humor
- **Tests:** none required
- **Treatment:** laser photocoagulation or cryotherapy is performed to halt tear progression; intraocular repair is performed to reattach the retina
- **Outcomes:** the degree of retinal involvement and the time until repair correlate with the degree of vision loss; vision may not be fully restored following retinal reattachment
- **Why eliminated from differential:** the findings of the fundoscopic examination and the gradual onset of the vision loss make this diagnosis unlikely

- **Retinal vessel occlusion**
  - Occlusion of a retinal artery or vein resulting in the sudden loss of vision
    - Most commonly occurs as a sequela to atherosclerosis, DM, HTN, or thromboembolic disease (Color Figures 8-2, 8-3, and 8-4)
  - **History:**
    - **Retinal artery occlusion:** sudden, painless loss of vision
    - **Retinal vein occlusion:** slow, painless loss of vision
  - **Physical examination:**
    - **Retinal artery occlusion:** fundoscopic examination shows a **cherry-red spot** in the fovea and poor arterial filling
    - **Retinal vein occlusion:** fundoscopic examination shows **cotton wool spots**, retinal edema, **retinal hemorrhages**, and dilated veins
  - **Tests:** none required
  - **Treatment:**
    - Thrombolysis of arterial occlusions should be performed within 8 hours of onset
    - Acetazolamide and oxygen administration are used to decrease retinal venous congestion and increase arterial perfusion
    - Laser photocoagulation may be useful for venous occlusion
  - **Outcomes:** the degree of vision loss correlates with the time until treatment occurs
  - **Why eliminated from differential:** the findings of the fundoscopic examination make these diagnoses less likely, but persistent vision deficits following lens replacement for the obvious cataracts should warrant a more extensive work-up given the patient's past medical history

CASE 8-3 "My son has a white eye"

A 3-year-old boy is brought to an ophthalmologist by his mother for evaluation of his right eye. The patient's mother says that when she took a photo of her son 2 weeks ago she noticed that one of his eyes had a white spot in the center of the pupil. When she looked at his eyes afterward she did not notice any abnormality but found that the white spot was reproduced when a light was shined in his eyes. She says that her son has not been complaining of pain in his right eye and has not been rubbing it. He has not been behaving strangely lately. He has met all of his developmental milestones and has no problem recognizing colors and objects. He is not accident prone and does not fall more than is expected for his age. He has not had any fevers, recent colds, or trauma to his right eye. He was the product of a full-term vaginal delivery that was uncomplicated. He has no medical problems and is up to date on his vaccinations. There is no family history of eye diseases. On examination, he is a well-appearing child in no distress. When light is shined in his eyes, the left eye has a normal red reflex, but the right eye has a central white appearance. His pupils react normally, and he is able to track objects well. His conjunctiva are pink, and his sclera are not injected. Fundoscopic slit lamp examination detects a small whitish growth involving the posterior wall of the retina. There are no corneal or lens defects.

There are no arteriovenous malformations or hemorrhages. There is no lymphadenopathy. The following vital signs are measured:

T: 98.5°F, HR: 85 bpm, BP: 114/73 mm Hg, RR: 18 breaths/min

Differential Diagnosis

- Retinoblastoma, uveitis, congenital cataract

Laboratory Data and Other Study Results

- Head computed tomography (CT): small mass of the posterior right eye globe without extension into the posterior orbit; normal cerebral and ventricular size; no hemorrhage
- Retinoblastoma (RB1) gene testing: mutation in the patient's *RB1* gene; no mutation found in either parent

Diagnosis

- Retinoblastoma

Treatment Administered

- Laser photocoagulation was performed on the lesion

Follow-up

- Examination confirmed complete destruction of the tumor
- As the child grew older, it was confirmed that he had a visual acuity deficit in the right eye that was treated with glasses and a small central visual field defect that created a blind spot
- The child was able to learn normally in school given his maintained left eye vision
- The family was counseled that the patient's genetic abnormality was a new defect and that future children were at no increased risk for the disease

Steps to the Diagnosis

- **Retinoblastoma**
  - Malignant tumor of the retina found most commonly in children
    - Most common intraocular tumor in children
    - Cases may be due to a new mutation in the *RB1* gene or a hereditary gene defect
  - **History:** patients are frequently initially asymptomatic but may have vision loss or eye inflammation
  - **Physical examination:** poor red reflex in the affected eye, possible white spot in the eye (i.e., **leukokoria**), fundoscopic examination may detect a white mass in the retina (Color Figure 8-5)
  - **Tests:** genetic testing is useful for detecting mutations in the *RB1* gene; CT, ultrasound (US), or magnetic resonance imaging (MRI) is needed to determine the full extent of the lesion and to detect any calcification of the tumor
  - **Treatment:**
    - **Enucleation** is performed for large tumors with no vision potential
    - External beam radiation may be used for bilateral tumors or those near the optic nerve but has been associated with stopping facial bone growth or causing other forms of cancer
    - Cryotherapy and laser photocoagulation may be used for smaller tumors in the posterior retina
    - Chemotherapy is used in metastatic disease and for large tumors

- **Outcomes:** overall survival is 85%, but this rate decreases with extension of the tumor posterior to the globe
- **Clues to the diagnosis:**
  - History: leukokoria in photo
  - Physical: leukokoria, white mass on fundoscopic examination
  - Tests: head CT demonstrating the lesion
- Uveitis
  - More thorough discussion in prior case
  - **Why eliminated from differential:** the absence of eye inflammation makes this diagnosis unlikely
- Congenital cataract
  - More thorough discussion in prior case
  - **Why eliminated from differential:** the slit lamp examination rules out this diagnosis

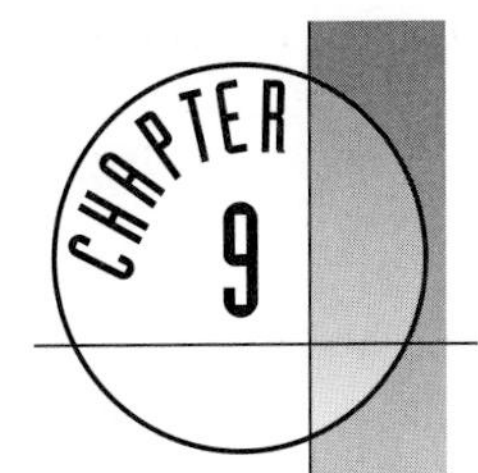

Orthopedics and Rheumatology

CASE 9-1 "My hands feel numb"

A 49-year-old woman presents to her primary care provider (PCP) with a 1-year history of progressive numbness and tingling in her hands. She says that she first noticed tingling in her hands during her work as a secretary about a year ago. Her symptoms have gradually worsened, and she now reports frequent numbness in her hands and weakness when gripping items. She says that her symptoms are typically mild at rest but become worse with activity. She says that she is right-handed and that her symptoms are slightly worse in this hand. She denies any numbness proximal to her hands. She denies any trauma to her upper extremities or neck and has no neck or back pain. She denies headaches and dizziness. She has a past medical history for type 2 diabetes mellitus (DM) and takes metformin for glucose regulation. She denies any allergies. She has an occasional alcoholic beverage but denies other substance use. On examination, she appears to be in no distress. Her face and body appear symmetrical. She has no lymphadenopathy. Examination of her upper extremities is notable for slight thenar muscle wasting in the right hand. She has 5/5 strength with all active ranges of motion in the upper extremities. She has subjectively decreased sensation to light touch in the palmar surface of both index fingers and the medial side of her palms, but her sensation is otherwise normal. She has strong pulses in both arms. Tapping her volar wrists elicits a sharp pain in both hands. Tapping on the medial side of her elbow does not elicit this response. Provocational maneuvers of her neck do not elicit such symptoms. When her wrists are held in a flexed position for over a minute, she reports numbness in both hands. She has no pain on palpation of her back and spine. No rashes or lesions are visible on her body. The following vital signs are measured:

Temperature (T): 98.6°F, heart rate (HR): 72 beats per minute (bpm), blood pressure (BP): 128/78 mm Hg, respiratory rate (RR): 14 breaths/min

Differential Diagnosis

- Carpal tunnel syndrome, cervical disc herniation, cervical spinal stenosis, brachial plexopathy, diabetic neuropathy, multiple sclerosis

Laboratory Data and Other Study Results

- 7-electrolyte chemistry panel (Chem7): sodium (Na): 138 mEq/L, potassium (K): 4.2 mEq/L, chloride (Cl): 106 mEq/L, carbon dioxide (CO_2): 27 mEq/L, blood urea nitrogen (BUN): 14 mg/dL, creatinine (Cr): 0.7 mg/dL, glucose (Glu): 75 mg/dL
- Electromyelogram (EMG)/nerve conduction studies (NCS): prolonged conduction latency, decreased amplitude of action potentials, and fibrillation potentials distal to the wrist only in both upper extremities

Diagnosis

- Carpal tunnel syndrome

Treatment Administered

- The patient was referred to an occupational therapist to be fit with wrist splints and to be instructed in activity modification to avoid inducing recurrent symptoms

Follow-up

- After 1 month, the patient reported no improvement with nonoperative treatments, so she was referred to an orthopedic surgeon to discuss surgical releases of the transverse carpal ligaments
- Following carpal tunnel releases the patient experienced a notable improvement in her symptoms, and her function improved

Steps to the Diagnosis

- **Carpal tunnel syndrome**
  - A syndrome of **median** nerve dysfunction, resulting from compression of the nerve at the wrist by the transverse carpal ligament (Figure 9-1)
    - More common in 30- to 55-year-olds
  - **Risk factors:** pregnancy, rheumatoid arthritis (RA), DM, acromegaly, hypothyroidism, obesity, overuse activity (e.g., typing, writing, piano playing), female gender
  - **History:** wrist pain that worsens with grip and hand flexion, numbness in thumb and index and long fingers
  - **Physical examination:** decreased grip strength, decreased radial-sided palmar two-point discrimination, positive **Tinel sign** (i.e., tapping over median nerve elicits tingling and shocking pain), positive **Phalen sign** (i.e., placing the dorsal surfaces of the hands together and flexing the wrists induces symptoms), thenar muscle atrophy
  - **Tests:** EMG and NCS will show increased conduction latency, fibrillation potentials, and a decreased conduction amplitude **below the wrist only**
  - **Treatment:**
    - Wrists splints, activity modification, and nonsteroidal anti-inflamatory drugs (NSAIDs) are the common first-line treatments
    - Corticosteroid injections through the transverse carpal ligament may help symptoms resolve in mild cases

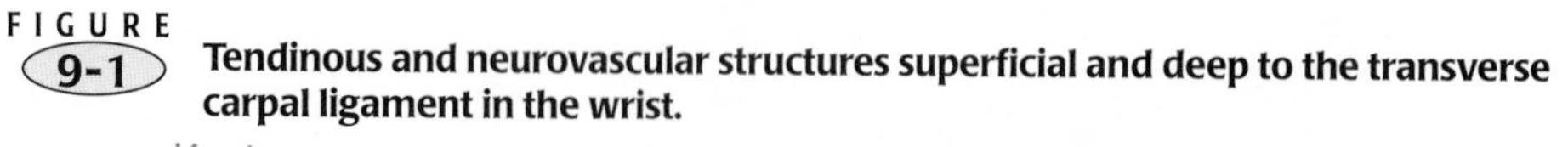

FIGURE 9-1 **Tendinous and neurovascular structures superficial and deep to the transverse carpal ligament in the wrist.**

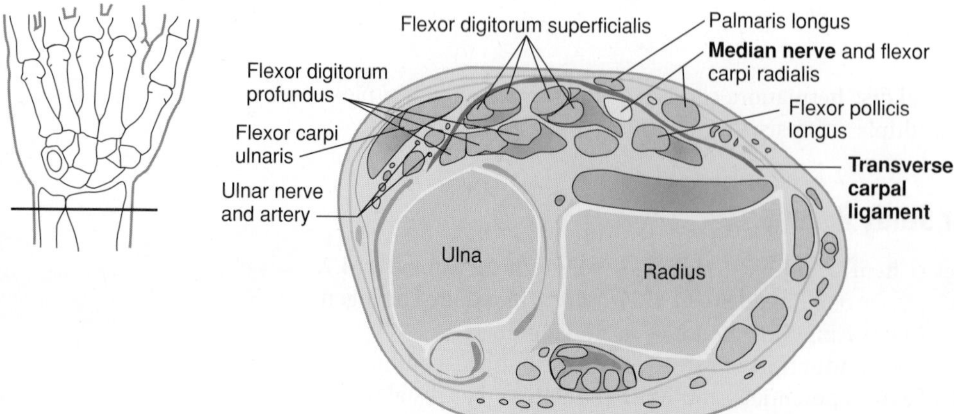

(Taken from Moore KL. *Clinically oriented anatomy.* 3rd ed. Baltimore: Williams & Wilkins, 1992. Used with permission of Williams & Wilkins.)

    - Surgical release of the transverse carpal ligament is required in cases that do not respond to nonoperative management
  - **Outcomes:** ninety percent of patients will experience an improvement in their symptoms following surgical release; complete restoration of strength and sensation may not occur in long-standing cases
  - **Clues to the diagnosis:**
    - History: numbness and weakness in hands, work as a secretary, history of DM, absence of symptoms above the wrist
    - Physical: thenar muscle atrophy, positive Tinel and Phalen signs
    - Tests: EMG/NCS findings
- **Spinal stenosis**
  - A generalized narrowing of the spinal foramina due to arthritic changes
    - Results in the symptomatic compression of exiting nerve roots
    - More common in middle-aged and older adults
  - **History:** radiating pain that corresponds with the distribution of the compressed nerve root (i.e., **radiculopathy**), pain may worsen with standing and walking
  - **Physical examination: chronic nerve compression** may result in motor and sensory deficits, abnormal gait and loss of lumbar lordosis are seen when occurring in the lumbar spine
  - **Tests:** x-ray or spinal magnetic resonance imaging (MRI) is used to confirm the diagnosis and to determine the degree of nerve impingement
  - **Treatment:**
    - NSAIDs and physical therapy are first-line treatments
    - Epidural injections of corticosteroids or anesthetic agents may be used in cases not responding to conservative treatment
    - Surgical decompression (e.g., laminectomy, foraminectomy) may be performed in patients not responding to nonoperative treatments
  - **Outcomes:** myelopathy may occur in patients with long-standing nerve compression; progression of nerve compression occurs in almost all patients with lumbar stenosis and one third of patients with cervical stenosis
  - **Why eliminated from differential:** the limitation to below the wrist for the patient's symptoms and the EMG/NCS abnormalities makes this diagnosis unlikely
- **Cervical disc herniation**
  - Degeneration of the vertebral discs, leading to herniation of the nucleus pulposus from the disc and subsequent nerve impingement
    - The normal disc is composed of a ring of dense fibrous tissue (i.e., **annulus fibrosis**) enclosing a gelatinous core (i.e., **nucleus pulposus**)
    - Disc herniation is most common in the lumbosacral region and second most common in the cervical spine
  - **History:** pain extending along the path of the compressed nerve, motor and sensory deficits with chronic compression (Table 9-1)
  - **Physical examination:** Valsalva maneuver causes a worsening of symptoms, patients with cervical herniations have a decreased neck range of motion and a positive **Spurling test** (i.e., compression, lateral bending, and extension of the neck produces radicular symptoms), patients with lumbosacral herniations have a reproduction of their symptoms with a **straight leg raise** and have an abnormal gait
  - **Tests:** MRI is used to confirm the presence of a herniation (Figure 9-2)
  - **Treatment:**
    - Some cases are self-limited and may be treated with analgesics, NSAIDs, and activity modification
    - Epidural injections of anti-inflammatory agents may be used in cases not resolving in a timely manner
    - Surgical discectomy and possible decompression may be performed in cases not responding well to nonsurgical treatment or in cases with an acute onset of significant neurologic deficits
  - **Outcomes:** many cases can be treated nonoperatively, but recurrence is more common in lumbosacral herniations; myelopathy can result from chronic nerve compression

TABLE 9-1 Neurologic Deficits Seen with Compression of Specific Cervical and Lumbosacral Nerve Roots

Nerve Root	Reflex	Motor Deficit	Sensory Deficit
C5	Biceps	Deltoid, biceps	Anterior/lateral shoulder
C6	Brachioradialis	Biceps, wrist extensors	Lateral forearm
C7	Triceps	Triceps, wrist flexors, finger extensors	Posterior forearm
C8	None	Finger flexors	4th and 5th fingers, medial forearm
T1	None	Finger interossei	Axilla
L4	Patellar	Tibialis anterior (foot dorsiflexion)	Medial leg
L5	None	Extensor hallucis longus (1st-toe dorsiflexion)	Lateral lower leg, 1st web space
S1	Achilles	Peroneus longus and brevis (foot eversion), gastrocnemius (foot plantar flexion)	Lateral foot

- **Why eliminated from differential:** symptoms related to nerve root compression would be expected to be manifested along the length of the nerve and not just below the wrist
- Brachial plexopathy
  - Traumatic injury of the brachial plexus, resulting in a peripheral neuropathy involving the distinct injured nerve roots (Figure 9-3)

FIGURE 9-2 **Magnetic resonance imaging of lumbar spine, demonstrating herniation of the L5–S1 disc (*arrows*) and the resulting compression of the spinal cord.**

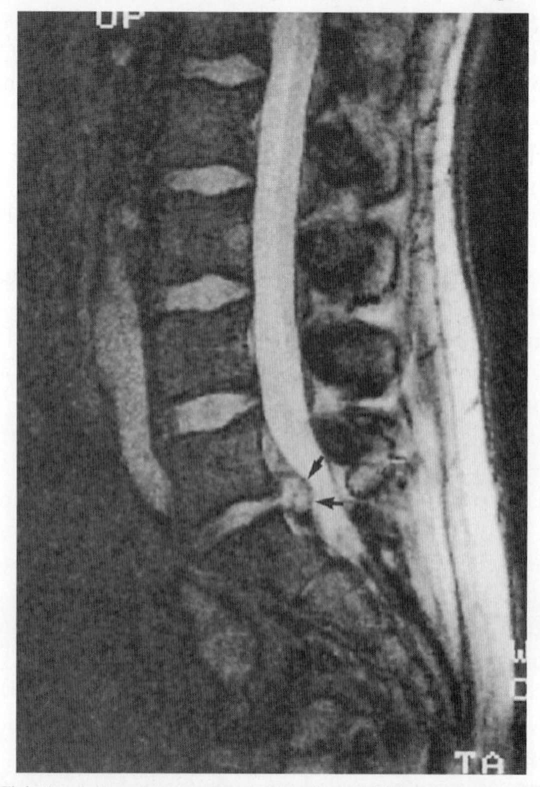

(Taken from Daffner RH. *Clinical radiology: the essentials.* 2nd ed. Philadelphia: Lippincott Williams & Wilkins, 1999. Used with permission of Lippincott Williams & Wilkins.)

Diagram of the major neural branches of the brachial plexus.

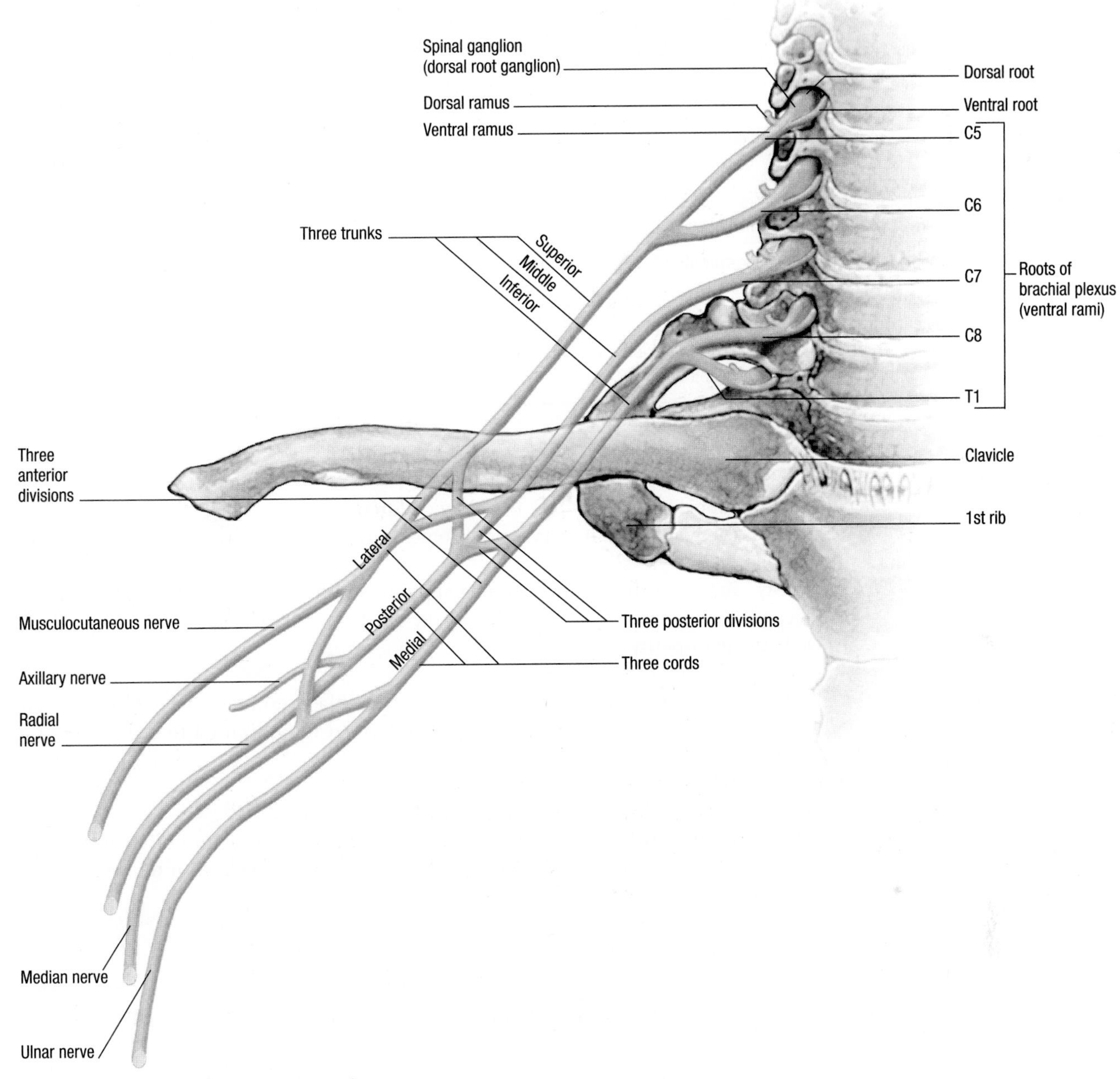

(Asset provided by Anatomical Chart Company.)

- **History:** pain, weakness, and paresthesias corresponding to the injured nerve roots (Table 9-2)
- **Physical examination:** motor and sensory deficits correspond to the injured nerve roots, contractures may develop from chronic denervation of muscular units
- **Tests:** EMG and NCS are useful to isolate the nerves affected and to determine the degree of injury; MRI may be able to detect sites of nerve rupture or compression
- **Treatment: physical therapy** is important to maximizing the degree of function attainable for a given nerve injury; tendon transfers, nerve grafting, or nerve transfers may be performed in hopes of improving the function of the affected limb
- **Outcomes:**
  - Recovery corresponds to the degree of nerve injury; traction injuries (i.e., neuropraxia) have the best chance of recovery, while nerve disruption (i.e., neurotmesis) is associated with a partial recovery of function at best

MNEMONIC

The organization of the brachial plexus may be remembered by the mnemonic "**R**eal **T**exans **D**rink **C**old **B**eer": **R**oots, **T**runks, **D**ivisions, **C**ords, **B**ranches (proximal to distal).

TABLE 9-2 Common Brachial Plexopathies

Condition	Site of Injury	Cause of Injury	Clinical Features
Erb-Duchenne palsy	Superior trunk	Hyperadduction of the arm causing widening of the humeral-glenoid gap (e.g., **birth**, **shoulder dystocia**)	**Waiter's tip** (i.e., arm extended and adducted with pronated forearm), lateral shoulder paresthesia
Claw hand	Ulnar nerve	Epiphyseal separation of medial epicondyle of humerus	Weak finger adduction, poor 4th/5th-finger flexion, clawed 4th/5th fingers from **lumbrical weakness**
Wrist drop	Posterior cord/radial nerve	Midhumerus fracture causes nerve impingement or tear	Inability to extend the wrist and fingers, loss of sensation from the dorsal hand
Deltoid paralysis	Axillary nerve	**Anterior shoulder dislocation** causes axillary nerve impingement or stretching	Impaired shoulder abduction and elevation, lateral shoulder paresthesia
Klumpke palsy	Posterior/medial cords	Hyperabduction of the arm places excess tension on the lower cords and nearby sympathetic chain	**Claw hand**, poor wrist and hand function, association with Horner syndrome

    - Functional recovery is best in young children
    - Nerve regeneration in nerves with some degree of integrity proceeds at about 1 mm per day
  - **Why eliminated from differential:** symptoms would be expected to occur along the length of the nerve and not just below the wrists
- **Diabetic neuropathy**
  - More thorough discussion in Chapter 5
  - **Why eliminated from differential:** hyperglycemia would be expected in a patient with DM, and symptoms would not be expected to be limited to only below the wrists
- **Multiple sclerosis**
  - More thorough discussion in Chapter 7
  - **Why eliminated from differential:** although the absence of any other neurologic complaints makes this diagnosis unlikely, it should be considered if the patient does not respond to any prescribed treatments

CASE 9-2 "I really hurt my ankle"

A 35-year-old woman presents to an emergency department after falling off a 6-foot ladder while painting a bedroom wall. The patient says that she landed on her left leg and immediately experienced severe ankle pain. She has been unable to bear weight on her ankle since her fall. She denies any numbness in her foot but is reluctant to move her ankle or toes because of the significant amount of pain. She denies having ever had a similar injury to her ankle in the past. She has no significant past medical history and only takes oral contraceptive pills. She drinks alcohol socially and denies other substance use. On examination, she appears to be in a significant amount of pain from her injury. Inspection of her ankle finds a large of amount of swelling and an abnormal position of the ankle. There are no lacerations around the site of injury. She has palpable dorsalis pedis and posterior tibial pulses and brisk capillary refill. She is able to detect light touch throughout her foot. With encouragement, she is able to flex and extend her toes, but she will not move her ankle due to pain. She has no pain with palpation or range of motion of her knee and hip, but palpation of her lateral lower leg and her medial malleolus is painful. The following vital signs are measured:

T: 98.9°F, HR: 110 bpm, BP: 130/90 mm Hg, RR: 14 breaths/min

Differential Diagnosis

- Fracture, dislocation, sprain

Laboratory Data and Other Study Results

- Ankle x-ray: displaced fractures of the distal tibia and fibula; no joint dislocation

Diagnosis

- Ankle fracture

Treatment Administered

- Closed reduction was performed, the patient was placed in a splint to immobilize her ankle, her leg was elevated, ice was applied to her ankle, and she was admitted to the hospital
- Open reduction and internal fixation of the patient's ankle was performed the following day

Follow-up

- The patient had an uncomplicated postoperative course and demonstrated good bony healing in her follow-up x-rays
- The patient was able to return to full weight-bearing by 2 months after surgery

Steps to the Diagnosis

- **Fracture**
  - Injury to the bone resulting in a discontinuity of the bony architecture (Table 9-3)
    - Most commonly results from trauma, but may also be due to pathologic instability
  - **History:** pain at the site of injury, inability to bear weight or resist a force
  - **Physical examination:** swelling at the site of injury, ecchymoses, pain with palpation or range of motion, crepitus at the site of injury, deformation of the extremity at the site of injury
  - **Tests:** x-rays are the standard test for detecting fractures; incomplete or nondisplaced fractures may be diagnosed with bone scan or MRI when x-rays are inconclusive
  - **Treatment:**
    - Nondisplaced fractures, fractures not extending into a joint, and fractures in non–weight-bearing locations may be treated with immobilization, protected activity, and analgesics
    - Displaced fractures and those extending into a joint require **surgical fixation** and reduction
    - **Open fractures** (i.e., fractures with a full-thickness soft tissue injury and exposure of bone to air) require urgent irrigation and debridement prior to surgical fixation
  - **Outcomes:**
    - The majority of fractures will heal with adequate stabilization
    - Nonunion or malunion of a fracture may result from inadequate stabilization or vascular insufficiency at the fracture site
    - Open fractures are associated with a significantly increased risk of **infection**
  - **Clues to the diagnosis:**
    - History: traumatic injury, ankle pain, inability to bear weight
    - Physical: ankle deformity, pain on palpation and movement
    - Tests: x-ray findings
- **Joint dislocation**
  - Incongruency of the articular surfaces of a joint due to **trauma**, deficient stabilizing structures, or ligamentous instability

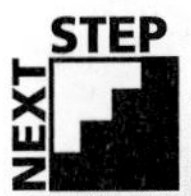

The Ottawa Ankle Rules should be applied to any blunt foot or ankle trauma. If there is ankle pain and bone tenderness in either malleoli, an ankle x-ray should be performed. If there is foot pain and tenderness at either the base of the fifth metatarsal or the navicular bone, get a foot x-ray.

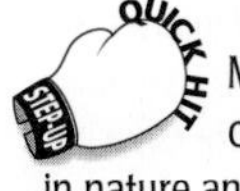

Most **shoulder** dislocations are **anterior** in nature and associated with trauma.

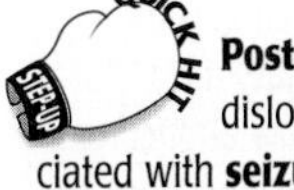

Posterior shoulder dislocations are associated with **seizures** and **electrical shock** injuries.

TABLE 9-3 Common Fractures, Their Mechanism of Injury, and Appropriate Treatment

Type	Bones Involved	H/P	Treatment	Clinical Pearls
Clavicle	Clavicle	Fall onto the shoulder	Immobilization in a sling; surgery is indicated for displaced fractures	**Most commonly fractured bone**
Humerus	Humerus	Trauma (e.g., motor vehicle accident, blunt trauma, etc.); more common in elderly patients	Closed reduction and immobilization; possible surgery	**Radial nerve** injuries may occur with midshaft fractures due to the proximity of the nerve to the bone
Colles	Distal radius +/− distal ulna	**Fall on an outstretched hand**; "dinner fork" deformity of the distal forearm	Closed reduction and immobilization; surgery is frequently required	Most common wrist fracture; particularly common in osteoporotic bone
Scaphoid	Scaphoid	Fall onto a radially deviated outstretched hand; "**snuff-box**" tenderness	Immobilization for nondisplaced fractures; surgery is frequently required	Possible avascular necrosis of the bone; **not seen on x-ray for 1–2 weeks after injury**; most common carpal fracture
Boxer	5th-metacarpal neck	Punching a hard object or surface with a strong force applied to 5th metacarpal	Closed reduction and immobilization; surgery is occasionally required	Beware the "**fight bite**," an open wound from impaction on a tooth that will need surgical exploration and debridement to prevent infection
Rib	Nonfloating ribs	Trauma; pain worse during deep breathing	Pain control	Multiple rib fractures may result in a "flail chest" with a significant impairment of breathing due to pain
Vertebral	Components of the spine	Trauma, osteoporosis (**compression fractures**)	Limited and stable fractures only require pain control; fractures causing instability of the spinal column require surgical fixation	Unstable fractures may be associated with spinal cord injury
Pelvic	Pelvis	Significant trauma	Pain control; surgery is required if in a weight-bearing portion of the pelvis or for unstable fractures	Risk of vascular injury increases with the severity of the fracture
Femur	Femur	Trauma	Surgical fixation	The thigh may be a site of significant blood loss that is not readily apparent on examination
Tibial	Tibia	Trauma	Immobilization for nondisplaced fractures; surgery for displaced fractures	Increased risk for **compartment syndrome**
Ankle	Medial, lateral, and/or posterior malleoli	Trauma; excessive twisting of the ankle	Immobilization or surgery depending on the degree of displacement and joint involvement	May lead to posttraumatic ankle arthritis; the Ottawa Ankle Rules are useful to making the diagnosis

H/P, history and physical.

QUICK HIT: Dashboard injuries are a frequent cause of hip dislocations in motor vehicle crashes.

NEXT STEP: Suspect an axillary nerve injury if a patient has difficulty abducting the arm (deltoid malfunction) following a shoulder dislocation.

- **History:** a history or trauma or prior joint laxity is associated with dislocations, joint pain, impaired ability to move a joint
- **Physical examination:** gross deformity of a joint, impaired range of motion, pain with attempted range of motion, possible motor or sensory deficits with an associated nerve injury
- **Tests:** x-ray or CT is useful to detect joint incongruency
- **Treatment:**
  - Prompt closed reduction under sedation or nerve block
  - Irreducible joints require a prompt open reduction
  - Recurrent instability frequently requires surgical intervention to prevent future dislocations

- **Outcomes:** failure to reduce a joint in a timely fashion increases the risk of a permanent neurologic injury; the risk of future dislocations increases significantly following an initial traumatic dislocation
- **Why eliminated from differential:** the appearance of the ankle x-ray rules out this diagnosis

- Sprains
  - Partial or complete tears of the **ligaments** and surrounding soft tissues in a joint
  - **History:** traumatic injury to a joint, joint pain, feeling of joint instability
  - **Physical examination:** increased joint laxity, pain with motion, joint swelling
  - **Tests:** MRI is the best means of detecting ligament injury and associated inflammation and should be performed for joints in which the physical exam is equivocal; x-ray may show joint subluxation in cases of complete ligament rupture
  - **Treatment:** activity modification, ice, compressive bandaging, and elevation are used to treat incomplete tears; surgical reconstruction may be required for completely torn ligaments and joint instability
  - **Outcomes:** partial tears will heal with adequate rest; complete tears with associated joint instability may lead to early arthritis
  - **Why eliminated from differential:** the finding of a boney injury on the x-ray makes this diagnosis less likely; MRI is rarely indicated to diagnose acute ankle sprains

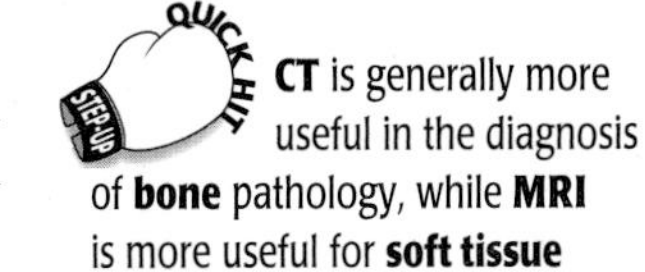

CT is generally more useful in the diagnosis of **bone** pathology, while **MRI** is more useful for **soft tissue** injuries.

MNEMONIC

The initial treatment for sprains may be remembered by the mnemonic **RICE**: **R**est, **I**ce, **C**ompression, **E**levation.

CASE 9-3 "My knee has been bothering me for a long time"

A 72-year-old man presents to his PCP with a complaint of chronic right knee pain that has gradually worsened over the past few years. The patient denies any significant trauma to his knee. He says that he feels minimal pain in the morning, but his knee pain worsens as the day passes. He particularly has pain with prolonged standing and walking. He says that his knee feels stiff, but he does not have any episodes of the joint locking or giving way. He says that the knee makes grinding sounds when he walks. He denies any fevers or erythema, but has swelling of the knee on days on which he does a considerable amount of walking. He has been taking ibuprofen for his pain, and he feels that this helps reduce his symptoms to some extent. He denies similar symptoms in other joints or any neurologic symptoms. He has a past medical history significant for hypertension (HTN), hypercholesterolemia, and benign prostatic hypertrophy and takes the medications enalapril, hydrochlorothiazide (HCTZ), simvastatin, and dutasteride. He smokes an occasional cigar and drinks three alcohol beverages per week. On examination, he is a well-appearing man in no distress. His right knee does not appear swollen or erythematous, and there is no effusion. He has dull pain along the tibial-femoral joint line. He has mild deep pain with range of motion that worsens at the extremes of flexion and extension. There is palpable crepitus during movement. Neurologic examination finds normal motor and sensory function.
The following vital signs are measured:

T: 98.5°F, HR: 68 bpm, BP: 125/84 mm Hg, RR: 16 breaths/min

Differential Diagnosis

- Osteoarthritis, rheumatoid arthritis, septic arthritis, meniscal tear, Lyme disease, gout, pseudogout

Laboratory Data and Other Study Results

- Knee x-ray: considerable loss of the tibial-femoral joint space with subchondral cyst and osteophyte formation

Diagnosis

- Osteoarthritis

Treatment Administered

- The patient was given an intra-articular injection of methylprednisolone and started on regular oral celecoxib

Follow-up

- The patient experienced an improvement in his symptoms for approximately 2 months; after that time he noted that his knee pain began to worsen
- The patient was referred to an orthopedic surgeon, who recommended total joint replacement
- The patient underwent a total knee replacement and had eradication of his knee pain following his recovery from surgery

Steps to the Diagnosis

- **Osteoarthritis (OA)**
  - Chronic, minimally inflammatory degeneration of joints through gradual deterioration of the **articular cartilage**
    - Can occur in any joint but most commonly occurs in the **hips**, **knees**, spine, hands, wrists, and shoulders
    - Degeneration of the spinal facet joints can lead to **spinal stenosis** and nerve compression symptoms
  - **Risk factors:** advanced age, family history, obesity, **previous joint trauma**, repetitive joint stress (e.g., heavy labor occupations)
  - **History:** insidious onset of joint stiffness and pain that **worsens with activity and weight-bearing** and improves with rest, pain tends to be worse at the end of the day, pain worsens following mild trauma to the joint
  - **Physical examination:** decreased and painful range of motion at the affected joint, mild joint swelling, joint crepitus, bony protuberances in the distal interphalangeal (DIP) (i.e., Heberden nodes) and proximal interphalangeal (PIP) (i.e., Bouchard nodes) joints with hand involvement
  - **Tests:**
    - X-rays will show **joint space narrowing**, **subchondral cyst formation**, **sclerotic subchondral bone**, and **osteophyte formation** (i.e., small periarticular outgrowths of bone in response to joint degeneration) (Figure 9-4)
    - Aspiration of the joint detects <2,000 white blood cells (WBC)/mm^3
    - Erythrocyte sedimentation rate (ESR), C-reactive protein (CRP), and serum WBCs are normal
  - **Treatment:**
    - Activity modification, physical therapy, and **NSAIDs** are used as the initial treatments
    - Patients with persistent symptoms or acute exacerbations of joint pain will have an improvement in their symptoms with an intra-articular corticosteroid injection
    - Some patients may have an improvement in their general symptoms with intra-articular injections of a **viscosupplement**
    - **Total joint replacement** is the definitive means of treating significant joint degeneration and has a high success rate of relieving joint pain
  - **Outcomes:**
    - Most patients will have worsening of their joint pain with time as joint degeneration progresses
    - Intra-articular injections provide temporary relief, but repeat injections are frequently due to the recurrence of pain
    - Joint replacement is associated with approximately a 95% satisfaction rate regarding pain relief and restoration of function
  - **Clues to the diagnosis:**
    - History: chronic, worsening knee pain that increases over the course of the day, joint stiffness, improvement of pain with NSAID use

MNEMONIC

Causes of joint pain may be remembered by the mnemonic **HOT INFARCTS**: **H**emarthrosis, **O**steoarthritis, **T**rauma (fracture), **I**nfection (septic joint, osteomyelitis), **N**europathy, **F**ibromyalgia, **A**vascular necrosis, **R**heumatic disease (RA, systemic lupus erythematosus [SLE], ankylosing spondylitis), **C**rystal disease (gout, calcium pyrophosphate dehydrate deposition [CPPD] disease), **T**umor, **S**oft tissue (tendon, ligament, meniscus).

QUICK HIT: A diagnosis of osteoarthritis is typically based on the history, physical examination, and x-rays, and joint aspiration and laboratory testing is rarely indicated in the diagnosis.

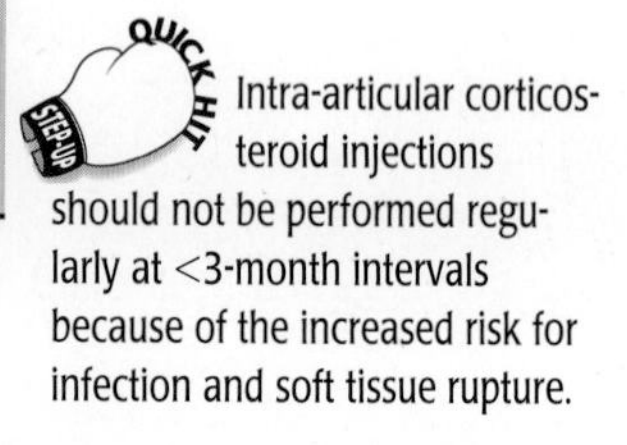

QUICK HIT: Intra-articular corticosteroid injections should not be performed regularly at <3-month intervals because of the increased risk for infection and soft tissue rupture.

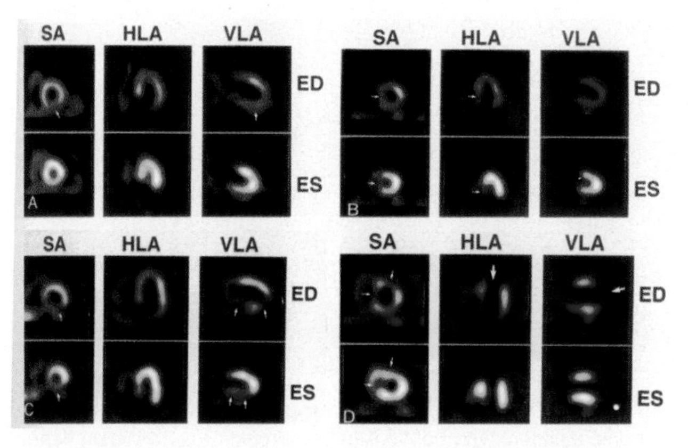

COLOR FIGURE 1-1 Four examples of patterns detected during technetium-99m-sestamibi nuclear stress testing with single-positron emission computed tomography imaging. (**A**) Normal patient. Homogenous thickening of the myocardium occurs during systole. Less uptake (*arrows*) is noted in the inferior wall in the end-diastolic short axis and vertical long axis views that is likely due to the spatial relationship of the heart to the diaphragm. (**B**) Patient with a septal infarct. Note the perfusion defects (*arrows*) in the ventricular septum in the short and horizontal long axis views in both the end-systolic and end-diastolic phases. (**C**) Patient with inferior wall ischemia. End-diastolic perfusion defects (*arrows*) are noted on the short and vertical long axis views. Slight signal increase occurs in the end-systolic views indicating reversible ischemia. (**D**) Patient with both ischemia and infarction. Septal and anteroapical perfusion defects are noted in the end-diastolic images. Only the septal region shows signal increase in the end-systolic images indicating reversible septal ischemia and anteroapical infarction. ED, end-diastolic; ES, end-systolic; HLA, horizontal long axis; SA, short axis; VLA, vertical long axis.

(Taken from Sandler MP, Gottschalk A, Patton JA, et al., eds. *Diagnostic nuclear medicine*. 4th ed. Philadelphia: Lippincott Williams & Wilkins, 2002. Fig. 15-16. Used with permission of Lippincott Williams & Wilkins.)

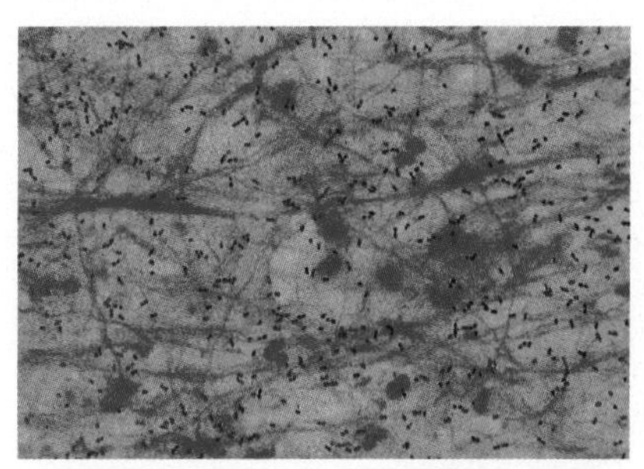

COLOR FIGURE 2-1 Paired Gram-positive cocci seen in sputum consistent with *Streptococcus pneumoniae* pneumonia.

(Taken from McClatchey KD. *Clinical laboratory medicine*. 2nd ed. Philadelphia: Lippincott Williams & Wilkins, 2002. Used with permission of Lippincott Williams & Wilkins.)

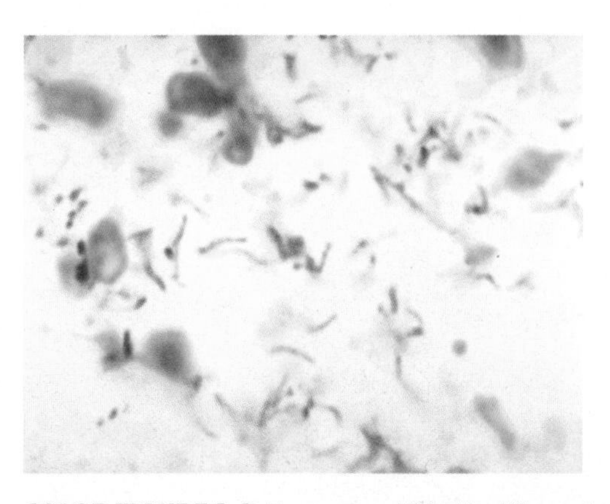

COLOR FIGURE 2-2 Numerous acid-fast bacilli seen in sputum specimen consistent with *Mycobacterium tuberculosis* infection.

(Taken from Rubin E, Farber JL. *Pathology*. 3rd ed. Philadelphia: Lippincott Williams & Wilkins, 1999. Used with permission of Lippincott Williams & Wilkins.)

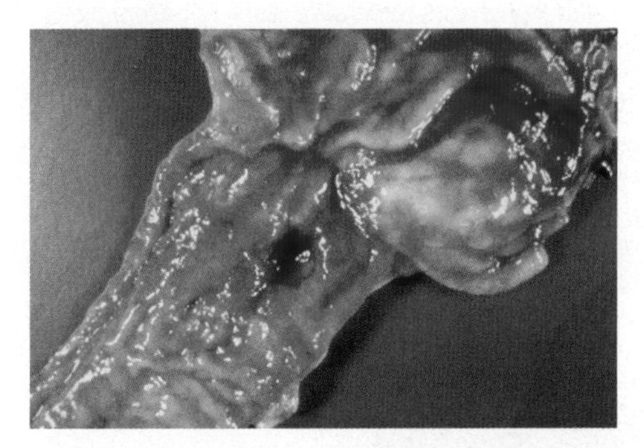

COLOR FIGURE 3-1 Duodenal ulcer in a tissue specimen. The ulcer is located distal to the musculature of the pyloric sphincter and demonstrates penetration of the mucosal surface.

(Taken from Rubin E, Farber JL. *Pathology*. 3rd ed. Philadelphia: Lippincott Williams & Wilkins, 1999. Fig. 13.19. Used with permission of Lippincott Williams & Wilkins.)

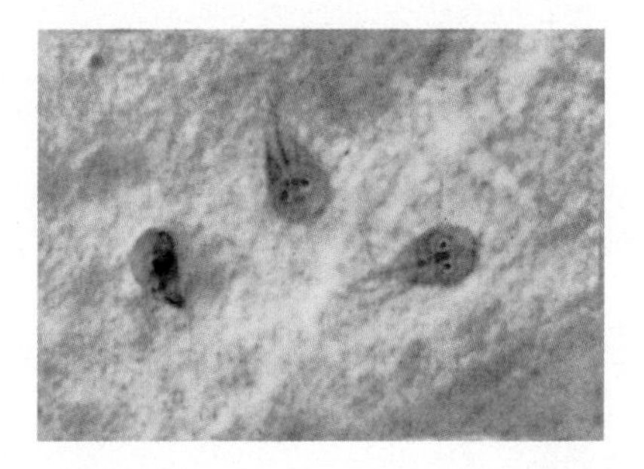

COLOR FIGURE 3-2 Giardiasis; several trophozoites are seen with characteristic pear shape and paired nuclei resembling owls' eyes.

(Taken from Fenoglio-Preiser CM, Lantz PE, Listrom MB, et al. *Gastrointestinal pathology. an atlas and text*. 2nd ed. Philadelphia: Lippincott Williams & Wilkins, 1999. Used with permission of Lippincott Williams & Wilkins.)

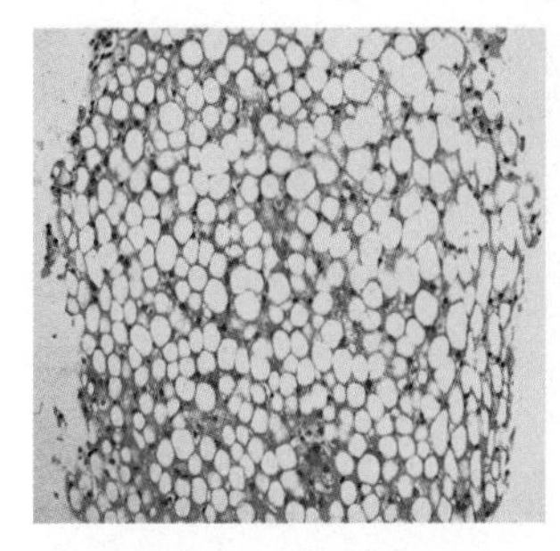

COLOR FIGURE 3-3 Hepatic steatosis due to chronic alcohol consumption. Numerous hepatocytes are distended due to cytoplasmic fat collections.

(Taken from Rubin E, Farber JL. *Pathology*. 3rd ed. Philadelphia: Lippincott Williams & Wilkins, 1999. Fig. 14.31. Used with permission of Lippincott Williams & Wilkins.)

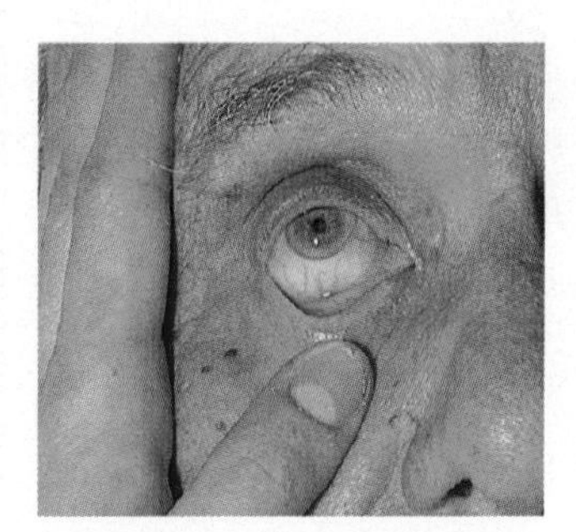

COLOR FIGURE 3-4 Jaundice in a patient with hyperbilirubinemia. Note the yellow sclera and skin compared to the normal hue of the examiner's hand.

(Taken from Bickley LS, Szilagyi P. *Bate's guide to physical examination and history taking*. 8th ed. Philadelphia: Lippincott Williams & Wilkins, 2003. Used with permission of Lippincott Williams & Wilkins.)

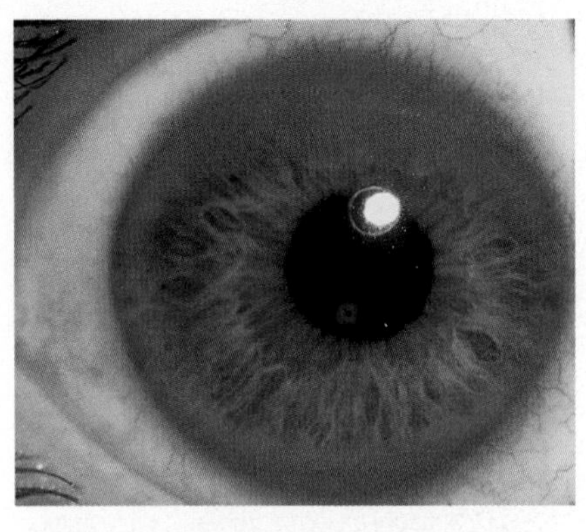

COLOR FIGURE 3-5 Photograph of a Kayser-Fleischer ring in a patient with Wilson disease. Note the brownish ring obscuring details of the peripheral iris.

(Taken from Gold DH, Weingeist TA. *Color atlas of the eye in systemic disease.* Baltimore: Lippincott Williams & Wilkins, 2001. Fig. 89.1. Used with permission of Lippincott Williams & Wilkins.)

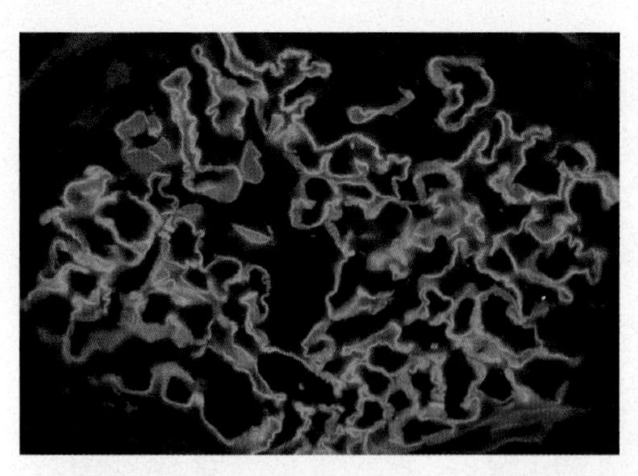

COLOR FIGURE 4-2 Immunofluorescence microscopy of a renal biopsy in a patient with Goodpasture syndrome. Note the linear deposition of anti-basement membrane IgG antibodies along the glomerular basement membrane. Ig, immunoglobulin.

(Taken from Rubin E, Farber JL. *Pathology.* 3rd ed. Philadelphia: Lippincott Williams & Wilkins, 1999. Fig. 16-50. Used with permission of Lippincott Williams & Wilkins.)

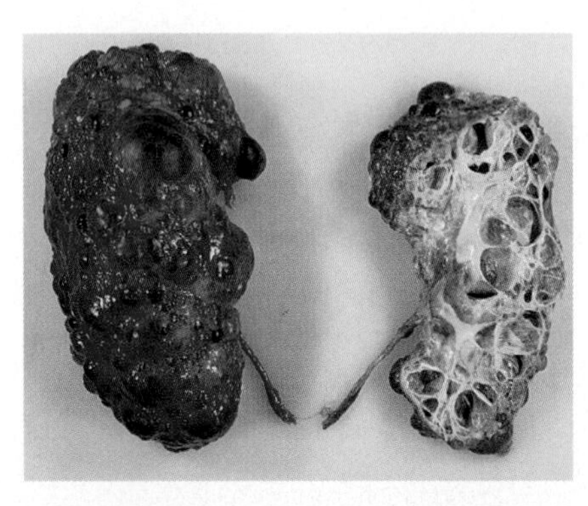

COLOR FIGURE 4-1 Autosomal dominant polycystic kidney disease; note enlargement of the kidney with many cysts of various sizes.

(Taken from Rubin E, Farber JL. *Pathology.* 3rd ed. Philadelphia: Lippincott Williams & Wilkins, 1999. Used with permission of Lippincott Williams & Wilkins.)

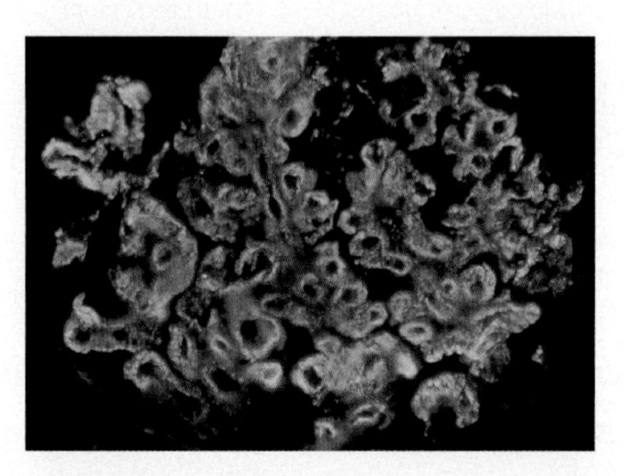

COLOR FIGURE 4-4 Immunofluorescence microscopy of a renal biopsy in a patient with membranoproliferative glomerulonephritis. Note the granular deposition of antibasement membrane IgG antibodies along the glomerular basement membrane. This granular appearance is more consistent with deposition of immune complexes along the basement membrane and may be contrasted with the linear appearance seen in Goodpasture syndrome. Ig, immunoglobulin.

(Taken from Rubin E, Farber JL. *Pathology.* 3rd ed. Philadelphia: Lippincott Williams & Wilkins, 1999. Fig. 16-39. Used with permission of Lippincott Williams & Wilkins.)

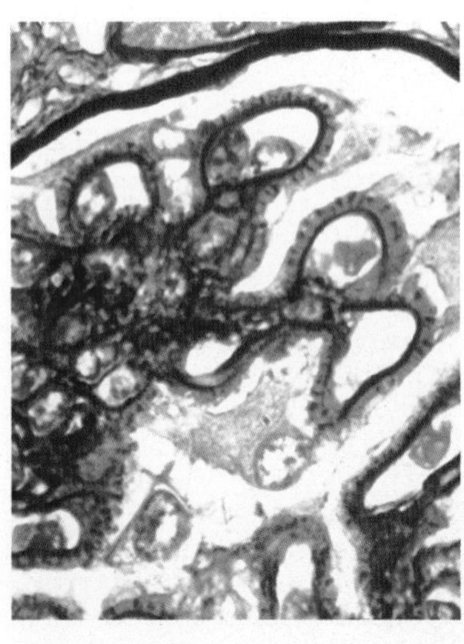

COLOR FIGURE 4-3 Renal biopsy with silver stain from a patient with membranous glomerulonephritis. Note the numerous "spikes" of immune complex deposition along the glomerular basement membrane.

(Taken from Rubin E, Farber JL. *Pathology.* 3rd ed. Philadelphia: Lippincott Williams & Wilkins, 1999. Fig. 16-20. Used with permission of Lippincott Williams & Wilkins.)

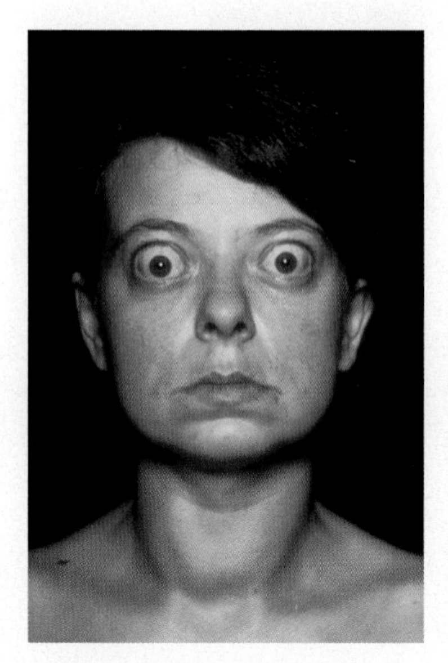

COLOR FIGURE 5-1 Photograph of a female patient with Graves disease. There is noticeable exophthalmos of both eyes, and a goiter is seen in the neck.

(Taken from Rubin E, Farber JL. *Pathology.* 3rd ed. Philadelphia: Lippincott Williams & Wilkins, 1999. Fig. 21-13. Used with permission of Lippincott Williams & Wilkins.)

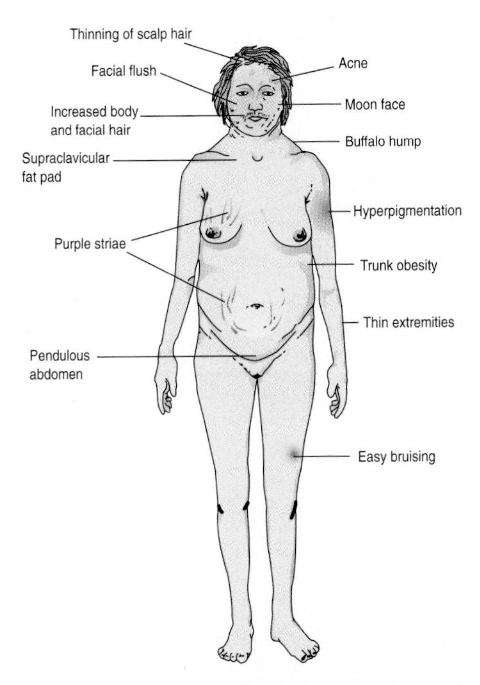

COLOR FIGURE 5-2 Diagram of the common physical characteristics seen in Cushing syndrome.

(Taken from Smeltzer SC, Bare BG. *Textbook of medical-surgical nursing*. 9th ed. Philadelphia: Lippincott Williams & Wilkins, 2000. Fig. 38-03.01. Used with permission of Lippincott Williams & Wilkins.)

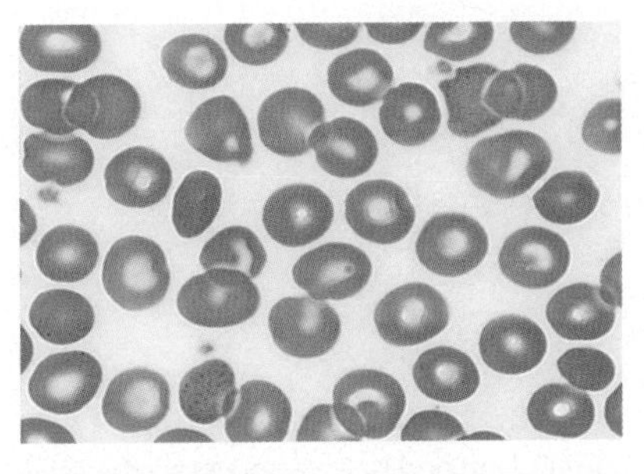

COLOR FIGURE 6-1 Lead poisoning anemia; note the hypochromic red blood cells and basophilic stippling seen in some cells.

(Taken from Anderson SC, Poulsen KB. *Anderson's atlas of hematology*. Philadelphia: Lippincott Williams & Wilkins, 2003. Fig. IIA2-18. Used with permission of Lippincott Williams & Wilkins.)

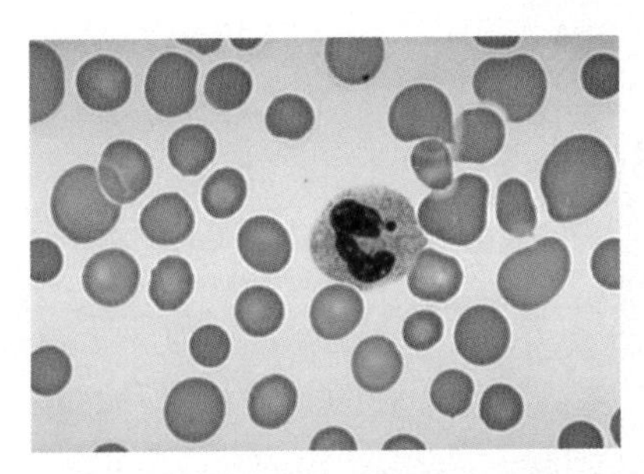

COLOR FIGURE 6-2 Hereditary spherocytosis; blood smear shows numerous spherocytes with decreased diameter, increased staining, and absence of central pallor.

(Taken from Rubin E, Farber JL. *Pathology*. 3rd ed. Philadelphia: Lippincott Williams & Wilkins, 1999. Fig. 20-27. Used with permission of Lippincott Williams & Wilkins.)

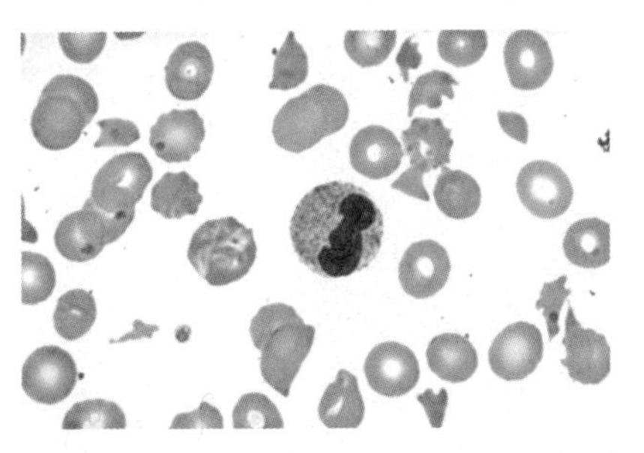

COLOR FIGURE 6-3 Microangiopathic hemolytic anemia demonstrating multiple schistocytes (fragmented red blood cells).

(Taken from Rubin E, Farber JL. *Pathology*. 3rd ed. Philadelphia: Lippincott Williams & Wilkins, 1999. Fig. 20-31. Used with permission of Lippincott Williams & Wilkins.)

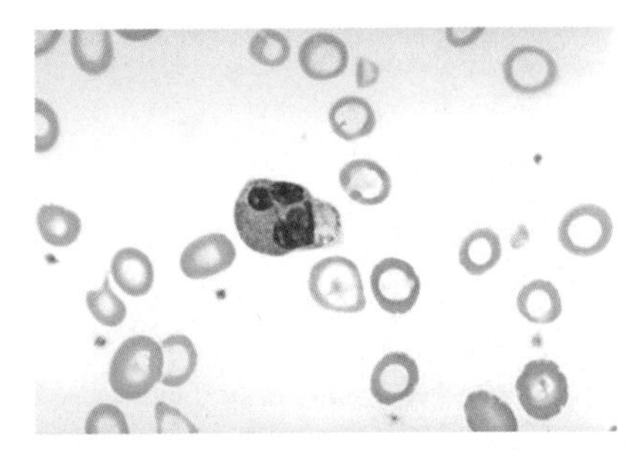

COLOR FIGURE 6-4 Microcytic hypochromic red blood cells characteristic of iron deficiency anemia.

(Taken from Rubin E, Farber JL. *Pathology*. 3rd ed. Philadelphia: Lippincott Williams & Wilkins, 1999. Fig. 20-22. Used with permission of Lippincott Williams & Wilkins.)

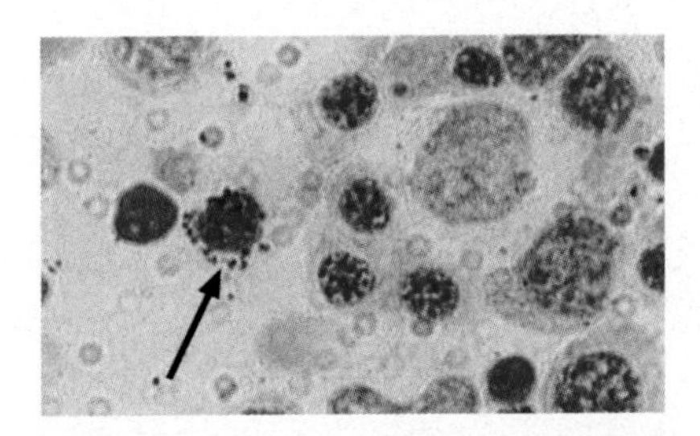

COLOR FIGURE 6-5 Blood smear in a patient with sideroblastic anemia; note several red blood cells surrounded by rings of iron granules (ring sideroblasts).

(Taken from Handin RI, Lux SE, Stossel TP. *Blood: principles and practice of hematology*. 2nd ed. Philadelphia: Lippincott Williams & Wilkins, 2003. Color Fig. 3-6D. Used with permission of Lippincott Williams & Wilkins.)

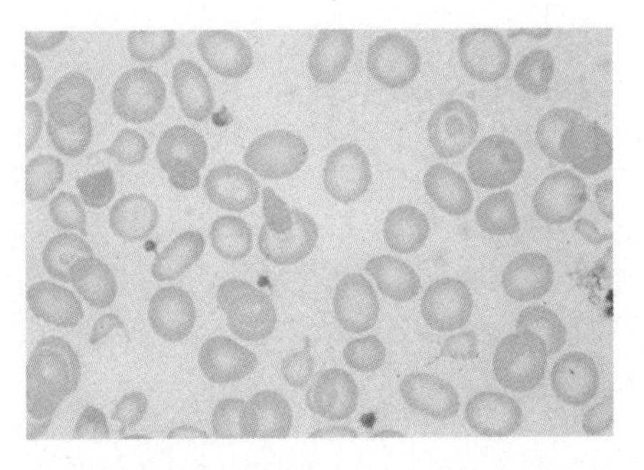

COLOR FIGURE 6-6 α-thalassemia, hemoglobin H type; note hypochromic red blood cells and occasional target cells.

(Taken from Anderson SC, Poulsen KB. *Anderson's atlas of hematology*. Philadelphia: Lippincott Williams & Wilkins, 2003. Fig. IIA2-2. Used with permission of Lippincott Williams & Wilkins.)

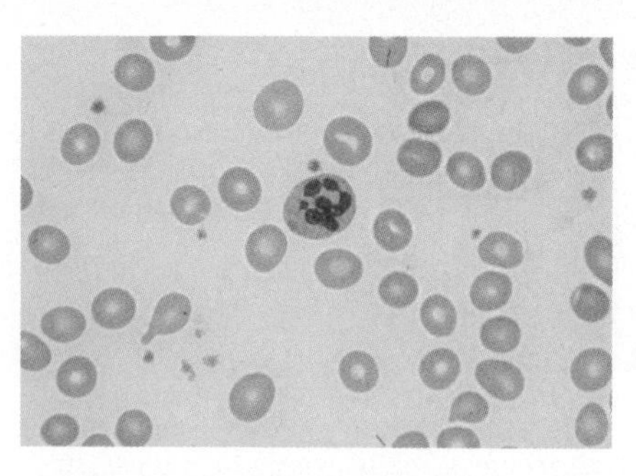

COLOR FIGURE 6-7 Anemia due to vitamin B_{12} deficiency; note the macrocytic red blood cells and presence of a hypersegmented neutrophil.

(Taken from Anderson SC, Poulsen KB. *Anderson's atlas of hematology.* Philadelphia: Lippincott Williams & Wilkins, 2003. Fig. IIA3-3. Used with permission of Lippincott Williams & Wilkins.)

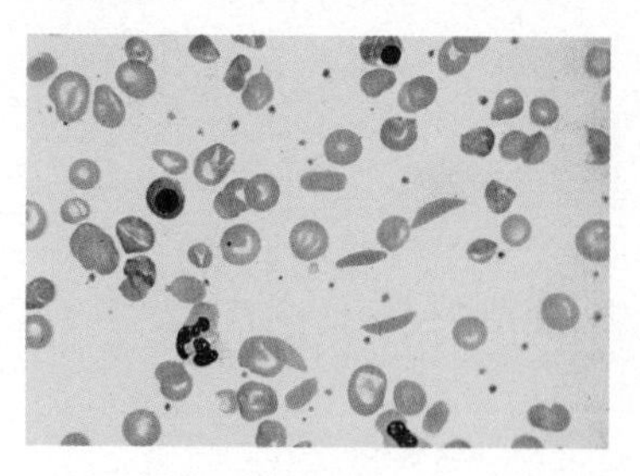

COLOR FIGURE 6-8 Sickle cell anemia; note multiple sickle cells and occasional target cells.

(Taken from Rubin E, Farber JL. *Pathology.* 3rd ed. Philadelphia: Lippincott Williams & Wilkins, 1999. Fig. 20-26. Used with permission of Lippincott Williams & Wilkins.)

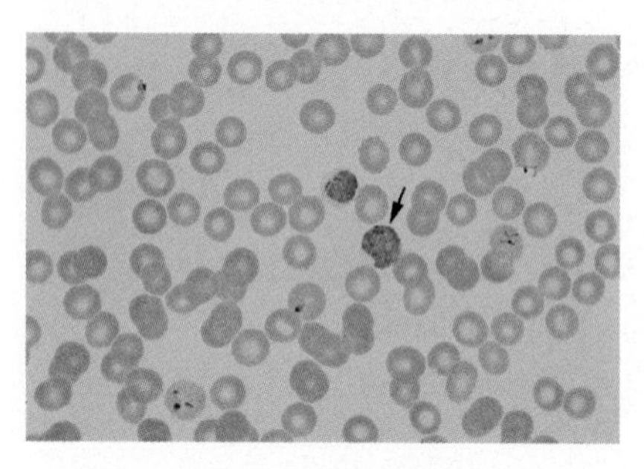

COLOR FIGURE 6-9 Blood smear from a patient with *Plasmodium* infection showing two microgametes with large nuclei and loose chromatin (*arrow*) and several red blood cells with intracellular rings and eosinophilic granules signifying infiltration.

(Taken from Sun T. *Parasitic disorders: pathology, diagnosis, and management.* 2nd ed. Baltimore: Lippincott Williams & Wilkins, 1999. Fig. 16.24. Used with permission of Lippincott Williams & Wilkins.)

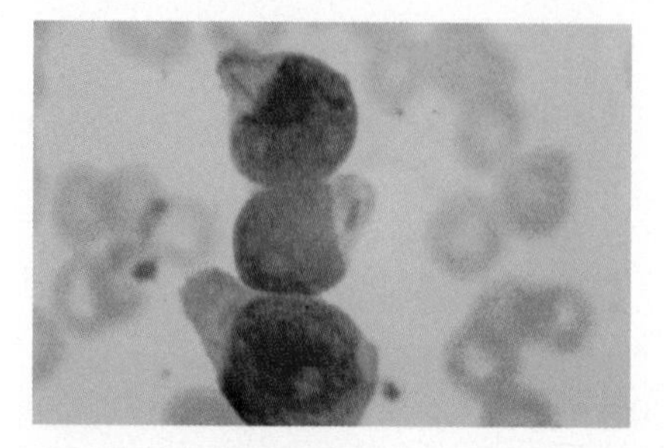

COLOR FIGURE 6-10 Acute myelogenous leukemia with monocytic differentiation. Note the prominent waxy nucleoli, large size of blasts, and presence of Auer rods.

(Taken from Handin RI, Lux SE, Stossel TP. *Blood: principles and practice of hematology.* 2nd ed. Philadelphia: Lippincott Williams & Wilkins, 2003. Color Fig. 15-1A. Used with permission of Lippincott Williams & Wilkins.).

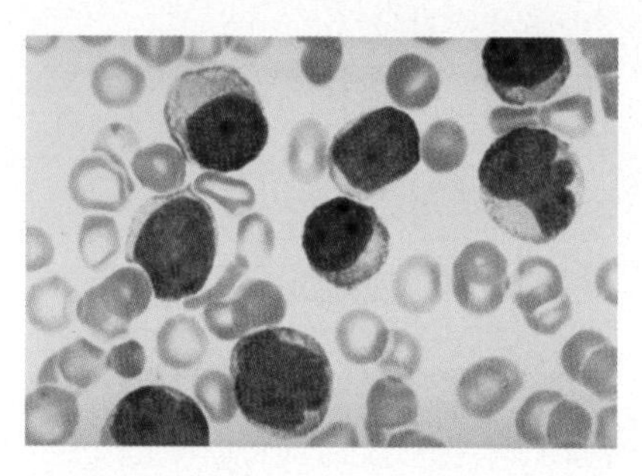

COLOR FIGURE 6-11 Acute lymphocytic leukemia. Note the lymphoblasts with irregular nuclei and prominent nucleoli.

(Taken from Rubin E, Farber JL. *Pathology.* 3rd ed. Philadelphia: Lippincott Williams & Wilkins, 1999. Fig. 20-59. Used with permission of Lippincott Williams & Wilkins.)

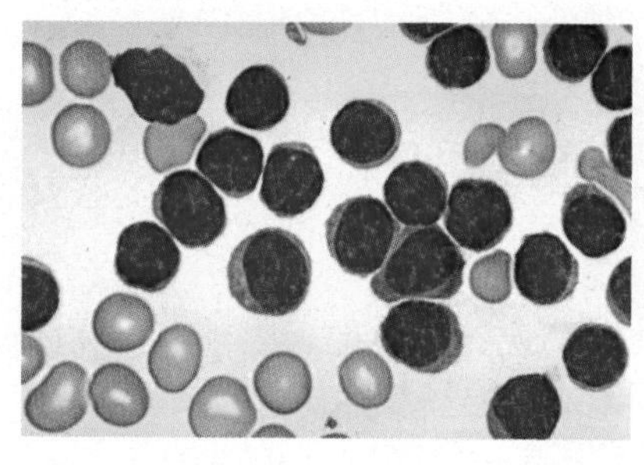

COLOR FIGURE 6-12 Chronic lymphocytic leukemia. Note the small lymphocytes of a comparable size to nearby red blood cells and the presence of smudge cells (fragile lymphocytes disrupted during smear preparation) in upper portion of image.

(Taken from Rubin E, Farber JL. *Pathology.* 3rd ed. Philadelphia: Lippincott Williams & Wilkins, 1999. Fig. 20-57. Used with permission of Lippincott Williams & Wilkins.)

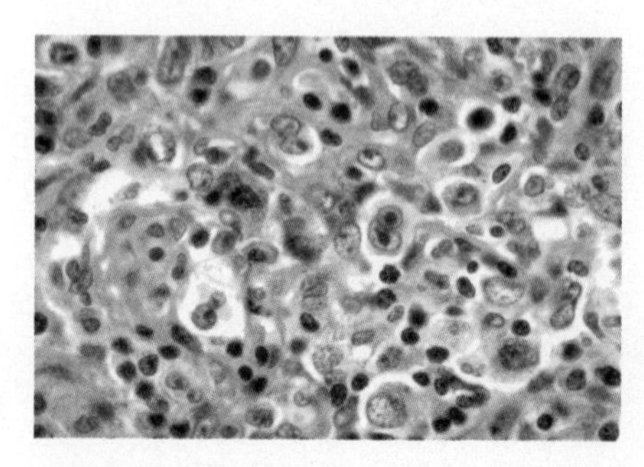

COLOR FIGURE 6-13 Hodgkin lymphoma. A histologic section of a lymph node demonstrates pathognomonic binucleated Reed-Sternberg cells that resemble owls' eyes.

(Taken from Rubin E, Farber JL. *Pathology.* 3rd ed. Philadelphia: Lippincott Williams & Wilkins, 1999. Fig. 20-72. Used with permission of Lippincott Williams & Wilkins.)

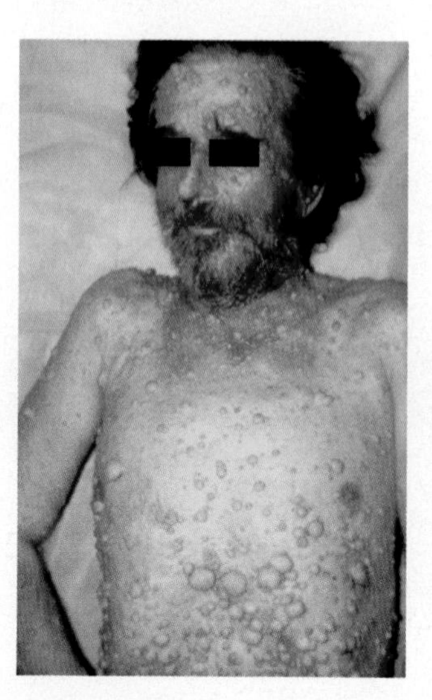

COLOR FIGURE 7-1 Patient with multiple neurofibromas on the face and chest consistent with neurofibromatosis type I.

(Taken from Rubin E, Farber JL. *Pathology.* 3rd ed. Philadelphia: Lippincott Williams & Wilkins, 1999. Fig. 6-19. Used with permission of Lippincott Williams & Wilkins.)

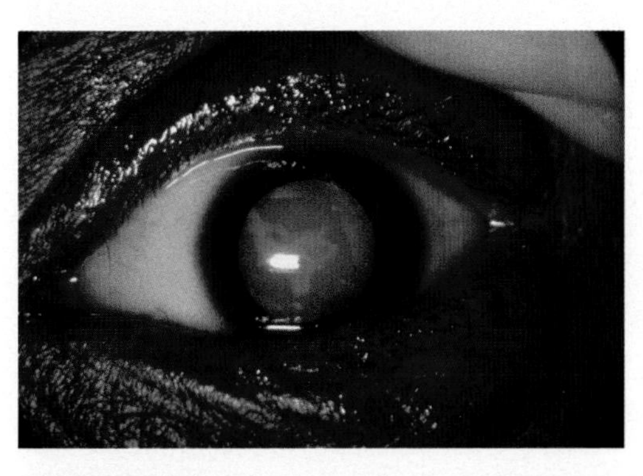

COLOR FIGURE 8-1 Patient with an age-related cataract, demonstrating complete opacification of the lens.

(Taken from Rubin E, Farber JL. *Pathology.* 3rd ed. Philadelphia: Lippincott Williams & Wilkins, 1999. Fig. 29-3. Used with permission of Lippincott Williams & Wilkins.)

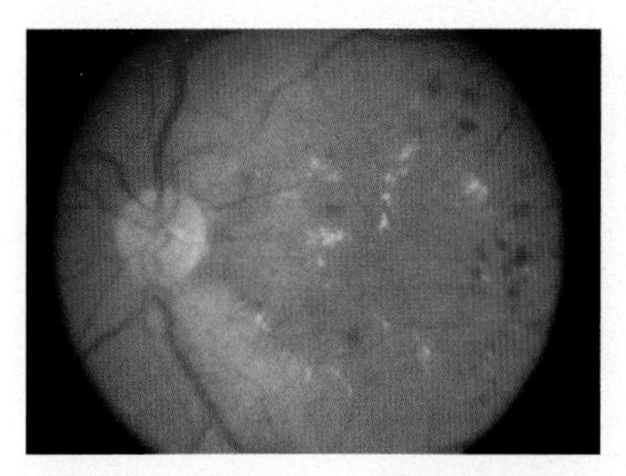

COLOR FIGURE 8-2 Fundoscopic view in a patient with diabetic retinopathy. Note the yellowish lipid exudates and multiple small retinal hemorrhages.

(Taken from Rubin E, Farber JL. *Pathology.* 3rd ed. Philadelphia: Lippincott Williams & Wilkins, 1999. Fig. 29-11A. Used with permission of Lippincott Williams & Wilkins.)

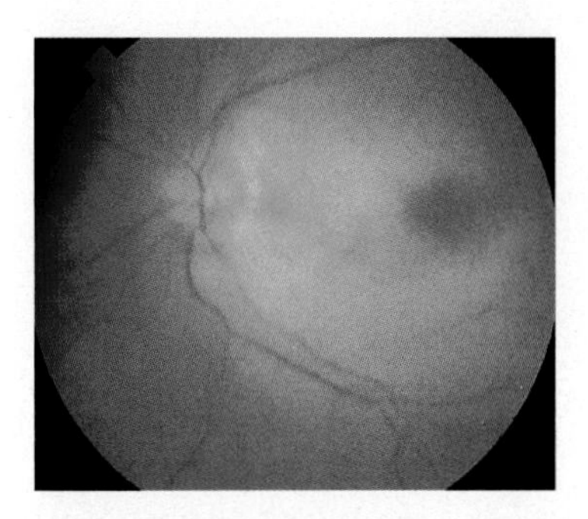

COLOR FIGURE 8-3 Fundoscopic view in a patient with retinal artery occlusion. Note the generalized retinal edema and the presence of a cherry-red spot.

(Taken from Gold DH, Weingeist TA. *Color atlas of the eye in systemic disease.* Philadelphia: Lippincott Williams & Wilkins, 2001. Fig. 75-2. Used with permission of Lippincott Williams & Wilkins.)

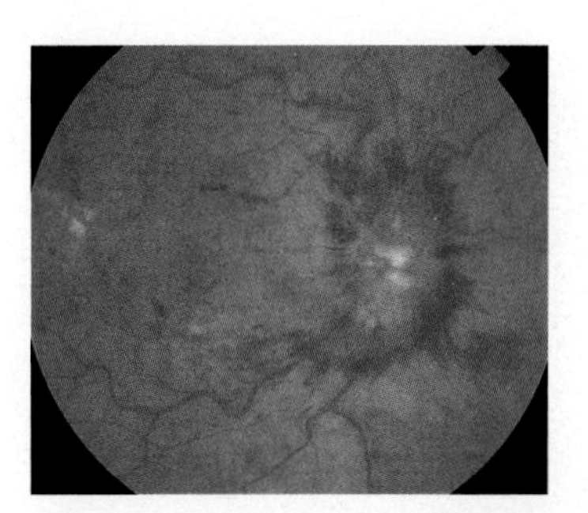

COLOR FIGURE 8-4 Fundoscopic view in a patient with retinal vein occlusion. Note the edematous retina, retinal hemorrhages, cotton wool spots, and venous dilation.

(Taken from Gold DH, Weingeist TA. *Color atlas of the eye in systemic disease.* Philadelphia: Lippincott Williams & Wilkins, 2001. Fig. 29-1. Used with permission of Lippincott Williams & Wilkins.)

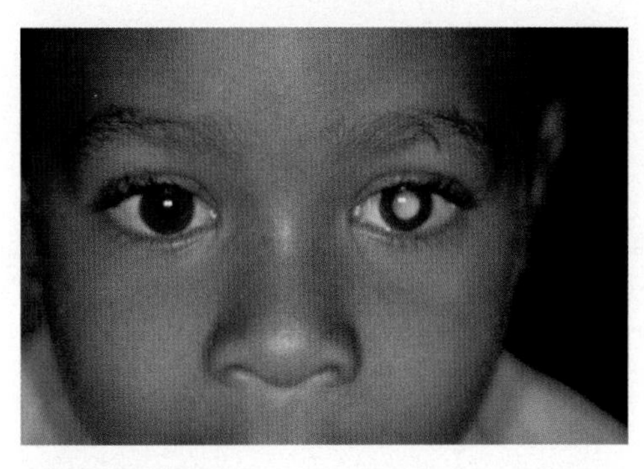

COLOR FIGURE 8-5 Leukokoria in a child with a left-eye retinoblastoma.

(Taken from Rubin E, Farber JL. *Pathology.* 3rd ed. Philadelphia: Lippincott Williams & Wilkins, 1999. Fig. 29-23A. Used with permission of Lippincott Williams & Wilkins.)

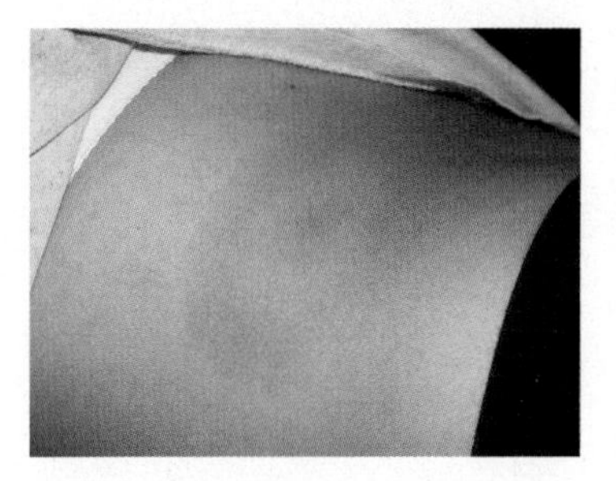

COLOR FIGURE 9-2 Patient with Lyme disease exhibiting erythema chronicum migrans (bull's eye rash).

(Taken from Goodheart HP. *Goodheart's photoguide of common skin disorders.* 2nd ed. Philadelphia: Lippincott Williams & Wilkins, 2003. Fig. 7-19. Used with permission of Lippincott Williams & Wilkins.)

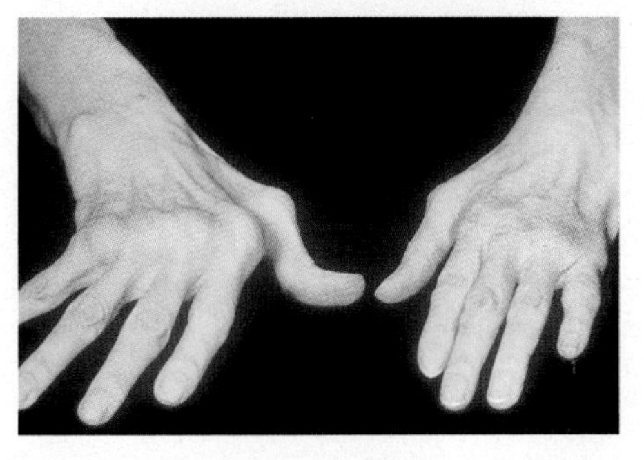

COLOR FIGURE 9-1 Photograph of the hands in a patient with rheumatoid arthritis. Note the ulnar deviation of the fingers and metacarpophalangeal hypertrophy.

(Taken from Smeltzer SC, Bare BG. *Textbook of medical-surgical nursing.* 9th ed. Philadelphia: Lippincott Williams & Wilkins, 2000. Fig, 50-4B. Used with permission of Lippincott Williams & Wilkins.)

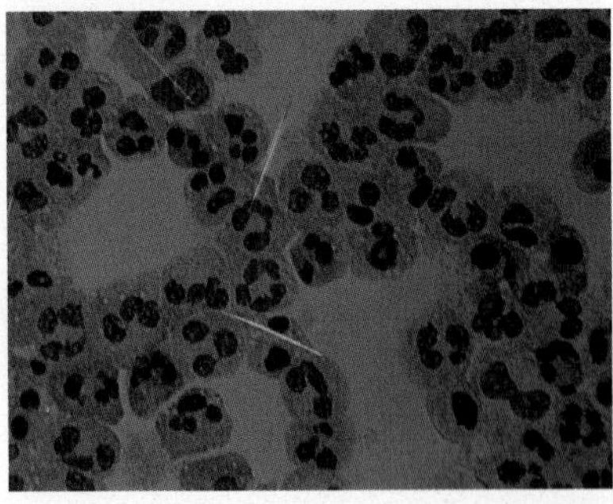

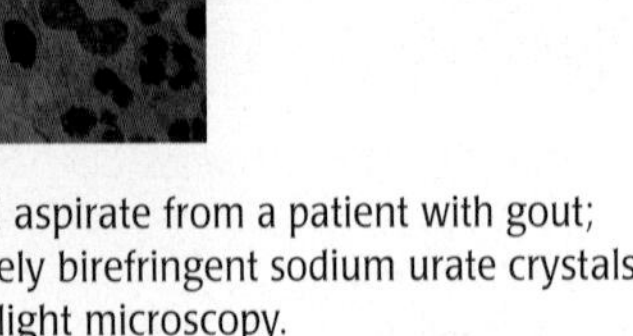

COLOR FIGURE 9-3 Synovial aspirate from a patient with gout; note the needle-shaped negatively birefringent sodium urate crystals that are visible under polarized light microscopy.

(Taken from McClatchey KD. *Clinical laboratory medicine.* 2nd ed. Philadelphia: Lippincott Williams & Wilkins, 2002. Fig. 27-17. Used with permission of Lippincott Williams & Wilkins.)

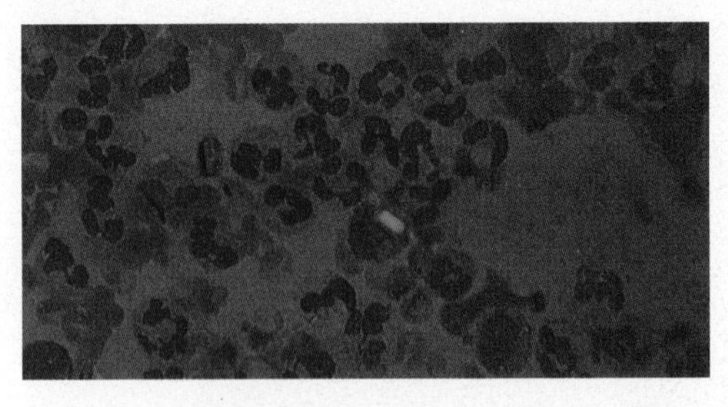

COLOR FIGURE 9-4 Synovial aspirate from patient with calcium pyrophosphate dehydrate deposition disease; under polarized light microscopy rhomboid-shaped calcium pyrophosphate dehydrate crystals appear positively birefringent.

(Taken from McClatchey KD. *Clinical laboratory medicine.* 2nd ed. Philadelphia: Lippincott Williams & Wilkins, 2002. Fig. 27-22. Used with permission of Lippincott Williams & Wilkins.)

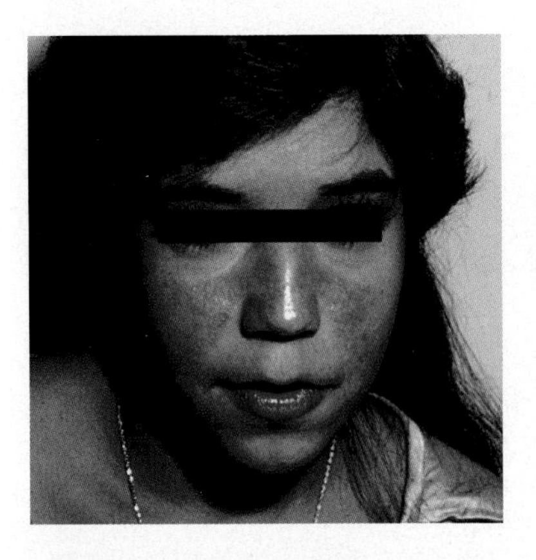

COLOR FIGURE 9-5 Patient exhibiting the classic malar rash of systemic lupus erythematosus.

(Taken from Goodheart HP. *Goodheart's photoguide of common skin disorders.* 2nd ed. Philadelphia: Lippincott Williams & Wilkins, 2003. Fig. 2-63. Used with permission of Lippincott Williams & Wilkins.)

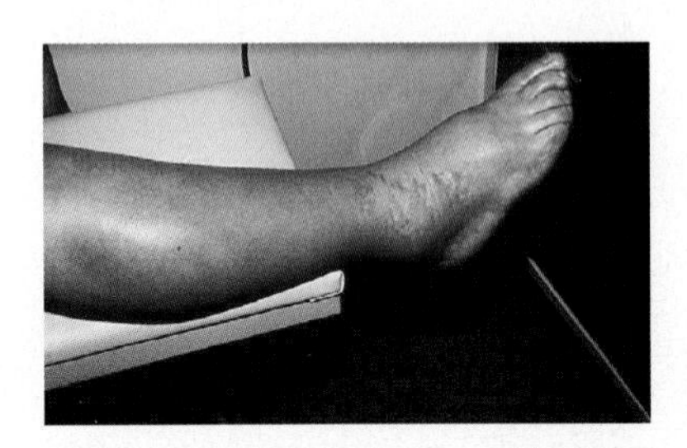

COLOR FIGURE 10-2 Cellulitis of the right pretibial region; note the erythematous, swollen skin with mild desquamation.

(Taken from Goodheart HP. *Goodheart's photoguide of common skin disorders.* 2nd ed. Philadelphia: Lippincott Williams & Wilkins, 2003. Fig. 2-69. Used with permission of Lippincott Williams & Wilkins.)

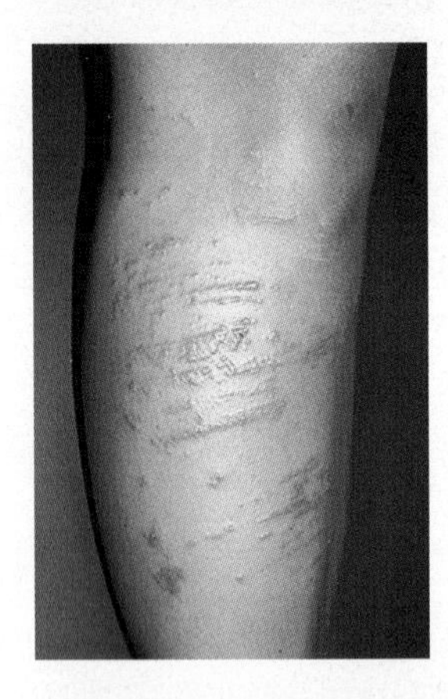

COLOR FIGURE 10-1 Allergic contact dermatitis due to exposure to poison ivy; note the linearity of the rash consistent with an outside-of-body cause.

(Taken from Goodheart HP. *Goodheart's photoguide of common skin disorders.* 2nd ed. Philadelphia: Lippincott Williams & Wilkins, 2003. Fig. 2-48. Used with permission of Lippincott Williams & Wilkins.)

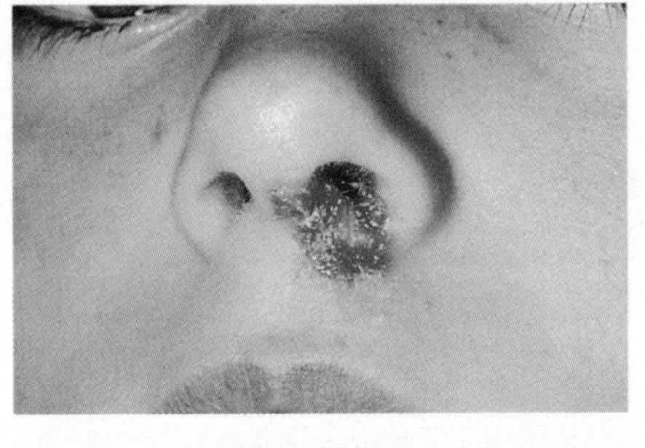

COLOR FIGURE 10-4 Impetigo involving left nostril due to *Staphylococcus aureus* infection; note presence of greasy yellow scales within lesion.

(Taken from Smeltzer SC, Bare BG. *Textbook of medical-surgical nursing.* 9th ed. Philadelphia: Lippincott Williams & Wilkins, 2000. Fig. 52-1. Used with permission of Lippincott Williams & Wilkins.)

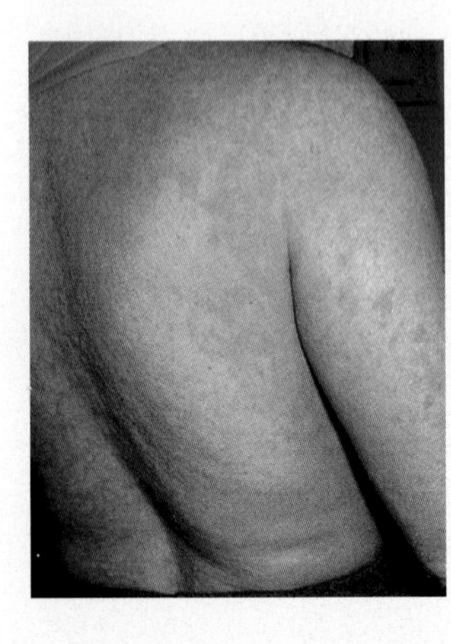

COLOR FIGURE 10-3 Adult atrophic dermatitis (eczema) characterized by erythematous patches of dry skin.

(Taken from Goodheart HP. *Goodheart's photoguide of common skin disorders.* 2nd ed. Philadelphia: Lippincott Williams & Wilkins, 2003. Fig. 2-8. Used with permission of Lippincott Williams & Wilkins.)

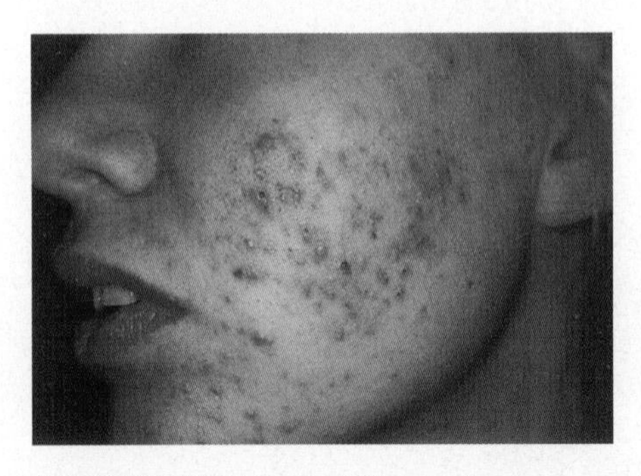

COLOR FIGURE 10-5 Multiple erythematous pustules on the face of an adolescent patient consistent with acne vulgaris.

(Taken from Sauer GC , Hall JC. *Manual of skin diseases.* 7th ed. Philadelphia: Lippincott-Raven Publishers, 1996, Fig. 32-6. Used with permission of Lippincott Williams & Wilkins.)

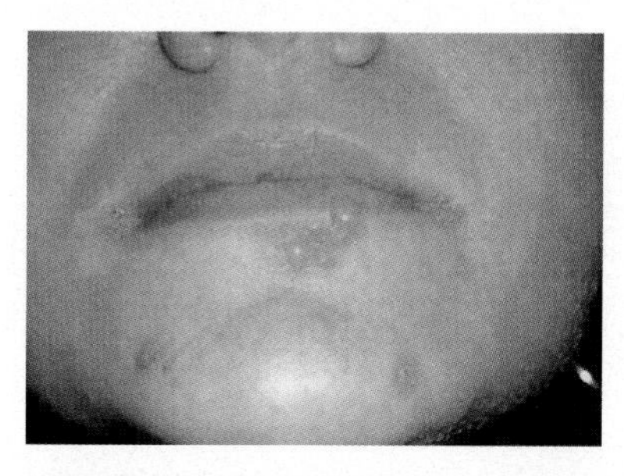

COLOR FIGURE 10-6 Herpes simplex; these perioral vesicles are more indicative of infection with herpes simplex virus type 1 than of type 2.

(Taken from Weber J, Kelley J. *Health assessment in nursing.* 2nd ed. Philadelphia: Lippincott Williams & Wilkins, 2003. Display 13-1a. Used with permission of Lippincott Williams & Wilkins.)

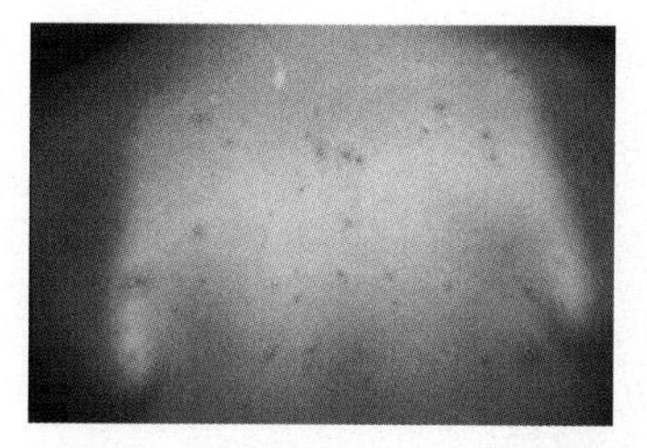

COLOR FIGURE 10-7 Chickenpox in a child due to varicella zoster infection. Although the small crusted vesicles are distributed across the body in the childhood form, reactivated infection in adults (shingles) occurs in a single dermatome.

(Taken from Goodheart HP. *Goodheart's photoguide of common skin disorders.* 2nd ed. Philadelphia: Lippincott Williams & Wilkins, 2003. Fig. 8-2. Used with permission of Lippincott Williams & Wilkins.)

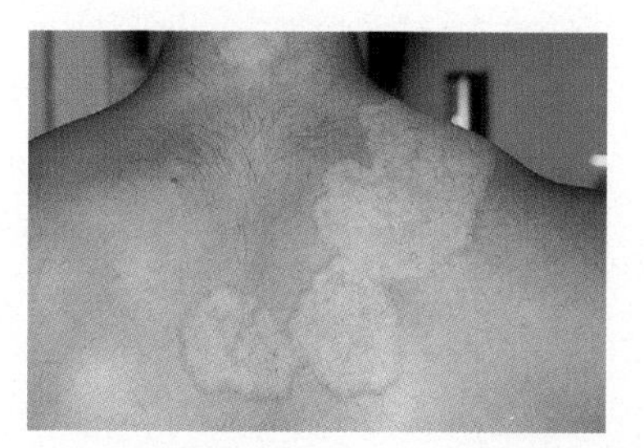

COLOR FIGURE 10-8 Tinea corporis; fungal infection of skin characterized by scaly rash on the body with central clearing and a papular border.

(Taken from Goodheart HP. *Goodheart's photoguide of common skin disorders.* 2nd ed. Philadelphia: Lippincott Williams & Wilkins, 2003. Fig. 4-12. Used with permission of Lippincott Williams & Wilkins.)

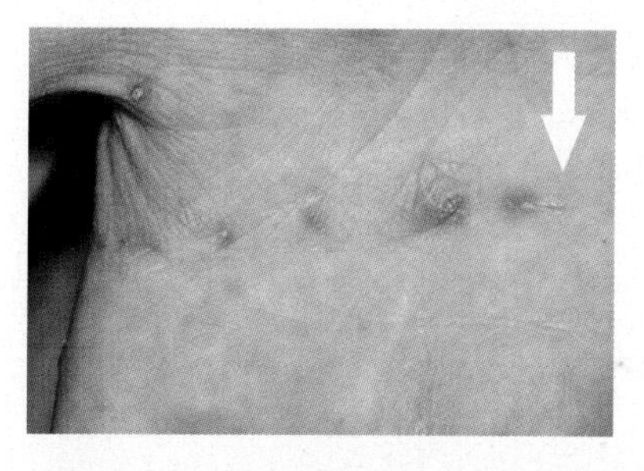

COLOR FIGURE 10-9 Palm of a patient with scabies. Note the multiple red papules and a visible mite burrow (*white arrow*).

(Taken from Goodheart HP. *Goodheart's photoguide of common skin disorders.* 2nd ed. Philadelphia: Lippincott Williams & Wilkins, 2003. Fig. 20-14. Used with permission of Lippincott Williams & Wilkins.)

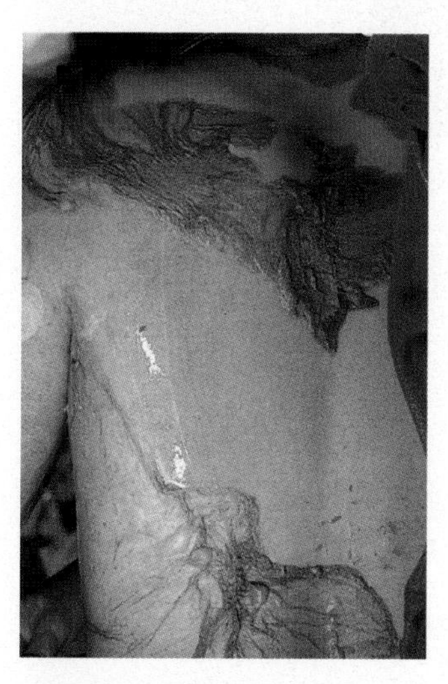

COLOR FIGURE 10-10 Toxic epidermal necrolysis. This severe dermatologic condition begins as a generalized erythematous rash that progresses into widespread desquamation and erosion formation.

(Taken from Elder D, Johnson B Jr, Ioffreda M, et al. *Synopsis and atlas of Lever's histopathology of the skin.* Philadelphia: Lippincott Williams & Wilkins, 1999. Clin. Fig. IVC2.c. Used with permission of Lippincott Williams & Wilkins.)

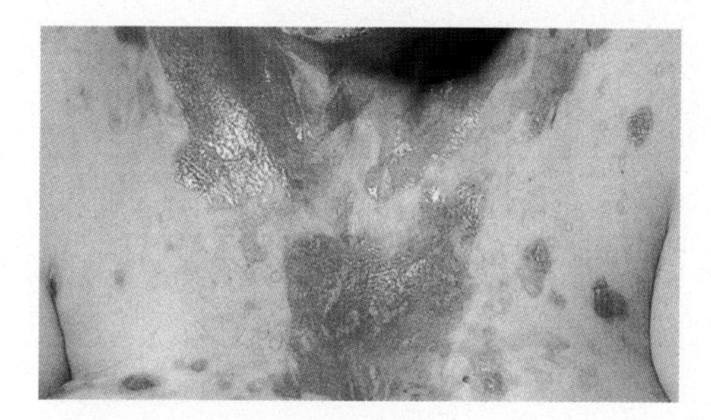

COLOR FIGURE 10-11 Pemphigus vulgaris. Fragile bullae develop which rupture easily leading to widespread erosions and desquamation.

(Taken from Elder D, Johnson B Jr, Ioffreda M, et al. *Synopsis and atlas of Lever's histopathology of the skin.* Philadelphia: Lippincott Williams & Wilkins, 1999. Clin. Fig. IVD3.b. Used with permission of Lippincott Williams & Wilkins.)

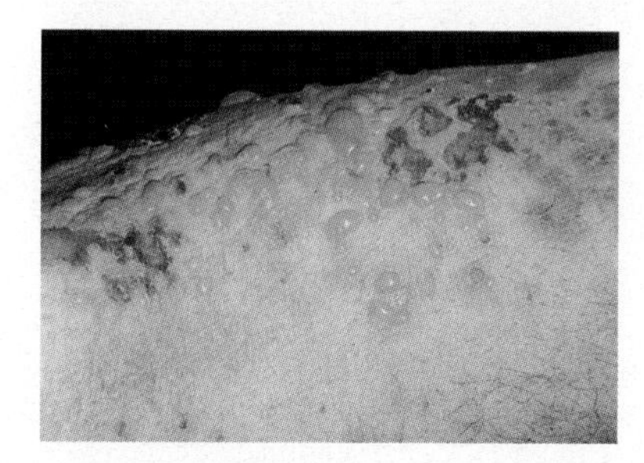

COLOR FIGURE 10-12 Bullous pemphigoid. Multiple large bullae form on an erythematous base leading to severe erosions.

(Taken from Elder D, Johnson B Jr, Ioffreda M, et al. *Synopsis and atlas of Lever's histopathology of the skin.* Philadelphia: Lippincott Williams & Wilkins, 1999. Clin. Fig. IVE3. Used with permission of Lippincott Williams & Wilkins.)

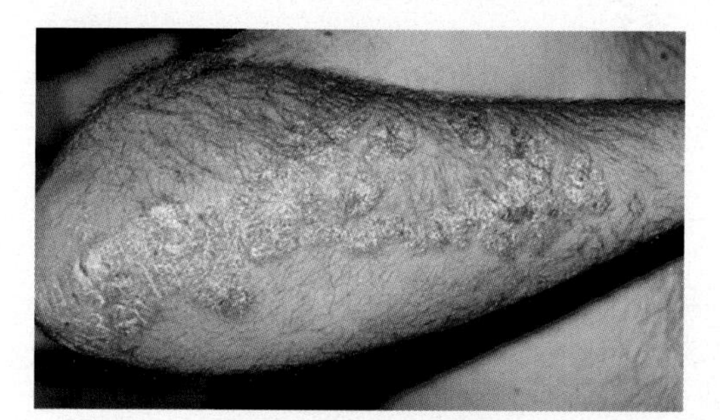

COLOR FIGURE 10-13 Red plaques with silver scales on the extensor forearm surface of a patient with psoriasis; similar lesions may also be seen on the extensor surfaces of the knee.

(Taken from Goodheart HP. *Goodheart's photoguide of common skin disorders.* 2nd ed. Philadelphia: Lippincott Williams & Wilkins, 2003. Fig. 2-23. Used with permission of Lippincott Williams & Wilkins.)

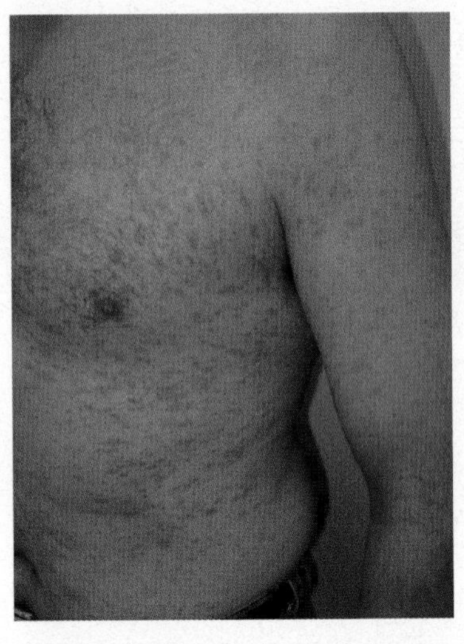

COLOR FIGURE 10-14 Pityriasis rosea. These scaled papules fan out across the chest or back to give the overall appearance of a Christmas tree pattern.

(Taken from Barankin B, Lin AN, Metelitsa AI. *Stedman's illustrated dictionary of dermatology eponyms.* Baltimore: Lippincott Williams & Wilkins, 2004. Used with permission of Lippincott Williams & Wilkins.)

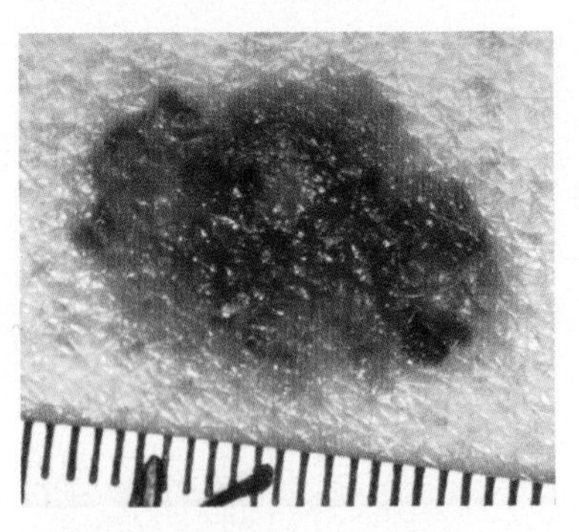

COLOR FIGURE 10-15 Melanoma, superficial spreading type; note the ABCDs of the lesion—**a**symmetry, irregular **b**order, inconsistent **c**olor, and large **d**iameter (>20 mm).

(Taken from Rubin E, Farber JL. *Pathology.* 3rd ed. Philadelphia: Lippincott Williams & Wilkins, 1999. Fig. 24-51. Used with permission of Lippincott Williams & Wilkins.)

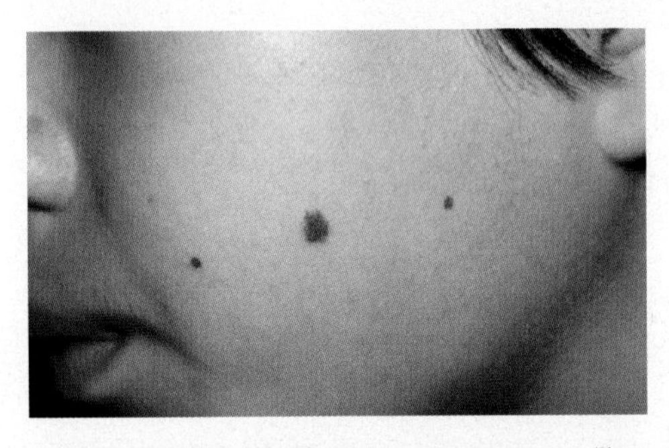

COLOR FIGURE 10-16 Melanocytic nevus; unlike melanoma, this lesion is near symmetrical, has better border regularity, is a more consistent color, and is a smaller diameter.

(Taken from Goodheart HP. *Goodheart's photoguide of common skin disorders.* 2nd ed. Philadelphia: Lippincott Williams & Wilkins, 2003. Fig. 21-1. Used with permission of Lippincott Williams & Wilkins.)

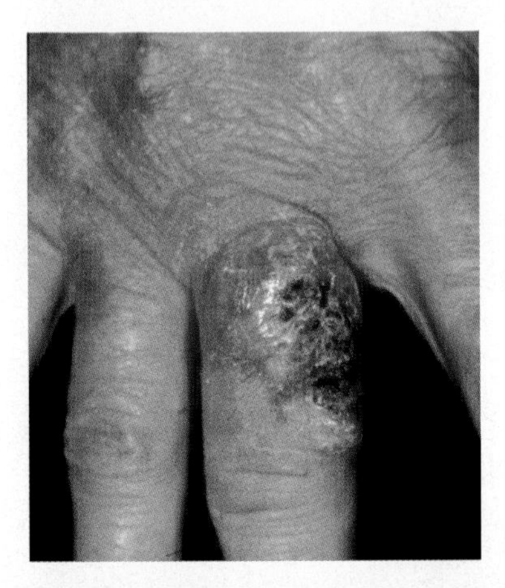

COLOR FIGURE 10-17 Squamous cell carcinoma with erythematous base and ulceration.

(Taken from Rubin E, Farber JL. *Pathology.* 3rd ed. Philadelphia: Lippincott Williams & Wilkins, 1999. Fig. 24-76A. Used with permission of Lippincott Williams & Wilkins.)

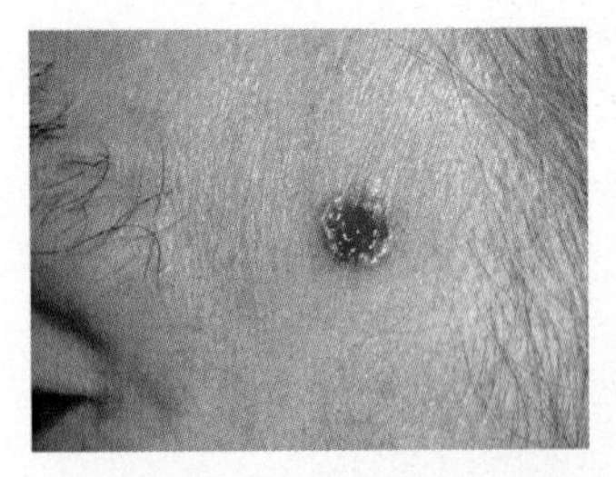

COLOR FIGURE 10-18 Basal cell carcinoma; note the pearly appearance of a papule with central ulceration.

(Taken from Goodheart HP. *Goodheart's photoguide of common skin disorders.* 2nd ed. Philadelphia: Lippincott Williams & Wilkins, 2003. Fig. 22-17. Used with permission of Lippincott Williams & Wilkins.)

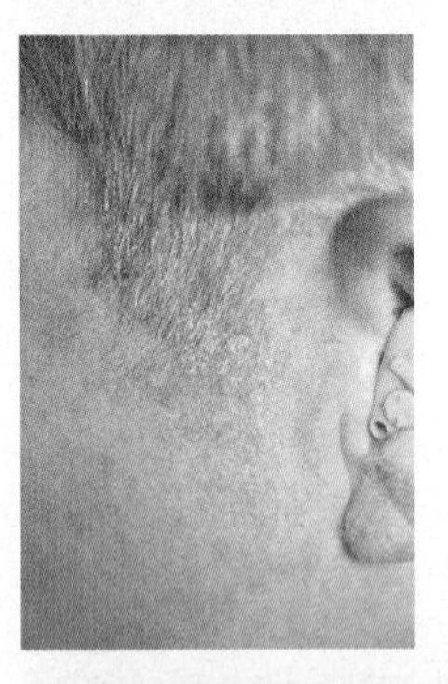

COLOR FIGURE 10-19 Actinic keratosis; these lesions are superficial papules covered by dry scales and are a result of sun exposure.

(Taken from Sauer GC. *Manual of skin diseases.* 5th ed. Philadelphia: JB Lippincott, 1985, Table 4-4. Used with permission of Lippincott Williams & Wilkins.)

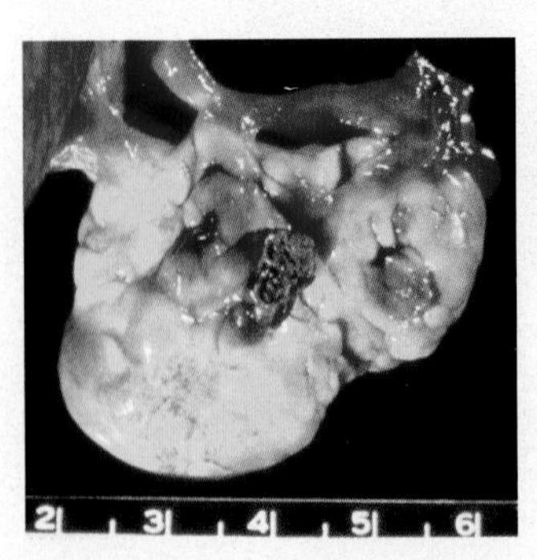

COLOR FIGURE 11-1 Pathology specimen of an ovary demonstrating the characteristic powder-burn lesions of endometriosis.

(Taken from Rubin E, Farber JL. *Pathology.* 3rd ed. Philadelphia: Lippincott Williams & Wilkins, 1999. Fig. 18-27A. Used with permission of Lippincott Williams & Wilkins.)

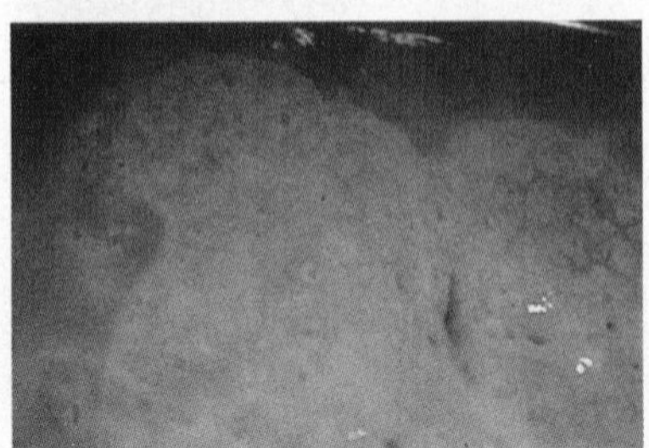

COLOR FIGURE 11-2 Colposcopy view of the cervix with multiple lesions consistent with human papilloma virus infection. Application of acetic acid to the cervix during the examination has made these lesions more apparent.

(Taken from Goodheart HP. *Goodheart's photoguide of common skin disorders.* 2nd ed. Philadelphia: Lippincott Williams & Wilkins, 2003. Fig. 19.6. Used with permission of Lippincott Williams & Wilkins.)

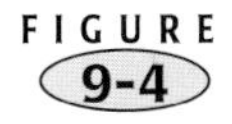

Osteoarthritis in a right hip joint; synovial cysts (*black arrows*) and osteophytes (*white arrow*) are evident.

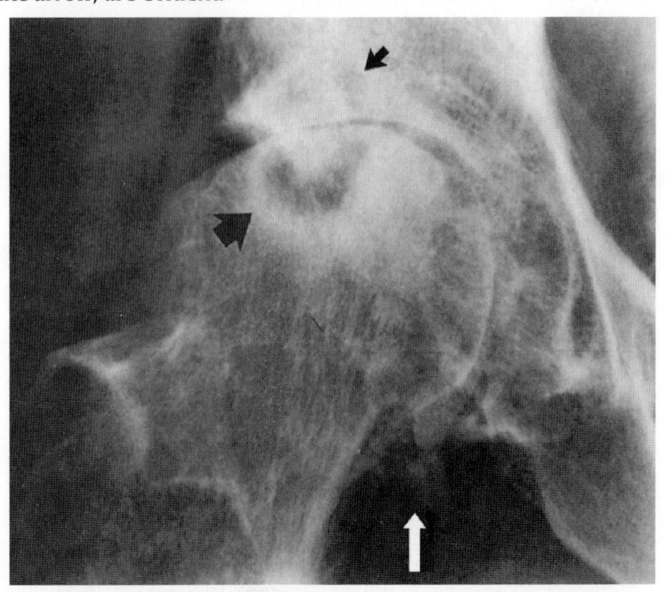

(Taken from Daffner RH. *Clinical radiology: the essentials.* 2nd ed. Philadelphia: Lippincott Williams & Wilkins, 1999. Used with permission of Lippincott Williams & Wilkins.)

  - Physical: joint crepitus, joint pain with range of motion
  - Tests: appearance of x-rays
- **Rheumatoid arthritis**
  - A chronic inflammatory arthropathy with infiltration of the synovial joint tissues by inflammatory cells and progressive erosion of both cartilage and bone
    - **Synovial hypertrophy** with the formation of granulation tissue on the articular cartilage (i.e., pannus formation) occurs due to chronic joint inflammation
    - Most commonly seen in middle-aged women and those with a human leukocyte antigen (HLA) **DR4** serotype
    - **PIP** and **metacarpophalangeal (MCP)** joints in the hands are frequently the first affected
    - A **symmetric polyarthropathy** involving the other major joints occurs after the initial joint development
  - **History**: malaise, weight loss, insidious onset of morning joint pain and stiffness that improves slightly over the day
  - **Physical examination**: decreased range of motion, joint warmth, joint swelling and hypertrophy, fever, ulnar deviation of the fingers, **swan neck deformities** (i.e., DIP held in a flexed position with a hyperextended PIP), **boutonniere deformities** (i.e., flexed PIP with a hyperextended DIP), subcutaneous nodules (Color Figure 9-1)
  - **Tests:**
    - **Rheumatoid factor (RF)** is positive in 75% of patients but is not specific for the disease
    - Antinuclear antibody (ANA) is positive in 40% of patients; ESR and anti–citrulline-containing protein immunoglobulin IgM antibodies are increased
    - Joint aspiration typically shows 5,000 to 50,000 WBC/mm^3
    - X-rays demonstrate soft tissue swelling, joint space narrowing, marginal bony erosions, and possible joint subluxation; MRI may be useful for detecting similar findings (Figure 9-5)
  - **Treatment:**
    - **NSAIDs** and physical therapy are the initial treatments to reduce pain and optimize function
    - Patients still mildly symptomatic following NSAID use may be started on sulfasalazine or hydroxychloroquine and analgesics as needed

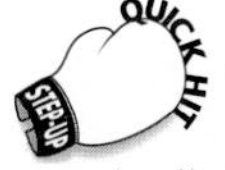

- **OA:** typically **asymmetrical** and may only affect one joint; the DIP joints are frequently involved in the hands.
- **RA:** affects joints on both sides of the body in a **symmetrical** distribution; the DIP joints are spared in the hands.

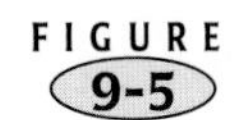
Hip x-ray in a patient with rheumatoid arthritis. Marginal erosions in the bone (*arrow*) are due to pannus formation (*arrowheads*).

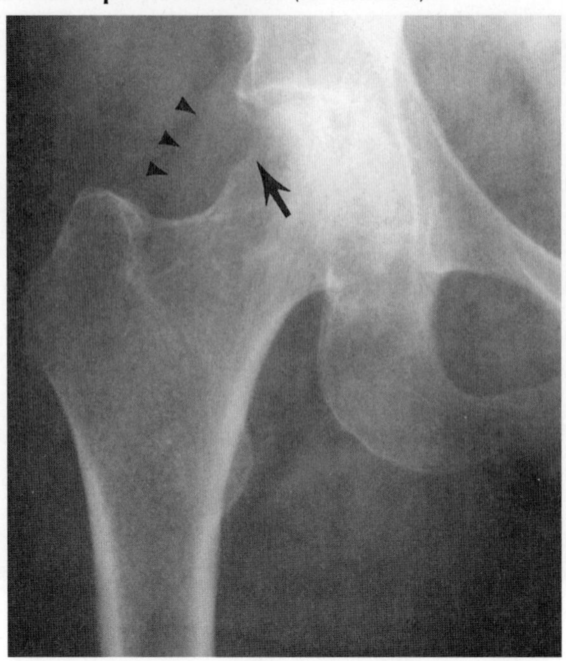

(Taken from Callaghan JJ, Rosenberg AG, Rubash HE. *The adult hip*. 2nd ed. Philadelphia: Lippincott Williams & Wilkins. 2007. Fig. 27-37. Used with permission of Lippincott Williams & Wilkins.)

- Moderate disease may be treated with methotrexate; anti-TNF (tumor necrosis factor) drugs (e.g., infliximab) or corticosteroids may also be utilized
- Severe disease is treated with **anti-TNF drugs** and corticosteroids
- Joint replacement is frequently required in patients with severe joint degeneration; soft tissue repairs are frequently performed for joint subluxations (particularly the hand)

- **Outcomes**: in the absence of antirheumatic medications the disease is progressive and occasionally debilitating
- **Why eliminated from differential**: the appearance of the x-rays is more consistent with OA, and the absence of any other joint involvement makes this diagnosis less likely

- **Meniscal tear**
  - Injury to the cartilaginous meniscus of the knee, causing altered knee mechanics
    - Results from repetitive meniscal microtrauma and degeneration or an acute forceful twisting of a planted knee
    - Frequently associated with tears of the **anterior cruciate ligament** (ACL) of the knee
  - **History**: deep knee pain, locking of the knee
  - **Physical examination**: joint line tenderness, clicking of the knee during range of motion
  - **Tests**: MRI is the modality of choice for detecting tears
  - **Treatment**: arthroscopic debridement or repair is performed to eliminate impingement of the torn meniscus; NSAIDs and physical therapy may be utilized in patients refusing surgery to help ease their symptoms
  - **Outcomes**: symptoms are typically eliminated following surgery; patients who have meniscal tears are at a higher risk for developing OA regardless of the treatment
  - **Why eliminated from differential** meniscal tears are fairly common in this age group, but the appearance of the x-ray suggests that joint degeneration is a much better explanation for the patient's symptoms
- **Septic arthritis**
  - More thorough discussion in later case
  - **Why eliminated from differential**: the lack of erythema, effusion, or micromotion pain makes this diagnosis unlikely

QUICK HIT: Meniscal tears are common in patients after the age of 60 years and are frequently asymptomatic in these patients.

QUICK HIT: A medially directed blow to the lateral side of the knee (i.e., a valgus stress) may cause the **unhappy triad: medial meniscus** tear, **medial collateral ligament (MCL)** tear, and **ACL** tear.

- **Lyme disease**
  - More thorough discussion in later case
  - **Why eliminated from differential:** the x-ray is highly suggestive of OA, and the absence of any dermatologic, neurologic, or cardiac symptoms make this diagnosis unlikely
- **Gout/pseudogout**
  - More thorough discussion in later case
  - **Why eliminated from differential:** the lack of erythema, an effusion, or signs of chondrocalcinosis on the x-ray makes this diagnosis unlikely

CASE 9-4 "This knee is killing me!"

A 44-year-old man presents to an emergency department with the complaint of severe left knee pain for the past day. He says that he has felt sick and fatigued for the past week, but that his knee only began to hurt last night. He denies any trauma to his knee over this time. He says that he woke up in the middle of the night with moderate knee pain and swelling that has steadily increased in severity. He says that he is unable to bear weight on his left leg because of the pain and that any movement causes severe pain. He denies that this has ever occurred previously. He also describes having chills at home prior to coming to the hospital. He denies any locking of the knee, lesions on the knee, or drainage from the knee. He has no symptoms in any other joint. He notes a history of multiple chlamydia infections that have been treated with antibiotics. He has had multiple human immunodeficiency virus (HIV) screenings (most recently 1 month ago) that have all been negative. He admits to drinking alcohol and smoking marijuana on a daily basis and started to inject cocaine intravenously about 3 months ago. On examination, he is an uncomfortable-appearing man in no respiratory distress. He is mildly diaphoretic. He has palpable inguinal lymph nodes on the left side. Auscultation of his lungs and heart detects clear breathing sounds and a regular heart beat without any abnormal sounds. His abdomen is nontender without any masses. His left knee is deeply erythematous and swollen. There is a palpable effusion in the knee, and the patella is easily ballottable. There do not appear to be any skin lesions over the knee, and there are no sites of drainage. Any range of motion causes significant discomfort in the patient. Palpation of his calf detects mild swelling, but the calf is generally soft. Neurovascular examination of the left leg detects normal motor and sensory function and a bounding dorsalis pedis pulse. The following vital signs are measured:

T: 102.1°F, HR: 110 bpm, BP: 140/95 mm Hg, RR: 14 breaths/min

Differential Diagnosis

- Septic arthritis, Lyme disease, osteomyelitis, fracture, gout, pseudogout, osteoarthritis, rheumatoid arthritis, compartment syndrome

Laboratory Data and Other Study Results

- Complete blood cell count (CBC): WBC: 21.2, hemoglobin (Hgb): 12.2, platelets (Plt): 312
- Chem7: Na: 146 mEq/L, K: 3.4 mEq/L, Cl: 104 mEq/L, CO_2: 32 mEq/L, BUN: 23 mg/dL, Cr: 1.2 mg/dL, Glu: 71 mg/dL
- ESR: 73 mm/hr
- CRP: 9.3 mg/dL
- Joint aspiration: 87,259 WBC/mm^3 (95% polymorphonuclear cells [PMNs]), 265 red blood cells [RBC]/mm^3; no crystals
- Knee x-ray: significant effusion; no fracture or dislocation; no signs of joint degeneration
- Blood cultures: Gram stain showing Gram-positive cocci in clusters

Diagnosis

- Septic arthritis

Treatment Administered

- The patient was taken urgently to the operating room by orthopedic surgery for an incision and drainage of the left knee
- The patient was placed on vancomycin awaiting the culture results for the aspiration fluid and the intraoperative cultures

Follow-up

- Following the initial surgical procedure, the patient noted improvement in his pain
- The patient was taken back to the operating room 2 days after his initial surgery for a repeat washout of the joint and examination of the tissues
- Both blood cultures and synovial fluid cultures from the knee grew methicillin-resistant *Staphylococcus aureus*
- Vancomycin was continued, and an infectious disease consultant recommended a 6-week course of treatment
- Following two consecutive negative blood cultures, the patient was transferred to a skilled nursing facility to continue the remainder of his antibiotic treatment

Steps to the Diagnosis

- **Septic arthritis**
  - Infection of a joint by bacteria or fungi, resulting in a significant host immune reaction
    - Damage to the joint occurs as a result of both bacterial toxins and the **host inflammatory response**
    - Occurs through the hematogenous spread of infection (e.g., bacteremia), extension of a local infection (e.g., cellulitis), or direct inoculation (e.g., open fracture)
    - ***S. aureus*** is the most common bacteria involved, and ***Neisseria gonorrhoeae*** is also common in sexually active patients
    - Patients with DM, vascular disease, and cancer may also be susceptible to Gram-negative rod infections
  - **History:** sudden onset of joint pain, refusal to bear weight or move the joint (particularly children)
  - **Physical examination**: significant joint swelling and erythema, warm skin overlying the joint, **micromotion pain** (i.e., significant pain with only a few degrees of movement), possible overlying skin lesions or draining sinus tracts
  - **Tests:**
    - Increased WBC, ESR, and **CRP**
    - Aspiration of synovial fluid demonstrates >50,000 WBC/mm^3 with a high percentage of PMNs (greater than 75%) (Table 9-4)
  - **Treatment:**
    - **Incision and drainage (I + D)** is required for any infection other than *N. gonorrhoeae*
    - Repeat washouts may be required to ensure removal of any diseased tissue
    - Long-term IV antibiotics (approximately 6 weeks) are prescribed once the offending organism has been identified
  - **Outcomes:** one third of cases will be complicated by chronic infection, early joint degeneration, or the need for surgical reconstruction
  - **Clues to the diagnosis:**
    - History: sudden and severe knee pain, history of IV drug use, and recurrent sexually transmitted diseases, inability to bear weight
    - Physical: swollen, erythematous knee, significant effusion, micromotion pain
    - Tests: increased ESR and CRP, increased WBCs, synovial fluid analysis results

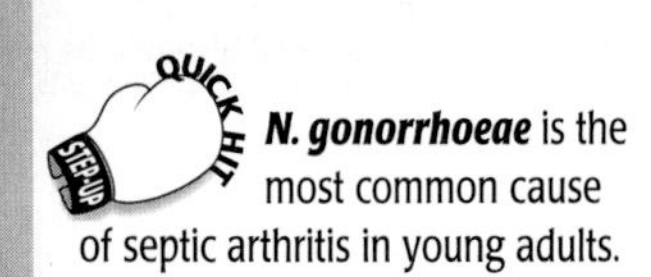

N. gonorrhoeae is the most common cause of septic arthritis in young adults.

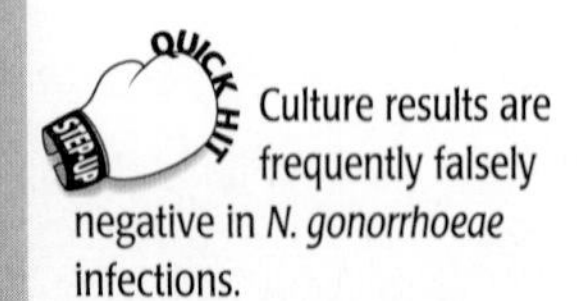

Culture results are frequently falsely negative in *N. gonorrhoeae* infections.

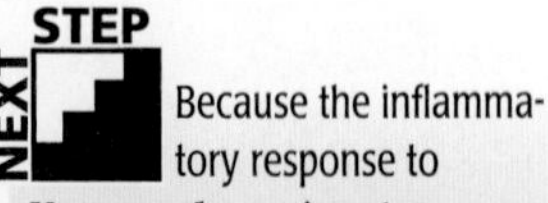

Because the inflammatory response to ***N. gonorrhoeae*** is not as severe as that for other bacteria, I + D is not required for treatment; treat these cases with intravenous (IV) ceftriaxone and doxycycline.

TABLE 9-4 Analysis of Synovial Fluid Aspiration

	Noninflammatory Arthropathy (e.g., OA, Trauma)	Inflammatory Arthropathy (e.g., RA, Gout)	Septic Arthritis
Appearance	Straw colored, viscous	Yellow, thin	Purulent
WBCs (WBC/mm^3)	<2,000	2,000–50,000	>50,000
PMNs (% of WBCs)	<25%	>50%	>75%
Fluid glucose	Similar to blood	Decreased	Decreased
Histology	Increased RBCs with trauma	Needle-shaped, negatively birefringent crystals in gout; rhomboid, positively birefringent crystals in pseudogout	Positive Gram stain and culture for the infectious pathogen

OA, osteoarthritis; PMNs, polymorphonuclear cells; RA, rheumatoid arthritis; RBCs, red blood cells; WBCs, white blood cells.

- Osteomyelitis
  - **Bone infection** due to pathogen exposure (e.g., hematogenous spread, local extension, direct inoculation)
    - ***S. aureus*** and *Pseudomonas* are the most common causes, but *Salmonella* is also common in **sickle cell** and asplenic patients
  - **History:** deep bone pain, difficulty bearing weight due to pain, chills
  - **Physical examination:** bone tenderness, fever, possible overlying cellulitis or a draining sinus tract
  - **Tests:**
    - Increased WBCs, ESR, and CRP
    - Bone culture provides a definitive identification of the infecting agents
    - **MRI** is the most sensitive means of detecting infection (Figure 9-6)
    - Bone scan will frequently show changes after the initial 72 hours of established infection; sensitivity is increased when performed as a **labeled-WBC scan** (using gallium or indium isotopes)
    - X-rays are usually not helpful for identifying infection in the initial 2 weeks of the disease
  - **Treatment:**
    - Long-term antibiotics are the primary form of treatment (initially empirically, then pathogen-specific after culture)
    - I + D is required for any abscess within the bone (i.e., sequestrum) or in the surrounding tissue
    - Debridement of affected bone in extensive cases may cause significant bone loss and disability and is avoided if possible
  - **Outcomes:** chronic infection is a problem in these patients, and the best chance of eradication correlates with a quick diagnosis and institution of treatment
  - **Why eliminated from differential:** the synovial aspirate confirms septic arthritis in this patient, but the long-term follow-up should consist of imaging (x-ray or MRI) to look for any development of infection beyond the joint itself
- Lyme disease
  - Systemic infection caused by *Borrelia burgdorferi*, a spirochete transmitted by the bite of the *Ixodes* tick
    - Progression of the disease is divided into early localized, early disseminated (i.e., spread of disease to the cardiac and neurologic systems), and late disseminated (i.e., establishment of chronic cardiac, neurologic, and joint infection) stages

QUICK HIT (STEP-UP): Although ***Salmonella*** should be considered in patients with sickle cell disease and ***Pseudomonas*** should be considered in intravenous drug abusers, ***S. aureus*** is still the **most common** cause of osteomyelitis in these patients.

FIGURE 9-6 **X-ray and magnetic resonance imaging (MRI) of the proximal tibia in a patient with osteomyelitis. (A) X-ray of the proximal tibia demonstrating a poorly defined lesion (*arrows*) involving much of the proximal tibia. (B) A T1-weighted MRI image of the same region demonstrates extensive involvement of the marrow from the epiphysis to the proximal diaphysis.**

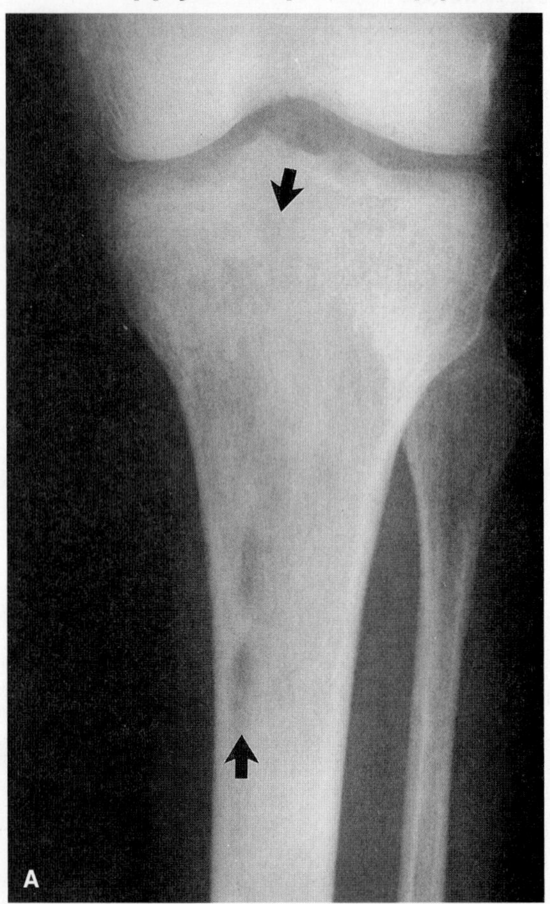

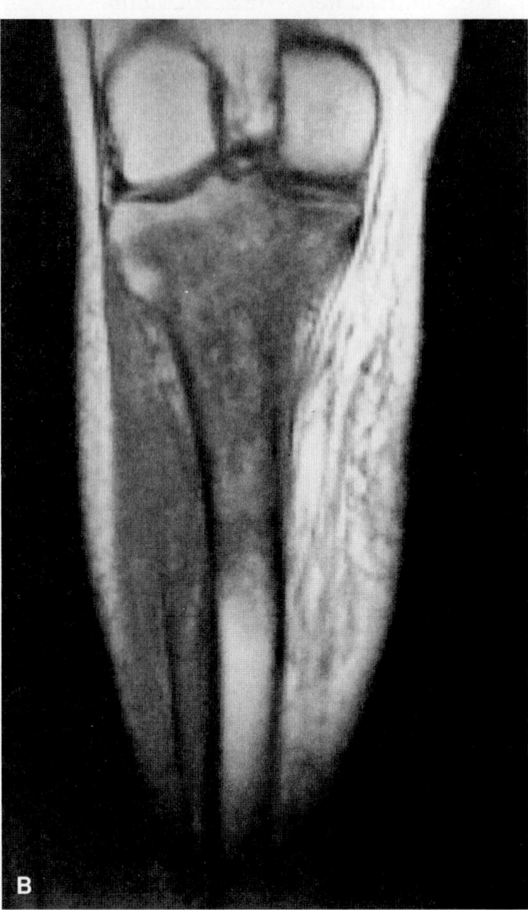

(Taken from Daffner RH. *Clinical radiology: the essentials.* 2nd ed. Philadelphia: Lippincott Williams & Wilkins, 1999. Figs. 11.2A, 11.11. Used with permission of Lippincott Williams & Wilkins.)

- History:
  - **Early localized**: chills, fatigue, arthralgias, headache
  - **Early disseminated**: chronic fatigue, headache, development of paresthesias
  - **Late disseminated**: chronic arthralgias
- Physical examination:
  - **Early localized: erythema chronicum migrans** (i.e., bull's eye rash), fever (Color Figure 9-2)
  - **Early disseminated**: arrhythmias from myocarditis, possible heart block, Bell's palsy
  - **Late disseminated**: signs of subacute encephalopathy (e.g., insomnia, mood disturbances, memory loss, ataxia), polyneuropathy
- **Tests**: enzyme-linked immunosorbent assay (ELISA) and Western blot tests for antibodies; joint aspiration is typically not helpful
- **Treatment: doxycycline**, amoxicillin, or cefuroxime (oral form is appropriate for early disease, but IV forms are needed for disseminated disease)
- **Outcomes**:
  - The long-term prognosis is variable, but Bell's palsy and carditis gradually resolve
  - Arthralgias and cognitive deficits appear to remain a chronic problem in disseminated cases
  - Recognizing the disease and treating it before it becomes disseminated appears to be the key to preventing long-term sequelae

- **Why eliminated from differential:** the sudden onset of severe symptoms in this patient and the synovial fluid results are more consistent with acute joint sepsis
- Gout
  - A peripheral monoarthritis due to the deposition of **sodium urate crystals** in joints
  - The **first metatarsophalangeal** joint is the most commonly affected (i.e., **podagra**), but other joints may be involved
  - **Risk factors:** renal disease, male gender, urate underexcretion, diuretic use, cyclosporine use, cancer, hemoglobinopathies, excessive alcohol consumption
  - **History:** sudden severe pain in one joint, chills, malaise
  - **Physical examination:** fever, warm and red joint, joint swelling
  - **Tests:**
    - Joint aspiration shows **needle-shaped, negatively birefringent crystals** and several WBCs (Color Figure 9-3)
    - Serum uric acid may be normal or increased and is not a reliable test for diagnosis
    - X-ray may show punched-out bone lesions in chronic cases
  - **Treatment:**
    - NSAIDs (especially **indomethacin**), colchicine, or corticosteroids may be used to treat acute flares
    - Decreasing alcohol and diuretic use and avoiding foods high in purines (e.g., red meats, fish) help to prevent exacerbations
    - Probenecid (inhibits renal uric acid resorption) and allopurinol (inhibits uric acid formation) are used in chronic cases to prevent flare-ups
  - **Outcomes:** long-standing, poorly controlled disease leads to chronic tophaceous gout with the formation of nodular tophi (i.e., large deposits of crystals in soft tissues) that cause permanent deformity
  - **Why eliminated from differential:** although the symptoms leading to presentation are consistent with this diagnosis, the results of the synovial fluid analysis rule it out

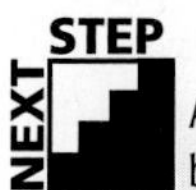

Allopurinol should **not** be administered in acute attacks of gout because it is only useful as prophylaxis in chronic cases.

- **Pseudogout (a.k.a. calcium pyrophosphate dehydrate deposition disease, CPPD)**
  - The deposition of calcium pyrophosphate dehydrate crystals in joints leading to an inflammatory reaction
    - Frequently associated with the presence of other endocrine conditions (e.g., DM, hyperparathyroidism)
    - The knee and wrist are most commonly affected
  - **History:** similar to gout but with less severe pain
  - **Physical examination:** joint swelling, erythema, and warmth
  - **Tests:** synovial fluid analysis detects **rhomboid, positively birefringent crystals** (Color Figure 9-4); x-ray may show **chondrocalcinosis** (i.e., calcification of articular cartilage)
  - **Treatment:** NSAIDs or colchicine are used to treat attacks
  - **Outcomes:** prognosis is fair with few extra-articular effects of the disease, but recurrent flares are possible
  - **Why eliminated from differential:** the results of the synovial fluid analysis rule out this diagnosis
- **Fracture**
  - More thorough discussion in prior case
  - **Why eliminated from differential:** the appearance of the x-ray rules out this diagnosis
- **Osteoarthritis**
  - More thorough discussion in prior case
  - **Why eliminated from differential:** the appearance of the x-ray and the synovial fluid analysis rule out this diagnosis
- **Rheumatoid arthritis**
  - More thorough discussion in prior case
  - **Why eliminated from differential:** the appearance of the x-ray and the synovial fluid analysis rule out this diagnosis

- **Compartment syndrome**
  - **Swelling** and an **increase of pressure** within a **fascial compartment**, leading to eventual compression of neurovascular structures and **ischemia** of tissues within the compartment and distal to the involved region; delayed reperfusion may worsen tissue ischemia
    - Most frequently occurs as a sequela of extremity trauma (especially **crush injuries**)
    - Occurs most commonly in the lower leg and forearm, but the hand, foot, and thigh are also potential sites of involvement
  - **History:** pain that does not respond to increasing doses of analgesia, numbness, weakness
  - **Physical examination:** pallor of the affected extremity, cool-feeling extremity (i.e., poikilothermia), paresthesia, motor weakness, eventual pulselessness, increased pain with **passive stretching** of the compartment
  - **Tests:** intracompartmental pressures (measured by inserting a needle attached to a manometer into the compartment of interest) will be elevated
  - **Treatment: emergent fasciotomies** are indicated for compartments with pressures >30 mm Hg or within 30 mm Hg of the diastolic blood pressure; delayed closure of the wounds is performed at a later date
  - **Outcomes:**
    - Tissue perfusion and neurologic function may be preserved with emergent fasciotomies
    - Patients undergoing fasciotomies are at an increased risk of infection due to the open wounds
    - Delays in treatment or missed compartment syndromes carry a devastating sequela of significant tissue necrosis and loss of function
  - **Why eliminated from differential:** the symptoms in this patient are more attributable to the knee than the calf, and examination of the calf carries a low clinical suspicion for this diagnosis

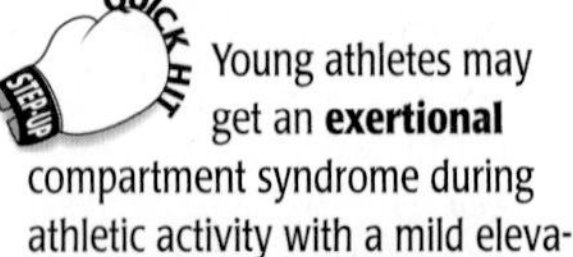

Young athletes may get an **exertional** compartment syndrome during athletic activity with a mild elevation of compartment pressures that **resolves following activity cessation** and that carries a **minimal risk** of significant tissue ischemia.

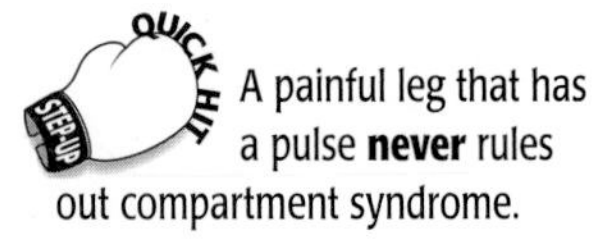

A painful leg that has a pulse **never** rules out compartment syndrome.

MNEMONIC

The signs of compartment syndrome may be remembered by the **six Ps**: **P**ain, **P**aresthesias, **P**aralysis, **P**allor, **P**oikilothermia, and **P**ulselessness.

CASE 9-5 "I can't control my bowels"

A 76-year-old man is brought to an emergency department by his wife after the acute onset of multiple neurologic symptoms. The patient said that he woke up in the middle of the night with low back pain. After he awoke he lost control of his bowels while in bed. He says that he now also feels numb around his groin. He denies ever having had these symptoms previously. He says that his legs feel weak and that he is having difficulty ambulating. He also has pain radiating down both legs. He denies numbness or weakness in his upper extremities. He also denies headaches or vision abnormalities. He states that a pulmonary nodule was detected 1 week ago on a chest x-ray being performed as part of a preoperative evaluation for a knee arthroscopy that he had scheduled to treat a torn meniscus. He was scheduled to have this lesion evaluated in the near future. He denies any shortness of breath or chest pain. He reports a past medical history of HTN, hypercholesterolemia, benign prostatic hypertrophy (BPH), and mild hyperglycemia. He takes the medications lisinopril, HCTZ, atorvastatin, aspirin, and terazosin. His hyperglycemia has been controlled with dietary modification. He reports smoking a pack of cigarettes per day for the past 60 years and drinks about six beers per week. On examination, he appears to be anxious but in no acute distress. Fundoscopic examination appears to be normal. He has no lymphadenopathy. Auscultation of his lungs detects clear breath sounds. Auscultation of his heart detects a regular rhythm with no extra heart sounds. His abdomen is nontender, but he has an easily palpable bladder. A rectal examination demonstrates poor rectal tone and incontinence of stool. He has decreased sensation in the perineal region. On neurologic examination he has normal function in his cranial nerves and upper extremities. He has generalized 3/5 strength in his lower extremities. On filament testing his sensory discrimination is worse in the legs than in his arms. He has negative Babinski signs bilaterally. Examination of his back detects no obvious step-offs or focal regions of pain. The following vital signs are measured:

T: 98.4°F, HR: 90 bpm, BP: 127/85 mm Hg, RR: 16 breaths/min

Differential Diagnosis

- Disc herniation, spinal stenosis, cauda equina syndrome, cerebral vascular accident, DM neuropathy, Guillain-Barre syndrome, multiple sclerosis

Laboratory Data and Other Study Results

- CBC: WBC: 11.3, Hgb: 12.4, Plt: 173
- 10-electrolyte chemistry panel (Chem10): Na: 141 mEq/L, K: 4.1 mEq/L, Cl: 105 mEq/L, CO_2: 30mEq/L, BUN: 13 mg/dL, Cr: 0.6 mg/dL, Glu: 98 mg/dL, magnesium (Mg): 2.0 mg/dL, calcium (Ca): 10.9 mg/dL, phosphorus (Phos): 3.3
- Head CT: no sign of intracranial lesion; no fractures; normal ventricles and cerebral volume
- Chest CT: 3 × 4 cm lesion in the right lung adjacent to a segmental bronchi
- Spine CT: no fractures; indiscrete mass involving the L_5 vertebral body
- Spine MRI: 3 × 3 cm mass in the L5 vertebra, with expansion into the spinal canal

Diagnosis

- Cauda equina syndrome

Treatment Administered

- A urethral catheter was placed into the patient's bladder to drain the volume of contained urine
- The patient was taken emergently to the operating room for decompression of his lumbar spine
- IV corticosteroids were started and administered for 48 hours to decrease spinal inflammation

Follow-up

- The patient recovered control of his bowels and sensation in his perineum
- A biopsy of the lung and spinal lesions confirmed the diagnosis of a pulmonary malignancy
- Radiation therapy was started to decrease the size of the vertebral lesion
- The patient's neurologic examination improved, and he was discharged to continue his tumor work-up with oncology as an outpatient

Steps to the Diagnosis

- **Cauda equina syndrome**
  - Compression of the cauda equina (i.e., an extension of the dural-arachnoid sac beyond the end of the spinal cord and the terminal nerve roots contained within it) following trauma or growth of a neoplasm
  - **History: urinary retention**, **incontinence of stool**, possible lower extremity weakness, low back pain
  - **Physical examination:** decreased rectal tone, **perineal anesthesia** (i.e., saddle anesthesia), possible decreased lower extremity sensation and strength
  - **Tests:** MRI or CT myelogram is used to locate the site of compression
  - **Treatment:**
    - Emergency surgical decompression is performed to relieve pressure on the terminal nerve roots
    - IV corticosteroids are frequently administered to decrease inflammation around the spinal cord
    - Radiation is used in cases of spinal neoplasm to decrease the size of the tumor
  - **Outcomes:** recovery of function is most likely with prompt treatment; delays in surgical decompression result in permanent neurologic deficits

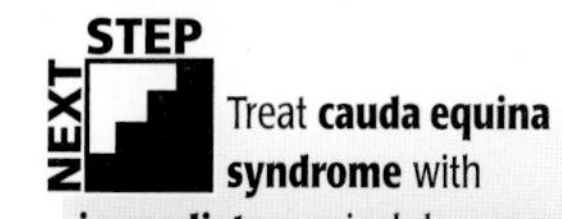

Treat **cauda equina syndrome** with **immediate** surgical decompression because it can quickly result in permanent neurologic injury.

- **Clues to the diagnosis:**
  - History: low back pain, bowel incontinence, radicular pain, recently detected pulmonary nodule
  - Physical: decreased rectal tone, palpable bladder, sensory and motor deficits in the legs
  - Tests: appearance of the MRI
- **Disc herniation**
  - More thorough discussion in prior case
  - **Why eliminated from differential:** the absence of a herniation on the MRI rules out this diagnosis
- **Spinal stenosis**
  - More thorough discussion in prior case
  - **Why eliminated from differential:** the sudden onset of symptoms makes this diagnosis unlikely, and the MRI rules it out
- **Cerebral vascular accident**
  - More thorough discussion in Chapter 7
  - **Why eliminated from differential:** the normal head CT rules out this diagnosis
- **Guillain-Barre syndrome**
  - More thorough discussion in Chapter 7
  - **Why eliminated from differential:** the pattern of neurologic findings makes this diagnosis unlikely
- **DM neuropathy**
  - More thorough discussion in Chapter 5
  - **Why eliminated from differential:** the normal serum glucose and sudden onset of symptoms rule out this diagnosis
- **Multiple sclerosis**
  - More thorough discussion in Chapter 7
  - **Why eliminated from differential:** the sudden onset of symptoms and lack of white matter lesions on the MRI make this diagnosis unlikely

The following additional Orthopedic and Rheumatology cases may be found online:

CASE 9-6 "There's a hole in my bone"

CASE 9-6 "I ache and I feel lousy"

CASE 9-6 "Why do I feel so dry all of the time?"

CASE 9-6 "I'm too young for chronic back pain"

CASE 9-6 "My son is having trouble walking"

CASE 9-6 "Our daughter's leg is very bowed"

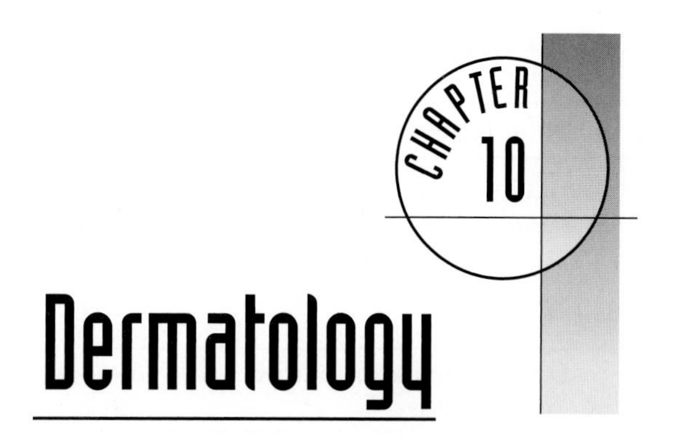

Dermatology

BASIC CLINICAL PRIMER

WOUNDS AND HEALING

- Wound types
  - **Clean**
    - Surgical incisions through disinfected skin
    - **No** gastrointestinal (GI) or respiratory contamination
    - Generally a 1%–3% infection risk for first-time procedures
  - **Clean-contaminated**
    - Surgical wounds with GI or respiratory tract **exposure**
    - A 2%–8% infection risk
  - **Contaminated**
    - Gross contact of a wound with GI or pulmonary **contents** or **environmental** exposure
    - Includes **traumatic** wounds
    - A 6%–15% infection risk
  - **Dirty**
    - **Established infection** in tissues prior to incision
    - The risk of continued infection following debridement ranges from 7%–40%
- **Wound healing**
  - Surgical wounds are typically covered for 48 hours following closure with dressing changes as needed following the removal of the initial bandage
  - **Open wounds** require debridement and **specialized dressings** (e.g., vacuum-assisted, Dakin solution, wet-to-dry dressings) designed to promote healing and reduce the risk of infection
  - Wound healing may be inhibited by **malnutrition**, corticosteroid use, smoking, hepatic or renal failure, or **diabetes mellitus (DM)**
  - **Types of wound healing**
    - **Primary intention**
      - Surgical closure of the wound (i.e., deep tissues and skin) performed to optimize the healing environment
      - **Low** risk of infection
      - Typically performed in clean and clean-contaminated wounds or in contaminated wounds following substantial cleaning
    - **Secondary intention**
      - Wound is left open and allowed to heal through epithelialization
      - Allowed to occur in infected wounds or with significant superficial skin loss preventing full wound closure
      - Incorporates various dressing techniques to promote successful healing
      - **Higher** risk of infection
    - **Delayed primary closure**
      - Wounds are left open for multiple days prior to a repeat cleansing and closure

TABLE 10-1 Common Types of Skin Grafts and Tissue Flaps Used in Wound Repair

Type	Description	Common Donor Sites	Indications
Split-thickness graft	Skin graft composed of epidermis and partial dermis	Abdomen, thighs, buttocks	Skin replacement in wounds; useful to cover an extensive surface area
Full-thickness graft	Skin graft composed of epidermis and full dermis	Above ears (for face), forearm, groin	Defects on face and hands
Composite graft	Skin grafts that also contain other tissues (e.g., cartilage, nail bed, fat)	Fingertip, ear, etc.	Site-specific anatomical reconstruction
Fasciocutaneous flap	Skin and subcutaneous tissue with an attached vascular supply	Forehead, groin, deltopectoral region, thighs	Large defects with a good vascular supply requiring padding
Muscle flap	Transferred muscle that either includes skin (i.e., myocutaneous flap) or that requires additional skin graft	Tensor fascia lata, gluteal muscles, sartorius, rectus abdominus, latissimus dorsi	Areas with inadequate vascularized tissue, exposed deep tissues, or severe radiation injury

- Performed in contaminated wounds in which closure is physically possible and in which serial debridement is able to provide a clean wound
- **Tissue transport**
  - Transfer of the cutaneous and/or deeper soft tissues (i.e., subcutaneous tissue, fascia, muscle) to a wound that cannot be physically closed where adequate protection of deeper neurovascular, visceral, or musculoskeletal structures cannot be provided (Table 10-1)
  - Skin grafts are most commonly **autografts** (i.e., from healthy tissue on the same patient), but may occasionally be allografts (i.e., donor tissue), or rarely xenografts (i.e., donor tissue from another species)
  - Flaps may be **rotational** or **transpositional** (i.e., left partially attached to the donor site) or may be **free flaps** (i.e., tissue completely removed from the donor site, transferred to the wounds, and revascularized at the wound)

CASE 10-1 "My skin has been red and blistered since the picnic"

A 23-year-old woman presents to her primary care provider (PCP) because of a 1-day history of erythema and pain in her face and hands. She says that she was at an all-day picnic 2 days ago and has had the above symptoms since that time. The picnic was held outdoors in a field. The patient says that it was a cloudy day and that she did not wear sunscreen. By the evening after the picnic she noticed pain in her face and hands. She found that both her face and the back of her hands were erythematous and that she had some small blisters on her forehead and nose. She denies any pruritus or numbness. She reports that she has had sunburns in the past but that they were not as severe as the current presentation. She admits that she was playing in the grass with her dog and both her face and hands were in contact with vegetation in the field. She has not noticed any insects on herself or her dog and denies finding any insect bites or sores on her body. She was wearing a long-sleeved shirt, jeans, and closed shoes, and her face and hands were the only part of her body exposed. She denies any past medical history and uses only oral contraceptives as a regular medication. She denies any known allergies. She drinks socially and denies other substance use. On examination, she is a well-appearing woman in no distress. Her face and the dorsum of both hands up to the wrist are quite erythematous. A few tiny blisters are notable on her forehead and on the bridge of her nose. Her skin is warm to the touch and blanches easily with pressure, but it is apparent that touching the inflamed regions is somewhat painful to the patient. No discrete lesions, patterns of inflammation, or wounds are noticeable. Examination of her arms above her wrists, her torso, and her legs finds normal-appearing skin without the characteristics of her hands and face. No flaking of the skin or dry patches are apparent. Examination of her eyes detects pink conjunctiva and white sclera. Her lips are inflamed, but her mouth appears normal without any swelling. She has no lymphadenopathy. The following vital signs are measured:

Temperature (T): 98.7°F, heart rate (HR): 84 beats per minute (bpm), blood pressure (BP): 122/81 mm Hg, respiratory rate (RR): 18 breaths/min

Differential Diagnosis

- Sunburn, contact dermatitis, cellulitis, atopic dermatitis, porphyria cutanea tarda, systemic lupus erythematosus

Laboratory Data and Other Study Results

- None performed

Diagnosis

- Mild second- and first-degree thermal burns due to sun exposure

Treatment Administered

- The patient was advised to take moderate-dose (600 mg) ibuprofen as needed, to maintain her fluid intake, and to use a skin moisturizer with a mild topical anesthetic as needed

Follow-up

- The patient's symptoms resolved over several days
- The patient was educated about the risks of sunburn and was provided with literature describing ways to prevent future burns

Steps to the Diagnosis

- Burns
  - Injury to the epithelium and dermis of the skin due to exposure to significant heat, radiation, caustic substances, or electrical shock
    - Classified by the depth of involvement
      - **First degree**: epidermis only
      - **Second degree**: partial thickness dermal involvement
      - **Third degree**: full epidermis and dermis and some fatty tissue involvement
    - Estimation of the surface extent of burns may be classified by the "**Rule of 9s**" (Figure 10-1)
  - **History:**
    - **First degree**: pain at the site of involvement
    - **Second degree**: moderate to severe pain at the site of involvement
    - **Third degree**: the site of true third-degree injury is typically painless
  - **Physical examination:**
    - **First degree**: erythema at the site of exposure
    - **Second degree**: erythema and blistering at the site of exposure
    - **Third degree**: charred, leathery, or gray skin at the site of involvement
    - **Electrical burns:** similar appearance to third-degree burns, possible cardiac arrhythmias and neurologic abnormalities (e.g., visual abnormalities, seizures, sensory or motor dysfunction)
  - **Tests:** burns are typically a clinical diagnosis, so additional testing is typically not required; serum carboxyhemoglobin should be measured in patients suspected of smoke inhalation to determine the risk of impaired tissue oxygenation
  - **Treatment:**
    - Any burning agents or chemicals should be **removed** from the skin (including affected clothing) to prevent further injury
    - Caustic substances should be **neutralized** or **diluted**

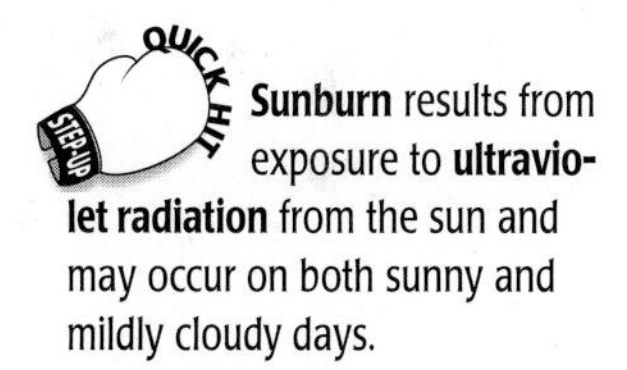

Sunburn results from exposure to **ultraviolet radiation** from the sun and may occur on both sunny and mildly cloudy days.

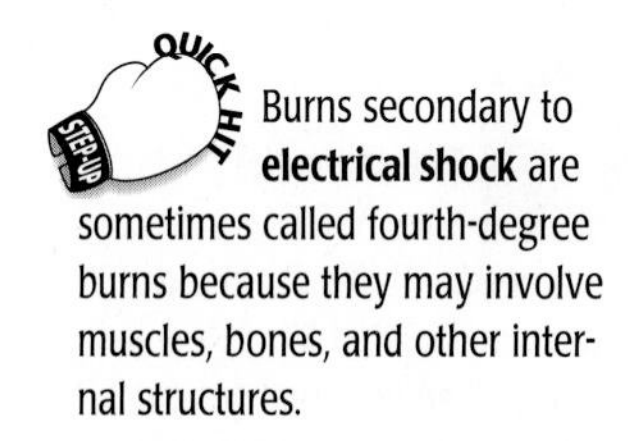

Burns secondary to **electrical shock** are sometimes called fourth-degree burns because they may involve muscles, bones, and other internal structures.

FIGURE 10-1 "Rule of 9s" for calculating the surface extent of burns. (A) The surface anatomy of the adult is divided into sections of 9% body surface area (genitals are considered 1% surface area). Note that the distribution considers both the front and back of the head and arms as single contributions. (B) Because of its greater relative size, the contribution of the head is increased in the child. Note that the front and back for the head, arms, and legs are considered as single contributions.

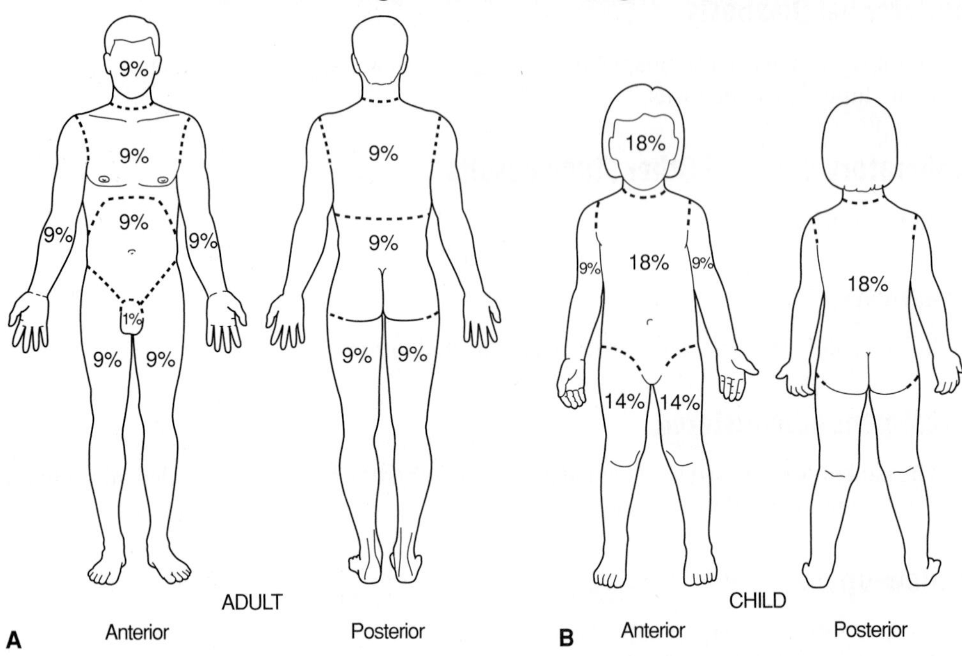

- First-degree and mild second-degree burns may be treated with cooling, cleansing, bandaging, topical antimicrobials, and topical agents intended to reduce rapid epidermal loss (e.g., moisturizers, emollients)
- Vigilant use of **sunscreen** is important to preventing sunburn (usually a first-degree or mild second-degree radiation burn)
- **Second-degree** burns involving more than **10%** body surface area (BSA) and **third-degree** burns involving more than **2%** BSA require inpatient treatment for intravenous (IV) hydration, wound care, and possible surgical escharectomy
- Second- and third-degree burns affecting the face, hands, genitalia, or major skin flexion creases must be considered for inpatient treatment because serious scarring or functional loss is a potential complication
- Second- or third-degree burns involving more than **25%** BSA or with significant face involvement require **airway management** (possible intubation), IV fluids, and careful body temperature regulation
- Patients with significant **smoke inhalation** should receive high-flow oxygen and close monitoring for respiratory distress
- Patients with electrical burns should be monitored until urine output is consistently normal, cardiac and neurologic examinations remain normal, and adequate perfusion is confirmed in all extremities; fasciotomies or escharotomies should be performed for any extremity demonstrating impaired perfusion from an impending compartment syndrome or constrictive eschar
- Cardiac and neurologic complications from shocks should be managed appropriately to reduce mortality

- **Outcomes:**
  - Prognosis is related to the depth of the burn and the BSA involved, with outcomes being worse as each increases
  - Potential complications of acute burns include significant fluid loss, infection, neurovascular impairment, and significant scarring that compromises function
  - Repetitive burns (e.g., **sunburn**) increase the overall risk of **skin cancers**

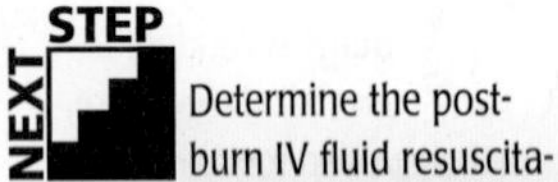

Determine the post-burn IV fluid resuscitation need with the **Parkland formula**: lactated Ringer's solution is given in a total volume of **[(4 mL) × (kg body weight) × (% body surface area burned)]**. Half of the volume is given during the initial 8 hours, and the remaining half is given over the following 16 hours.

- **Clues to the diagnosis:**
  - History: prolonged outdoor exposure, lack of sunscreen use, involvement only on exposed areas
  - Physical: erythema, blistering
  - Tests: nonapplicable
- **Contact dermatitis**
  - An allergic reaction in the skin due to cutaneous contact (e.g., plants, animal dander) with a given allergen
    - A somewhat similar but more diffuse reaction is seen with ingestion of the allergen
    - An allergic reaction occurs through one of two general mechanisms
      - **Type I:** due to mast cell degranulation; light diffuse rash (i.e., **urticaria**) appears shortly after exposure and lasts several hours
      - **Type II:** due to lymphocyte activity; measleslike (i.e., **morbilliform**) rash appears several days after a second exposure to the allergen (most contact dermatitis cases)
  - **History:** pruritus, history of contact or ingestion of an allergen, history of a previous similar reaction
  - **Physical examination:** erythematous rash in a distinct pattern (e.g., lines, shapes) in contact dermatitis, rash in a characteristic location or poorly defined area following ingestion of an allergen (Color Figure 10-1)
  - **Tests:** application testing (i.e., a small amount of the allergen is applied to the skin to elicit a reaction) is useful to identify culprit allergens
  - **Treatment:**
    - Stop use of the offending agent or remove contact with the allergen
    - Mild cases may be treated with topical corticosteroids and antihistamines
    - Oral corticosteroids may be required in severe case
  - **Outcomes:** an inability to identify the causative allergen may lead to repeat exposures; secondary bacterial infection is an uncommon complication
  - **Why eliminated from differential:** the diffuse nature of the erythema without a pattern makes this diagnosis less likely

QUICK HIT STEP-UP: Common causes of allergic contact dermatitis include plants (e.g., poison ivy, poison oak, etc.), nickel, soaps, and **latex**.

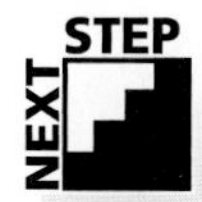

NEXT STEP: Use the pattern of a rash to distinguish an **external** cause (**defined** shape) from an **internal** cause (**nondefined** distribution) of the rash.

- **Cellulitis**
  - Acute skin infection most commonly due to ***Staphylococcus aureus*** or **group A streptococcus**
    - **Methicillin-resistant *S. aureus*** (MRSA) has evolved as a cause of cellulitis that is difficult to treat because of antibiotic resistance
  - **Risk factors: IV drug use**, **DM**, immunocompromise, skin penetration, previous cellulitis, vascular or lymphatic dysfunction
  - **History:** pain at the site of involvement, myalgias, chills
  - **Physical examination:** erythema, swollen skin, lymphadenopathy (Color Figure 10-2)
  - **Tests:** increased serum white blood cells (WBC), C-reactive protein (CRP), and erythrocyte sedimentation rate (ESR); occasionally magnetic resonance imaging (MRI) or ultrasound (US) may be used to rule out deeper infection
  - **Treatment:**
    - Oral cephalosporins or penicillinase-resistant β-lactam for 10 to 14 days in mild cases
    - IV antibiotics are required for more severe cases or for bacteremia
    - Diabetic patients should receive broad coverage because of the increased risk of multiorganism infections
    - Patients with MRSA will require treatment with vancomycin, TMP-SMX, doxycycline, or linezolid
  - **Outcomes:**
    - Complications include the extension of the infection into joint spaces, fascia, muscle, or other deeper tissues
    - Abscess formation may result in severe infections
    - Recurrent cases may result in lymphedema
    - Prognosis is usually very good when the appropriate antibiotic therapy is utilized
  - **Why eliminated from differential:** although this diagnosis should be considered, the limitation of the findings to the exposed areas makes sunburn more likely; a lack of improving findings within days should lead to a full cellulitis work-up

QUICK HIT STEP-UP: Although MRSA was initially limited to nosocomial transmission, the rates of **community-acquired MRSA** have increased significantly in recent years.

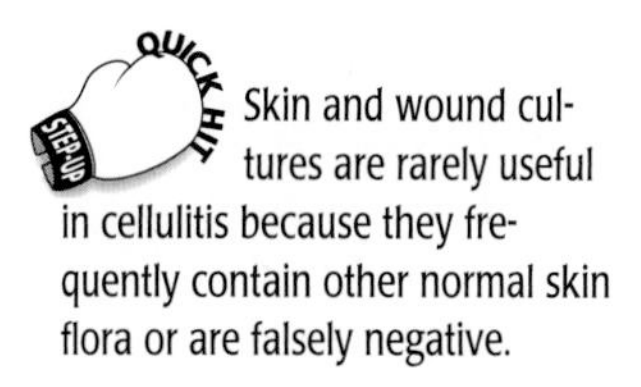

QUICK HIT STEP-UP: Skin and wound cultures are rarely useful in cellulitis because they frequently contain other normal skin flora or are falsely negative.

- **Atopic dermatitis (a.k.a. eczema)**
  - A chronic inflammatory skin rash characterized by **dry skin patches** with papules
    - Both **infantile** (resolves in the initial few years of life) and **adult** (recurrent history) forms exist
  - **Risk factors: asthma**, allergic rhinitis, family history
  - **History**: pruritus, recurrent lesions in adults
  - **Physical examination:** erythematous patches of dry skin with possible blisters on the flexor surfaces, dorsal hands and feet, chest, back, or face (face and scalp more common in infants) (Color Figure 10-3)
  - **Tests:** typically not needed to make the diagnosis
  - **Treatment:**
    - Avoidance of precipitating factors
    - Use of moisturizing creams, emollients, or topical corticosteroids or tacrolimus may help to improve the lesions
    - Severe cases may be treated with oral corticosteroids and antihistamines
  - **Outcomes:** prognosis is generally good, although a small portion of patients will develop asthma or allergic rhinitis
  - **Why eliminated from differential:** the absence of dry skin in this patient makes this diagnosis unlikely
- **Porphyria cutanea tarda**
  - A disease resulting from a deficiency of hepatic uroporphyrinogen decarboxylase, an enzyme involved in heme metabolism
    - Exposure to a hepatotoxic substance (e.g., alcohol, tobacco) or history of a hepatic disease (e.g., viral hepatitis, HIV, hemochromatosis, Wilson's disease) results in the excessive production of sun-sensitive porphyrins
  - **Risk factors: alcohol use**, hepatitis C, iron overload, estrogen use, tobacco use
  - **History**: blistering on sun-exposed areas
  - **Physical examination:** blistering and erosions on chronic sun-exposed areas, hypopigmented scars, hyperpigmented patches of skin, dark urine
  - **Tests:** decreased serum uroporphyrinogen decarboxylase; increased porphyrins in the serum, urine, and feces
  - **Treatment:**
    - Avoidance of excessive sunlight exposure helps to prevent the lesions
    - Chloroquine is used to bind porphyrins and improve their excretion
    - Periodic phlebotomy is performed to decrease the body's excessive iron stores and reduce the excess porphyrins
  - **Outcomes:** chronic excessive iron stores from porphyrin accumulation increases the risk of cirrhosis and hepatocellular carcinoma
  - **Why eliminated from differential:** since blistering does not appear to be a consistent occurrence in this patient with sun exposure, this diagnosis is unlikely
- **Systemic lupus erythematosus**
  - More thorough discussion in Chapter 9
  - **Why eliminated from differential:** the absence of any other significant symptoms makes this diagnosis unlikely

CASE 10-2 "My child has sores around his mouth"

A 5-year-old boy is brought to his pediatrician by his mother with a 2-day history of blistering around the mouth. The patient's mother says that she noticed a single tiny blister near his lips 2 days ago, but now there are multiple small blisters around his mouth and nostrils. Several of the blisters have broken and have become encrusted. She has not noticed any other lesions elsewhere on his face or on his body. She says that he has never had these lesions previously. She says that her son has been complaining about his mouth hurting and itching and has been rubbing his lips. He has not complained of any congestion, ear or throat pain, or cough. She has not noticed any shortness of breath or abnormal activities besides the lip rubbing. The child has not consumed any new foods recently or used any new personal hygiene products. She adds that he is in kindergarten, and when she talked to another student's mother the day prior to presentation, the other parent reported that her daughter had a similar finding. The patient is an only child. He has no past medical history. The family history is significant for adult-onset hypertension, hypercholesterolemia, breast cancer, and cervical cancer. The patient takes children's vitamins and has no known allergies. He is up to date on his vaccinations. On examination, the patient is a well-appearing boy in no distress. He has multiple yellow-crusted lesions around his lips and nostrils. A few small (1 to 2 mm) pustules are also near his lips. There are no scars, telangiectasias, or dry skin patches. No lesions are found on his forehead, around his eyes, across his nose, on his cheeks, or on his neck. Examination of his eyes detects white sclera, pink conjunctiva, and no exudates. Examination of his ears detects translucent tympanic membranes with normal motion to air. Examination of his oropharynx detects no inflammation or exudates. He has mild cervical lymphadenopathy bilaterally. Auscultation of his heart and lungs finds clear breath sounds, normal heart sounds, and no extra sounds. Examination of his torso and extremities does not detect any abnormal lesions. The following vital signs are measured:

T: 98.7°F, HR: 90 bpm, BP: 110/70 mm Hg, RR: 16 breaths/min

Differential Diagnosis

- Acne vulgaris, impetigo, herpes simplex, varicella, atopic dermatitis, cutaneous fungal infection, scabies, molluscum contagiosum, pemphigus vulgaris, seborrheic dermatitis, Stevens-Johnson syndrome

Laboratory Data and Other Study Results

- Complete blood cell count (CBC): white blood cells (WBC): 12.2, hemoglobin (Hgb): 14.1, platelets (Plt): 234
- Urinalysis (UA): straw colored, pH: 6.9, specific gravity: 1.010, no nitrates/leukocyte esterase/glucose/ketones/hematuria/proteinuria
- Gram stain and culture of pustule contents: Gram-positive cocci in clusters, culture pending
- Tzanck smear of lesions: no multinucleated giant cells
- Potassium hydroxide (KOH) preparation of lesions: no hyphae or pseudohyphae
- Hematoxylin and eosin microscopy: small collections of purulent and necrotic material in the stratum corneum of the epidermis; many neutrophils; occasional collections of cocci in clusters

Diagnosis

- Impetigo

Treatment Administered

- The patient was prescribed dicloxacillin for 10 days
- The patient's mother was instructed to wash her child's face with a chlorhexidine antimicrobial solution daily until the lesions appeared to be nearly resolved
- The child was kept home from school during his treatment

Follow-up

- Culture results indicated methicillin-sensitive *S. aureus* and multiple potential contaminant bacteria but no evidence of MRSA
- The child's lesions appeared much improved at a 1-week follow-up appointment
- The child's lesions resolved completely in <2 weeks, and he was allowed to return to school

Steps to the Diagnosis

- Impetigo
  - A **highly contagious** skin infection caused by *S. **aureus*** or **group A streptococci**
    - Most common in infants and **school-aged children**
  - **History:** facial pruritus and pain, no symptoms of otitis media or pharyngitis
  - **Physical examination:** erythematous vesicles or pustules around mucosal surfaces that eventually break and become **yellow crusted**, lymphadenopathy (Color Figure 10-4)
  - **Tests:** Gram stain and culture of exudates beneath the yellow crusting or within the pustules may be helpful to identify an organism (although contamination is possible) but is more useful to rule out MRSA as a causative organism
  - **Treatment:**
    - Topical antibiotics may be used for limited cases with only a few pustules
    - Oral antibiotics are indicated for more extensive lesions
    - Lesions should be washed with a antimicrobial soap or solution until they have resolved

> NEXT STEP: Children with impetigo should be held out of school until the lesions have resolved to prevent transmission to other students.

  - **Outcomes:** streptococcal glomerulonephritis and scarring are rare complications; lesions rarely resolve without treatment, but the prognosis is good once treatment is initiated
  - **Clues to the diagnosis:**
    - History: evolution of lesions from a few pustules to yellow-crusted lesions, evidence of other children at school with similar findings, facial itching
    - Physical: yellow-crusted lesions and small pustules around the mouth and nose, lymphadenopathy
    - Tests: evidence of Gram-positive bacteria on microscopy
- Acne vulgaris
  - Inflammation of hair follicles and sebaceous glands associated with ***Propionibacterium acne*** infection
  - **Risk factors:** adolescence, androgens (use or elevated levels), obstruction of skin pores (e.g., exfoliated skin, cosmetic products, personal care products)
  - **History:** possible pain at the site of lesions
  - **Physical examination:** erythematous pustules or cystic lesions on the face, neck, chest, or back (Color Figure 10-5)

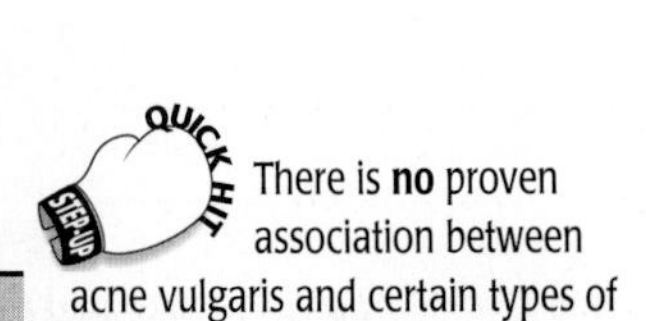

> QUICK HIT: There is **no** proven association between acne vulgaris and certain types of food.

  - **Tests:** typically a clinical diagnosis; outbreaks in adult patients may warrant a workup for androgen excess
  - **Treatment:**
    - **Topical retinoids** decrease sebaceous gland activity and are the recommended first-line treatment
    - Oral or topical antibiotics may inhibit bacterial growth

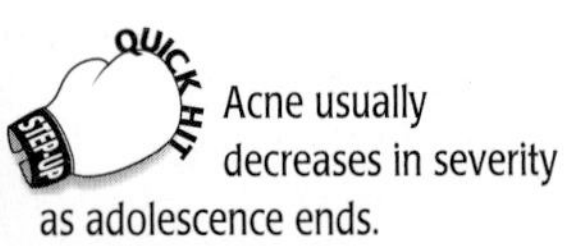

> QUICK HIT: Acne usually decreases in severity as adolescence ends. **Corticosteroid use** and **androgen** production disorders are common causes of outbreaks in **adulthood**.

    - Benzoyl peroxide helps prevent follicular obstruction by decreasing skin oiliness (second-line therapy)
    - Oral contraceptives may be useful in women with excess androgen production to help in hormone regulation
    - Oral **isotretinoin** may be prescribed for severe cases but requires close monitoring of liver enzymes and **mandatory pharmacologic contraception** (high teratogenic risks)

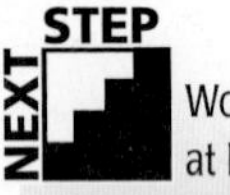

> NEXT STEP: Women should have at least two **negative urine pregnancy tests** before being prescribed oral isotretinoin.

  - **Outcomes:** prognosis is generally excellent, and most cases resolve by the end of adolescence; scarring may result from severe cases of cystic acne
  - **Why eliminated from differential:** the age of the patient and the limit of the lesions to only the mouth and nose make this diagnosis unlikely
- Herpes simplex
  - A recurrent viral infection of **mucocutaneous** surfaces caused by herpes simplex virus 1 or 2 (HSV-1, HSV-2)
    - Transmitted through contact with **oral** or **genital** fluids
    - HSV-1 causes primarily **oral** disease; HSV-2 causes primarily **genital** disease
    - Following primary infection, viral genetic material remains dormant in the sensory ganglia but becomes reactivated during periods of stress

- **History:** painful vesicles around the mouth or genitals lasting several days, possible dysphagia and odynophagia with esophageal involvement
- **Physical examination:** small vesicles around mucosal surfaces, possible vision deficits if lesions are periocular (Color Figure 10-6)
- **Tests: Tzanck smear** of the lesions will show multinucleated giant cells; viral culture may be used to confirm the diagnosis
- **Treatment:**
  - The condition is essentially incurable, so therapy is directed toward minimizing the severity and frequency of flare-ups
  - Acyclovir, famciclovir, or valacyclovir shorten the duration and frequency of recurrences
  - Sexual partners should use barrier contraception consistently and should avoid sexual contact during exacerbations to avoid transmission
- **Outcomes:** herpes meningitis, ocular infection, and bacterial infection of sores are uncommon complications; **maternal transmission** to a neonate during delivery can result in severe central nervous system infection in the child
- **Why eliminated from differential:** the negative Tzanck smear and the yellow-crusted appearance of the lesions rule out this diagnosis

QUICK HIT: The primary demonstration of herpes simplex infection is typically more severe than subsequent flares.

- Varicella
  - Infection by varicella zoster virus (a.k.a. herpes zoster) that may present as a primary disease (i.e., **chickenpox**) or recurrent presentation (i.e., **shingles**) (Table 10-2)
  - **History:** an eruption of vesicles that differ between the primary and recurrent forms
  - **Physical examination:** numerous small vesicles in a wide distribution (i.e., chickenpox) or limited to a single dermatome (i.e., shingles) (Color Figure 10-7)
  - **Tests:** typically a clinical diagnosis; Tzanck smear may show giant cells
  - **Treatment:** supportive care; acyclovir may be used to shorten the course of the disease or prevent worsening in immunocompromised patients

TABLE 10-2 Characteristics of Primary (Chickenpox) and Recurrent (Shingles) Varicella

Varicella Condition	Chickenpox (primary)	Shingles (recurrent)
Patients affected	More common in **children**	Patient with a prior history of varicella zoster infection
Timing of presentation	Symptoms 2 or more weeks after infection occurs; symptoms of headache, malaise, myalgias, and fever precede the development of lesions by <3 days	Myalgias, fever, and malaise preceding lesions by approximately 3 days
Type of lesion	Small red macules that evolve into papules and then vesicles that eventually become crusted	Small red macules that evolve into papules and then vesicles that eventually become crusted
Distribution of lesions	**Wide** distribution	Limited to a single or few distinct **dermatomes**; involvement of multiple dermatomes indicates **disseminated** disease
Course of disease	Lesions may develop for up to 1 week and resolve a few days after appearing; infective until lesions crust over	Lesions exist for a week and may be **painful**; infective until lesions crust over
Treatment	Antipruritics aid symptoms; acyclovir used in severe cases or in immunocompromised patients; **vaccination** has reduced disease incidence significantly	Analgesics and possible corticosteroids; acyclovir is used in immunocompromised patients and with trigeminal nerve distribution
Complications	More severe course in older and pregnant patients (increased risk of varicella pneumonia); may have severe consequences if passed from **infected mother to unborn fetus**	Postinfectious neuralgia (i.e., long-lasting pain at site of eruption), trigeminal neuropathy

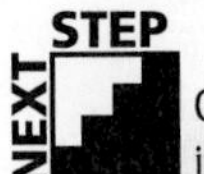

Check the varicella immunity status (i.e., prior vaccination or disease history) in all **pregnant** women; **varicella immune globulin** should be given to all nonimmune pregnant women who contract the disease.

Immunocompromised patients are at an increased risk for developing **encephalopathy** or **retinitis** as complications from varicella infection.

- **Outcomes:** the prognosis is good in most primary cases; refer to Table 10-2 for more potential complications
- **Why eliminated from differential:** the limited distribution of the lesions is not consistent with primary disease, and shingles in a vaccinated child is highly unlikely

- **Atopic dermatitis**
  - More thorough discussion in prior case
  - **Why eliminated from differential:** although the appearance of the lesions for atopic dermatitis and impetigo may be similar, the presence of lymphadenopathy is more indicative of an infectious process in this case
- **Cutaneous fungal infection**
  - More thorough discussion in Table 10-3 (Color Figure 10-8)
  - **Why eliminated from differential:** the negative KOH preparation makes this diagnosis less likely
- **Scabies**
  - Cutaneous infestation by the *Sarcoptes scabiei* mite
  - **Risk factors: crowded living conditions**, poor hygiene
  - **History:** severe pruritus at the site of involvement, pruritus worsens after soaking in hot water
  - **Physical examination:** visible **mite burrows**, papular rash around burrows (Color Figure 10-9)
  - **Tests:** microscopic examination of skin scraping may detect mites and eggs
  - **Treatment:**
    - Permethrin cream or oral ivermectin is used to kill the existing mites
    - Diphenhydramine is useful to control itching
    - All clothing, towels, and linens used by the patient must be washed in hot water
  - **Outcomes: infection of close contacts** is common; prognosis is excellent with the proper treatment and cleansing
  - **Why eliminated from differential:** the absence of mite burrows on inspection and mites on microscopy rule out this diagnosis
- **Molluscum contagiosum**
  - A viral skin infection most frequently seen in children and in patients with immunodeficiencies
  - **History:** painless papules
  - **Physical examination: shiny papules** with a **central umbilication**
  - **Tests:** Giemsa and Wright stains will help demonstrate large inclusion bodies on histology of the lesions
  - **Treatment:** frequently self-limited; chemical, laser, or cryotherapy may be considered for removal

Lesions of molluscum contagiosum are found on the face, torso, and extremities in children and in the **perineal** region in adults.

DERMATOLOGY

TABLE 10-3 Common Cutaneous Fungal Infections

Condition	Fungus	Lesions	Diagnosis	Treatment
Tinea versicolor	*Malassezia furfur*	Small scaly macules most frequently on chest and back	KOH prep shows short hyphae, Wood's lamp examination shows extent of disease	Topical antifungal agent for several weeks or oral ketoconazole for 1–5 days
Tinea not due to *M. furfur* Described by location: corporis (body), cruris (groin), pedis (feet), unguium (nail beds), capitis (scalp)	*Microsporum, Trichophyton, Epidermophyton*	Pruritic, erythematous, scaly plaques with central clearing	KOH prep shows hyphae	Topical antifungal agent for multiple weeks Oral antifungal agent for resistant cases
Intertrigo	*Candida albicans*	Pruritic, painful, erythematous plaques with pustules most commonly in skin creases	KOH prep shows pseudohyphae	Topical antifungal agent Topical corticosteroid

KOH, potassium hydroxide.

- **Outcomes:** prognosis is excellent
- **Why eliminated from differential:** yellow crusting and pustule formation are not typically seen in this diagnosis

- **Pemphigus vulgaris**
  - More thorough discussion in later case
  - **Why eliminated from differential:** the age of the patient and limited extent of the lesions are not typical for this diagnosis
- **Seborrheic dermatitis**
  - Chronic hyperproliferation of the epidermis most commonly on the **scalp** or face
    - Most common in infants and adolescents
  - **History:** pruritus at the site of involvement
  - **Physical examination:** erythematous plaques with **greasy, yellow scales**
  - **Tests:** the diagnosis is typically clinical
  - **Treatment:** shampoo containing selenium, tar, or ketoconazole may be used on the scalp; topical corticosteroids or antifungals may be used on other regions of the body
  - **Outcomes:** recurrences are common
  - **Why eliminated from differential:** although the lesions for this diagnosis and impetigo may appear somewhat similar, the location of the lesions in this case would be unusual for this diagnosis
- **Stevens-Johnson syndrome**
  - More thorough discussion in later case
  - **Why eliminated from differential:** the limited extent of the lesions and the absence of systemic symptoms make this diagnosis unlikely

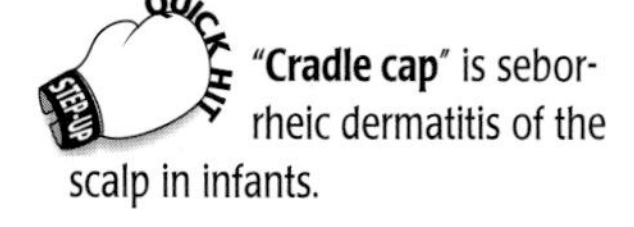

"Cradle cap" is seborrheic dermatitis of the scalp in infants.

CASE 10-3 "My arm is turning black"

A 57-year-old man presents to an emergency department with the complaint that his left arm is swollen and turning a darker color. The patient says that he has chronic sores on his arms and in his left axilla. He says that he scratches his left armpit often because it itches and occasionally has scratched open the lesions located there. He says that while he was fishing on the river bank 2 days ago he slipped and fell into the water. He has not bathed since this event. He feels that his axilla looked worse than normal when he awoke today, and his left arm has become progressively swollen over the course of the morning. He says that the upper arm has become erythematous over the past few hours and that it feels "funny." He has not noticed any drainage from his axilla. At the same time he has begun to feel fatigued and generally not well. He has had chills for part of today. It is painful to move his left shoulder because of the swelling. He states that his symptoms have never been this bad previously. He describes a past medical history of diabetes mellitus and hypertension (HTN). He has not taken any medications for several months but says that he was prescribed a few drugs for his "heart and blood sugar." He denies any allergies. He is homeless and generally lives outdoors. He drinks alcohol on multiple days per week but denies tobacco or other substance use. On examination, he is an unkempt man in mild distress. Both of his arms are notable for a few 2-mm sores that are in various states of healing. His left arm is quite swollen from the axilla to the elbow. It is warm to the touch, and palpation elicits a subtle popping sensation under the skin near the axilla. He has several 1-cm palpable masses in the axilla. When his shoulder is abducted to better visualize the undersurface, purulent material begins to drain from a small wound in his armpit. His skin is a dark red proximally and fades to a light red by the elbow, and multiple small blisters are notable proximally. His right arm appears normal other than the aforementioned small sores. Auscultation of his lungs and heart find clear lung and heart sounds and no abnormal sounds. He has full strength in both arms, although movement of his left shoulder is painful. Sensory testing reveals a subjective decrease in upper arm light touch sensitivity compared to the right. The following vital signs are measured:

T: 102.5°F, HR: 105 bpm, BP: 108/75 mm Hg, RR: 20 breaths/min

Differential Diagnosis

- Necrotizing fasciitis, gangrene, cellulitis, skin abscess, hidradenitis suppurativa

Laboratory Data and Other Study Results

- CBC: WBC: 27.1, Hgb: 12.4, Plt: 319
- 7-electrolyte chemical panel (Chem7): sodium (Na): 145 mEq/L, potassium (K): 4.1 mEq/L, chloride (Cl): 100 mEq/L, carbon dioxide (CO_2): 24 mEq/L, blood urea nitrogen (BUN): 15 mg/dL, creatinine (Cr): 0.9 mg/dL, glucose (Glu): 302 mg/dL
- Coagulation panel (Coags): protime (PT): 12.1, international normalized ratio (INR): 1.0, partial thromboplastin time (PTT): 31.1
- ESR: 24 mm/h
- CRP: 12.4 mg/dL
- Shoulder x-ray: no fracture or dislocation; significant soft tissue swelling in the axilla and visible upper arm; subcutaneous air in the axilla tracking down to the mid-portion of the upper arm

Diagnosis

- Necrotizing fasciitis

Treatment Administered

- The patient was taken emergently to the operating room where an extensive irrigation and debridement of the left upper arm was performed (significant purulent material was found along the fascial planes of the medial upper arm)
- Operative Gram stain and culture of diseased tissue was performed
- The patient's wound was packed following debridement and bandaged without primary closure
- IV vancomycin was started until culture results were reported
- The patient was placed on an insulin regimen to better control his blood glucose levels

Follow-up

- The patient was returned to the operating room every 2 days for additional irrigation and debridement procedures
- Partial closure was achieved after the third irrigation and debridement, and the remainder of the wound was covered with a skin graft
- Cultures indicated an infection by MRSA, and vancomycin was continued
- Successful control of the patient's glucose was achieved, and he was transitioned to oral medication
- The patient was discharged to a skilled nursing facility to continue his wound management and IV antibiotics

Steps to the Diagnosis

- Necrotizing fasciitis
  - A **quick-spreading** infection of the **fascial planes** of an extremity, leading to extensive soft tissue destruction and systemic infection
    - ***S. aureus*** and **group A streptococci** are the most common causative organisms
  - **History**: significant pain at the site of involvement that evolves into numbness; history of a recent surgery or wound
  - **Physical examination**: significant **spreading erythema**, warm and swollen skin, decreased sensation near the affected area, fever, **subcutaneous crepitus**, **vesicles** or **bullae** around the affected region, purulent drainage

- **Tests:**
  - Increased WBC, ESR, and CRP
  - Intraoperative cultures are important for determining the causative organism
  - Subcutaneous collections of air are seen on x-ray or computed tomography (CT)
- **Treatment:**
  - **Emergent surgical debridement** is required; amputation is a frequent definitive procedure
  - Multiple repeat surgeries are frequently required to eliminate all necrotic material; skin grafts or tissue flaps may be needed to achieve adequate wound coverage
  - IV antibiotics are used to treat any extended or systemic infection
- **Outcomes:** complications include renal failure, sepsis and septic shock, and scarring; **acute mortality is 70%**
- **Clues to the diagnosis:**
  - History: rapidly evolving arm swelling and erythema, chronic sores with an acute exposure to river water
  - Physical: significant erythema, arm swelling, subcutaneous crepitus, purulent drainage
  - Tests: increased WBC, ESR, and CRP, intraoperative cultures

- Gangrene
  - Tissue necrosis due to a **poor vascular supply** or severe infection
    - May be classified as either **wet** or **dry**, depending on the appearance
    - ***Clostridium*** is the bacteria most commonly implicated in cases due to infection
  - **History**: prior skin infection or wound, severe skin pain
  - **Physical examination**: fever, hypotension, subcutaneous crepitus, **rotten-smelling skin**
  - **Tests:**
    - Ankle-brachial indices will demonstrate asymmetry between the limbs
    - WBC, ESR, and CRP are elevated in infectious cases
    - Culture is useful to identify a pathogen in cases due to infection
    - Subcutaneous collections of air are seen on x-ray or CT in cases due to infection
    - Angiography or magnetic resonance angiography (MRA) is used to demonstrate vascular insufficiency
  - **Treatment**: debridement and antibiotic therapy are required; **amputations** are frequently indicated for nonviable extremities
  - **Outcomes:**
    - Prompt treatment carries the best chance for limb salvage
    - The need for distal amputations in vascular disease is usually a harbinger for the eventual need of additional, more proximal amputations
    - Cases due to infections can result in systemic involvement
  - **Why eliminated from differential**: although this diagnosis and necrotizing fasciitis may appear very similar, the rapid onset of symptoms and limb compromise in this case is more consistent with the process of necrotizing fasciitis

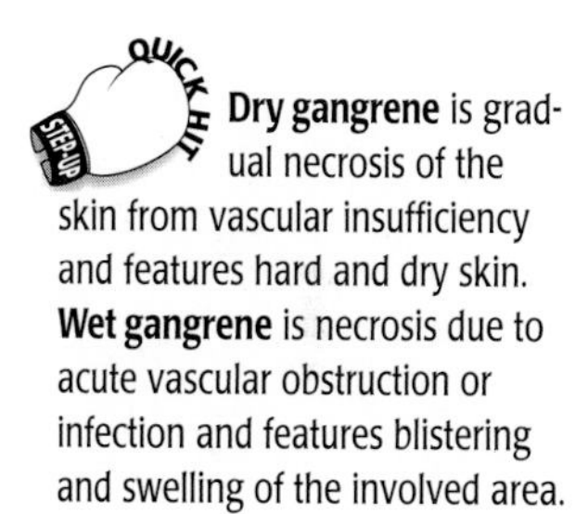

Dry gangrene is gradual necrosis of the skin from vascular insufficiency and features hard and dry skin. **Wet gangrene** is necrosis due to acute vascular obstruction or infection and features blistering and swelling of the involved area.

- Cellulitis
  - More thorough discussion in prior case
  - **Why eliminated from differential**: the extensive involvement of the upper arm, obvious collections of purulent material, and rapid evolution are suggestive of a process much more severe than cellulitis
- Skin abscess
  - A subcutaneous collection of pus most commonly due to staphylococcal bacteria
    - May occur as a collection of multiple infected hair follicles (i.e., carbuncle)
  - **History**: painful region of focal cutaneous swelling
  - **Physical examination**: erythema, **fluctuant subcutaneous mass**, tenderness to palpation
  - **Tests**: possibly increased WBC, ESR, and CRP; cultures of abscess contents can determine the pathogen but carry high false-positive rates if not performed under sterile conditions
  - **Treatment: irrigation and debridement** with healing by secondary intention; antibiotic therapy (oral or IV depending on the extent of the abscess)

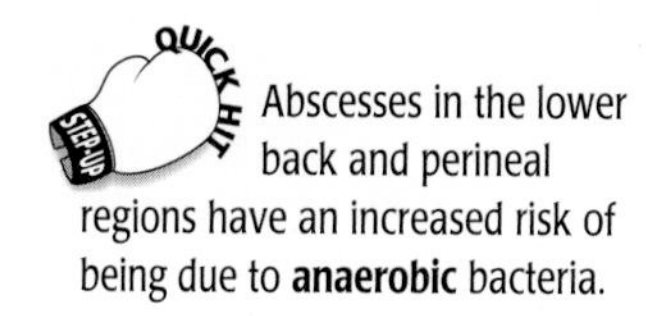

Abscesses in the lower back and perineal regions have an increased risk of being due to **anaerobic** bacteria.

- **Outcomes:** the prognosis is good if treated in a timely fashion; large abscesses may erode into adjacent areas (e.g., joint spaces, fascial planes), leading to worsening infection that requires additional treatment
- **Why eliminated from differential:** the rapidly evolving nature of this case is suggestive of a more advanced infection

- **Hidradenitis suppurativa**
  - A condition of chronic follicular occlusion and **apocrine gland** inflammation, resulting in recurrent abscesses in the axilla, groin, and perineum
  - **History:** pruritus at the site of involvement, recurrent abscesses in the above-mentioned regions
  - **Physical examination:** multiple fluctuant subcutaneous masses, tenderness to palpation, evidence of significant scarring from earlier abscesses, skin tethering
  - **Tests:** culture of abscess material may be useful for identifying a pathogen; CT is useful to determine the extent of the disease prior to surgery
  - **Treatment:**
    - Antibiotics should be given for any abscess formation
    - Corticosteroid injections into nonpurulent collections may help them to resolve before becoming infected
    - Irrigation and debridement of abscesses, excision of sinus tracts, and extensive resection are all surgical options, depending on the extent of the disease
  - **Outcomes:** fistula formation, chronic infection, and significant soft tissue fibrosis are potential complications; recurrences are extremely common without some type of wide resection of the involved area
  - **Why eliminated from differential:** this diagnosis is a chronic condition, while the presentation in the case is an acute, rapidly worsening process

The following additional Dermatology cases may be found online:

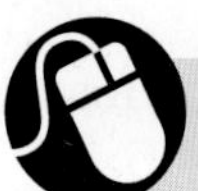

CASE 10-4 "My skin is falling off!"

CASE 10-5 "My arms and legs are scaly"

CASE10-6 "The mole on my back is growing"

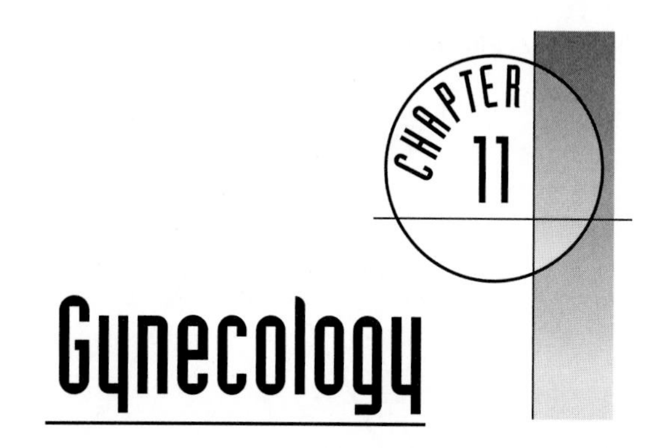

Gynecology

BASIC CLINICAL PRIMER

MENSTRUAL PHYSIOLOGY

- **Gynecologic development**
  - Follicle-stimulating hormone (FSH), luteinizing hormone (LH), and estrogens are the key hormones that drive reproductive development (Figure 11-1, Table 11-1)
  - Androgens also play a role in the development of secondary sexual characteristics
  - The Tanner stages are used to describe the development of the genitalia, breasts, and pubic hair growth in growing children (Table 11-2)
- **Normal menstrual cycle**
  - The primary hormones involved in the menstrual cycle are LH, FSH, estrogen, progesterone, and human chorionic gonadotropin (hCG) (Figure 11-2, Table 11-3)
  - **Follicular phase**
    - Begins at the first day of menstruation (i.e., menses)
    - **FSH** stimulates the growth of the **ovarian follicle**
    - **Granulosa** cells of the ovarian follicle secrete **estradiol**
    - Estradiol induces **endometrial proliferation** and further increases FSH and LH secretion due to positive feedback of the pituitary
  - **Luteal phase**
    - A sudden rise in LH (i.e., LH surge) induces **ovulation**
    - The residual follicle (i.e., **corpus luteum**) secretes estradiol and **progesterone** to maintain the **endometrium** and to induce the development of secretory ducts
    - High estradiol levels inhibit FSH and LH secretion
    - If the ovum is **not** fertilized, the corpus luteum degrades, progesterone and estradiol levels decrease, and the **endometrial lining degrades** (i.e., menses)
  - **Fertilization**
    - If the ovum is fertilized, it will implant in the endometrium
    - The endometrial tissue secretes **hCG** to **maintain the corpus luteum**
    - The corpus luteum continues to secrete progesterone until a sufficient production is achieved by the developing **placenta** (approximately 8 to 12 weeks)

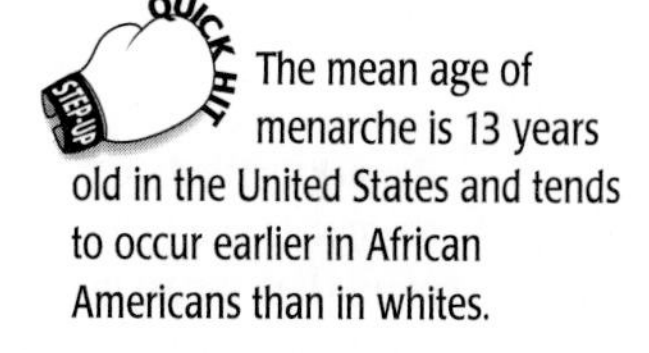

The mean age of menarche is 13 years old in the United States and tends to occur earlier in African Americans than in whites.

CONTRACEPTION

- Behaviors, medicines, instruments, or procedures designed to prevent pregnancy from occurring (Table 11-4)
- **Method activity**
  - Methods may alter menstrual physiology (e.g., preventing ovulation), prevent fertilization (e.g., barrier contraception), or prevent implantation and development of the fertilized ovum (e.g., some intrauterine devices)

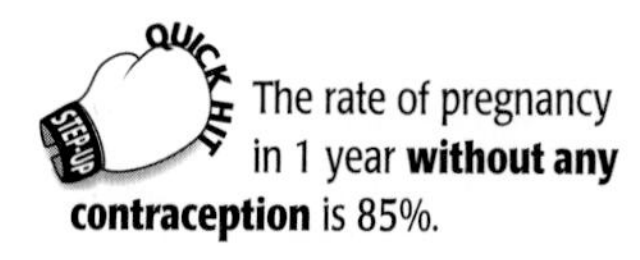

The rate of pregnancy in 1 year **without any contraception** is 85%.

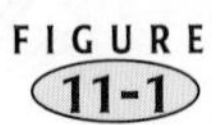

FIGURE 11-1 Changes in hormone and oogonia (egg) levels with gestation and age. DHEA, dehydroepiandrosterone; FSH, follicle-stimulating hormone; hCG, human chorionic gonadotropin; LH, luteinizing hormone.

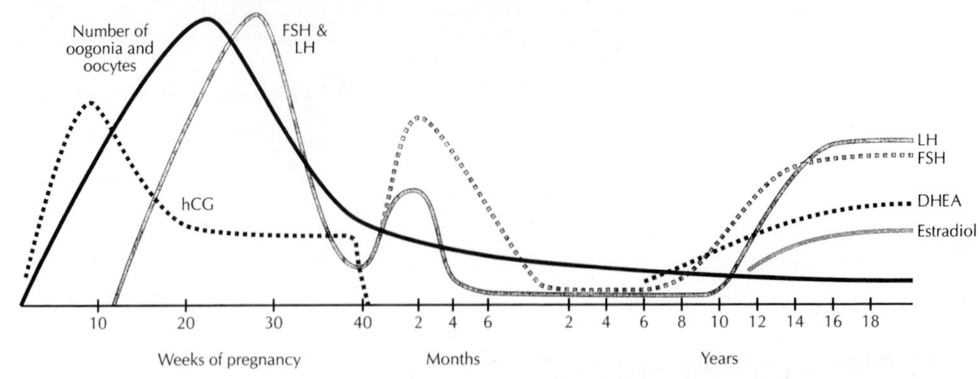

(Taken from Speroff L, Glass RH, Kase NG. *Clinical gynecologic endocrinology and infertility.* 7th ed. Baltimore: Williams & Wilkins, 1991. Used with permission of Williams & Wilkins.)

QUICK HIT: **Barrier methods** (not spermicide alone) are the only contraception shown to reduce the spread of sexually transmitted diseases.

- Method selection
  - The physician and patient must consider the likelihood of compliance; patients who are more at risk for noncompliance should use a method requiring less responsibility (e.g, progestin implants or injections)
  - The patient must be able to tolerate certain side effects (e.g., possible nausea or headaches with OCPs)
  - Some medical conditions may be contraindications for certain methods (e.g., DVT and OCP use)
  - Some sexual behaviors or the risk of transmission of sexually transmitted diseases may affect selection (e.g., barrier methods to reduce STD risk)

TABLE 11-1 Gynecologic Development by Age

Age	Hormone Levels	Characteristics
Fetal–4 yr old	• High intrauterine FSH and LH that peak at 20 weeks gestation and decrease until birth • FSH and LH increase again from birth until 6 months of age and then gradually decrease to low levels by 4 years old	• All oocytes are formed and partially matured by 20 weeks gestation • Tanner stage 1 characteristics
4–8 yr old	• Low FSH, LH, and androgen levels due to GnRH suppression	• Tanner stage 1 characteristics • Any sexual development is considered precocious
8–11 yr old	• LH, FSH, and androgen levels begin to increase	• Initial pubertal changes including early breast development and pubic and axillary hair growth
11–17 yr old	• Further increase of LH, FSH, and androgens to mature levels • Hormones secreted in a pulsatile fashion (higher at night) due to a sleep-associated increase in GnRH secretion	• Puberty • Progression through Tanner stages • Development of secondary sexual characteristics and growth spurt • Menarche in females (beginning of menstrual cycles) and further oocyte maturation
17–50 yr old (females)	• LH and FSH levels vary during the menstrual cycle • Gradual increase in FSH and LH as ovarian insensitivity increases	• Menstrual cycles • Mature sexual characteristics
≥ 50 yr old (females)	• LH and FSH levels increase with the onset of ovarian failure	• Perimenopause: menstrual cycles become inconsistent (oligomenorrhea) • Menopause: menstrual cycles cease (amenorrhea)

FSH, follicle stimulating hormone; GnRH, gonadotropin-releasing hormone; LH, luteinizing hormone.

TABLE 11-2 Tanner Stages for Sexual Characteristic Development

	Female		Male	
Tanner Stage	Breast Development	Pubic Hair Development	Penile/Testicular Development	Pubic Hair Development
1	Prepubertal; raised papilla (nipple) only	Prepubertal; no hair growth	Prepubertal; small genitals	Prepubertal; no hair growth
2	Breast budding, areolar enlargement	Slight growth of fine labial hair	Testicular and scrotal enlargement with skin coarsening	Slight growth of fine genital and axillary hair
3	Further breast and areolar enlargement	Further growth of hair	Penile enlargement and further testicular growth	Further growth of hair
4	Further breast enlargement—areola and papilla form a secondary growth above the level of the breast	Hair becomes coarser and spreads over much of the pubic region	Further penile glans enlargement and darkening of scrotal skin	Hair becomes coarser and spreads over much of the pubic region
5	Mature breast—areola recedes to the level of the breast while the papilla remains extended	Coarse hair extends from the pubic region to the medial thighs	Adult genitalia	Coarse hair extends from the pubic region to the medial thighs

CASE 11-1 "My daughter is growing up too fast"

A 6-year-old girl is brought to her pediatrician by her mother who is concerned about the patient's early breast development. It has been almost 1 year since the patient's previous pediatric check-up, and the patient was in good health at that time. The patient's mother says that she first noticed breast budding in her daughter 8 months ago while clothes shopping. She assumed it was related to recent rapid growth and did nothing at the time. She

TABLE 11-3 Roles of Hormones Involved in the Menstrual Cycle

Hormone	Effects
Luteinizing hormone (LH)	• Midcycle **surge** induces **ovulation** • Regulates cholesterol conversion to pregnenolone in ovarian theca cells as the initial step in estrogen synthesis
Follicle-stimulating hormone (FSH)	• Stimulates the **development** of the **ovarian follicle** • Regulates ovarian granulosa cell activity to control estrogen synthesis
Estrogens (estradiol, estriol)	• Stimulates **endometrial proliferation** • Aids in follicle growth • Induces the LH surge • High levels inhibit FSH secretion • A **decrease** in levels leads to **menstruation** • Principal role in sexual development
Progesterone	• Stimulates **endometrial gland development** • Inhibits uterine contraction • Increases the thickness of cervical mucus • **Increases basal body temperature** • Inhibits LH and FSH secretion and maintains pregnancy • A **decrease** in levels leads to **menstruation**
Human chorionic gonadotropin (hCG)	• Acts like LH after the implantation of the fertilized egg • **Maintains corpus luteum viability** and progesterone secretion

FIGURE 11-2 **Hormone levels during the menstrual cycle with appropriate ovarian, endometrial, and basal body temperature responses. FSH, follicle-stimulating hormone; LH, luteinizing hormone.**

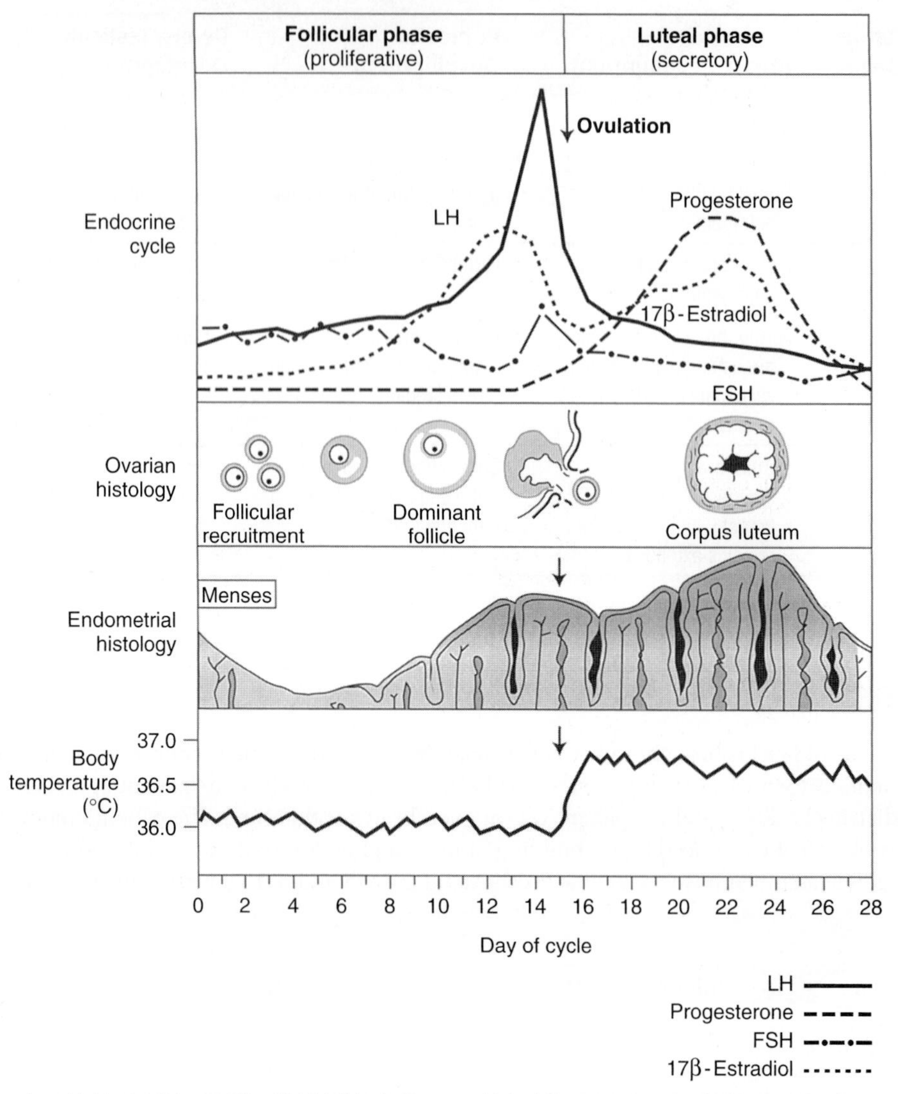

(Taken from Mehta S, Milder EA, Mirachi AJ, Milder E. *Step-up: a high-yield, systems-based review for the USMLE step 1.* 2nd ed. Philadelphia: Lippincott Williams & Wilkins, 2003. Used with permission of Lippincott Williams & Wilkins.)

says that since that time her daughter's breasts have continued to develop and enlarge. There has been no point at which her breasts have decreased in size. The mother denies the presence of any nipple discharge or breast erythema. The mother also says that she began to notice the growth of pubic hair in her daughter after a bath 2 months ago. This hair growth has not receded since the discovery. The patient's mother denies any vaginal bleeding in her daughter. The patient denies any breast or genital pain or headaches. The mother says that she chose to bring her daughter to the pediatrician at this time because the breast and pubic hair growth were continuing to evolve and not reverse. She says that her daughter is a happy child and is doing well in her first grade class. She is active and likes to draw pictures. Her mother denies any physical limitations. She denies any prior medical problems, and her daughter only takes children's vitamins. The patient was the product of a full-term uncomplicated pregnancy and vaginal delivery. The mother denies any medical conditions during her pregnancy and is only aware of hypertension (HTN), hypercholesterolemia, and ischemic heart disease in the family history. Neither parent smokes or uses any illicit substances. On examination, the patient is a happy appearing child in no distress. She is able to participate well in the examination. She appears tall for her age. She has minimal

TABLE 11-4 Methods of Contraception

Method	Description	Effectiveness[1] Ideal (%)	Effectiveness[1] Typical (%)	Side Effects
HORMONAL METHODS				
Oral contraceptive pills (combined formulation)	• Estrogen-progestin combination pills that inhibit follicle development and ovulation, change endometrial quality, and increase cervical mucus viscosity to prevent fertilization and implantation	99	92	• Possible nausea, headache, weight gain • Increased risk of DVT • Contraindicated for heavy smokers, or women with a history of DVT, estrogen-related cancer, liver disease, or hypertriglyceridemia
Oral contraceptive pills (progestin formulation)	• Progestin-only pills that change endometrial quality and increase cervical mucus viscosity to prevent fertilization and implantation • May be option for women with contraindication for estrogen	98	92	• Increased breakthrough bleeding • Less nausea and vomiting than combination pills • Must be taken at same time every day to maximize efficacy
Medroxyprogesterone acetate (e.g., Depo-Provera)	• Progestin analogue injected by health care provider every 3 months that inhibits ovulation and endometrial development	99	97	• Nausea, headache, weight gain • Irregular bleeding
Progestin implant	• Subcutaneous implant that slowly releases progestin over approximately 3 years (similar activity to progestin-only pill)	100[2]	100[2]	• Irregular bleeding, breast pain
Transdermal contraceptive patch	• Transdermal delivery of estradiol and progestin analogue to act in similar manner to OCPs • Patch must be changed weekly	99	92	• Risk of patch detachment • Nausea, headache, weight gain • Irregular bleeding, breast pain • Less effective in heavier women because of diffusion into adipose tissue • Increased risk of DVT
Intravaginal ring	• Ring inserted intravaginally that releases ethinyl estradiol over 3 weeks to prevent ovulation (less estrogen than OCP) • Replaced each month	99	92	• Withdrawal bleeding, device-related discomfort, headache • Increased risk of DVT
Emergency contraception	• Regimen of estradiol and progestin or progestin alone taken within 72 hours of unprotected intercourse or intercourse with failed contraception method (e.g., poor withdrawal, broken condom) to prevent ovulation, inhibit fertilization, or interrupt new pregnancy	—[3]	—[3]	• Nausea, headache more severe than that seen with OCPs • Menstrual bleeding expected within 1 week of administration
BARRIER METHODS				
Condom	• Barrier (most frequently latex) placed over penis and left in place until withdrawal following ejaculation • Frequently used with spermicide • Polyurethane condoms are produced for those with latex allergy	98	85	• Risk of condom breakage • Latex significantly more effective than other materials (with possible exception of polyurethane) • Risk of latex allergy
Diaphragm/ cervical cap	• Barrier inserted into vagina before intercourse to cover cervix • Used with spermicide and left in place for several hours after intercourse	94	84	• Inconvenient • Frequent poor compliance • Increased risk of UTI
Contraceptive sponge	• Polyurethane sponge implanted with spermicide that releases spermicide over 24 hours after insertion to inhibit fertilization	91[4]	80[4]	• Possible increased risk of toxic shock syndrome
Spermicide alone	• Insertion of spermicidal jelly or cream into vagina immediately before intercourse	82	71	• Correct usage and quantity is difficult to achieve consistently

(continued)

TABLE 11-4 Methods of Contraception (*Continued*)

Method	Description	Effectiveness[1] Ideal (%)	Typical (%)	Side Effects
SEXUAL PRACTICE METHODS				
Abstinence	• Not engaging in intercourse	100	100	• None
Rhythm method	• Recording the occurrence of menses, daily basal body temperature, and cervical mucus viscosity to determine the timing of the cycle, the occurrence of ovulation, and the period of fertility	95	83	• May be useful in diagnosing infertility
Withdrawal method	• Withdrawal of penis from vagina immediately before ejaculation	96	73	• Decreased pleasure • Difficult to conduct in an effective manner
Lactation	• Unprotected intercourse during the active postpartum lactation period	98	95	• Only able to be performed if actively breast feeding, <6 months postpartum, and amenorrheic (pregnancy rate equals no contraception rate otherwise)
INTRAUTERINE DEVICES				
Copper intrauterine device	• Object inserted into the uterus by a physician with a slow release of copper to prevent fertilization and interfere with sperm transportation • Left in place approximately 10 years • May be placed soon after intercourse as emergency contraception (90% decrease in pregnancy rate)	99	99	• Small risk of spontaneous abortion and uterine perforation • Menorrhagia
Progestin-releasing IUD	• Object inserted into the uterus by a physician with a slow release of progestin to prevent fertilization, interfere with sperm transportation, and inhibit ovulation • Left in place approximately 5 years	99	99	• Small risk of spontaneous abortion and uterine perforation
SURGICAL METHODS				
Sterilization	• Cutting of the vas deferens in men (vasectomy) or tubal ligation in women to prevent fertilization	~100	~100	• May be difficult to reverse • Increased risk of ectopic pregnancy in cases of failure or after voluntary ligation reversal

DVT, deep venous thrombosis; HTN, hypertension; IUD, intrauterine device; OCPs, oral contraceptive pills; UTI, urinary tract infection.

[1]As defined by pregnancy rate with 1 year of use (6 months for lactation).

[2]Only one efficacy study performed; no pregnancies occurred in study.

[3]Rate of pregnancy decreased 75%–90% with timely use.

[4]Effectiveness decreases to 80% and 60%, respectively, in women with prior vaginal birth history.

acne on her face but not on her trunk. Her ears appear clear. Examination of her eyes finds them equally reactive with no asymmetry. Her oropharynx appears normal. She has no lymphadenopathy. Auscultation of her lungs and heart detects clear and equal breath sounds, a normal heart rate, and no extra heart sounds. Her abdomen is nontender with no masses. Her extremities are symmetric, and her motor and sensory function is normal. She has Tanner stage 3 breast development and Tanner stage 2 pubic hair development. She does not appear to have any signs of vaginal bleeding or clitoromegaly. The following vital signs are measured:

Temperature (T): 98.5°F, heart rate (HR): 85 beats per minute (bpm), blood pressure (BP): 112/78 mm Hg, respiratory rate (RR): 18breaths/min

Differential Diagnosis

- Central precocious puberty, ovarian tumor, congenital adrenal hyperplasia, McCune-Albright syndrome, hypothyroidism

Laboratory Data and Other Study Results

- Height and weight: 54″(>97th percentile), 60 lb (94th percentile)
- Skeletal survey x-ray: ossification of multiple cartilage growth centers prior to what is expected for the patient's age; no closure of growth plates; no fractures of any age; no skeletal lesions
- FSH: 8.1 U/L
- LH: 7 U/L
- Gonadotropin-releasing hormone (GnRH) stimulation test: FSH: 32 U/L, LH: 73 U/L
- Estradiol: 23 pg/mL
- Cortisol (afternoon): 7 μg/dL
- Dehydroepiandrosterone (DHEA): 2.7 ng/mL
- Thyroid-stimulating hormone (TSH): 1.2 μU/mL

After the review of these test results, the additional following studies are ordered:

- Abdominal ultrasound (US): no renal, adrenal, or ovarian mass
- Brain magnetic resonance imaging (MRI): normal ventricular size; normal cerebral volume for age; no areas of ischemia or cerebral masses

Diagnosis

- Idiopathic central precocious puberty

Treatment Administered

- The patient was referred to a pediatric endocrinologist to direct further care
- The patient was placed on histrelin at monthly intervals to decrease her serum FSH and LH levels

Follow-up

- By 2 months after starting histrelin therapy, the patient's FSH and LH had returned to prepubertal levels
- The patient was maintained on monthly histrelin therapy until she was 11 years old, at which time therapy was stopped, and she was allowed to progress through normal puberty

Steps to the Diagnosis

- **Central precocious puberty**
  - Premature development of the sex-appropriate pubertal process in boys or girls (Table 11-5)
    - Due to the premature activation of the hypothalamic-pituitary-gonadal axis
    - The majority of cases are due to idiopathic causes
  - **History**: premature development of sexual characteristics in prepubertal-aged children
  - **Physical examination**: premature breast development, genital enlargement, pubic hair growth, possible mild acne
  - **Tests:**
    - **FSH** and **LH** will be elevated from age-appropriate levels; administration of GnRH (i.e., **GnRH stimulation test**) will cause an **additional** increase in FSH and LH levels

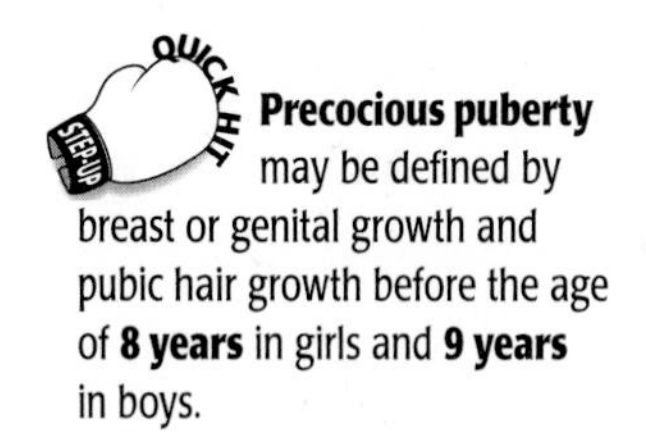

Precocious puberty may be defined by breast or genital growth and pubic hair growth before the age of **8 years** in girls and **9 years** in boys.

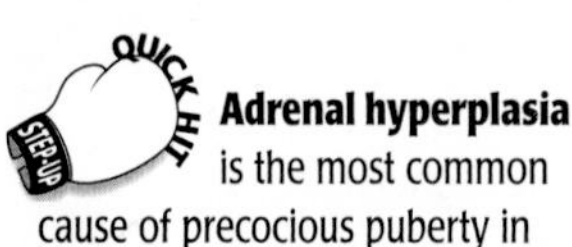

Adrenal hyperplasia is the most common cause of precocious puberty in boys.

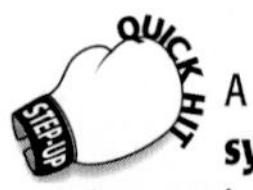

A **central nervous system (CNS) lesion** or **trauma** is the cause of central (isosexual) precocious puberty in approximately 10% of cases.

TABLE 11-5 Classification of Precocious Puberty

Heterosexual	Isosexual	
• Virilization of girls or feminization of boys • In girls most commonly due to CAH, exogenous androgen exposure, or an androgen-secreting neoplasm	• Gender-appropriate premature sexual development	
	Complete	**Incomplete**
	• Normal pubertal changes occur at a premature age for all sexual characteristics	• Isolated premature breast development (i.e., thelarche) or pubic hair growth (i.e., pubarche)

CAH, congenital adrenal hyperplasia.

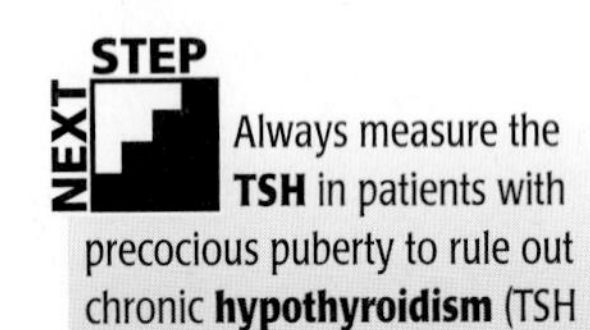

Always measure the **TSH** in patients with precocious puberty to rule out chronic **hypothyroidism** (TSH is increased).

- Low FSH and LH or a poor response to GnRH are more consistent with a direct overproduction of androgens or estrogens (e.g., ovarian neoplasm, congenital adrenal hyperplasia)
- An abdominal US may be used to rule out any adrenal or ovarian tumors
- **Brain MRI** should be performed to determine if a cerebral mass is the cause of the activated hypothalamic-pituitary-gonadal axis
- **Treatment:**
  - **GnRH agonists** (e.g., leuprolide acetate) or **LH-releasing hormone agonists** (e.g., histrelin) are used to decrease FSH and LH levels and prevent further sexual maturation
  - FSH and LH inhibition is stopped at the age of normal pubertal onset to allow sexual maturation to continue
  - Children near the age of the appropriate onset of puberty are frequently allowed to progress through puberty at the slightly early age
- **Outcomes:**
  - Children undergoing puberty inhibition develop normal sexual characteristics once inhibition is stopped
  - Short stature may result if bone maturity has advanced significantly by the time treatment has been initiated
  - Parents and physicians should be aware of the social and emotional adjustment issues in school-aged children that begin premature sexual maturation
- **Clues to the diagnosis:**
  - History: young age, observation of both breast and pubic hair growth, period of rapid growth
  - Physical: Tanner stage 3 breast and Tanner stage 2 pubic hair growth in a 6-year-old child, minimal acne
  - Tests: increased FSH and LH, positive GnRH stimulation test

- **Ovarian tumor**
  - More thorough discussion in later case
  - **Why eliminated from differential:** the negative abdominal US, absence of excessive elevation in the estradiol level, and elevated LH and FSH levels in the presence of a normal estradiol level combine to rule out this diagnosis
- **Congenital adrenal hyperplasia**
  - More thorough discussion in Chapter 5
  - **Why eliminated from differential:** the normal cortisol and DHEA levels and the negative abdominal US make this diagnosis unlikely
- **McCune-Albright syndrome**
  - A syndrome of precocious puberty, multiple sites of fibrous skeletal dysplasia, and multiple café-au-lait lesions of the skin
    - Precocious puberty occurs as a result of excessive gonadal activity in the presence of normal hypothalamic-pituitary function
    - Secondary Cushing syndrome may result from an associated overproduction of cortisol

- **History:** premature breast development, premature menarche in the absence of pubic hair growth
- **Physical examination:** greater height than expected for age, premature labial and clitoral maturation, inconsistent development of pubic hair, multiple café-au-lait spots, possible gross deformity of extremities due to fibrous skeletal dysplasia
- **Tests:**
  - **Increased estradiol and testosterone**; **prepubertal** FSH and LH levels
  - Possible increased alanine aminotransferase (ALT), aspartate aminotransferase (AST), and bilirubin
  - Cortisol is frequently elevated and does not decrease following the administration of either low-dose or high-dose dexamethasone
  - Abdominal US or computed tomography (CT) will detect ovarian cysts and possible adrenal enlargement
  - X-rays will detect multiple skeletal lesions consistent with fibrous dysplasia
- **Treatment:**
  - **Aromatase inhibitors** (e.g., testolactone, fadrozole) or tamoxifen help to prevent the conversion of testosterone into estrogens
  - Lesions of fibrous dysplasia are observed unless fracture occurs (necessitating fixation); bisphosphonates may help to heal lesions more quickly
  - Adrenalectomy is considered in patients with Cushing syndrome due to adrenal enlargement
- **Outcomes:** complications include short stature due to premature growth plate closure, pathologic fractures, failure to thrive, acromegaly, and sudden death; the prognosis depends on the timeliness of the initiation of treatment
- **Why eliminated from differential:** the absence of café-au-lait spots and skeletal lesions and an abnormal cortisol level rule out this diagnosis

- **Hypothyroidism**
  - More thorough discussion in Chapter 5
  - **Why eliminated from differential:** the normal TSH level rules out this diagnosis

CASE 11-2 "I still haven't gotten my period"

An 18-year-old female presents to a gynecologist because she has never undergone menses. She feels that she has never fully grown up. Her parents told her that she "must just be a late-bloomer." She reports that she has never had a single menstrual period or ever developed breasts. She has grown pubic hair. She has had vaginal intercourse as an adolescent without any difficulties. She denies any difficulty eating, abnormal eating behaviors, or any heat or cold intolerance. She says that she looked similar to the other girls in her primary school grades as a younger child. Once she reached high school, she did not grow as much as the other girls and was the shortest girl in her grade. She says that she was a healthy child and is unaware of any medical history. She does not take any medications. Her family history is significant for breast and pancreatic cancer, HTN, coronary artery disease (CAD), hypercholesterolemia, and stroke. She smokes a quarter-pack of cigarettes each day and drinks alcohol on some weekends. On examination, she is a short, well-nourished female in no distress. She has a mild ptosis of both eyes. Gross and fundoscopic examination of her eyes detects normal vasculature and color. Her ear canals and oropharynx appear normal. She has no lymphadenopathy. Her neck is short and broad. Auscultation of her lungs and heart detects clear breath sounds, an extra heart sound between a normal S_1 and S_2, and a faint systolic murmur. Her abdomen is soft and nontender with normal bowel sounds and no masses. Her extremities are symmetric although both of her elbows bow slightly inward. She has Tanner stage 1 breast development and Tanner stage 5 pubic hair development. A manual and speculum vaginal examination detects a perforate narrow vaginal canal and a visible but small cervix without any discharge. She has no vaginal or cervical tenderness. A neurologic examination detects normal motor and sensory function. The following vital signs are measured:

T: 98.4°F, HR: 90 bpm, BP: 132/83 mm Hg, RR: 18 breaths/min

Differential Diagnosis

- Genital tract abnormality, anorexia nervosa, hypothyroidism, sex chromosome abnormality (e.g., Turner syndrome), polycystic ovarian syndrome, pregnancy, congenital adrenal hyperplasia, prolactinoma

Laboratory Data and Other Study Results

- Height and weight: 4′ 11″, 128 lbs, BMI 25.9
- Serum pregnancy test: negative
- TSH: 2.6 μU/mL
- FSH: 75 U/L
- LH: 81 U/L
- Estradiol: 2 pg/mL
- Cortisol (afternoon): 9 μg/dL
- DHEA: 3.5 ng/mL
- Prolactin: 3 ng/mL
- Progestin challenge: no vaginal bleeding in the week following progestin administration

Following receipt of these test results, the following tests are ordered:

- Abdominal US: no renal, adrenal, or ovarian masses
- Karyotype: 45XO
- Y chromosome genetic probe: negative
- Echocardiogram: bicuspid aortic valve with mild stenosis and increased flow velocity; minimal concentric left ventricle hypertrophy; normal left atrial and right-heart chamber size and motion

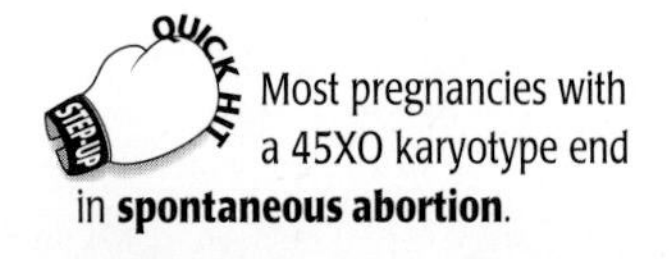

Most pregnancies with a 45XO karyotype end in **spontaneous abortion**.

Diagnosis

- Turner syndrome

MNEMONIC

Causes of amenorrhea may be remembered by the mnemonic **NO CATCHUP**: **N**utrition (e.g., anorexia, malnutrition), **O**varian disease (e.g., failure, cysts), **C**ushing syndrome, **A**natomic abnormalities, **T**hyroid disease, **C**hromosome abnormalities, **H**ypothalamic-pituitary dysfunction, **U**terine disease, **P**regnancy.

Treatment Administered

- The patient was started on estrogen and progesterone replacement therapy
- The patient was referred to a cardiologist to monitor her bicuspid aortic valve and the development of any related cardiac sequelae

Follow-up

- The patient was able to achieve pharmacologic-driven menstrual cycles and developed breasts after the initiation of hormone replacement therapy

MNEMONIC

Causes of short stature may be remembered by the mnemonic **ABCDEFGHIJKL**: **A**buse, **B**ad cancers, **C**hromosomal (Turner), **D**elayed growth (constitutional), **E**ndocrine (growth hormone deficiency, hypothyroidism), **F**amilial short stature, **G**astrointestinal disease (irritable bowel syndrome, celiac), **H**eart (congenital disease), **I**mmune disorders, **J**oint and bone dysplasias, **K**idney failure, **L**ung disease (asthma, cystic fibrosis).

Steps to the Diagnosis

- **Turner syndrome**
  - A sex chromosome abnormality in which patients carry only one full X chromosome in their genome (Table 11-6)
    - The patient's karyotype is 45XO
    - It is an uncommon cause of **primary amenorrhea**, **short stature**, and **infertility** and is typically detected during the work-up for one of these findings (Figure 11-3)
  - **History: primary amenorrhea**, failure to have a pubertal growth spurt, **infertility**
  - **Physical examination: little or no breast development**, **normal pubic hair growth**, **short stature**, possible nail deformities, ptosis, strabismus, low-set ears, broad neck, numerous nevi, cubitus valgus (i.e., lateral angulation of the forearms at the elbow), abnormal heart sounds, or lymphedema

TABLE 11-6 The Most-Common Sex Chromosome Disorders

Condition	Karyotype	H/P
Turner syndrome	45XO or mosaicism	Female with **short stature**, **infertility**, and **primary amenorrhea**; increased incidence of renal and cardiac defects, craniofacial abnormalities, and lymphedema
Klinefelter syndrome	47XXY	Male with **testicular atrophy**, tall and thin body, gynecomastia, infertility, mild mental retardation, and psychosocial adjustment abnormalities
XYY	47XYY	Male with tall body, significant acne, and mild mental retardation
XXX	47XXX	Female with increased incidence of mental retardation and menstrual abnormalities

H/P, history and physical.

- **Tests:**
  - **Karyotyping** is the definitive test for diagnosing the condition
  - LH and FSH will be elevated to menopausal levels; estradiol will be at prepubertal levels
  - An echocardiogram and abdominal US should be performed to detect renal and cardiac abnormalities

FIGURE 11-3 **Approach to the patient with amenorrhea. GnRH, gonadotropin-releasing hormone; FSH, follicle-stimulating hormone; β-hCG, human chorionic gonadotropin; LH, luteinizing hormone. Neg, negative; PCOS, polycystic ovary syndrome; Pos, positive.**

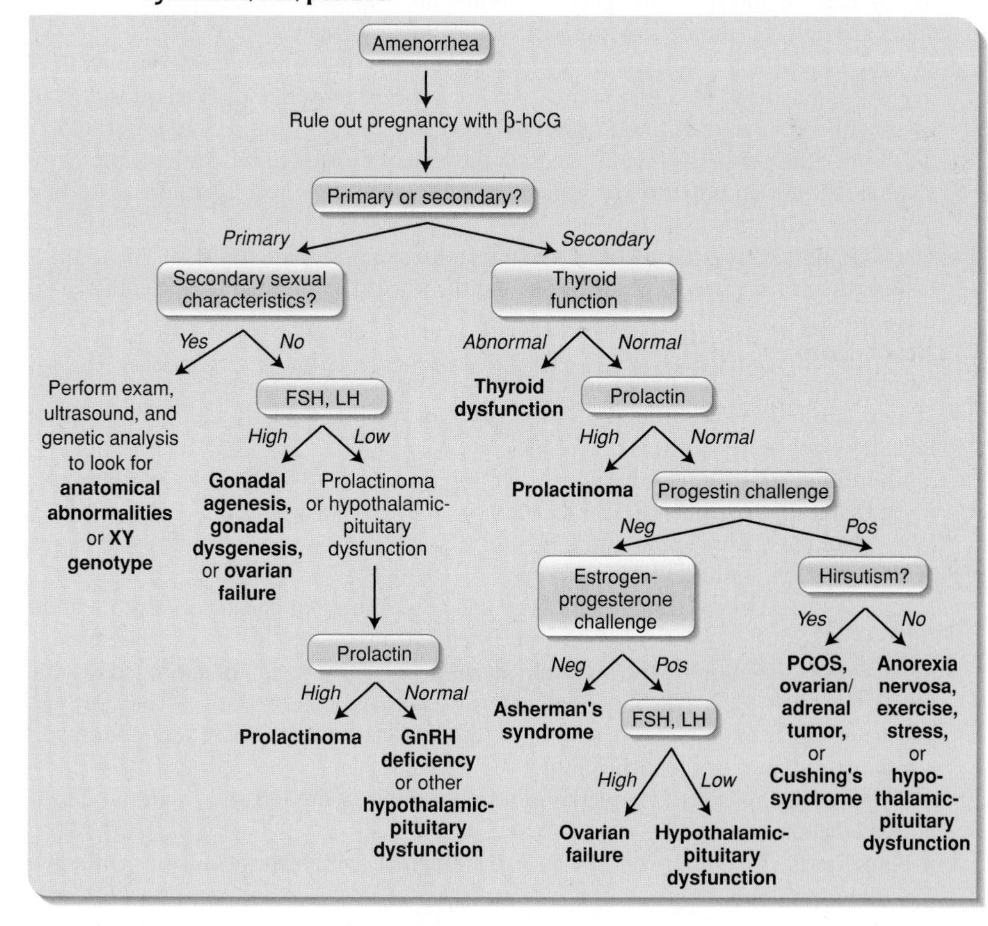

Patients with Turner syndrome taking hormone replacement therapy are not at a significantly increased risk of breast cancer or cardiovascular disease because of their preexisting hormone deficiencies.

  - **Treatment:**
    - Estrogen and progesterone replacement therapy is indicated to achieve menses and breast growth
    - Donor ovum implantation and fertilization is required for pregnancy
    - Good cardiac and renal follow-up is required to detect any evolving complications for those systems
  - **Outcomes:**
    - The prognosis is generally good with adequate hormone replacement therapy until the age of menopause
    - Permanent short stature is typical unless the diagnosis is made at a young age
    - Infertility is almost universal
    - Cardiac anomalies (e.g., coarctation of the aorta, aortic valve abnormalities), renal abnormalities (e.g., collecting duct anomalies), hearing loss, osteoporosis, hypothyroidism, and lymphedema are possible comorbid conditions and complications
  - **Clues to the diagnosis:**
    - History: primary amenorrhea, absence of growth spurt
    - Physical: short stature, no breast development, ptosis, broad neck, extra heart sounds, normal pubic hair growth
    - Tests: 45XO karyotype, elevated LH and FSH, low estradiol
- **Genital tract abnormality**
  - Abnormal development of the genital tract, resulting in the inability to have normal menses
    - Variations include vaginal septa, imperforate hymen, uterine agenesis, or intrauterine adhesions
    - Androgen insensitivity is a rare condition in 46XY individuals who fail to develop a male genital tract due to nonfunctional hormone signaling pathways
  - **History:** amenorrhea, periodic pelvic pain
  - **Physical examination:** possible visualization or detection of the anatomic abnormality during manual and speculum pelvic examination
  - **Tests:** pelvic US is the best means of detecting an abnormality
  - **Treatment:** surgical treatment is required to recreate the normal uterine-vaginal tract in cases amenable to reconstruction; hormone replacement therapy is administered in cases with inadequate hormone production or in androgen insensitivity syndrome
  - **Outcomes:** the prognosis is contingent on the ease of treating the condition; cases with vaginal septa or an imperforate hymen typically regain the greatest degree of normal genital tract function
  - **Why eliminated from differential:** the history of successful attempts at vaginal intercourse, the normal pelvic examination, and the normal abdominal US make this diagnosis unlikely
- **Anorexia nervosa**
  - More thorough discussion in Chapter 13
  - **Why eliminated from differential:** the patient's weight (actually mildly overweight for her height) rules out this diagnosis
- **Hypothyroidism**
  - More thorough discussion in Chapter 5
  - **Why eliminated from differential:** the normal TSH rules out this diagnosis
- **Polycystic ovary syndrome (PCOS)**
  - A disease of the hypothalamic-pituitary axis with androgen and LH overproduction that leads to **amenorrhea**, **infertility**, and **virilization**
    - Excess LH secretion by the pituitary causes an overproduction of androgens by the ovaries
    - The excessive androgens are converted into estrogens that further induce androgen production and lead to virilization
    - The high estrogen levels cause an inhibition of FSH secretion and result in infertility and amenorrhea
    - Some cases are associated with hyperinsulinemia, which causes further androgen overproduction

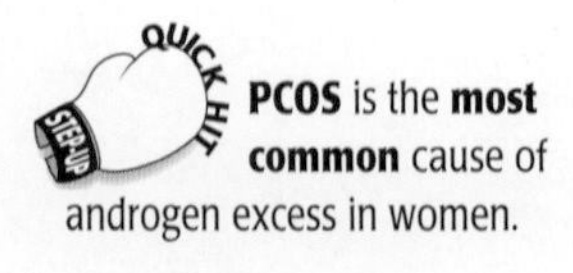

PCOS is the **most common** cause of androgen excess in women.

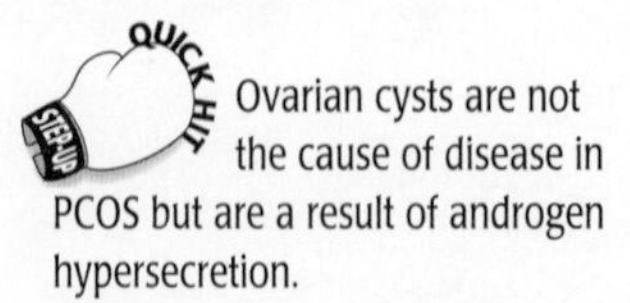

Ovarian cysts are not the cause of disease in PCOS but are a result of androgen hypersecretion.

- **History: amenorrhea** or oligomenorrhea, breakthrough bleeding, **infertility**
- **Physical examination:** obesity, **hirsutism** (e.g., excess facial, chest, and abdominal hair), **virilization** (e.g., pattern baldness, clitoral enlargement, voice deepening), palpable bilateral ovarian enlargement
- **Tests:**
  - **Increased LH**; LH/FSH ratio >3
  - Increased DHEA and androstenedione
  - Positive progestin challenge (i.e., administration of progestin causes uterine bleeding within 5 days of administration)
  - Abdominal US will show **enlarged ovaries** with **multiple cysts**
- **Treatment:**
  - Clomiphene may be used to induce follicle maturation to allow pregnancy
  - Estrogen-progesterone oral contraceptives may be used to regulate the menstrual cycles and decrease the androgen unbalance to lessen hirsutism and virilization
  - Metformin and rosiglitazone may be used to control glucose intolerance and assist in inducing ovulation
- **Outcomes:** glucose intolerance with subsequent diabetes mellitus (DM) and an increased risk of endometrial cancer from chronic hormone stimulation are the main complications
- **Why eliminated from differential:** the elevation of both FSH and LH, the normal DHEA level, and the normal US rule out this diagnosis

- **Pregnancy**
  - More thorough discussion in Chapter 12
  - **Why eliminated from differential:** the negative pregnancy test rules out this diagnosis
- **Congenital adrenal hyperplasia**
  - More thorough discussion in Chapter 5
  - **Why eliminated from differential:** the normal cortisol and DHEA levels make this diagnosis unlikely
- **Prolactinoma**
  - A pituitary tumor that produces excess prolactin and is related to the occurrence of amenorrhea
    - Effects of the tumor are a result of both the overproduction of prolactin and the mass effect of the tumor
  - **History:** amenorrhea or oligomenorrhea, headache, vaginal dryness, dyspareunia (i.e., painful intercourse)
  - **Physical examination:** galactorrhea (i.e., ability to express milk from the breast) in the absence of pregnancy, possible vision abnormalities
  - **Tests:** increased serum prolactin level; brain MRI may be performed to detect the pituitary tumor
  - **Treatment:** bromocriptine is used to decrease prolactin secretion; surgical resection is indicated for large tumors and in women desiring pregnancy
  - **Outcomes:**
    - Microscopic tumors have an excellent prognosis, but larger tumors have more complications
    - Large tumors can cause permanent vision deficits due to impingement upon the optic nerve
    - Surgical resection is associated with possible hypopituitarism and a small risk of death
  - **Why eliminated from differential:** the normal prolactin level and absence of breast tissue makes this diagnosis unlikely

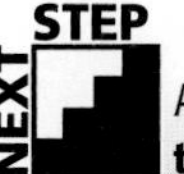

A **β-hCG pregnancy test** is always the first step in the work-up of any type of amenorrhea.

QUICK HIT: Although a prolactinoma is the most common pituitary tumor, any hypothalamic or pituitary tumors can disturb the normal hypothalamic-pituitary-gonadal signaling pathway and cause abnormal menstrual function.

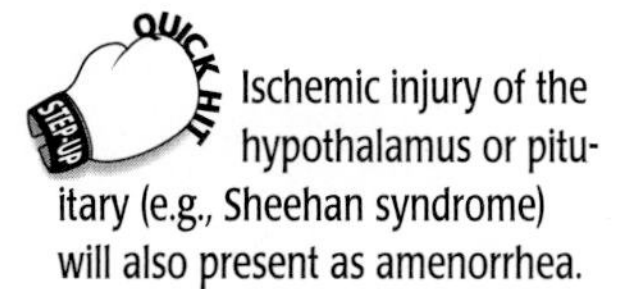

QUICK HIT: Ischemic injury of the hypothalamus or pituitary (e.g., Sheehan syndrome) will also present as amenorrhea.

GYNECOLOGY

CASE 11-3 "My periods are disappearing"

A 49-year-old woman presents to her gynecologist and reports that she has had few menses in the past year. She has not had menses in consecutive months within the past year, and she has not had a menstrual period at all in the past 6 months. Two of her menstrual periods in the past year have been heavier than normal. She denies any breakthrough bleeding between menstrual periods. She denies any abdominal pain and has had mild pelvic cramping during menses that has been similar to that experienced in the past during her menstrual periods. Sexual intercourse has been painful at times because she has felt "dry," and she has lost interest in sex recently. She says that she has felt worn down and has been irritable at work. She feels very warm at times and occasionally breaks out into a sweat when she feels too warm. She denies pain during urination, urinary frequency, or vaginal discharge. She reports having a good appetite and denies any recent significant weight loss. She has a past medical history significant for three full-term vaginal child births, HTN, and controlled atrial flutter. She takes atenolol and lisinopril. She drinks five alcohol drinks per week and denies any other substance use. On examination, she is a well-appearing woman in no distress. Her face appears symmetric, and her eyes appear grossly normal. She has no lymphadenopathy or neck masses. Auscultation of her lungs and heart detects normal breath sounds and heart sounds. Her abdomen is soft and nontender. A neurovascular examination is normal. A breast examination detects mild diffuse bilateral breast tenderness. A pelvic examination finds a dry and minimally irritated vaginal wall, no cervical or adnexal tenderness, and no cervical discharge. No masses on her uterus or ovaries are palpated. The following vital signs are measured:

T: 98.5°F, HR: 80 bpm, BP: 122/82 mm Hg, RR: 16 breaths/min

Differential Diagnosis

- Menopause, pregnancy, premature ovarian failure, polycystic ovarian syndrome, hypothyroidism, anorexia nervosa

Laboratory Data and Other Study Results

- Height and weight: 5′ 8″, 150 lbs, BMI 22.8
- Serum pregnancy test: negative
- TSH: 3.1 μU/mL
- FSH: 120 U/L
- LH: 100 U/L
- Estradiol: 29 pg/mL
- DHEA: 3.1 ng/mL
- Abdominal US: no masses of the kidneys, adrenals, or ovaries; normal uterine appearance

Diagnosis

- Perimenopause (i.e., early menopause)

Treatment Administered

- The patient was started on calcium, vitamin D, and alendronate to prevent osteopenia
- Lubricating agents were recommended for use during intercourse

Follow-up

- The patient continued to not have menstrual periods and was amenorrheic for 18 months at the time of last follow-up
- The patient reported to have some improvement in her mood and libido over time
- The patient reported the elimination of pain during intercourse when lubricating agents were utilized

Steps to the Diagnosis

- Menopause
  - The permanent end of menstruation due to the **cessation of regular ovarian function**
    - Occurs typically around 50 years of age
    - Requires **12 consecutive months** without a menstrual period; the period of time leading up to this point is the **perimenopausal period**
    - During the evolution of menopause, the ovarian response to FSH and LH decreases, FSH and LH levels increase, and the serum estrogen level gradually decreases
  - **History: hot flashes** (i.e., periods of feeling excessively warm due to thermoregulatory dysfunction), diaphoresis, breast pain, **menstrual irregularity** with eventual **amenorrhea**, fatigue, anxiety, irritability, depression, **dyspareunia** (i.e., pain during sexual intercourse due to vaginal wall atrophy and decreased lubrication), urinary frequency or dysuria
  - **Physical examination:** breast tenderness, vaginal wall atrophy
  - **Tests:** FSH and LH are increased; estrogen is decreased
  - **Treatment:**
    - Calcium and vitamin D supplementation and bisphosphonates are indicated to prevent **osteopenia**
    - Selective estrogen receptor modulators (e.g., raloxifene, tamoxifen) may help to reduce osteoporosis and cardiovascular risks
    - Regular cardiologic follow-up is important to detect evolving ischemic disease
    - Lubricating agents or topical vaginal estrogen may be used to treat dyspareunia
  - **Outcomes:** postmenopausal women are at a higher risk for **CAD**, **osteoporosis**, and cognitive deterioration
  - **Clues to the diagnosis:**
    - History: hot flashes, secondary amenorrhea, irritability, dyspareunia
    - Physical: breast tenderness, vaginal dryness
    - Tests: increased FSH and LH, decreased estradiol
- Pregnancy
  - More thorough discussion in Chapter 12
  - **Why eliminated from differential:** the negative serum pregnancy test rules out this diagnosis
- Premature ovarian failure
  - Onset of menopausal changes **prior to the age of 40 years**
    - Although several etiologies exist, they typically involve either premature ovarian follicle loss or follicle dysfunction
    - Unlike menopause, patients retain infrequent menstrual activity during the course of the process
  - **Risk factors:** tobacco use, pelvic radiation, chemotherapy, autoimmune disease, prior abdominal or pelvic surgery
  - **History:** similar to menopause except that patients may occasionally have menses
  - **Physical examination:** similar to menopause
  - **Tests:**
    - Increased FSH and LH; decreased estradiol
    - Gonadotropin and estrogen levels during the periods of residual ovarian activity may be normal and warrant repeat periodic testing
    - Karyotyping and ovarian antibody screening may be helpful for determining an underlying cause
  - **Treatment:**
    - Estrogen and progesterone replacement therapy is indicated until menopausal age is reached to reduce symptomatology
    - Donor ovum may be required to achieve pregnancy
    - Treatment of an underlying disorder may help prevent further ovarian deterioration
  - **Outcomes:** the prognosis for fertility is poor with few patients being able to achieve an unaided pregnancy; because the complications are the same as for menopause but

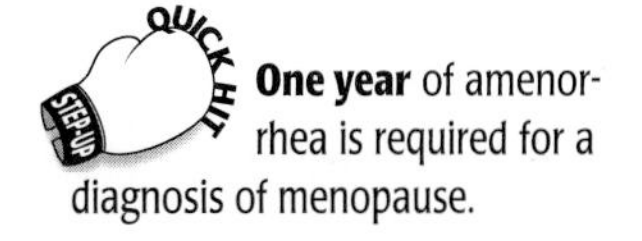

One year of amenorrhea is required for a diagnosis of menopause.

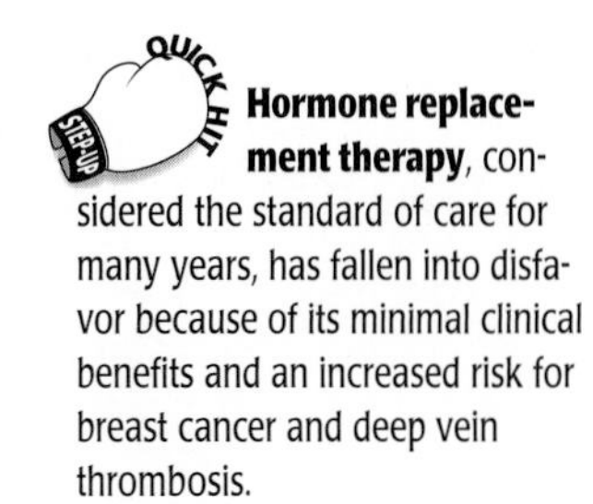

Hormone replacement therapy, considered the standard of care for many years, has fallen into disfavor because of its minimal clinical benefits and an increased risk for breast cancer and deep vein thrombosis.

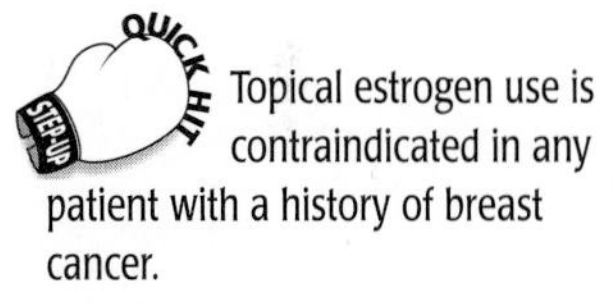

Topical estrogen use is contraindicated in any patient with a history of breast cancer.

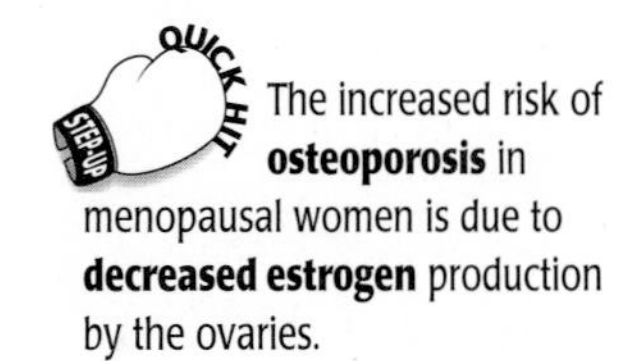

The increased risk of **osteoporosis** in menopausal women is due to **decreased estrogen** production by the ovaries.

occur at a younger age, attention to maintaining cardiac and bone health is important to avoid related sequelae
  - **Why eliminated from differential:** the age of the patient rules out this diagnosis
- **Polycystic ovarian syndrome**
  - More thorough discussion in prior case
  - **Why eliminated from differential:** the normal DHEA level and the similarity in FSH and LH levels rule out this diagnosis
- **Hypothyroidism**
  - More thorough discussion in Chapter 5
  - **Why eliminated from differential:** the normal TSH makes this diagnosis unlikely
- **Anorexia nervosa**
  - More thorough discussion in Chapter 13
  - **Why eliminated from differential:** the normal weight for height in this patient makes this diagnosis unlikely

CASE 11-4 "I've been spotting a little"

A 57-year-old woman presents to her gynecologist with a complaint of occasional vaginal bleeding. She says that she has experienced occasional bleeding about two to three times per week for the past 3 months. She has been wearing absorbent pads in her underwear consistently because she is unable to predict when this bleeding will occur. The amount of blood is small she says; but she estimates that she finds approximately one tablespoon of blood on her absorbent pads a couple of times each week. She has some mild pelvic cramping around the time of these bleeding episodes. She reports that she thought that she went through menopause 5 years ago and has had no menstrual periods since she was 52 years old. She says that she is married and only has intercourse with her husband. She denies any pain during urination or urinary frequency. She says that her urine is typically light yellow in color. She has a past medical history of morbid obesity, noninsulin-dependent DM, hypercholesterolemia, and HTN. She had two children through full-term vaginal births. She takes metformin, simvastatin, ezetimibe, hydrochlorothiazide (HCTZ), and losartan. She denies any substance use. On examination, she is a morbidly obese woman in no distress. She has no lymphadenopathy. Her abdomen is soft and nontender, but it is difficult to palpate any viscera due to her body habitus. A rectal examination detects no gross blood. A pelvic examination detects a small amount of blood within the vagina and at the os of the cervix. The cervix is nontender to palpation but is relatively fixed in place. It is difficult to palpate her ovaries or uterus, but the posterior uterine wall near the cervix feels firm. The following vital signs are measured:

T: 98.7°F, HR: 85 bpm, BP: 140/84 mm Hg, RR: 20 breaths/min

Differential Diagnosis

- Uterine fibroids, endometrial cancer, cervical cancer, urinary tract infection, pelvic inflammatory disease, bladder cancer, pregnancy with threatened abortion, menopausal atrophic vaginitis

Laboratory Data and Other Study Results

- Complete blood cell count (CBC): white blood cells (WBC): 6.9, hemoglobin (Hgb): 12.2, platelets (Plt): 294
- 7-electrolyte chemistry panel (Chem7): sodium (Na): 145 mEq/L, potassium (K): 4.2 mEq/L, chloride (Cl): 102 mEq/L, carbon dioxide (CO_2): 28 mEq/L, blood urea nitrogen (BUN): 24 mg/dL, creatinine (Cr): 1.2 mg/dL, glucose (Glu): 132 mg/dL
- Serum pregnancy test: negative
- UA: straw colored, pH: 6.9, specific gravity: 1.015, no glucose/ketones/nitrites/leukocyte esterase/hematuria/proteinuria

- Papanicolaou (Pap) smear: atypical squamous cells of undetermined significance; numerous red blood cells (RBCs)
- Transvaginal US: no cervical masses; significant thickening of the posterior uterine wall; no distinct masses within the uterine cavity

Following these studies, a dilation and curettage of the endometrium is scheduled and performed, and the following results are noted:

- Endometrial cytology: hyperplastic glandular tissue with significant neovascularization

The following imaging studies are then performed:

- Chest CT: normal lung volumes with no atelectasis, infiltrates, or effusions; no pulmonary masses; normal appearance of the heart and pericardium
- Abdomen/pelvis CT: enlargement of the uterus with significant thickening of the posterior and right lateral walls; close approximation of the right ovary to the uterus; normal size and shape of both ovaries; normal appearance of all remaining viscera; no discrete abdominal or pelvic fluid collections

Diagnosis

- Endometrial cancer

Treatment Administered

- Hysterectomy and bilateral salpingo-oophorectomy was performed with regional lymph node biopsies; extension of a uterine mass to the right-sided broad ligament was noted at the time of surgery
- A chemotherapeutic regimen using cisplatin was initiated following surgery

Follow-up

- The patient recovered well from surgery without any complications
- Lymph node cytology did not detect any presence of metastases
- Surgical pathology found negative margins surrounding the surgical specimen
- At 5 years following surgery and chemotherapy, the patient was doing well and considered to be disease free

Steps to the Diagnosis

- **Endometrial carcinoma**
  - **Adenocarcinoma** of the endometrial lining of the uterus
    - Most frequently associated with **exposure to high estrogen levels**
    - Squamous cell carcinomas of the endometrium occur but are far less common than adenocarcinoma
  - **Risk factors: postmenopausal** women, **unopposed exogenous estrogen use**, **obesity**, PCOS, nulliparity, DM, HTN, family history, high fat diet, hereditary nonpolyposis colorectal cancer (HNPCC)
  - **History:** heavy menses, midcycle bleeding, or **postmenopausal** uterine bleeding, possible abdominal pain
  - **Physical examination:** possible visualization of blood at the cervical os, possible pelvic mass or decreased mobility of the uterus or ovaries
  - **Tests:**
    - **Transvaginal US** may be able to detect uterine masses or uterine wall thickening and is frequently the first test performed because it is noninvasive
    - **Endometrial biopsy** (performed in the clinic or as part of a dilation and curettage procedure) will show hyperplastic glandular tissue with vascular invasion; while office-based biopsies may be performed for most postmenopausal bleeding, abnormal US findings necessitate a dilation and curettage

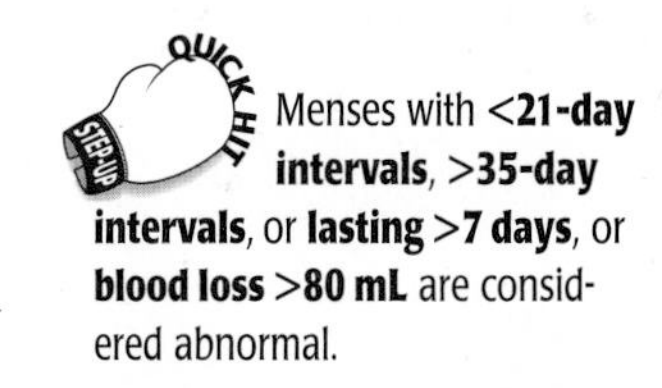

Menses with **<21-day intervals**, **>35-day intervals**, or **lasting >7 days**, or **blood loss >80 mL** are considered abnormal.

MNEMONIC

Common causes of abnormal female genital tract bleeding may be remembered by the mnemonic **PANAMA CUTIE**: **P**regnancy, **A**novulation, **N**eoplasm (benign or malignant), **A**natomic abnormality, **M**edications, **A**trophy (uterine), **C**oagulation disorders, **U**rinary tract disorders (infection, prolapse), **T**rauma, **I**nfection, **E**ndocrine disorders (PCOS, thyroid disease).

- Chest x-ray (CXR) or chest CT may be used to look for the presence of metastases; abdominal/pelvic CT is not imperative to the diagnosis but may be useful in surgical planning
- **CA125** tumor marker may be increased and can be used for monitoring the response to therapy
- **Treatment:**
  - **Total abdominal hysterectomy** and **bilateral salpingo-oophorectomy (TAH-BSO)** with lymph node sampling are the primary treatments
  - Radiation therapy is frequently performed for any tumors with extension to the pelvic contents
  - Chemotherapy may be used in addition to or in place of radiation therapy for tumors extending beyond the uterus
  - Surgical debulking should be performed for extensive tumors unable to be fully resected
  - Hormone therapy (e.g., progesterone, tamoxifen) may be beneficial to treating extensive tumors not responding to other treatments
- **Outcomes:**
  - Tumors typically metastasize to the peritoneum, aortic and pelvic lymph nodes, lungs, and vagina
  - The 5-year survival rate is 87% for tumors limited to the endometrial lining, 76% for tumors with extension to the cervix, 63% for tumors extending to the vagina, ovaries, or regional lymph nodes, and 37% for tumors extending to the gastrointestinal (GI) viscera or with distant metastases
  - Endometrial cancer **not related** to excess endogenous or exogenous estrogen exposure carries a **worse** prognosis than estrogen-related tumors
- **Clues to the diagnosis:**
  - History: postmenopausal bleeding, mild abdominal pain
  - Physical: bleeding from the cervical os, fixed cervix, firm uterine wall
  - Tests: endometrial thickness on transvaginal US, endometrial biopsy results

- **Uterine fibroids (a.k.a. uterine leiomyoma)**
  - Benign uterine masses composed of smooth muscle
    - Masses vary in size with the menstrual cycle and generally shrink following menopause
  - **Risk factors:** nulliparity, alcohol consumption, African American heritage, diet high in meat consumption, family history
  - **History:** patient may be asymptomatic or may have abdominal pain, menorrhagia (i.e., heavy periods), or abnormal uterine bleeding
  - **Physical examination:** a uterine mass may be palpable
  - **Tests:**
    - Transvaginal US or hysteroscopy may be used to detect and visualize uterine masses
    - MRI is useful to determine the size and extent of uterine masses
    - Biopsy is typically required to rule out a malignant neoplasm
  - **Treatment:**
    - **Asymptomatic** fibroids may be followed with serial US to look for any abnormal growth
    - **GnRH agonists** reduce uterine bleeding and the size of the fibroid but should be considered a temporary therapy
    - **Hysterectomy** is performed for women with symptomatic fibroids
    - **Myomectomy** may be considered for the resection of symptomatic fibroids in women wishing to maintain fertility
    - **Uterine artery embolization** following a pelvic MRI to rule out other soft tissue pathology may be performed to selectively infarct small fibroids in women wishing to avoid surgery (carries a high likelihood of infertility)
  - **Outcomes:** although most fibroids are asymptomatic, those that do cause symptoms typically require treatment; infertility is the most common complication
  - **Why eliminated from differential:** the results of the endometrial biopsy rule out this diagnosis

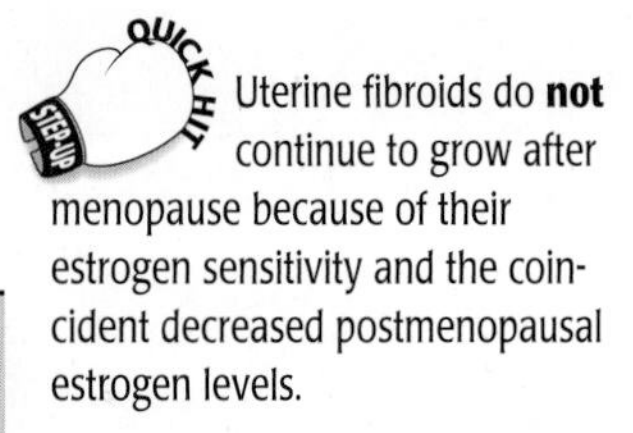

Uterine fibroids do **not** continue to grow after menopause because of their estrogen sensitivity and the coincident decreased postmenopausal estrogen levels.

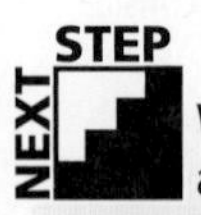

While menopausal atrophic vaginitis and **uterine fibroids** are the **most common causes** of vaginal **bleeding** in postmenopausal women (80% cases), endometrial cancer must be ruled out for any postmenopausal woman presenting with this complaint (i.e., perform an **endometrial biopsy**).

TABLE 11-7 Bethesda Classification of Cervical Squamous Cell Dysplasia and Appropriate Therapy

Grade	Characteristics	Treatment
Atypical squamous cells of undetermined significance (ASCUS)	Cellular abnormalities not explained by reactive changes; not suggestive of intraepithelial lesions	HPV screening; repeat Pap smear in 6 and 12 months; repeat HPV testing in 12 months
Atypical squamous cells, cannot exclude HSIL (ASCH)	Cellular abnormalities not explained by reactive changes; HSIL cannot be excluded	HPV screening; endocervical biopsy; repeat Pap smear in 6 and 12 months; repeat HPV testing in 12 months
Low-grade squamous intraepithelial lesion (LSIL) (a.k.a. CIN 1)	Mild cellular dysplasia	Repeat Pap smear in 6 and 12 months; repeat HPV testing in 12 months; excision by LEEP or conization or laser ablation may be performed
High-grade squamous intraepithelial lesion (HSIL) (a.k.a. CIN 2 or 3)	Moderate or severe cellular dysplasia including carcinoma *in situ*	Excision by LEEP or conization or laser ablation; repeat cervical cytology every 6 months
Squamous cell carcinoma	Highly atypical cells with stromal invasion	Varies with degree of invasion and extent of involvement

ASCUS, atypical squamous cells of undetermined significance; ASCH, atypical squamous cells, cannot exclude HSIL; CIN, cervical intraepithelial neoplasia; HPV, human papilloma virus; HSIL, high-grade squamous intraepithelial lesion; LEEP, loop electrocautery excision procedure; LSIL, low-grade squamous intraepithelial lesion; Pap smear, Papanicolaou smear.

- Cervical cancer
  - Cancer of the **cervix** that results from the malignant transformation of **cervical dysplasia**
    - The majority of cases are **squamous cell carcinomas** (80%), but adenocarcinoma (15%) and adenosquamous carcinoma (5%) are possible
    - **Cervical dysplasia**
      - Precancerous squamous cell lesions of the cervix that may progress to invasive cervical cancer in up to 22% of cases depending on the cellular grade
      - The cellular grade is classified by the Bethesda system (Table 11-7)
  - **Risk factors:** young age at first vaginal intercourse, **human papilloma virus (HPV) types 16, 18, 31, and 33**, multiple sexual partners, high-risk sexual partners, history of prior sexually transmitted diseases (STDs)
  - **History:** although typically asymptomatic in the early stages, vaginal bleeding (spontaneous or following intercourse), pelvic pain, or cervical discharge may occur in more progressed disease
  - **Physical examination:** possible palpable or visible cervical mass, possible decreased cervical mobility
  - **Tests:**
    - **Pap smear** is the primary screening tool for detecting cervical dysplasia or cancer
    - Biopsy of concerning lesions (punch or cone) is required to make a formal histologic diagnosis
    - CT, MRI, or transvaginal US may be useful for determining the extent of neoplasms
  - **Treatment:**
    - Cervical dysplasia is treated with observation or excision depending on the histologic grade (Table 11-7)
    - Malignant neoplasms with <5 mm of invasion may be treated with **conization** if the patient desires to maintain fertility and are treated with hysterectomy otherwise
    - Chemotherapy is administered for any cancer with close surgical margins
    - A combination of hysterectomy, lymph node excision, radiation therapy, and chemotherapy is used for any invasive lesions that do not extend to abdominal viscera or the distal vagina
    - Neoplasms with extension to pelvic contents or the distal vagina or those with metastases are treated with radiation therapy and chemotherapy

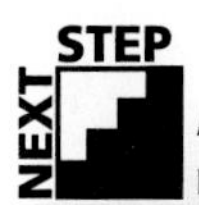

All women should receive **annual Pap smears** beginning approximately 3 years after the onset of vaginal intercourse or no later than 21 years of age. In those who have never engaged in intercourse, Pap smears may be deferred because of the low risk of cervical cancer related to HPV.

- **Outcomes:** the 5-year survival is >90% for microscopic lesions confined to the cervical epithelium, 65%–85% for visible lesions limited to the uterus, 50% for lesions extending beyond the uterus, and <30% for metastatic lesions
- **Why eliminated from differential:** the endometrial biopsy results are more indicative of endometrial cancer; the hysterectomy performed in this case eliminates the need for further work-up of the cervical dysplasia

- **Pelvic inflammatory disease**
  - More thorough discussion in later case
  - **Why eliminated from differential:** the absence of cervical motion tenderness makes this diagnosis unlikely
- **Urinary tract infection**
  - More thorough discussion in Chapter 4
  - **Why eliminated from differential:** the normal UA makes this diagnosis unlikely
- **Bladder cancer**
  - More thorough discussion in Chapter 4
  - **Why eliminated from differential:** the absence of hematuria on the UA makes this diagnosis unlikely
- **Pregnancy/threatened abortion**
  - More thorough discussion in Chapter 12
  - **Why eliminated from differential:** the negative serum pregnancy test rules out these diagnoses
- **Atrophic vaginitis (due to menopause)**
  - More thorough discussion in prior case (refer to section on menopause/perimenopause)
  - **Why eliminated from differential:** although vaginal irritation commonly occurs in menopause, this diagnosis would not account for the uterine bleeding or biopsy abnormalities

The following additional Gynecology cases may be found online:

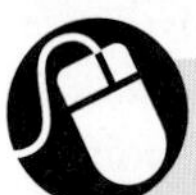

CASE 11-5 "My belly hurts so bad!"

CASE 11-6 "I've got a weird bump down there"

CASE 11-7 "I think there is a lump on my ovary"

CASE 11-8 "I found a lump on my breast"

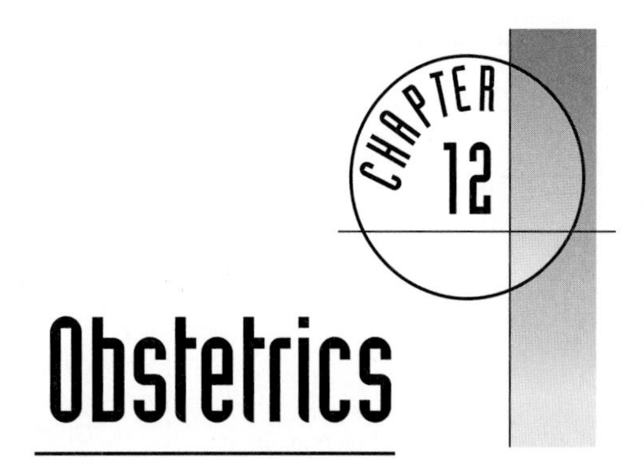

Obstetrics

BASIC CLINICAL PRIMER

MATERNAL PHYSIOLOGY IN PREGNANCY

- **Fetal development**
  - Following fertilization of the ovum, the newly created zygote begins mitotic cell division
  - Implantation of the zygote in the endometrium occurs approximately 6 days following fertilization, and the placenta begins to develop as the supporting conduit for maternal-fetal circulation
  - Fetal maturity occurs through a developmental process taking approximately 38 weeks (Figure 12-1)
- **Changes in maternal physiology**
  - Physiologic changes occur in every maternal organ system in response to the need to maintain fetal viability (Table 12-1)

PRENATAL CARE

- **Nutrition**
  - Maternal nutrition demands change with the beginning of pregnancy in order to fully support both the mother and the developing fetus (Table 12-2)
  - Some nutrients are important to **reduce the risk of birth defects** (e.g., folate, iron)
  - The ideal maternal weight gain during pregnancy is dependent on the mother's preexisting body mass index (BMI) (Table 12-3)
  - Consumption of fish (due to methylmercury contamination) and caffeine (due to an increased risk of spontaneous abortion) should be limited during pregnancy
- **Prenatal obstetrics care**
  - **Thorough prenatal care** should be considered a vital component of pregnancy because its goals are to prevent or manage any conditions that may be harmful to the mother or fetus
  - The initial prenatal visit includes a detailed history, physical, and **risk assessment**
  - Maternal weight, urinalysis (to detect urinary tract infections [UTI] and gestational diabetes mellitus [DM]), blood pressure, fundal height (to estimate fetal growth), and fetal heart sounds (to confirm fetal viability) are evaluated at each visit
  - Patients should be educated about weight gain, nutrition, drug and substance abstinence, animal handling or avoidance, seat belt use, symptoms and signs for risks to the mother or fetus, scheduling of care and tests, childbirth and breast feeding classes, and confidentiality issues
  - Labs and ultrasound (US) are performed at certain time points during gestation to screen for infection and fetal abnormalities (Table 12-4)
  - Screening tests that are not routinely performed at the first prenatal visit but should be considered in **at-risk populations** include a purified protein derivative (PPD) (for

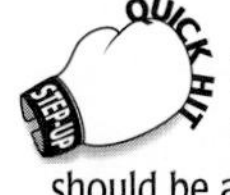

Daily caloric intake during pregnancy should be approximately **2,500** kcal.

QUICK HIT: **Exercise** is **encouraged** during pregnancy to improve maternal feelings of well-being, improve symptoms due to positional effects of the fetus, and promote healthy blood sugar levels.

QUICK HIT: Work and travel may be continued throughout pregnancy as long as fatigue and excessive stress are avoided; airline travel is permitted up to 36 weeks of gestation.

QUICK HIT: Sexual intercourse may be continued during pregnancy unless the mother is considered a high risk for spontaneous abortion, premature labor, or placenta previa.

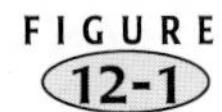

FIGURE 12-1 Time line of fetal development during gestation. CNS, central nervous system; hCG, human chorionic gonadotropin.

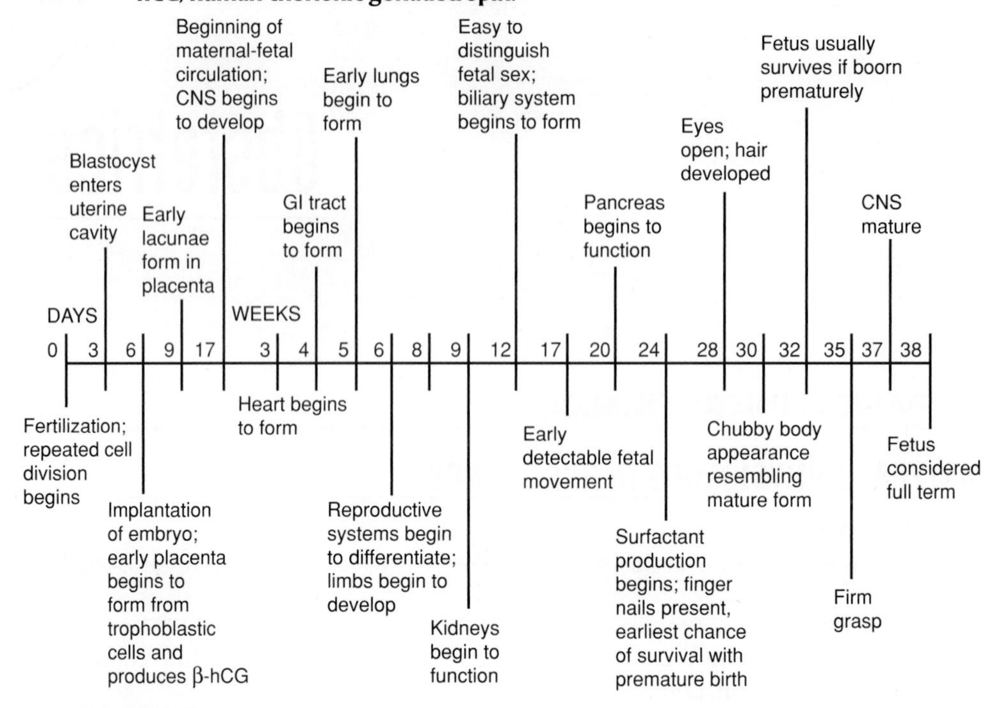

TABLE 12-1 Normal Changes in Maternal Physiology during Pregnancy

Anatomy/System	Changes
Cardiovascular	• Cardiac output increases 40% with associated increases in SV (10%–30%) and HR (12–18 bpm) • A systolic murmur may be heard due to the increased cardiac output • Myocardial O_2 demand increases • Systolic and diastolic blood pressures decrease slightly • The uterus displaces the heart slightly superiorly
Respiratory	• The uterus displaces the diaphragm superiorly and causes a decrease of residual volume, functional residual capacity, and expiratory reserve volume • Total body O_2 consumption increases 20% • Tidal volume increases 40% with an associated increase in minute ventilation due to stimulation by progesterone • P_{CO_2} decreases to approximately 30 mm Hg; dyspnea is a frequent complaint despite the increased minute ventilation and normal breathing rate
Renal	• Renal plasma flow and the glomerular filtration rate increase 40% • Decrease in BUN and creatinine • Increased renal loss of bicarbonate to compensate for respiratory alkalosis • Blood and interstitial fluid volumes increase
Endocrine	• Nondiabetic hyperinsulinemia with an associated mild glucose intolerance • Production of human placental lactogen contributes to the glucose intolerance by interfering with insulin activity • Fasting triglycerides increase • Cortisol increases
Hematologic	• Increased RBC production • Hematocrit decreases due to increased blood volume • Hypercoagulable state
Gastrointestinal	• Increased salivation • Decreased gastric motility

BUN, blood urea nitrogen; HR, heart rate; O_2, oxygen; P_{CO_2}, partial pressure of carbon dioxide; RBC, red blood cell; SV, stroke volume.

TABLE 12-2 Increased Nutritional Demands during Pregnancy

Substance	Increased Need	Reason for Need	Effects of Insufficiency
Calcium	1,000–1,300 mg/day (50% increase)	Lactation reserves, increased utilization by the fetus	Impaired maternal bone mineralization, HTN, premature birth, low birth weight
Fluids	Adequate hydration is important	Increased total maternal-fetal fluid volume	Relative dehydration
Folate	0.8–1 mg/day (should be started 4 weeks before attempted conception)	Normal fetal neural tube development	Neural tube defects
Iron	30 mg/day (100% increase)	RBC production	Maternal anemia, premature birth, low birth weight, maternal cardiac complications
Protein	60 g/day (30% increase)	Additional needs of maternal, fetal, and placental tissue	Impaired fetal and placental growth

HTN, hypertension; RBC, red blood cell.

TABLE 12-3 Ideal Weight Gain during Pregnancy

Prepregnant BMI	Ideal Weight Gain (lb)
<19.8	28–40
19.8–26	25–35[1]
>26	15–25

BMI, body mass index; lb, pounds.

[1]Weight gain should be approximately 2 lb in the first trimester and 0.75 to 1 lb/week in the remainder of the pregnancy.

TABLE 12-4 Common Screening Labs Performed during Pregnancy

Length of Gestation	Labs or Study Performed
Initial visit	• CBC • Blood antibody and Rh typing • Pap smear • Gonorrhea/chlamydia screening • Urinalysis • RPR or VDRL • Rubella antibody titer • Hepatitis B surface antigen • HIV screening (with maternal consent)
6–11 weeks	• US to determine gestational age
16–18 weeks	• Quadruple screen (maternal serum α-fetoprotein, hCG, unconjugated estradiol, maternal serum inhibin A) to look for trisomies 21 and 18 and neural tube defects
18–20 weeks	• US for detecting gross fetal and placental abnormalities
24–28 weeks	• 1-hour glucose challenge to screen for gestational DM
32–37 weeks	• Cervical culture for *Neisseria gonorrhoeae* and *Chlamydia trachomatis* (selected populations) • Group B streptococcus screening

CBC, complete blood count; DM, diabetes mellitus; hCG, human chorionic gonadotropin; Pap, Papanicolaou; PPD, purified protein derivative of tuberculin; Rh, rhesus factor; RPR, rapid plasma reagin; US, ultrasound; VDRL, Venereal Disease Research Laboratories.

TABLE 12-5 Prenatal Assessment for Congenital Diseases in High-Risk Pregnancies

Test	Description	Indications
Quadruple screen	Maternal serum α-fetoprotein, estradiol, hCG, and maternal serum inhibin A levels are measured to assess the risk for neural tube defects and trisomies 18 and 21	Performed in all pregnant women between 16–18 weeks of gestation; frequently the initial marker for fetal complications
Full integrated test	US measurement of nuchal translucency and serum measurement of PAPP-A in the first trimester and a quadruple screen in the second trimester; lowest false-positive rate for noninvasive tests	Women who present in the first trimester who desire noninvasive testing with the lowest false-positive risk
Amniocentesis	Transabdominal needle aspiration of amniotic fluid from the amniotic sac after 16 weeks of gestation to measure amniotic α-fetoprotein and determine the fetal karyotype; detects neural tube defects and chromosome disorders with greater sensitivity than triple screen alone	Abnormal quadruple screen, women >35 years old, risk of Rh sensitization; carries an excess 1% risk of spontaneous abortion over the normal risks for abortion
Chorionic villi sampling	Transabdominal or transcervical aspiration of chorionic villus tissue between 9–12 weeks of gestation to detect chromosomal abnormalities	Early detection of chromosomal abnormalities in higher-risk patients (e.g., advanced age, history of children with genetic defects)
Percutaneous umbilical blood sampling	Blood collection from the umbilical vein after 18 weeks of gestation to identify chromosomal defects, fetal infection, Rh sensitization	Late detection of genetic disorders, pregnancies with high risk for Rh sensitization

hCG, human chorionic gonadotropin; PAPP-A, pregnancy-associated plasma protein A; Rh, rhesus factor.

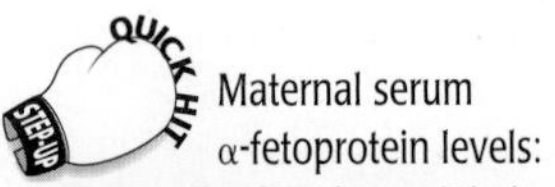

Maternal serum α-fetoprotein levels:
- **Only valid** if performed during the correct gestational window **(16 to 18 weeks' gestation)**
- **High** levels are associated with an increased risk of **neural tube defects** or multiple gestation
- **Low** levels are associated with increased risk of **trisomies 21** and **18**.

tuberculosis [TB]), red blood cell (RBC) indices and hemoglobin electrophoresis (for anemias), hexosaminidase A (for Tay-Sachs disease), phenylalanine levels (for phenylketonuria), hepatitis C serology, toxoplasmosis screening, and cystic fibrosis genetic screening

- Women considered to be at a **higher risk** for **congenital fetal defects** (e.g., older than 35 years, prior spontaneous abortion, teratogen exposure, DM, prior fetal demise) may be screened for fetal complications using more complex or invasive testing (Table 12-5)
- **Leopold maneuvers** (i.e., external abdominal examination) are performed in the third trimester to determine the fetal presentation

LABOR AND DELIVERY

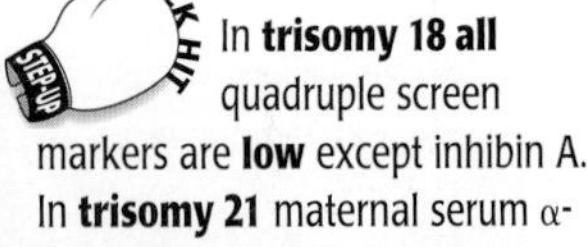

In **trisomy 18 all** quadruple screen markers are **low** except inhibin A. In **trisomy 21** maternal serum α-fetoprotein and unconjugated estradiol are low, while **human chorionic gonadotropin (hCG)** and **inhibin A** are **high**.

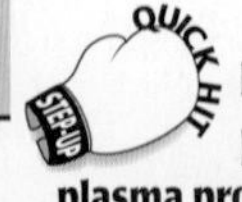

Low maternal pregnancy-associated plasma protein A (PAPP-A) levels are associated with an increased risk of **trisomies 21** and **18**.

- **Assessment of fetal well-being**
  - Tests of fetal activity, heart rate, and responses to stress are used to confirm fetal well-being and to detect fetal distress
    - **Nonstress test**
      - Performed during the **prenatal** assessment and in early labor
      - The mother reclines in the left lateral decubitus position and the fetal heart rate is monitored externally; uterine contractions are also monitored externally
      - The mother reports each fetal movement, and the **effects of fetal movement** on the **fetal heart** rate are noted
      - A normal (i.e., "**reactive**") test is considered to be two or more 15-beat-per-minute accelerations of the fetal heart rate that each last 15 seconds during a 20-minute monitoring period
      - A vibroacoustic stimulator can be applied to the mother's abdomen to encourage fetal activity and shorten the time of the test
      - A **nonreactive** test should prompt the performance of a **biophysical profile**
    - **Biophysical profile**
      - A nonstress test is repeated with the addition of an US assessment
      - A transabdominal US is performed to measure the **amniotic fluid index** (i.e., total linear measurement in centimeters of the largest amniotic fluid pocket

TABLE 12-6 Scoring of the Biophysical Profile

Measurement	Criteria	Score[1]
Nonstress test	Reactive	0 or 2
Amniotic fluid index	5–23 cm	0 or 2
Fetal breathing rate	One or more episodes of rhythmic breathing lasting at least 20 seconds in a 30-minute time period	0 or 2
Fetal movement	Two or more discrete spontaneous movements in a 30-minute time period	0 or 2
Fetal tone	One or more episodes of spine and limb extension with a return to flexion	0 or 2

[1]Satisfaction of the criteria equals a score of 2; failure to satisfy the criteria equals a score of 0 (no scores of 1).

detected in each of four quadrants of the amniotic sac), **fetal breathing rate**, **fetal movement**, and **fetal tone** (i.e., active extension of the fetal spine or limb with a return to flexion)
- A scoring system is applied to the nonstress test and the US measurements (Table 12-6)
- A **reassuring** profile is a score of **8** or **10** and suggests a minimal risk of fetal asphyxia; a **lower** score suggests **fetal distress**

- **Contraction stress test**
  - Performed late in pregnancy or during labor to assess uteroplacental dysfunction
  - The fetal heart rate is recorded with an external fetal monitor or scalp electrode
  - **Beat-to-beat variability** of approximately 5 beats per minute, **long-term heart rate variability**, and occasional **heart rate accelerations** (i.e., two or more accelerations of 15 beats per minute lasting at least 15 seconds within a 20-minute period) are **reassuring** signs
  - **Decelerations** of the fetal heart rate and their relationship to uterine contractions may be indicative of normal activity during labor or possible fetal distress (Figure 12-2, Table 12-7)
- **Fetal scalp blood sampling**
  - Performed when a consistently abnormal fetal heart rate tracing is measured or when a significant amount of meconium is detected in the amniotic fluid
  - A normal fetal blood pH is reassuring; a **decreased pH**, **hypoxemia**, or **increased lactate** level indicates **fetal distress**
- **Fetal scalp monitoring**
  - A monitor is attached to the fetal scalp to track pulse oximetry and to perform continuous fetal heart rate monitoring and an electrocardiogram (ECG)

QUICK HIT: Although the full integrated test is the most sensitive screening test for trisomies with the lowest false-positive rate, it is not routinely performed because abnormal first trimester results frequently prompt the decision to abandon the second trimester tests and perform a more invasive test to find a definitive answer.

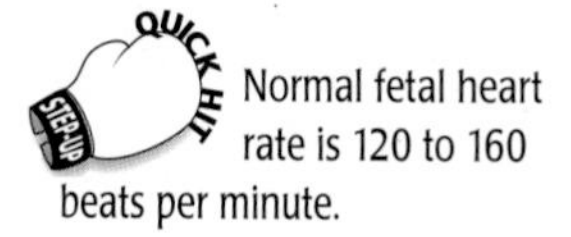

Normal fetal heart rate is 120 to 160 beats per minute.

TABLE 12-7 Types of Decelerations Seen on Fetal Heart Rate Tracings

Deceleration	Appearance	Cause	Treatment
Early	Decelerations begin and end **with** uterine contractions	Head compression	None required; **not a sign of fetal distress**
Late	Begin **after** the initiation of uterine contraction and end **after** a contraction has finished	**Uteroplacental insufficiency**, maternal venous compression, maternal hypotension, or abruptio placentae; **may suggest fetal hypoxia**	Test fetal blood from a scalp sample to diagnose hypoxia or acidosis; recurrent late decelerations or fetal hypoxia direct a **prompt delivery**
Variable	**Inconsistent** onset, duration, and degree of decelerations	Umbilical cord compression	Change the mother's position

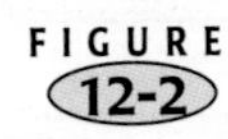

Examples of fetal heart and uterine tone tracings for early, late, and variable decelerations of the fetal heart rate (FHR) following uterine contraction (UC).

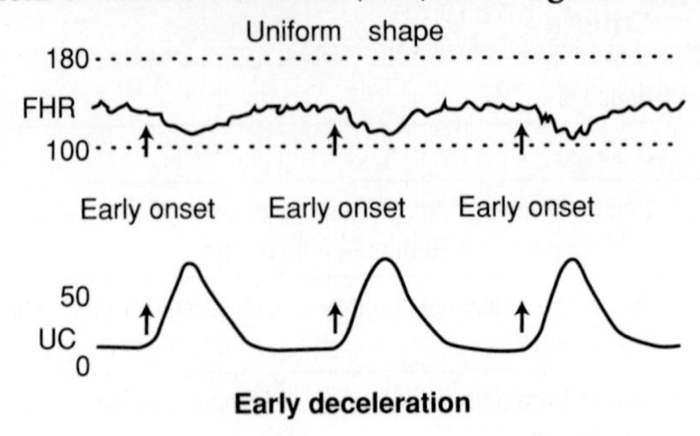

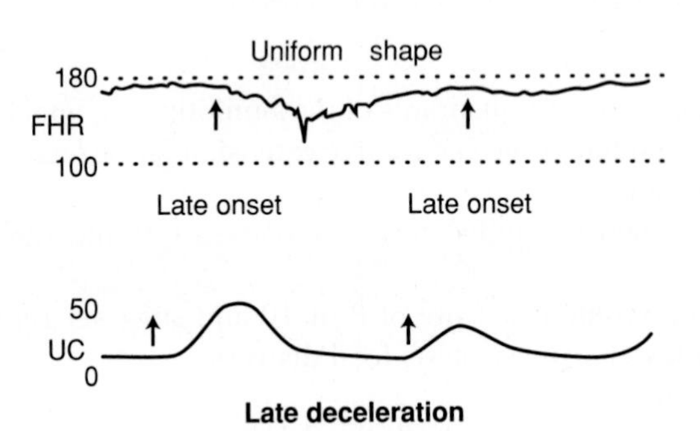

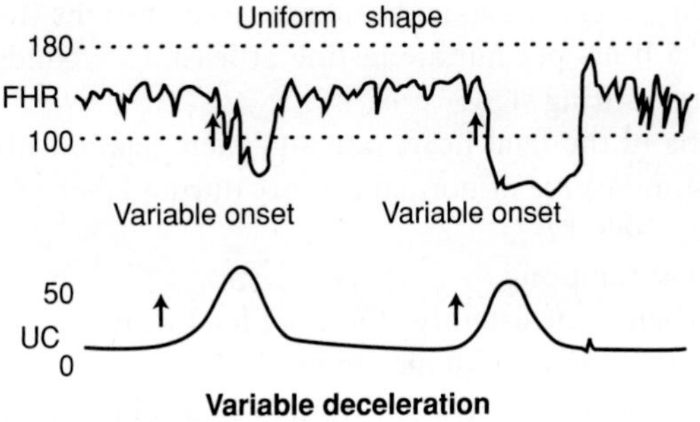

(Modified from Hon E. *An introduction to fetal heart rate monitoring*. Los Angeles; University of Southern California, 1973, with permission. Also see Feibusch KC, Breaden RS, Badr CD, Gomperts SN. *Prescription for the boards: USMLE step 2*. 3rd ed. Philadelphia; Lippincott Williams & Wilkins, 2002.)

OBSTETRICS

- Monitoring should be started in the first stage of labor to determine an accurate baseline ECG
- It should only be performed in pregnancies beyond 36 weeks of gestation with a vertex presentation to avoid tangling of the wires around the fetus

- **Stages of labor**
  - Labor (i.e., contractions and cervical effacement) typically begins at 38 to 42 weeks of gestation and involves four stages of progression (Table 12-8)
  - Nulliparous and multiparous women proceed through labor at different rates
  - **Induction of labor**
    - **Oxytocin** is administered to initiate uterine contractions or to speed the progress of labor
    - Indications include pre-eclampsia, DM, stalled stage of labor, chorioamnionitis, prolonged pregnancy (i.e., >40 to 42 weeks), intrauterine growth restriction (IUGR), premature rupture of membranes (PROM), and some congenital defects

QUICK HIT: During the last few weeks of gestation a woman may experience multiple **false** (i.e., Braxton-Hicks) **contractions** not associated with true labor.

TABLE 12-8 Stages of Labor

Stage	Beginning/End	Activity	Management	Nulliparous	Multiparous
1	• Latent phase—start of uterine contractions until 4 cm cervical dilation • Active phase—4 cm cervical dilation until near 10 cm cervical dilation with consistent progression • Deceleration phase—transition from active phase to second stage of labor	• Latent phase—cervical effacement and gradual dilation • Active phase—regular uterine contractions, quick progression of cervical dilation (1.5 cm/hr if nulliparous, 1 cm/hr if multiparous) and effacement • Deceleration phase—slow down of dilation and effacement shortly before engagement of fetal head in pelvis	Monitor fetal heart rate and uterine contractions, assess progression of cervical changes periodically during active phase	6–20 hr (latent, active)	2–10 hr
2	Full (10 cm) cervical dilation until delivery	Fetal descent through the birth canal driven by uterine contractions	Monitor fetal heart rate and movement through birth canal	30 min–3 hr	5–30 min
3	Delivery of neonate until placental delivery	Placenta separates from uterine wall up to 30 minutes after delivery of neonate and emerges through birth canal, uterus contracts to expel placenta and prevent hemorrhage	Uterine massage, examination of placenta to confirm no intrauterine remnants	0–30 min	0–30 min
4	Initial postpartum hour	Hemodynamic stabilization of mother	Monitor maternal pulse and blood pressure, look for signs of hemorrhage	1 hr	1 hr

- Contraindications to induction include prior uterine surgery, fetal lung immaturity, malpresentation, acute fetal distress, active maternal herpes infection, placenta or vasa previa
- The likelihood of vaginal delivery following induction is predicted by measuring fetal station and cervical dilation, effacement, consistency, and position (i.e., **Bishop score**) (Table 12-9)
- A higher Bishop score is associated with a greater chance of vaginal delivery, while a lower score is associated with a higher likelihood of cesarian delivery
  - The rate of cesarian delivery is 30% if the Bishop score following induction is <3 and 15% if >3

TABLE 12-9 Bishop Scoring System

Score	0	1	2	3
Dilation (cm)	0	1–2	3–4	5–6
Effacement (%)	0–30	40–50	60–70	>70
Station (cm)[1]	−3	−2	−1, 0	+1, +2
Cervical Consistency	Firm	Medium	Soft	
Cervical Position	Posterior	Middle	Anterior	

[1]Distance of presenting body part above (−) or below (+) ischial spines.
(Taken from Bishop, *Obstet Gynecol*, 1964.)

- **Cesarian section**
  - Surgical delivery of the fetus through an incision in the uterine wall
  - **Vertical type**
    - A **vertical** incision is made in the anterior portion of the uterus (i.e., classical) or lower uterine segment (i.e., low vertical)
    - Utilized when the fetus lies in a transverse presentation, if adhesions or fibroids prevent access to the lower uterus, if hysterectomy is scheduled to follow delivery, if cervical cancer is present, or in a postmortem delivery to remove a living fetus from a mother who has just died
  - **Low transverse type**
    - A **transverse** incision is made in the lower anterior portion of the uterus
    - It carries a decreased risk of uterine rupture, bleeding, bowel adhesions, and infection and is **preferred** to and performed more commonly than the vertical type
  - Indications include **eclampsia**, **prior uterine surgery**, **prior classic cesarean section**, maternal cardiac disease, birth canal obstruction, maternal death, cervical cancer, active maternal herpes simplex infection, **acute fetal distress**, **malpresentation**, umbilical cord prolapse, macrosomia, **failure to progress in labor**, placenta previa, abruptio placentae, and cephalopelvic disproportion
  - In subsequent pregnancies, vaginal delivery may be attempted only if a **transverse** cesarean section was performed
  - If a **vertical** incision has been utilized previously, repeat cesarean delivery **must** be performed due to an increased risk of **uterine rupture** during attempted vaginal delivery
  - Potential **complications** include maternal hemorrhage, infection and sepsis, thromboembolism, and injury to surrounding structures

QUICK HIT: Risk of maternal mortality is similar for elective cesarean section and vaginal delivery, but emergency cesarian section carries a higher risk of mortality.

NORMAL PUERPERIUM AND POSTPARTUM ACTIVITY

- **Care of the newborn**
  - Following delivery, the neonate's mouth and nose are suctioned to aid in breathing and to prevent aspiration
  - The neonate is dried and wrapped in a blanket to prevent heat loss
  - The umbilical cord is clamped and cut, and a cord blood sample is used to measure blood type and blood gases
  - If spontaneous respiration does not begin within 30 seconds of birth, resuscitation must be initiated
  - Tracheal injection of a synthetic or exogenous surfactant may be administered in cases of lung immaturity
  - **Apgar scores** are performed at 1 and 5 minutes after birth (Table 12-10)
    - Scores of at least 7 at 1 minute and 9 at 5 minutes are reassuring
- **Maternal changes after delivery**
  - The uterus decreases in size, and the cervix becomes firm over 3 weeks; the vaginal wall also gradually becomes more firm

TABLE 12-10 Apgar Scoring System for Determining Neonatal Well-Being

	Score		
Sign	0	1	2
Heart rate	None	<100 bpm	>100 bpm
Respirations	None	Poor, weak cry	Good, strong cry
Muscle tone	Poor	Some movement	Active movement
Response to stimulation	None	Grimace	Strong cry
Color	Blue, pale	Pink torso, blue extremities	Pink

bpm, beats per minute.
(Taken from Apgar, *Curr Res Anesth Analg*, 1953.)

- Uterine discharge (i.e., lochia) is red during the initial days after birth but becomes paler and white by the 10th postpartum day
- Total peripheral resistance increases rapidly due to the elimination of uteroplacental circulation, diuresis of the excess fluid volume causes a significant weight loss in the first postpartum week, and cardiac output gradually returns to normal
- Postpartum depression is common for a few days after delivery, but most cases resolve without complications
- Menses return 6 to 8 weeks following delivery in **nonnursing** mothers, but may not occur for several months in **nursing** mothers

QUICK HIT: Breast milk is considered the ideal infant nutrition because it contains important **immunoglobulin (Ig) A antibodies** for the newborn, is in **sufficient supply**, is **cost-free**, and enhances mother-infant bonding.

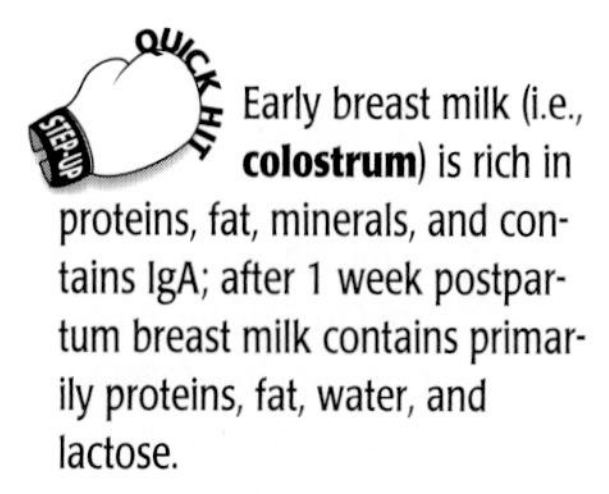

QUICK HIT: Early breast milk (i.e., **colostrum**) is rich in proteins, fat, minerals, and contains IgA; after 1 week postpartum breast milk contains primarily proteins, fat, water, and lactose.

CASE 12-1 "Does pregnancy give you bad headaches?"

A 26-year-old woman, who is G1P0000 (i.e., one pregnancy, no prior deliveries, premature births, spontaneous abortions, or current living children), presents to her obstetrician at 34 weeks of gestation for a scheduled prenatal visit. She says that she has developed fairly significant headaches within the past week. She gets these headaches on a daily basis. They are dull and poorly defined, and she describes the severity as a 4/10. She claims that she has slight tunnel vision when the headaches are at their worst. The headaches last for a few hours and then self-resolve. She has also experienced epigastric abdominal pain and nausea and has vomited four times this past week. Her emesis has not been bilious or bloody. She denies any numbness or weakness in her extremities. She denies having had any seizures at any point in her life including this past week. She denies any vaginal bleeding. She denies any significant past medical history. She is taking prenatal vitamins but no other medication. She denies any substance use. On examination, she is a well-appearing woman in no distress. Her face and eyes appear symmetric, not swollen, and not inflamed. Auscultation of her heart and lungs is normal. Her abdomen is gravid and nontender. Pelvic examination detects a closed cervical os with no discharge and no cervical tenderness. A neurovascular examination is normal. She has some mild swelling of her hands. She has no rashes. Her fundal height is 32 cm, and a regular fetal heart rate is easily detected. The following vital signs are measured:

Temperature (T): 98.7°F, heart rate (HR): 90 beats per minute (bpm), blood pressure (BP): 165/90 mm Hg, respiratory rate (RR): 18 breaths/min

Differential Diagnosis

- Eclampsia, pre-eclampsia, hyperemesis gravidarum, abruptio placentae, migraine headache, tension headache, cerebral vascular accident

Laboratory Data and Other Study Results

- Height and weight: 5′ 6″ 159 lb (initial weight 140 lb, BMI 22.6)
- Complete blood cell count (CBC): white blood cells (WBC): 6.4, hemoglobin (Hgb): 12.5, platelets (Plt): 189
- 7-electrolyte chemistry panel (Chem7): sodium (Na): 142 mEq/L, potassium (K): 4.1 mEq/L, chloride (Cl): 104 mEq/L, carbon dioxide (CO_2): 28 mEq/L, blood urea nitrogen (BUN): 17 mg/dL, creatinine (Cr): 1.0 mg/dL, glucose (Glu): 105 mg/dL
- Liver function tests (LFTs): alkaline phosphatase (AlkPhos): 87 U/L, alanine aminotransferase (ALT): 71 U/L, aspartate aminotransferase (AST): 50 U/L, total bilirubin (TBili): 0.9 mg/dL, direct bilirubin (DBili): 0.2 mg/dL
- Urinalysis (UA): straw colored, pH: 7.1, specific gravity: 1.025, 2+ protein, no glucose/ketones/nitrites/leukocyte esterase/hematuria
- Biophysical profile: score of 8 (fetal tone criteria not satisfied); intact placenta seen on US

Diagnosis

- Pre-eclampsia

Treatment Administered

- The patient was admitted to the labor and delivery floor
- Hydralazine and magnesium sulfate were administered to control the patient's blood pressure and to serve as seizure prophylaxis
- The patient was permitted restricted activity but was maintained on constant cardiac and external fetal monitoring

Follow-up

- The patient's blood pressure was reduced to 125/80, and no seizures occurred
- Delivery was induced once the patient reached 37 weeks of gestation, and an uncomplicated vaginal delivery ensued
- Medications were continued and weaned over 3 weeks after delivery to ensure that seizures did not occur and that the patient's blood pressure returned to the normal levels

QUICK HIT: In the GP notation used to describe pregnant women, the number following "G" notes the historical number of gestations in the patient and the four numbers following "P" refer to the number of deliveries (any type), premature births, spontaneous abortions, and living children.

Steps to the Diagnosis

- Pre-eclampsia
  - Pregnancy-induced **hypertension (HTN)**, **proteinuria**, and **edema** that develops after 20 weeks of gestation
    - Occurs in 5% of pregnancies and is due to an unknown cause
    - **HELLP syndrome** is a subtype of pre-eclampsia characterized by **hemolysis**, **elevated liver** enzymes, and **low platelets** (note the mnemonic!)
  - **Risk factors:** HTN, nulliparity, **prior history** of pre-eclampsia, younger than 15 years or older than 35 years, multiple gestations, vascular disease, chronic renal disease, DM, obesity, African heritage
  - **History**: although it is asymptomatic in mild cases, patients may experience rapid weight gain, headaches, epigastric abdominal pain, and visual disturbances as the severity increases
  - **Physical examination**: hand and face **edema**, hyperreflexia, **blood pressure >140/90**
  - **Tests:**
    - UA will demonstrate 2+ proteinuria or >4 g protein in a 24-hour collection
    - Decreased platelets, normal or mildly increased creatinine, decreased glomerular filtration rate, increased ALT and AST
    - A fetal nonstress test should be performed to confirm fetal well-being
  - **Treatment:**
    - If at 37 weeks of gestation or longer, **induce delivery**
    - If the patient is at <37 weeks of gestation and has mild symptoms, prescribe restricted activity and re-examinations, proteinuria assessments, and fetal nonstress tests twice per week
    - If the patient is at <37 weeks of gestation and has significant symptoms, admit the patient to the hospital for inpatient fetal and maternal health monitoring, maintain the maternal blood pressure at <155/105 with hydralazine or labetalol, administer intravenous (IV) magnesium sulfate as seizure prophylaxis, and induce delivery as soon as the fetus is considered viable
    - Antihypertensives and magnesium sulfate should be continued postpartum until the patient remains consistently normotensive
    - Patients with preexistent HTN should be treated with labetalol, hydralazine, or a long-acting calcium channel blocker to keep their blood pressure <140/95
  - **Outcomes:**
    - Potential complications include **eclampsia** with seizures, cerebral vascular accident, IUGR, pulmonary edema, **maternal organ failure**, oligohydramnios, and preterm delivery
    - HELLP syndrome is associated with abruptio placentae, renal insufficiency, encephalopathy, and disseminated intravascular coagulation (DIC); it is associated with a 1% maternal mortality

MNEMONIC

Findings suggestive of pre-eclampsia may be remembered by the mnemonic **HELP HER**: **H**TN, **E**dema (hands and face), **L**iver enzymes increased, **P**roteinuria, **H**eadache, **E**ye disturbances, **R**enal impairment (decreased glomerular filtration rate).

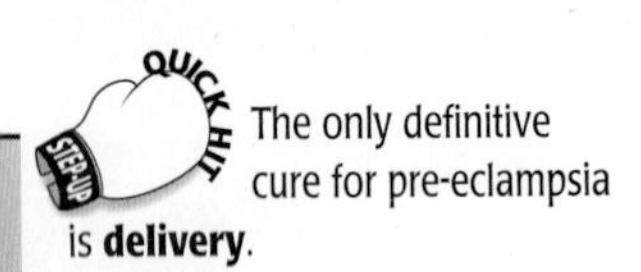

The only definitive cure for pre-eclampsia is **delivery**.

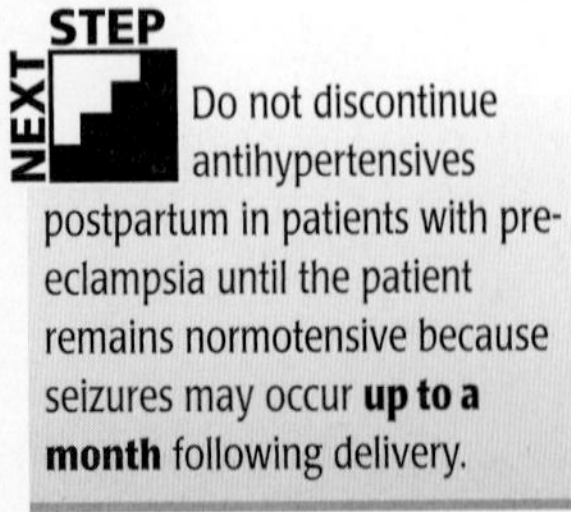

STEP NEXT: Do not discontinue antihypertensives postpartum in patients with pre-eclampsia until the patient remains normotensive because seizures may occur **up to a month** following delivery.

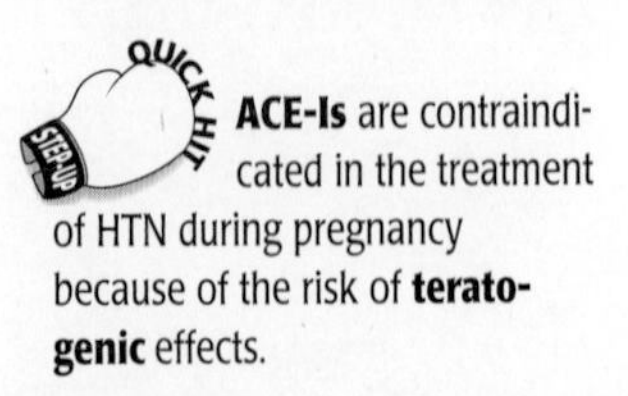

ACE-Is are contraindicated in the treatment of HTN during pregnancy because of the risk of **teratogenic** effects.

- The **recurrence** rate is 5% in patients with mild symptoms and up to 70% in patients with severe symptoms
- **Clues to the diagnosis:**
  - History: headaches, epigastric pain
  - Physical: HTN, hand edema
  - Tests: proteinuria, increased ALT and AST

- **Eclampsia**
  - The progression of pre-eclampsia, leading to **maternal seizures** that may be severe and fatal for both the mother and fetus if not treated promptly
  - **History:** similar to pre-eclampsia with the addition of **seizure activity**
  - **Physical examination:** similar to pre-eclampsia
  - **Tests:** similar to pre-eclampsia
  - **Treatment:**
    - **Delivery** is the definitive treatment, and the mother should be induced following the conclusion of any seizures and when she is medically stable
    - **Magnesium sulfate** with phenytoin (short-term use only) and diazepam as second-line agents should be used to control seizures
    - Supplemental oxygen should be supplied to the patient, and blood pressure should be carefully controlled
    - Magnesium sulfate and antihypertensives must be continued for at least 48 hours postpartum because **25% of seizures** occur within 24 hours following delivery
  - **Outcomes:**
    - The maternal and fetal mortality rates are 1% and 12%, respectively
    - There is up to a 70% risk of pre-eclampsia and 2% risk of eclampsia in future pregnancies
    - More than half of mothers who have eclampsia will have temporary neurologic deficits following seizures
  - **Why eliminated from differential:** the absence of seizures in this patient rules out this diagnosis

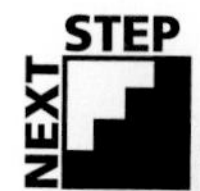

Patients with preexisting epilepsy who become pregnant should be treated with a **single** anticonvulsant, **valproic acid** and carbamazepine should be avoided because of the increased teratogenic risks, and supplemental **vitamin K** and **folate** should be administered to reduce the risk of teratogeny.

- **Hyperemesis gravidarum**
  - Severe persistent nausea and vomiting in pregnancy that leads to dehydration, weight loss, and electrolyte abnormalities
    - The cause is poorly understood but likely involves a combination of psychological, hormonal, and gastrointestinal factors
  - **History: persistent nausea and vomiting**, dizziness, fatigue
  - **Physical examination:** signs of dehydration (e.g., dry mucous membranes, decreased skin turgor, altered mental status) may be present
  - **Tests:**
    - UA will show the presence of ketones
    - Sodium, potassium, BUN, and creatinine abnormalities are common; ALT and AST are increased
    - Increased T_4 and decreased thyroid-stimulating hormone (TSH) are common
  - **Treatment:**
    - Eating small frequent meals and avoiding foods that are spicy or high in fat may decrease nausea
    - Adequate hydration must be maintained to avoid dehydration
    - Antiemetics (e.g., promethazine), antihistamines, and vitamin B_6 have been shown to improve symptoms in severe cases
    - IV correction of dangerous electrolyte abnormalities should be performed in an inpatient setting
  - **Outcomes:** complications include seizures, encephalopathy, renal failure, pancreatitis, and hepatic dysfunction; symptoms rarely last beyond the first trimester
  - **Why eliminated from differential:** the gestational age of the patient and the presence of significant HTN make this diagnosis unlikely

QUICK HIT

Although the **majority** of pregnant women have nausea and vomiting in the **first trimester**, it does not lead to the volume depletion and electrolyte abnormalities seen in hyperemesis gravidarum.

- **Abruptio placentae**
  - More thorough discussion in later case
  - **Why eliminated from differential:** the absence of vaginal bleeding and the appearance of the placenta on the US rule out this diagnosis

- **Migraine/tension headache**
  - More thorough discussion in Chapter 7
  - **Why eliminated from differential:** the presence of significant HTN and hand edema make these diagnosis less likely
- **Cerebral vascular accident**
  - More thorough discussion in Chapter 7
  - **Why eliminated from differential:** the normal neurologic examination reduces the concern for this diagnosis, and computed tomography (CT) should be avoided, if possible, during pregnancy; the development of more significant neurologic findings or worsening headaches would necessitate a more significant work-up

CASE 12-2 "I'm here for my normal prenatal appointment"

A 34-year-old woman, who is G4P2012 (i.e., four pregnancies, two deliveries, one spontaneous abortion, two living children), presents to her obstetrician at 26 weeks of gestation for a scheduled prenatal visit. All of her prenatal examinations and tests have been normal in her previous visits. The patient says that she has been doing relatively well. She says that she occasionally becomes fatigued. She denies any headaches, visual disturbances, numbness, or weakness. She says that the occasional nausea and vomiting that she had earlier in the pregnancy has completely resolved. She says that she feels minimally out of breath after prolonged walking but usually has no problems breathing. She reports urinating multiple times per day without any significant urgency. She has mild swelling in her feet and ankles after standing for prolonged periods of time. She walks two miles four times per week. She has continued to work as a producer for a local television news program without any difficulty other than occasional fatigue. She is taking prenatal vitamins and supplemental folate, calcium, and iron. She has no significant past medical history. She denies any substance use. On examination, she is a well-appearing woman in no distress. Her face is symmetrical and nonedematous. She has no lymphadenopathy. Auscultation of her heart and lungs detects normal breath sounds and a soft systolic murmur. Her abdomen is gravid and nontender with normal bowel sounds. A pelvic examination finds a closed cervical os, no cervical discharge, and no cervical or adnexal tenderness. Her fundal height is 26 cm, and fetal heart sounds are detectable with a Doppler. She has minimal edema in her feet. Her neurovascular examination is normal. The following vital signs are measured:

T: 98.7°F, HR: 87 bpm, BP: 105/70 mm Hg, RR: 17 breaths/min

Laboratory Data and Other Study Results

- Height and weight: 5′ 7″ 143 lb (initial weight 132 lb, BMI 20.7)
- UA: light yellow colored, pH: 7.4, specific gravity: 1.000, trace glucose, no ketones/nitrites/leukocyte esterase/hematuria/proteinuria
- 1-hour glucose tolerance test: 172 mg/dL

Following receipt of these results, the following test is ordered:

- 3-hour glucose tolerance test: fasting glucose: 127 mg/dL, 1-hour glucose: 173 mg/dL, 2-hour glucose: 159 mg/dL, 3-hour glucose: 147 mg/dL

Differential Diagnosis

- Gestational diabetes mellitus, preexisting diabetes mellitus

Diagnosis

- Gestational diabetes mellitus

Treatment Administered

- The patient was placed on a 2,400 kcal/day diet and encouraged to continue her exercise regimen

Follow-up

- Repeat glucose testing 1 week following initiation of the diet detected a fasting glucose of 113 mg/dL and a 1-hour postprandial glucose of 153 mg/dL
- A low-dose insulin regimen with daily self-monitoring of glucose levels was initiated
- Following the start of insulin therapy, the patient was able to maintain a fasting glucose of <90 mg/dL
- The patient's pregnancy proceeded with no further events, and she was able to have an uncomplicated vaginal delivery of a healthy child; her glucose levels remained normal off her insulin regimen following her recovery

Steps to the Diagnosis

- **Gestational diabetes mellitus**
  - **New onset** glucose intolerance that begins during pregnancy
  - **Risk factors:** family history of DM, older than 25 years, obesity, prior polyhydramnios, recurrent abortions, prior stillbirth, prior macrosomia, HTN, African or Pacific Islander heritage, corticosteroid use, polycystic ovary syndrome (PCOS)
  - **History:** usually asymptomatic
  - **Physical examination:** there are typically no significant physical findings for new onset DM
  - **Tests:** fasting glucose >126 mg/dL or an abnormal **1-hour glucose tolerance test** performed between 24 and 28 weeks of gestation; any abnormal 1-hour glucose tolerance test should indicate the need for a **3-hour glucose tolerance test** (Figure 12-3)
  - **Treatment:**
    - The initial treatments are directed at control through **diet** and **exercise**
      - Women with a prepregnant BMI of <22 should be placed on a 40 kcal/kg/day diet
      - Women with a prepregnant BMI of 22 to 27 should be placed on a 30 kcal/kg/day diet
      - Women with a pre-pregnant BMI of 27 to 29 should be placed on a 24 kcal/kg/day diet
      - Women with a pre-pregnant BMI of >29 should be placed on a 12 to 15 kcal/kg/day diet
    - Patients who continue to have abnormal fasting and 1-hour postprandial glucose levels 1 week after initiating the decreased caloric diet should be started on **insulin** therapy
    - Self-monitoring of glucose levels is prescribed to maintain tight control and to keep **fasting** levels below **90 mg/dL** and **1-hour postprandial** levels below **120 mg/dL**
    - Periodic fetal nonstress tests and US should be performed to assess fetal well-being
  - **Outcomes:**
    - Several complications of pregnancy are associated with gestational diabetes including polyhydramnios, pre-eclampsia, renal insufficiency, diabetic ketoacidosis (DKA), hyperosmolar hyperglycemic nonketotic coma (HHNC), retinopathy, fetal hypoglycemia, **macrosomia**, IUGR, neural tube defects, fetal cardiac defects, and intrauterine fetal demise
    - Macrosomia is associated with increased rates of birth trauma and cesarian delivery
    - Mothers who develop gestational DM are at an increased risk of developing nongestational DM later in life; 70% of women requiring insulin during pregnancy will develop DM during their lifetimes
    - Children from a pregnancy complicated by gestational DM are at a higher risk of being obese during childhood or adulthood
  - **Clues to the diagnosis:**
    - History: noncontributory (gestational DM is typically asymptomatic, and the patient's minor complaints are typical for pregnancy)
    - Physical: noncontributory
    - Tests: presence of glucose in the UA, results of both the 1-hour and 3-hour glucose tolerance tests

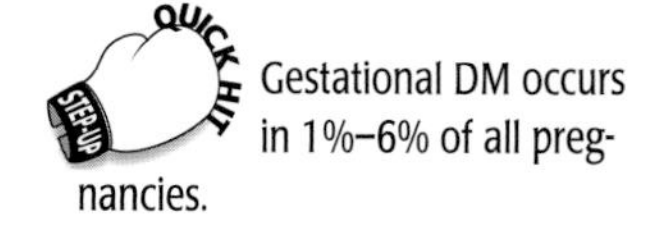

Gestational DM occurs in 1%–6% of all pregnancies.

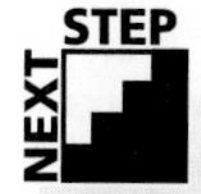

Continue glucose assessments after delivery because maternal glucose needs will change suddenly in patients with gestational DM and because it is uncertain if the mother will remain diabetic following delivery.

FIGURE 12-3 Screening for gestational diabetes mellitus performed at 24 to 28 weeks of gestation using the glucose tolerance tests.

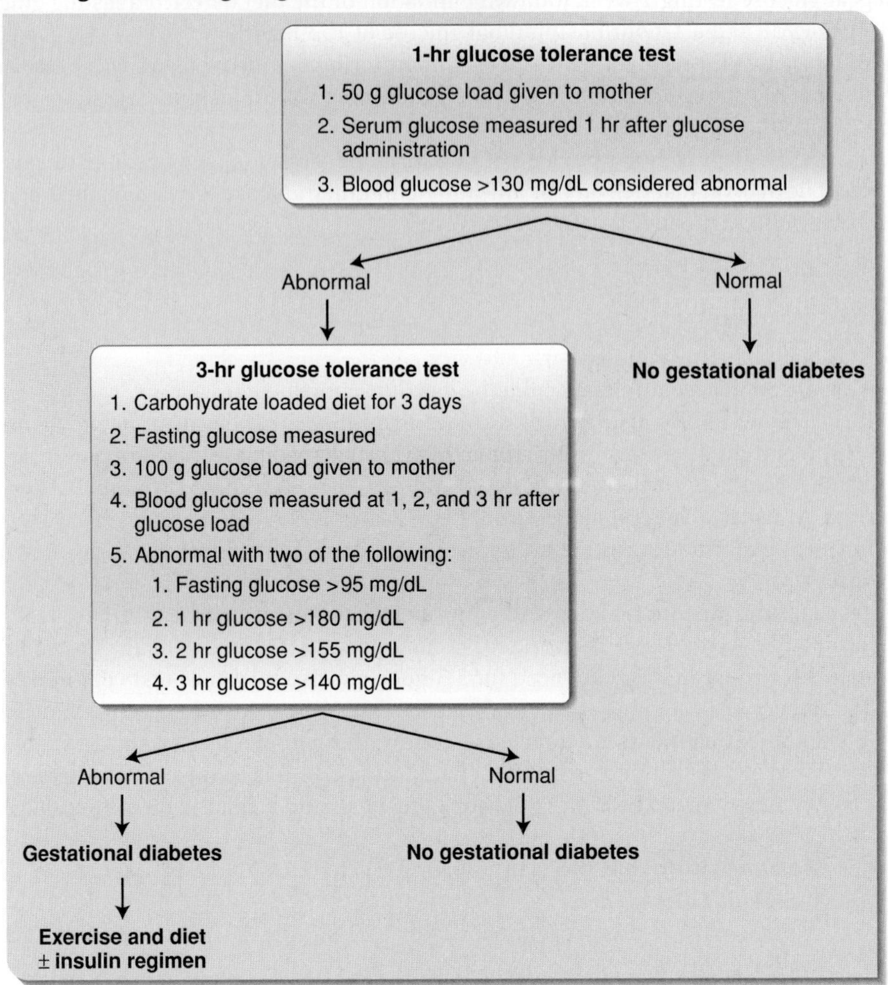

- **Diabetes mellitus (preexisting)**
  - More thorough discussion in Chapter 5
  - **Why eliminated from differential:** the absence of glucose intolerance in the patient's past medical history and the normal prior prenatal testing suggest that preexisting DM was not present in this patient

NEXT STEP Gestational DM occurs most frequently in the **second** or **third trimester**. If the mother presents with signs of DM earlier in pregnancy, suspect nongestational (type 1 or 2) DM.

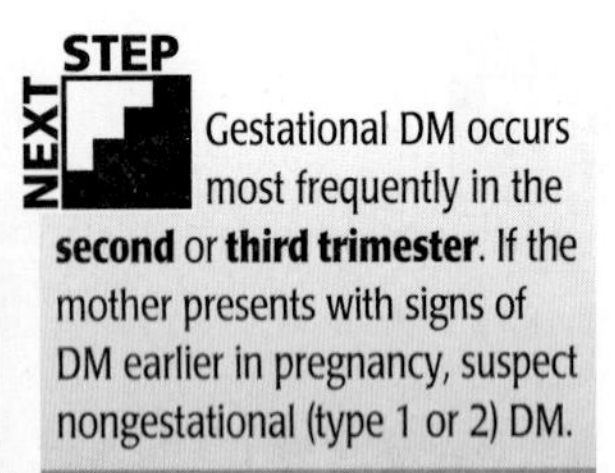

Insulin is used preferentially over the oral hypoglycemics during pregnancy because of the better safety profile.

CASE 12-3 "I'm pregnant and bleeding"

A 31-year-old woman who is G3P1011 presents to an emergency department at 35 weeks of gestation with the complaint of vaginal bleeding. She says that she noticed the bleeding earlier in the day and denies any bleeding prior to this time. She says that the bleeding has been light and she has only worn one absorbent pad today to absorb the blood. She reports mild-to-moderate abdominal pain and pelvic cramping. The pain radiates into her lower back. She denies any nonbloody vaginal discharge or seeing any expelled clots or tissue. She says that she tripped over a cat and fell down two stairs last evening but did not feel any abdominal pain or notice any bleeding until this morning. She denies any nausea, vomiting, diarrhea, dizziness, or shortness of breath. Although she feels crampy, she also says that she feels like she is having uterine contractions. She has not noticed much movement by the fetus since this morning. She says that she had a spontaneous abortion at 12 weeks of gestation during her last pregnancy for an unknown reason. Her first pregnancy was uncomplicated, and she delivered vaginally at 40 weeks of gestation. She has a history of chronic low back pain. She currently takes prenatal vitamins and no other medications. She admits that she smokes one to two cigarettes per day. She denies any alcohol or illicit drug use. On examination, she is an anxious-appearing pregnant woman. Auscultation of her heart and lungs detects normal breath sounds and a soft systolic murmur. Her abdomen is gravid and mildly tender in the lower portion. Lower abdominal palpation detects a firm uterus. She has normal bowel sounds. A pelvic speculum examination detects a small amount of blood at her cervical os, which is nearly closed. A bimanual examination is not performed. Her fundal height is 33 cm, and fetal heart sounds are detected with a Doppler. The following vital signs are measured:

T: 98.8°F, HR: 98 bpm, BP: 124/72 mm Hg, RR: 17 breaths/min

Differential Diagnosis

- Abruptio placentae, placenta previa, spontaneous abortion, ectopic pregnancy, preterm labor, pre-eclampsia, appendicitis, hydatidiform mole, choriocarcinoma

Laboratory Data and Other Study Results

- CBC: WBC: 8.9, Hgb: 12.3, Plt: 231
- Chem7: Na: 141 mEq/L, K: 3.9 mEq/L, Cl: 100 mEq/L, CO_2: 26 mEq/L, BUN: 16 mg/dL, Cr: 0.8 mg/dL, Glu: 91 mg/dL
- Coagulation panel (Coags): protime (PT) 12.1 sec, international normalized ratio (INR): 1.0, partial thromboplastin time (PTT): 27.2 sec
- Serum β-hCG: 74,318 U/L
- Biophysical profile: score of 6 (fetal tone criteria and fetal movement not satisfied); placental implantation on the upper posterior wall of the uterus seen on US; small hyperechoic signal adjacent to the placenta consistent with hemorrhage seen on US; single fetus visualized with no abnormal appearance of the ovaries or fallopian tubes

Diagnosis

- Abruptio placentae

Treatment Administered

- The patient was admitted to the labor and delivery floor and placed on modified bedrest
- Constant maternal and fetal monitoring was initiated
- IV fluids were started to maintain maternal intravenous volume
- Magnesium sulfate was administered to prevent further contractions

Follow-up

- Under monitoring, the fetal heart rate remained stable, as did maternal hemodynamic monitoring
- A repeat biophysical profile 12 hours later was found to have a score of 8 (fetal tone criteria not met)
- The lecithin/sphingomyelin ratio of the amniotic fluid was measured and found to be consistent with fetal lung maturity; the decision was made to proceed with delivery
- Magnesium sulfate was stopped, and the patient rapidly entered labor
- Both the mother and the fetus remained stable during labor, and an uncomplicated vaginal delivery was performed

Steps to the Diagnosis

- **Abruptio placentae**
  - Premature separation of the placenta from the uterine wall, leading to **maternal hemorrhage**

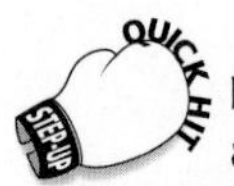

Placenta previa and **abruptio placentae** are the most common causes of vaginal bleeding **after 20 weeks** gestation. Bleeding in **placenta previa** is **painless**, and bleeding in **abruptio placentae** is **painful**.

MNEMONIC

Causes of abdominal pain during pregnancy may be remembered by the mnemonic **CRUEL CRAMP**: **C**onstipation, **R**ound ligament stretching, **U**TI, **E**ctopic pregnancy, **L**abor (preterm or term), **C**holestasis, **R**upture (ectopic or uterine), **A**bruptio placentae, **M**iscarriage, **P**re-eclampsia.

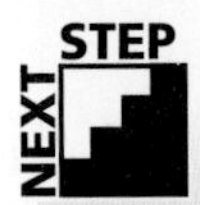

Delivery should be delayed until at least **34 weeks of gestation** if the mother and fetus remain stable during abruptio placentae.

- **Risk factors:** HTN, prior abruptio placentae, trauma, tobacco use, cocaine use, PROM, multiple gestations, multiparity
- **History: painful** vaginal bleeding in the **third** trimester, **abdominal pain** radiating to the back, **uterine contractions, decreased fetal activity**
- **Physical examination:** pelvic and abdominal tenderness, **increased uterine tone**, possible maternal HTN, and increased fundal height with significant hemorrhage
- **Tests:**
  - Decreased hemoglobin and fibrinogen and increased PT, INR, and PTT are seen with significant hemorrhage
  - Abdominal US **inconsistently** shows separation of the placenta from the uterus; it may also show a **maternal hemorrhage**
  - A biophysical profile is important to assess fetal well-being
- **Treatment:**
  - Mild cases with stable maternal hemodynamics and fetal assessments may be treated with **modified bedrest** (i.e., bedrest except for bathroom privileges and necessary mobilization) and close maternal and fetal monitoring
  - Delivery typically proceeds rapidly due to uterine irritation
  - Delivery may be delayed using tocolytic therapy (e.g., magnesium sulfate) in cases in which greater fetal maturity is desired
  - **Cesarian delivery** is indicated in cases of **maternal hemodynamic instability** or **fetal distress**
- **Outcomes:**
  - Potential complications include DIC, severe maternal hemorrhage, maternal or fetal death, and the need for a hysterectomy to control uterine bleeding
  - The fetal mortality rate is 12%
  - The risk of abruptio placentae in future pregnancies is 12%
- **Clues to the diagnosis:**
  - History: painful uterine bleeding in the third trimester, uterine contractions, recent trauma, tobacco use
  - Physical: abdominal tenderness, uterine bleeding, uterine firmness
  - Tests: abdominal US results

- **Placenta previa**
  - Implantation of the placenta **near the cervical os**
    - Frequently associated with uterine bleeding during pregnancy
    - **Variations** (Figure 12-4)
      - **Low implantation:** the placenta implants in the lower uterus but does not infringe upon the cervical os until full dilation occurs during labor
      - **Partial** placenta previa: the placenta partially covers the cervical os
      - **Complete** placenta previa: the placenta completely covers the cervical os
  - **Risk factors:** multiparity, maternal age >30 years, prior placenta previa, multiple gestations, uterine fibroids, prior abortion, **tobacco use**
  - **History: painless** vaginal bleeding in the **third** trimester
  - **Physical examination:** speculum examination detects bleeding from the cervical os
  - **Tests:** US is performed to determine the location of the placenta (transvaginal is most accurate)
  - **Treatment:**
    - Mild, periodic bleeding should be treated with modified bedrest
    - Active bleeding requires an inpatient admission for maternal and fetal monitoring
    - Delivery by **cesarian section** should be performed once fetal lung maturity has occurred
    - **Tocolytics** (e.g., magnesium sulfate, ritodrine, terbutaline, indomethacin, nifedipine) may be used to delay delivery and to reduce the maternal bleeding risk in cases of a preterm fetus with **immature lungs** and **mild maternal bleeding**
    - Vaginal delivery may be attempted in cases of a **low-lying placenta**
  - **Outcomes:**
    - Potential complications include severe maternal hemorrhage, IUGR, malpresentation, PROM, and vasa previa (i.e., fetal vessels overlying the cervical os)

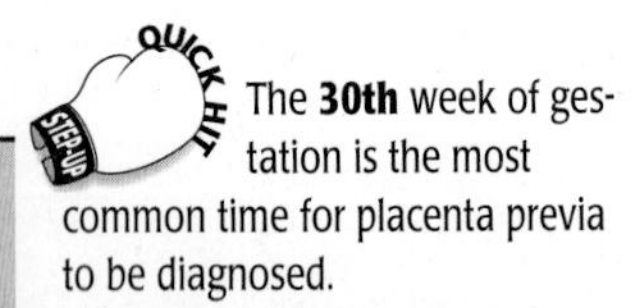

The **30th** week of gestation is the most common time for placenta previa to be diagnosed.

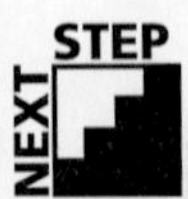

Do not perform a **manual** vaginal examination in a pregnant patient with vaginal bleeding until placenta previa can be ruled out with an US; manual examination increases the risk of inducing **greater hemorrhage**.

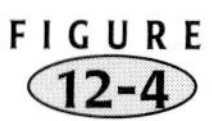

FIGURE 12-4 **Uterine profiles and cross-sections demonstrating normal placental implantation and examples of low-lying placental implantation, partial placenta previa, and complete placenta previa.**

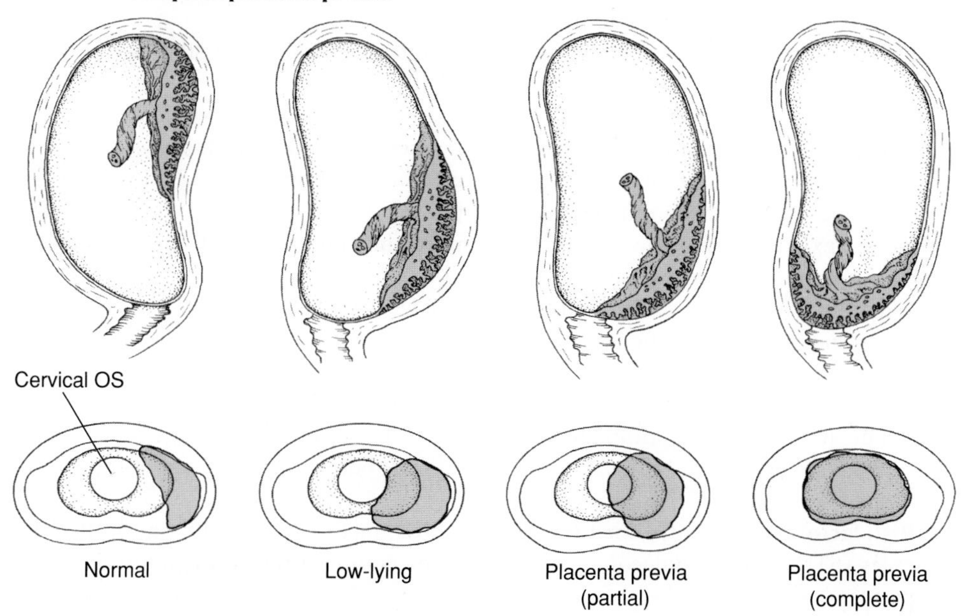

(Taken from *OB-GYN scenes and procedures.* LifeART Nursing Collection, with permission.)

- Preterm delivery occurs in 50% of patients
- Fetal mortality occurs in 3% of cases; maternal mortality occurs in <0.5% of cases
- **Why eliminated from differential:** the painful nature of the bleeding and the location of the placenta indicated by the US rule out this diagnosis

- **Spontaneous abortion (a.k.a. miscarriage)**
  - **Nonelective** termination of a pregnancy prior to **20 weeks** of gestation (Table 12-11)
    - **First trimester** spontaneous abortions are usually due to **fetal chromosomal abnormalities**
    - **Second trimester** spontaneous abortions are usually due to infection, **cervical incompetence, uterine abnormalities**, hypercoagulable states, poor maternal health, or **drug use**

QUICK HIT: Spontaneous abortions occur in up to 25% of pregnancies.

MNEMONIC

Causes of recurrent spontaneous abortion may be remembered by the mnemonic **CUPID'S SIGHT**: **C**oagulopathy, **U**terine issues (fibroids, cervical incompetence), **P**COS, **I**mmunologic causes, **D**M, **S**ubstance use (tobacco, alcohol), **S**tress, **I**nfection, **G**enetic issues (chromosome abnormalities), **H**yperprolactinemia, **T**hyroid disorder.

TABLE 12-11 Types of Spontaneous Abortions

Abortion Type	Threatened	Inevitable	Incomplete	Complete	Missed
SIGN/SYMPTOMS					
Uterine bleeding	In the initial 20 weeks of gestation	Initial 20 weeks plus pain	Initial 20 weeks	Initial 20 weeks	Present or with pain
Cervical os	Closed	Open	Open	Open	Closed
Uterine contents expelled	None	None	Some	All	None
DIAGNOSIS	US detects viable fetus	Possible detection of fetus by US	Based on history of expelled products of conception	Based on history of expelled products of conception	US detects nonviable intrauterine fetus
TREATMENT	Bedrest, limited activity	Misoprostol or D&C to remove uterine contents	Misoprostol or D&C	None	Misoprostol or D&C

D&C, dilation and curettage; US, ultrasound.

- **Risk factors: increased maternal age**, multiparity, **uterine abnormalities**, **tobacco use**, alcohol use, nonsteroidal anti-inflammatory drugs (NSAIDs), cocaine, caffeine, low folate levels, and congenital infections
- **History**: abdominal pain, crampy vaginal bleeding
- **Physical examination**: visualization of blood at the cervical os, possible open cervical os, possible abdominal tenderness
- **Tests**: β-hCG levels may be used to determine fetal viability and estimate the gestational age; US is used to detect a fetus and to assess viability (via a biophysical profile)
- **Treatment**: dependent on the type of spontaneous abortion (Table 12-11)
- **Outcomes**: fetal demise is inevitable in all but threatened abortions; unless other risk factors exist, patients should not have any further increased risk for spontaneous abortion in future pregnancies
- **Why eliminated from differential**: the time of gestation is beyond what is considered consistent with a spontaneous abortion

QUICK HIT: The most common causes of vaginal bleeding in **early** pregnancy are **ectopic pregnancy**, threatened or inevitable **spontaneous abortion**, **physiologic** bleeding (related to implantation), and **uterine-cervical pathology**.

- **Ectopic pregnancy**
  - Implantation of a fertilized ovum **outside** of the uterus
    - The **ampulla** of the **fallopian tube** is the most common location of implantation (95% of cases), but the ovary, cervix, and the abdominal cavity are also potential sites
  - **Risk factors: pelvic inflammatory disease (PID)**, history of sexually transmitted diseases (STDs), prior gynecologic surgery, **prior ectopic pregnancy**, multiple sexual partners, tobacco use
  - **History**:
    - **Abdominal pain**, nausea, amenorrhea or known pregnancy, mild vaginal bleeding
    - Abdominal pain becomes severe if rupture occurs
  - **Physical examination**:
    - Abdominal tenderness, visualized vaginal bleeding, possible palpable pelvis mass
    - Abdominal guarding, rebound tenderness, hypotension, and tachycardia develop if rupture occurs
  - **Tests**:
    - **Elevated β-hCG** in the presence of an US that is **unable** to locate an **intrauterine** pregnancy
      - β-hCG for an intrauterine pregnancy should double every 48 hours, so a β-hCG level that is low for the time of gestation should raise the suspicion for an ectopic pregnancy
    - Transabdominal and transvaginal US should be able to visualize a pregnancy once the β-hCG reaches 6,500 mIU/mL and 1,500 mIU/mL, respectively
  - **Treatment**: an unruptured ectopic pregnancy of **<6 weeks** duration is treated with methotrexate to induce an abortion; longer term or ruptured ectopic pregnancies require **surgical excision** with an attempt to preserve the fallopian tube
  - **Outcomes**: complications include inevitable fetal death, severe maternal hemorrhage, increased risk of future ectopic pregnancies, infertility, Rh (rhesus factor) sensitization, and maternal death; the risk of future ectopic pregnancy is up to 25%
  - **Why eliminated from differential**: based on the US findings and despite the small possibility of multiple gestations with one gestation being ectopic, it is much more likely that the patient has a single pregnancy complicated by abruption

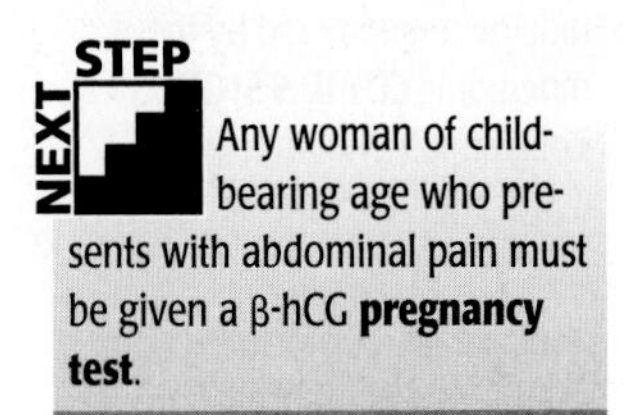
Any woman of childbearing age who presents with abdominal pain must be given a β-hCG **pregnancy test**.

- **Preterm labor**
  - Onset of labor before 37 weeks of gestation
  - **Risk factors: multiple gestation**, infection of genital tract, **PROM**, placenta previa, abruptio placentae, previous preterm labor, polyhydramnios, cervical incompetence, poor nutrition, stressful environment, tobacco use, substance abuse, lower socioeconomic status
  - **History**: low back pain, abdominal cramping, more than eight uterine contractions per hour
  - **Physical examination**: cervical dilation and effacement prior to 37 weeks of gestation
  - **Tests**: US may be helpful to assess the cervical length, amniotic fluid volume, fetal well-being, and to verify gestational age

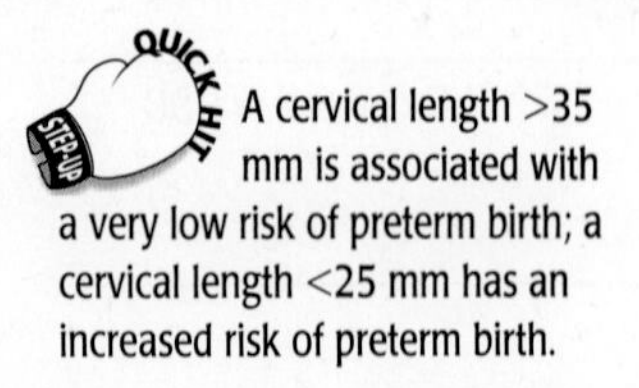
A cervical length >35 mm is associated with a very low risk of preterm birth; a cervical length <25 mm has an increased risk of preterm birth.

- Treatment:
  - Patients should be supplied with adequate hydration and restricted in their activity
  - **Tocolytics** can be used to inhibit contractions and delay delivery if the patient is at <34 weeks of gestation
  - Corticosteroids may be given to the mother to **hasten fetal lung maturity** if the pregnancy is at <34 weeks of gestation
  - Antibiotics should be given for group B streptococcus prophylaxis or if there is evidence of an active infection
  - Expectant management may proceed once the pregnancy has reached 34 weeks
- **Outcomes:** the rates of fetal demise, fetal sepsis, respiratory distress of the newborn, and necrotizing enterocolitis increase with the degree of prematurity before 34 weeks
- **Why eliminated from differential:** although the patient is at only at 35 weeks of gestation, the presence of vaginal bleeding and the US appearance signify that preterm labor is not a complete explanation for the current presentation and that there is an underlying etiology

- **Pre-eclampsia**
  - More thorough discussion in prior case
  - **Why eliminated from differential:** the normal maternal blood pressure rules out this diagnosis
- **Appendicitis**
  - More thorough discussion in Chapter 3
  - **Why eliminated from differential:** this diagnosis is unlikely because it would not account for the vaginal bleeding
- **Hydatidiform mole**
  - A **benign** neoplasm of **trophoblastic** cells (i.e., placental cells) that carries a risk of malignant transformation
    - Types:
      - **Complete:** 46,XX genotype; completely derived from the father (i.e., an empty egg is penetrated by sperm)
      - **Incomplete:** 69,XXY genotype; fertilization of an egg by two sperm simultaneously
  - **Risk factors:** low socioeconomic status, age >40 years during pregnancy, prior molar pregnancy, Asian heritage, tobacco use
  - **History:** heavy or irregular painless vaginal bleeding during the **first** or **second** trimester of a suspected pregnancy, severe nausea and vomiting, dizziness, anxiety
  - **Physical examination:** large fundal height for gestational age, expulsion of **"grape-like" vesicles** from the vagina, no detectable fetal movement or heart tones
  - **Tests:** β-hCG is higher than expected for the gestational age; US detects a **"snow storm"** pattern in the uterus without the presence of a gestational sac (Figure 12-5)

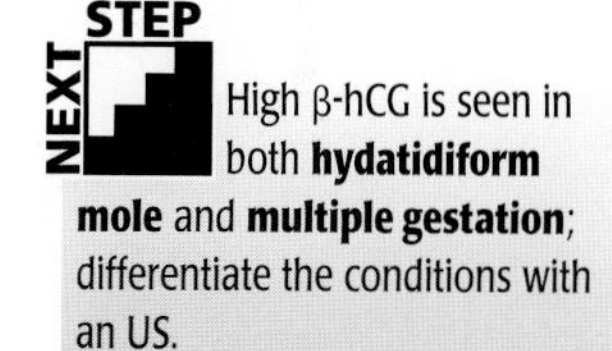

High β-hCG is seen in both **hydatidiform mole** and **multiple gestation**; differentiate the conditions with an US.

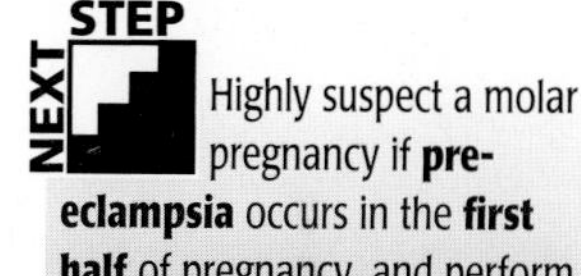

Highly suspect a molar pregnancy if **pre-eclampsia** occurs in the **first half** of pregnancy, and perform an US to confirm the diagnosis.

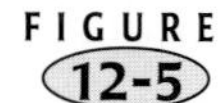

Ultrasound of the uterus demonstrating the "snow storm" appearance consistent with a hydatidiform mole.

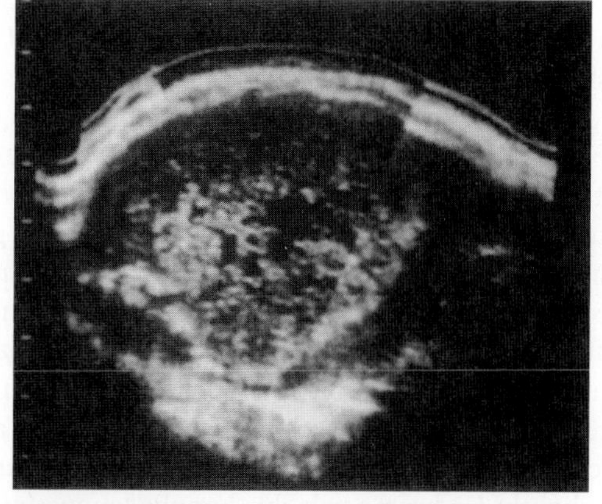

(Taken from Beckmann CRB, Ling FW, Laube DW, et al. *Obstetrics and gynecology*. 4th ed. Baltimore: Lippincott Williams & Wilkins, 2002. Fig. 42.2. With permission of Lippincott Williams & Wilkins.)

- **Treatment:**
  - **Dilation and curettage** is performed to remove the neoplasm
  - Pregnancy should be avoided for 6 months to a year to avoid recurrences
  - **β-hCG** levels should be followed for a year to confirm a decreasing level
- **Outcomes:** a malignant trophoblastic neoplasm develops in 20% of cases but carries an excellent prognosis
- **Why eliminated from differential:** the appearance of the US rules out this diagnosis

- Choriocarcinoma
  - A malignant trophoblastic neoplasm that arises from hydatidiform moles (in 50% of cases) or following a spontaneous abortion, ectopic pregnancy, or normal pregnancy
  - **History:** vaginal bleeding, hemoptysis, dyspnea, headache, dizziness, rectal bleeding
  - **Physical examination:** enlarged uterus, visualized bleeding from the cervical os
  - **Tests:**
    - Increased β-hCG (usually >100,000 U/L)
    - US will detect a uterine mass with a mix of hemorrhagic and necrotic areas and possible parametrial invasion
    - CT is useful to detect metastases
  - **Treatment:**
    - Chemotherapy is administered routinely
    - Pregnancy should be avoided for a year to avoid recurrences
    - **β-hCG** levels should be followed for a year to confirm a decreasing level
    - **Hysterectomy** is performed in women older than 40 years if the disease is limited to the uterus
  - **Outcomes:** potential sites of metastases include the lungs, brain, liver, kidneys, and gastrointestinal tract; the prognosis is good in the absence of brain or liver metastases
  - **Why eliminated from differential:** although the US in this case and that for this diagnosis may be similar appearing, the β-hCG is not consistent with choriocarcinoma

CASE 12-4 "My baby's not right"

A 6-day-old neonate boy is a patient in the neonatal intensive care unit (NICU) after developing respiratory distress. His mother is a 16-year-old girl who received no prenatal care. She says that she was trying to hide the fact that she was pregnant from other people. She says that she has had multiple sexual partners and is unsure who is the father of the child. She denies any previous pregnancies. She says that she was treated for a *Neisseria gonorrhoeae* infection 1 year ago but denies any other past medical history. She denies any medication or substance use. She says that she has a family history of HTN and DM. Dating based on the mother's last menstrual period estimates that the pregnancy was at 37 weeks of gestation at the time of delivery. The child was delivered via an uncomplicated vaginal delivery. Apgar scores were 5 at 1 minute and 9 at 5 minutes. No meconium was visible at the time of delivery. Initially, the neonate appeared to be doing well. The child's mother says that she was unsuccessful in breast feeding him and that any attempts made him cry. Attempts to formula feed the child were also unsuccessful in all but a couple of attempts. He had two nonbloody bowel movements after eating. Because of the child's poor feeding, he was kept as an inpatient when his mother was discharged on the second day following the delivery. On the fourth day after his birth the child experienced a grand mal seizure and exhibited respiratory distress. He was urgently intubated and transferred to the NICU. This morning he was weaned from the ventilator and extubated but has remained lethargic, despite receiving IV fluids and parenteral nutrition. No additional seizures have been witnessed. On examination, the child is an ill-appearing neonate with little spontaneous activity. He is mildly jaundiced. His right eye conjunctiva is inflamed and there is a cluster of small blisters at the corner of the eye. A few similar vesicles are seen on his scalp. His fontanelles are bulging slightly. He has no palpable lymphadenopathy. Auscultation of his lungs detects mild rhonchi. Auscultation of his heart detects no abnormal heart sounds.

His abdomen is soft with few bowel sounds. He has little spontaneous movement but withdraws and grimaces to pinching. The following vital signs are measured:

T: 98.5°F, HR: 153 bpm, BP: 65/45 mm Hg, RR: 31 breaths/min
(Normal for neonate: HR: 100–170 bpm, BP: 65–95/30–60, RR: 30–50 breaths/min)

Differential Diagnosis

- Hemolytic disease of the newborn, congenital infection, maternal substance use during pregnancy, necrotizing enterocolitis, congenital heart disease, meconium aspiration syndrome

Laboratory Data and Other Study Results

- CBC: WBC: 12.5, Hgb: 19.5, Plt: 97
- Neonatal blood type: A+
- Maternal blood type: A+
- Chem7: Na: 138 mEq/L, K: 4.3 mEq/L, Cl: 100 mEq/L, CO_2: 28 mEq/L, BUN: 12 mg/dL, Cr: 0.6 mg/dL, Glu: 79 mg/dL
- LFTs: AlkPhos: 178 U/L, ALT: 121 U/L, AST: 156 U/L, TBili: 10 mg/dL, DBili: 0.2 mg/dL
- Chest x-ray (CXR): mild diffuse infiltrates; normal lung size; no focal lesions or effusions; no fractures
- Abdominal x-ray (AXR): sparse bowel air; no air-fluid levels; no apparent organomegaly
- Head CT: increased signal in both temporal lobes with associated edema; mild to moderate ventricular compression; no focal masses
- Echocardiogram: normal blood flow and chamber size; normal valve, vessel, and chamber anatomy
- Lumbar puncture: cloudy appearance, opening pressure 89 mm Hg, WBC: 37/μL, Glu: 45 mg/dL, protein: 60 mg/dL
- Neonatal cytomegalovirus (CMV) IgM: negative
- Neonatal varicella IgM: negative
- Maternal human immunodeficiency virus (HIV) enzyme-linked immunosorbent assay (ELISA): negative
- Maternal herpes simplex virus (HSV)-1 and -2 antibodies: positive HSV-2 antibodies
- Maternal rapid plasma reagin (RPR): negative
- Maternal urine toxicology screen: negative
- Maternal group B streptococcus antigen: negative
- Maternal *N. gonorrhoeae* and *Chlamydia trachomatis* immunoassays: negative
- Maternal rubella IgM antibodies: negative
- Maternal rubeola IgM antibodies: negative

The following confirmatory tests are ordered:

- Tzanck smear of neonatal vesicles: multinucleated giant cells
- Neonatal cerebral spinal fluid (CSF) HSV-2 polymerase chain reaction (PCR): positive

Diagnosis

- Neonatal herpes simplex-2 infection with encephalopathy

Treatment Administered

- Acyclovir was started in the neonate
- Parenteral feeding and supportive measures were continued

Follow-up

- Despite the administration of acyclovir, the neonate experienced an additional seizure on the eighth day of life but did not experience respiratory distress

TABLE 12-12 Congenital Infections and Their Effects on the Fetus and Neonates

Maternal Infection	Possible Fetal/ Neonatal Effects	Diagnosis	Treatment
Cytomegalovirus	IUGR, chorioretinitis, **CNS abnormalities**, mental retardation, vision abnormalities, deafness, hydrocephalus, seizures, hepatosplenomegaly	• Possible mononucleosislike illness • IgM antibody screening or PCR of viral DNA within first few weeks of life	• No treatment if infection develops during pregnancy • Ganciclovir may decrease effects in neonates • **Good hygiene** reduces risk of transmission
Gonorrhea/ chlamydia	Increased risk of spontaneous abortion; neonatal sepsis, **conjunctivitis**	• Cervical culture and immunoassays	• Erythromycin given to mother or neonate
Group B streptococcus	Respiratory distress, pneumonia, **meningitis,** sepsis	• Antigen screening after 34 weeks gestation	• IV β-lactams or clindamycin during labor or in infected neonates
Hepatitis B	Increased risk of prematurity and IUGR; increased risk of neonatal death if acute disease develops	• Prenatal surface antigen screening	• Maternal **vaccination**; vaccination of neonate and administration of immune globulin shortly after birth
Herpes simplex	Increased risk of prematurity, IUGR, and spontaneous abortion; high risk of **neonatal death** or **CNS abnormalities** if disease transmission occurs	• Clinical diagnosis confirmed with viral culture or immunoassays	• Delivery by **cesarean section** to avoid disease transmission if active lesions present or if primary outbreak • Acyclovir may be beneficial in neonates
HIV	Viral transmission in utero (5% risk), **rapid progression** of disease to AIDS	• Early prenatal maternal blood screening (consent required)	• **AZT** significantly reduces vertical transmission risk • Continue prescribed antiviral regimen but avoid efavirenz, didanosine, stavudine, and nevirapine
Rubella	Increased risk of spontaneous abortion, skin lesions ("**blueberry muffin baby**"), **congenital rubella syndrome** (i.e., IUGR, deafness, cardiovascular abnormalities, vision abnormalities, CNS abnormalities, hepatitis) if disease transmission occurs	• Early prenatal IgG screening	• Mother should be immunized before attempting to become pregnant • No treatment if infection develops during pregnancy • No proven benefit from rubella immune globulin
Rubeola (measles)	Increased risk of prematurity, IUGR, and spontaneous abortion; **high risk** (20% if term birth, 55% if preterm) **of neonatal death** if disease transmission occurs	• Clinical diagnosis in mother confirmed by IgM or IgG antibodies after rash develops	• Mother should be immunized before attempting to become pregnant • Immune serum globulin given to mother if infection develops during pregnancy
Syphilis	Neonatal anemia, deafness, hepatosplenomegaly, pneumonia, hepatitis, osteodystrophy; 25% neonatal mortality	• Early prenatal RPR or VDRL	• Maternal or neonatal penicillin
Toxoplasmosis	Hydrocephalus, intracranial calcifications, chorioretinitis, microcephaly, spontaneous abortion, seizures	• Possible mononucleosislike illness • Amniotic fluid PCR for *Toxoplasma gondii* or serum antibody screening may be helpful for the diagnosis	• Pyrimethamine, sulfadiazine, and folinic acid • Mother should avoid gardening, raw meat, cat litter boxes, and unpasteurized milk
Varicella zoster	Prematurity, **encephalitis**, **pneumonia**, IUGR, **CNS abnormalities**, limb abnormalities, blindness; high risk of neonatal death if birth occurs during active infection	• IgG titer screening in women with **no known history of disease** • IgM and IgG antibody titers can confirm diagnosis in neonates	• Varicella immune globulin given to nonimmune mother within 96 hours of exposure and to neonate if born during active infection • Vaccine is contraindicated during pregnancy (live attenuated virus carries risk of fetal infection)

AIDS, acquired immune deficiency syndrome; AZT, zidovudine; CNS, central nervous system; Ig, immunoglobulin; IUGR, intrauterine growth restriction; IV, intravenous; PCR, polymerase chain reaction; RPR, rapid plasma reagin; VDRL, Venereal Disease Research Laboratories.

- The neonate entered status epilepticus the following day and subsequent cardiopulmonary collapse; despite resuscitative efforts, he was unable to be revived

Steps to the Diagnosis

- **Congenital infections**
  - Maternal infections during pregnancy that can have significant deleterious effects on fetal development or viability (Table 12-12)
  - **History:** the mother may exhibit findings consistent with each disease, neonatal symptoms and findings are also disease dependent
  - **Physical examination:** disease dependent (Table 12-12)
  - **Tests: prenatal screening** is vital to the early detection of these infections; diagnostic tests following delivery are disease dependent (Table 12-12)
  - **Treatment:** frequently maternal therapies are available to prevent fetal infection or to reduce the severity of the disease effects; treatment of infected neonates is disease dependent (Table 12-12)
  - **Outcomes:** generally these infections carry **significant long-term sequelae** that may result in life-long disabilities and a decreased lifespan (Table 12-12)
  - **Clues to the diagnosis:**
    - History: lack of prenatal care, previous maternal STD infection, poor feeding, child lethargy, neonatal seizures, respiratory distress
    - Physical: lethargy, jaundice, bulging fontanelles, vesicles on scalp and near eye, conjunctivitis
    - Tests: CSF analysis consistent with infection, positive HSV serology, head CT appearance
- **Maternal substance use during pregnancy**
  - Several **medicinal** and **illicit** substances carry **teratogenic** risks during pregnancy (Tables 12-13 and 12-14)
  - **History:** the mother should be able to provide a list of any medications that she is taking
  - **Physical examination:** dependent on the abnormalities caused by the substance

MNEMONIC

Congenital infections are frequently referred to as the **TORCHS** infections: **T**oxoplasmosis, **O**ther (varicella-zoster, group B streptococcus, *Chlamydia*, *Neisseria*), **R**ubella/Rubeola, **C**ytomegalovirus, **H**erpes simplex/Hepatitis B/HIV, **S**yphilis.

TABLE 12-13 Recreational Drug Use and Associated Risks to Mother and Fetus during Pregnancy

Drug	Maternal Risks	Fetal Risks
Cocaine	**Arrhythmia**, myocardial infarction, subarachnoid hemorrhage, seizures, stroke, abruptio placentae	IUGR, prematurity, facial abnormalities, delayed intellectual development, **stroke**
Ethanol	Minimal	**Fetal alcohol syndrome** (i.e., mental retardation, IUGR, sensory and motor neuropathy, facial abnormalities), spontaneous abortion, intrauterine fetal demise
Hallucinogens	Personal endangerment (poor decision-making)	Possible developmental delays
Marijuana	Minimal	IUGR, prematurity
Opioids	**Infection** (from needles), narcotic withdrawal, premature rupture of membranes	Prematurity, IUGR, meconium aspiration, neonatal infections, **narcotic withdrawal** (may be fatal)
Stimulants	Lack of appetite and **malnutrition**, arrhythmia, withdrawal depression, HTN	IUGR, congenital heart defects, cleft palate
Tobacco	**Abruptio placentae**, **placenta previa**, premature rupture of membranes	Spontaneous abortion, prematurity, **IUGR**, intrauterine fetal demise, impaired intellectual development, higher risk of neonatal respiratory infections

HTN, hypertension; IUGR, intrauterine growth restriction.

TABLE 12-14 Common Medications that Carry Teratogenic Risks

Medication	Teratogenic Risks
ACE-I	Renal abnormalities, decreased skull ossification
Aminoglycosides	CN VIII damage, skeletal abnormalities, renal defects
Carbamazepine	Facial abnormalities, IUGR, mental retardation, cardiovascular abnormalities, neural tube defects
Chemotherapeutics (all drug classes)	Intrauterine fetal demise (approximately 30% of pregnancies), severe IUGR, multiple anatomical abnormalities (e.g., palate, bones, limbs, genitals, etc.), mental retardation, spontaneous abortion, secondary neoplasms
Diazepam	Cleft palate, renal defects, secondary neoplasms
Diethylstilbestrol	Vaginal and cervical cancer later in life (e.g., adenocarcinoma)
Fluoroquinolones	Cartilage abnormalities
Heparin	Prematurity, intrauterine fetal demise; considered much safer than warfarin
Iodide	Goiter, hypothyroidism, mental retardation
OCPs	Spontaneous abortion, ectopic pregnancy
Phenobarbital	Neonatal withdrawal
Phenytoin	Facial abnormalities, IUGR, mental retardation, cardiovascular abnormalities
Retinoids	CNS abnormalities, cardiovascular abnormalities, facial abnormalities, spontaneous abortion
Sulfonamides	Kernicterus (i.e., bile infiltration of brain)
Tetracycline	Skeletal abnormalities, limb abnormalities, teeth discoloration
Thalidomide	Limb abnormalities
Valproic acid	Neural tube defects (approximately 1% of pregnancies), facial abnormalities, cardiovascular abnormalities, skeletal abnormalities
Warfarin	Spontaneous abortion, IUGR, CNS abnormalities, facial abnormalities, mental retardation, Dandy-Walker malformation

ACE-I, angiotensin converting enzyme inhibitors; CN, cranial nerve; CNS, central nervous system; IUGR, intrauterine growth restriction; OCPs, oral contraceptive pills.

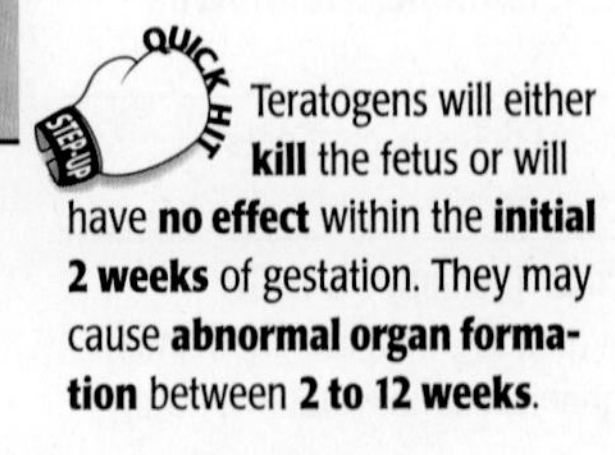

Teratogens will either **kill** the fetus or will have **no effect** within the **initial 2 weeks** of gestation. They may cause **abnormal organ formation** between **2 to 12 weeks**.

- **Tests:** toxicology screening may be useful to determine traces of any substances in the mother's system (legal or illicit) but must be obtained with the mother's consent
- **Treatment:**
  - Honest disclosure must be encouraged for all mothers-to-be in order to make any necessary adjustments to current medication regimens or to provide counseling and education for nonprescribed substance use
  - In some cases the cessation of a medication may be more harmful than the teratogenic risks, and proper counseling about these risks should be provided
- **Outcomes:** the risks of teratogen use to the fetus are directly associated with the ability to avoid the use of such substances during pregnancy; teratogenic birth defects often carry significant lifelong sequelae
- **Why eliminated from differential:** the negative urine toxicology screen makes this diagnosis less likely, but this diagnosis must still be considered in any mother who voluntarily forgoes prenatal care

- **Hemolytic disease of the newborn**
  - More thorough discussion in Chapter 6
  - **Why eliminated from differential:** the lack of disparity between the maternal and neonatal blood types rules out this diagnosis

- **Necrotizing enterocolitis**
  - More thorough discussion in Chapter 3
  - **Why eliminated from differential:** the absence of bloody vomiting or diarrhea, abdominal distention, and excessive bowel gas on the AXR make this diagnosis less likely
- **Congenital heart diseases**
  - More thorough discussion in Chapter 1
  - **Why eliminated from differential:** the absence of extra heart sounds and the normal echocardiogram rule out these diagnoses
- **Meconium aspiration syndrome**
  - More thorough discussion in Chapter 2
  - **Why eliminated from differential:** the absence of meconium during the delivery, neonatal cyanosis, and lung hyperinflation on the CXR make this diagnosis unlikely

The following additional Obstetrics cases may be found online:

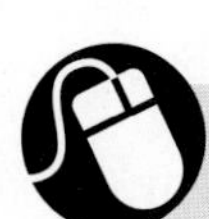

CASE 12-5 "I don't think that my belly is getting any bigger"

CASE 12-6 "I can't seem to stop bleeding"

CASE 12-7 "My cousin is going to have a baby"

Psychiatry

BASIC CLINICAL PRIMER

INITIAL PSYCHIATRIC EVALUATION

- **Patient history**
  - The patient's **chief complaint** (i.e., what he or she perceives as wrong) may not be the only issue that needs to be addressed
  - A **review of systems** and discussion of any **past medical history** should occur to help determine if any **medical conditions** are contributing to a psychiatric disturbance
  - A **family history** is useful to determining if any psychiatric behaviors are inherited
  - The **social history** should address substance use, employment history, legal issues, relationships, education, sexual history, and any precipitating social factors for behaviors; the effects of these issues on daily function should be discussed
  - It may be helpful to involve family members or friends in the evaluation to help obtain a more complete history (with the **patient's permission**)
- **Physical examination**
  - The physical examination should be used to detect any contributory medical conditions (frequently performed by another provider prior to the psychiatric evaluation)
- **Diagnostic tests**
  - Blood or urine analysis is useful for identifying any medical conditions or substance use
  - A head computed tomography (CT) or magnetic resonance imaging (MRI) may be used to detect brain lesions
- **Classification**
  - Psychiatric disorders are organized by the multiaxis classification system (Table 13-1)

MNEMONIC

The components of the mental status examination may be remembered by the mnemonic **ABC STAMP LICKER**: **A**ppearance, **B**ehavior, **C**ooperation, **S**peech, **T**hought processes and content, **A**ffect, **M**ood, **P**erceptions, **L**evel of consciousness, **I**nsight and judgment, **C**ognition, **K**nowledge base, **E**ndings, **R**eliability.

MENTAL STATUS EXAMINATION

- **Appearance, behavior, and cooperation**
  - Patient appearance and behavior help define the **ability to function** and the patient's mental state (e.g., depression, mania, psychosis)
  - Patient gait, coordination, posture, and facial expressions are considered to be components of appearance
  - The patient's ability to cooperate with the evaluation helps to suggest the impact of his or her mental state on the ability to function with others
- **Speech**
  - The tone, rate, rhythm, articulation, and volume of the patient's speech should be noted
  - Excessive or exaggerated qualities may suggest mania or aggressive behavior
  - Impoverished qualities may suggest a depressed mood, social withdrawal, or impaired consciousness

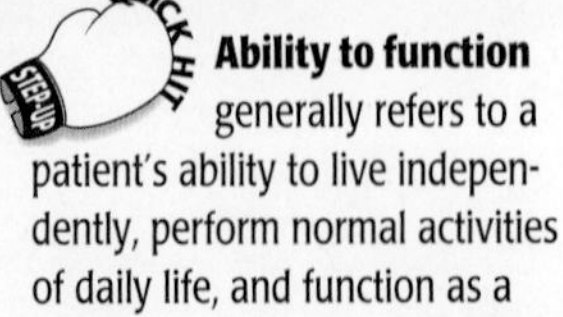

Ability to function generally refers to a patient's ability to live independently, perform normal activities of daily life, and function as a contributing member of society.

TABLE 13-1 Multiaxis Classification of Psychiatric Disorders

Axis	Category	Examples
I	Clinical psychiatric disorders	Mood disorders, anxiety disorders, substance abuse, delirium
II	Personality and development disorders	Borderline personality disorder, mental retardation
III	Medical conditions	Encephalopathy, neoplasm, HIV
IV	Psychosocial stresses	Support structures, social environment, occupational factors
V	Global assessment of functioning	(100-point scale that describes how well the patient has functioned in society)

HIV, human immunodeficiency virus.

(From *Diagnostic and Statistical Manual of Mental Disorders*. 4th ed. Washington DC: American Psychiatric Association, 1994, with permission.)

- Thought process and content
  - **Production** of thought abnormalities include **impoverished** thoughts (i.e., decreased interaction with others or difficulty reasoning), **blocked** thoughts (i.e., sudden stops in the thought process), or "**flight of ideas**" (i.e., rapid transitions between incomplete thoughts)
  - **Form** of thought abnormalities include **circumstantiality** (i.e., unnecessary detail en route to a conclusion), **tangentiality** (i.e., deviations from the original topic to another), **loose associations** (i.e., illogical jumps between different subjects), "**word salad**" (i.e., use of individual words without logical sense or sentence form), or **neologisms** (i.e., invented words)
  - Abnormal **thought content** may include **phobias** (i.e., abnormal fears), **obsessions** (i.e., persistent and pervading thoughts), **compulsions** (i.e., urges to perform a particular task), and **delusions** (i.e., false beliefs without a realistic basis)
- Mood and affect
  - **Mood** is the patient's **subjective** emotional state
  - **Affect** is the way a patient **expresses** his or her state of mood
- Perception
  - Involves the processing of sensory information
  - **Hallucinations** are the abnormal processing of sensory information or the self-creation of a sensory experience
- Level of consciousness
  - Level of alertness and any variability during an evaluation
- Insight and judgment
  - **Insight** is the patient's awareness of any problems and his or her effect on daily life
    - A patient may not realize the effect of a psychiatric problem on his or her ability to function or may not be aware that treatment can improve function
    - A patient's insight into his or her condition will progress through stages of **precontemplation** (i.e., denial), **contemplation** (i.e., thought of addressing the problem), **preparation** (i.e., forming a plan to deal with the problem), **action** (i.e., implementing the plan), and **maintenance** (i.e., making sure that changes are maintained)
  - **Judgment** is a patient's response to a given situation
- Cognition
  - **Orientation** is the awareness of time, place, and identity
  - **Memory** is the ability to retrieve mentally stored information
  - **Concentration** is the ability to maintain attention to a task
- Knowledge base
  - Any logical or chronological gaps in common knowledge should be noted
  - The patient's **intelligence** (i.e., the ability to learn, process, and retain new information) must be taken into account

- **Endings**
  - Suicidal or homicidal ideations must be taken seriously, and a proper risk assessment must be performed in these cases
- **Reliability**
  - Any information gathered during an evaluation must be reassessed to determine if it is reliable
  - The ability of the patient to participate in the evaluation should be considered

CASE 13-1 "My wife is very moody"

A 34-year-old woman presents to a psychiatrist for an initial evaluation for moodiness. She is accompanied by her husband. She says that her moods have fluctuated significantly since she was in her mid-20s, and she currently feels that she is unable to cope with the daily demands on her life. Her husband was concerned for her well-being and finally convinced her to see a psychiatrist. She says that she has been "in a funk" for the past month and that she feels tired and "down" all of the time. There have been some days in the past month that she has stayed in bed almost the entire day. She is upset that she has stopped keeping the house clean and cooking in the past few weeks. She says that she is more of a burden than a help to her husband and two teenaged children, and that she cannot see this situation ever getting better. She denies having visions or hearing voices or having thoughts of harming herself. She says that she is fatigued but denies any significant weight gain. She denies headaches, chest pain, or abdominal pain. Her husband confirms most of her story. He says that she has been very lethargic in the past month and that she spends most of her time in bed. He has absorbed most of the duties of running the household during this time. He must convince her to eat because she says that she never has an appetite. He denies that she has ever discussed harming herself or others. He says that his wife goes through these episodes of feeling down once or twice per year and that they usually last between a few weeks to a month. They then seem to resolve over the course of a few days, and she is able to function normally as a stay-at-home mother. When she is functionally normal, it seems as that the down episodes had never happened and that she does not seem to recall the extent of her previous behavior. On three occasions in the past 10 years she has emerged from one of her down periods and become extremely active. She tends to undertake multiple jobs at these times that are not always completed because she switches between tasks. He remembers coming home from work on one occasion to find that she had repainted every bedroom in the house in one day. On these few occasions she is unable to sleep and performs housework through the night because she has so much excess energy. He says that the last time one of these energetic episodes occurred was a year ago and that it lasted 1 week before she became "more normal." The patient denies having any medical problems or taking medications. She says that she occasionally drinks alcohol but denies other substance use. Her husband says that she tends to drink more when she is in a down period. On further mental status examination, the patient appears slightly disheveled. Her hair appears unwashed and uncombed. She is wearing a clean sweat suit. She answers questions appropriately but otherwise volunteers little information beyond what is pertinent to the current question. She is able to complete her sentences and thoughts. She has no abnormal patterns of speech. Her affect appears to be depressed based on her speech and lack of activity. She remains alert throughout the interview. She is oriented to her name, the current place, and the date. When given the name of three objects, she is able to repeat the names of the objects but can only remember two of them 5 minutes later. A brief physical examination is normal and does not detect any abnormal cardiopulmonary findings, masses, sites of tenderness, or neurologic abnormalities. The following vital signs are measured:

Temperature (T): 98.5°F, heart rate (HR): 78 beats per minute (bpm), blood pressure (BP): 122/81 mm Hg, respiratory rate (RR): 17 breaths/min

Differential Diagnosis

- Bipolar disorder, major depressive disorder, dysthymia, cyclothymia, alcohol abuse, schizoaffective disorder, hypothyroidism, Cushing syndrome

Laboratory Data and Other Study Results

- Complete blood cell count (CBC): white blood cells (WBC): 7.7, hemoglobin (Hgb): 14.1, platelets (Plt): 248
- 7-electrolyte chemistry panel (Chem7): sodium (Na): 139 mEq/L, potassium (K): 3.8 mEq/L, chloride (Cl): 102 mEq/L, carbon dioxide (CO_2): 27 mEq/L, blood urea nitrogen (BUN): 17 mg/dL, creatinine (Cr): 0.8 mg/dL, glucose (Glu): 79 mg/dL
- Thyroid-stimulating hormone (TSH): 3.1 μU/mL
- Urinalysis (UA): straw colored, pH: 6.7, specific gravity: 1.010, no glucose/ketones/nitrites/leukocyte esterase/hematuria/proteinuria
- Urine toxicology screen: negative

Diagnosis

- Bipolar disorder, type I

Treatment Administered

- The patient was started on lithium and paroxetine
- The patient was referred to psychotherapy to help identify stressors and precipitating events for her depression

Follow-up

- By report of the patient's husband, the patient's mood improved 2 weeks later
- The patient and her husband reported a more consistent mood over the next 2 years with no recurrent "high" episodes and only three episodes of minor depression with no major depressive episodes

Steps to the Diagnosis

- **Bipolar disorder (a.k.a. manic depression)**
  - **Cyclic depression** and **mania** (or hypomania) that impairs a patient's ability to function during episodes of significant depression and elation
    - The patient is able to function normally between the episodes
    - Types:
      - **Type I** (i.e., manic): periodic depression with the history of at least one manic episode
      - **Type II** (i.e., hypomanic): periodic depression with the occurrence of at least one hypomanic episode
      - The **diagnosis** requires a history of **at least one** manic or hypomanic episode and **recurrent** major depressive episodes
  - History:
    - **Depression** is consistent with that seen in major depressive disorder
    - **Mania**
      - **Elation** or **irritability** lasting at least 1 week
      - Three or more of the following findings: grandiosity, pressured speech, **decreased need for sleep**, flight of ideas, **easy distractibility**, **increased goal-oriented activity**, or increased risky pleasurable activity
      - Episodes cause a **significant impairment** in the ability to function
    - **Hypomania**
      - **Elation** or **irritability** lasting at least 3 days
      - At least three of the following findings: grandiosity, pressured speech, **decreased need for sleep**, flight of ideas, **easy distractibility**, psychomotor agitation, engaging in risky pleasurable activity
      - The ability to perform daily functions is maintained and not impaired significantly

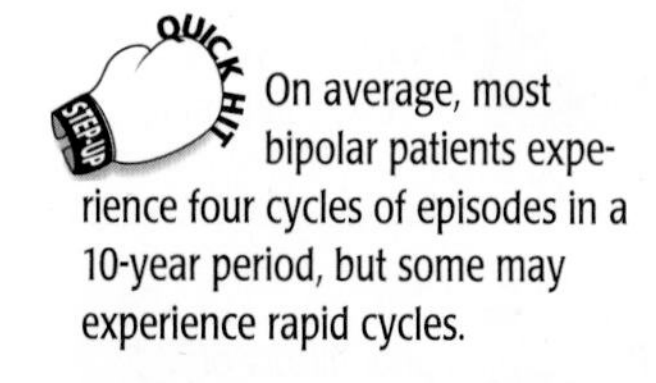

On average, most bipolar patients experience four cycles of episodes in a 10-year period, but some may experience rapid cycles.

MNEMONIC

The characteristics of manic episodes may be remembered with the mnemonic **DIGFAST: D**istractibility, **I**nsomnia, **G**randiosity (feelings of), **F**light of ideas, **A**ctivity (increase in goal-oriented), **S**peech (pressured), **T**aking risks.

- **Physical examination:**
  - **Depression**
    - Decreased activity, disheveled or unkempt appearance, poor eye contact, depressed affect
  - **Mania and hypomania**
    - Excessive activity, agitation, outlandish appearance
- **Tests:** typically noncontributory but may help to rule out other diagnoses
- **Treatment:**
  - Any patient considered to be psychotic or at risk to him- or herself or others should be admitted for inpatient treatment until his or her mood can be stabilized
  - **Mood stabilizers** (e.g., lithium, anticonvulsants atypical antipsychotics) are used to control and prevent manic and hypomanic episodes
    - **Lithium** has long been the first-line treatment for maintenance therapy but is associated with multiple adverse effects, including hypothyroidism, polyuria, tremors, weight gain, renal insufficiency, teratogenesis, and decreased cognitive function
    - Some of the **atypical antipsychotics** are now also considered initial medications because of a similar degree of effectiveness and a better side effect profile
    - Rapid cycling may respond better to carbamazepine and valproate than lithium
  - **Antidepressants** are used to treat depression
- **Outcomes:**
  - Full control of episodes is difficult to achieve, and 50% of patients will have additional episodes of mania or major depression
  - In patients who are successfully treated, the minority will never have a recurrent episode, and many will have recurrent, but less frequent, episodes
  - Substance abuse, prolonged depression, psychotic features, frequent manic episodes, and suicidal or homicidal ideation are all associated with a worse prognosis
  - Suicide or homicide is considered the worst potential complication
- **Clues to the diagnosis:**
  - History: recurrent major depressive elements (e.g., depressed mood, fatigue, poor appetite, difficulty performing normal activities), occurrence of manic behaviors (e.g., increased goal-oriented activity, decreased sleep need, easy distractibility)
  - Physical: unkempt appearance of patient, paucity of speech, depressed affect, forgetfulness
  - Tests: noncontributory

MNEMONIC

The characteristics of major depressive disorder may be remembered with the mnemonic **SIG E CAPS: S**leep disturbances (insomnia), **I**nterest loss, **G**uilt, **E**nergy reduction (fatigue), **C**oncentration impairment, **A**ppetite changes, **P**sychomotor disturbances, **S**uicidal ideation.

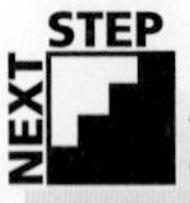

Always assess the depressed patient for suicidal risk.

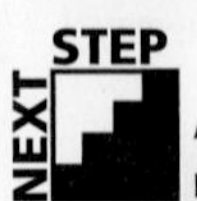

A prior history of **mania** must be ruled out by a thorough history in a patient suspected of having major depressive disorder before antidepressants are prescribed. **Antidepressants** given to a patient with **bipolar disorder** who is **not** taking mood stabilizers can induce a **manic episode**.

- **Major depressive disorder**
  - **Significant depression** that impairs the patient's ability to function, lasts at least 2 weeks, and is not attributable to substance use, medical comorbidities, or bereavement
    - The patient is able to function normally between episodes
    - Psychotic features are rare but may occur
    - The causative pathology is not fully understood but may be related to serotonin, norepinephrine, or dopamine activity
    - The **diagnosis** requires the presence of **five depressive historical findings** including either depressed mood or anhedonia lasting **>2 weeks**
  - **History: depressed mood, anhedonia** (i.e., a loss of interest in previously pleasurable activity), changes in sleep patterns (e.g., insomnia, hypersomnia), feelings of worthlessness, fatigue, inability to concentrate, changes in appetite, psychomotor retardation (i.e., decreased motor activity), **suicidal ideation**
  - **Physical examination:** frequently noncontributory, although the patient's appearance may be disheveled
  - **Tests:** noncontributory
  - **Treatment:**
    - **Antidepressants** are the mainstay of pharmacologic therapy (Table 13-2)
    - **Psychotherapy** consists of cognitive or behavioral counseling and instruction designed to provide insight into the depressive condition and to modify exacerbating behaviors and environments

TABLE 13-2 **Antidepressant Medications**

Drug/Class	Mechanism	Indications	Adverse Effects
SSRIs (e.g., fluoxetine, sertraline, paroxetine, citalopram, escitalopram)	Block presynaptic serotonin reuptake to increase synaptic free-serotonin concentration and postsynaptic serotonin receptor occupancy	**First-line** treatment for depression	Require **3–4 weeks** of administration before they take effect; sexual dysfunction, decreased platelet aggregation, possible increased risk of suicidal ideation in **adolescents**
SNRIs (e.g., venlafaxine, duloxetine)	Inhibit reuptake of both serotonin and norepinephrine in similar fashion to TCAs	First-line treatment for depression with comorbid neurologic pain; second-line treatment for patients failing SSRIs	Nausea, dizziness, insomnia, sedation, constipation, **HTN**; side effects more benign than TCAs
TCAs (e.g., imipramine, amitriptyline, desipramine, nortriptyline)	Block norepinephrine and serotonin reuptake to potentiate postsynaptic receptor activity	Second-line treatment for depression; may be useful in patients with comorbid neurologic pain	Easy to overdose and may be **fatal at only five times the therapeutic dose** (due to cardiac QT interval prolongation that causes arrhythmias), sedation, weight gain, sexual dysfunction, **anticholinergic symptoms**
MAOIs (e.g., phenelzine, isocarboxazid, tranylcypromine, selegiline)	Block monoamine oxidase activity to inhibit deamination of serotonin, norepinephrine, and dopamine and increase levels of these substances	Second-line treatment for depression; may be particularly useful in treatment of depression with neurologic symptoms or in refractory cases	Dry mouth, indigestion, fatigue, headache, **dizziness**; consumption of foods containing **tyramine** (e.g., cheese, aged meats, beer) may cause **hypertensive crisis**
Bupropion	Poorly understood but may be related to inhibition of dopamine reuptake and augmentation of norepinephrine activity	Depression with **fatigue** and difficulty concentrating or comorbid ADHD	Headache, insomnia, weight loss
Trazodone	Poorly understood but related to serotonin activity	Depression with significant insomnia	Hypotension, nausea, **sedation**, priapism; seizure risk at high doses
Mirtazapine	Blocks α_2 receptors and serotonin receptors to increase adrenergic neurotransmission	Depression with insomnia	Dry mouth, weight gain, sedation
St. John's wort (*Hypericum perforatum*)	Decreases reuptake of serotonin and to a lesser extent norepinephrine and dopamine	Used as first-line agent in Europe but only considered an **alternative therapy** in the United States	GI distress, dizziness, sedation; drug interactions are common

ADHD, attention-deficit hyperactivity disorder; HTN, hypertension; GI, gastrointestinal; MAOIs, monoamine oxidase inhibitors; SNRIs, selective serotonin/norepinephrine-reuptake inhibitors; SSRIs, selective serotonin-reuptake inhibitors; TCAs, tricyclic antidepressants.

 - **Electroconvulsive therapy (ECT)** may be used to treat refractory or severe cases to decrease the frequency of episodes
- **Outcomes:** up to 80% of patients will have an improvement in their symptoms with treatment; suicide is considered the most concerning complication
- **Why eliminated from differential:** the description by the patient's husband of multiple manic episodes in the patient makes a bipolar mood disorder more likely than a depressive disorder alone

- **Dysthymia**
  - Feelings of a **depressed mood** that occur on **more days than not** for **more than 2 years**
    - The patient must have **no prior history** of any **major depressive episodes**
    - A **diagnosis** requires a **depressed mood** and **at least two historical findings** for a **majority of days** for **at least 2 years**

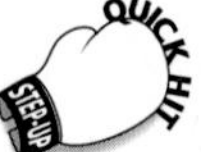

Risks for a **successful** suicide attempt include age >45 years, violent behavior, **drug use**, prior suicidal attempts, existence of a suicide plan, male gender, recent significant loss, **depression**, unemployment, or being single, widowed, or divorced.

- **History:** depressed mood, feelings of hopelessness, changes in sleep patterns, changes in appetite, fatigue, inability to concentrate, or low self-esteem
- **Physical examination:** typically noncontributory
- **Tests:** noncontributory
- **Treatment:** psychotherapy is frequently the initial approach to treatment; antidepressants may be added for persistent symptoms
- **Outcomes:** these cases are much milder than major depressive disorder but may be more chronic in nature; dysthymia in children or younger adults may be a precursor to other mood disorders
- **Why eliminated from differential:** the significant impact of the patient's symptoms upon her daily life and the occurrence of multiple manic episodes rule out this diagnosis

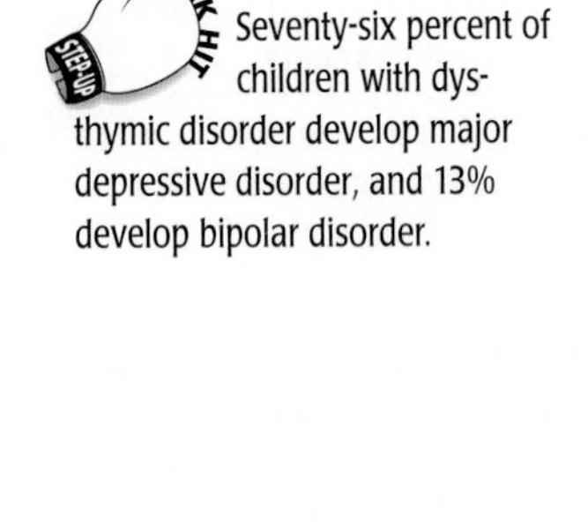

Seventy-six percent of children with dysthymic disorder develop major depressive disorder, and 13% develop bipolar disorder.

- Cyclothymia
  - **Rapid cycling** of **hypomanic** and **mild depressive** episodes for **>2 years** with **no period of normal mood** lasting **>2 months**
    - Patients retain the ability to function normally despite their mood
  - **History:** alternating symptoms of dysthymia (e.g., depressed mood, feelings of hopelessness, etc.) and hypomania (e.g., irritability, grandiosity, etc.)
  - **Physical examination:** typically noncontributory
  - **Tests:** noncontributory
  - **Treatment:** a combination of antidepressants, mood stabilizers, and psychotherapy is utilized to optimize mood control
  - **Outcomes:** the prognosis is similar to that for bipolar disorder, with recurrences being common despite therapy
  - **Why eliminated from differential:** the significant impact of the patient's symptoms upon her ability to function and the absence of rapid cycles rule out this diagnosis
- Alcohol abuse
  - More thorough discussion in later case
  - **Why eliminated from differential:** although the husband's report of the patient's alcohol use is of concern and substance abuse is very common in patients with mood disorders, the patient's alcohol use does not sound as if it is a constant significant problem, and the significant fluctuations and inconsistency of the patient's mood are unlikely to be due to alcohol alone
- Schizoaffective disorder
  - More thorough discussion in later case
  - **Why eliminated from differential:** the absence of psychotic symptoms makes this diagnosis unlikely
- Hypothyroidism
  - More thorough discussion in Chapter 5
  - **Why eliminated from differential:** the normal TSH rules out this diagnosis
- Cushing syndrome
  - More thorough discussion in Chapter 5
  - **Why eliminated from differential:** the absence of any significant physical findings decreases the concern for this diagnosis

CASE 13-2 "I hate talking to people"

A 36-year-old woman presents to a psychiatrist because she is frustrated with her persistent discomfort in talking to people. She says that she has always been a shy person and that this has affected many aspects of her life. As part of this shyness, she has the frequent fear that she will do something to embarrass herself around others. She says that when she was a teenager she never felt comfortable in social situations because she was afraid of how people perceived her. Whenever she was invited to a dance or out on a date, she would become dizzy and would have palpitations and shortness of breath. When she went to college, she chose to remain in her dorm room most of the time not spent in class for the same reason.

She never went out with people at night or on the weekends because of not feeling comfortable around others. She says that she rationalized that her studies should take precedence over any social activity. Following college, she began to work as an actuary for an insurance company. She has performed well at her work, in part, she believes, because she rarely has to interact with people outside of the office. Recently, she was passed over for a promotion because she became extremely nervous before her interview and performed poorly. On that occasion, she began to feel short of breath and lightheaded during the conversation with her boss. She is extremely frustrated over this event because she says that she was the most qualified person interviewing for the job. She says that she has never been in a committed relationship because of her concern over meeting new people. She would like to meet someone, but when she has been set up for dates by other people, she has consistently had the feelings of dizziness and shortness of breath on the night of the date and has canceled them. She has had a few close friendships over the years but typically has few general acquaintances. She says that she enjoys talking to people via email or on Internet chat rooms and does not have symptoms in these situations. Likewise, she says that she never has had a problem working with classmates in college or interacting with people at work within the work setting. She says that when she is at home or alone at her desk at work she feels fine and does not experience the feeling of uneasiness. She denies feeling sad, but is very frustrated over the perceived limitation of her behavior. She denies any hallucinations or suicidal ideation. She says that she realizes that this behavior is not normal but feels incapable of changing. She denies any past medical history and only takes a multivitamin. She is unaware of a similar history in any family members. She occasionally drinks wine at home but uses no other substances. On the mental status examination, she is well groomed and dressed professionally. She is anxious-appearing during the entire interview but is able to answer questions appropriately and volunteers her history. Her speech is rapid and slightly pressured, and she chews her fingernails occasionally when not talking. She is able to fully describe her concerns and problems without deviating from the subject. There are no abnormalities in her phrasing of statements. She remains alert and focused throughout the interview. She is oriented to name, place, and time. She is able to repeat the names of three listed objects and recalls all three objects later in the conversation. The following vital signs are measured:

T: 98.6°F, HR: 105 bpm, BP: 135/86 mm Hg, RR: 18 breaths/min

Differential Diagnosis

- Panic disorder, social phobia, specific phobia, generalized anxiety disorder, schizoid personality disorder, avoidant personality disorder

Laboratory Data and Other Study Results

- None performed

Diagnosis

- Social phobia

Treatment Administered

- The patient was placed on paroxetine
- The patient was referred to behavioral psychotherapy to focus on a gradual progressive exposure to social situations and to evaluate her perceptions of others in such situations

Follow-up

- By 2 months after the onset of therapy, the patient reported feeling more comfortable in social situations and was no longer having any physical symptoms during interactions with others

- By six months, the patient continued to report feeling generally "shy," but was able to interact with acquaintances on a regular basis and was able to begin dating other people

Steps to the Diagnosis

- **Social phobia**
  - Excessive fear of **social situations** and **anxiety** that results when the patient encounters such situations
    - The onset is typically in childhood
    - The anxiety cannot be associated with any medical conditions or substance use
  - **History: anxiety** that consistently occurs in **certain social settings** (e.g., performances, conversations), severe anxiety that may lead to panic attacks (i.e., multiple physical symptoms that accompany the anxiety), persistent **fear of being embarrassed**, **avoidance of social situations** because of anxiety, difficulty functioning normally or in forming relationships because of the anxiety, realization that the feelings of anxiety are abnormal
  - **Physical examination:** the patient frequently appears anxious during the interview
  - **Tests:** typically noncontributory
  - **Treatment:**
    - Selective serotonin reuptake inhibitors (SSRIs) are frequently effective at reducing anxiety and improving social interactions
    - Benzodiazepines and monoamine oxidase inhibitors (MAOIs) are alternative treatments but carry more side effects than SSRIs; benzodiazepines may be particularly helpful for reducing acute anxiety (Table 13-3)
    - β-blockers may be useful in mild cases to decrease palpitations, tachycardia, and diaphoresis
    - Psychotherapy is useful for instructing the patient not to focus on others' perceptions and to desensitize him- or herself to social interactions
  - **Outcomes:** mild cases have a good prognosis, but more disabling cases may not improve to the same extent
  - **Clues to the diagnosis:**
    - History: anxiety in social situations with occasional panic attacks, fear of embarrassment, difficulty forming new relationships, realization that behavior is abnormal
    - Physical: anxious affect
    - Tests: none performed
- **Panic disorder**
  - The experience of **recurrent**, spontaneous **panic attacks** with the associated fear of recurrence
    - Typically begins in adolescence
    - Anxiety cannot be explained by a comorbid medical condition or substance use
    - Severe panic disorder may lead to **agoraphobia** (i.e., a severe fear of public places)

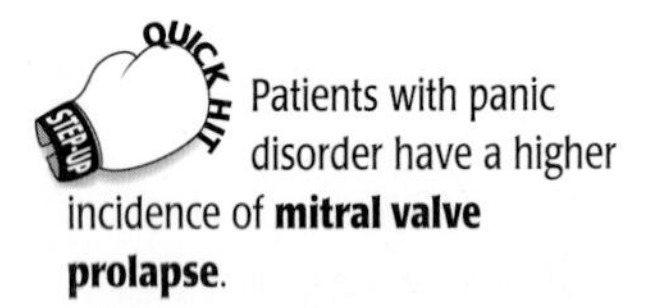

Patients with panic disorder have a higher incidence of **mitral valve prolapse**.

TABLE 13-3 Anxiolytic Medications

Drug	Mechanism	Indications	Adverse Effects
Benzodiazepines (e.g., alprazolam, clonazepam, diazepam, lorazepam)	Increase GABA inhibition of neuronal firing	Alprazolam has a rapid onset and short half-life and is particularly useful to break panic attacks; clonazepam and diazepam are more useful for prolonged therapy	Sedation, confusion; stopping alprazolam usage is associated with withdrawal symptoms of restlessness, confusion, and insomnia (especially with frequent use)
Buspirone	Unclear, but related to serotonin and dopamine receptors	Anxiety disorders in which abuse or sedation is a concern	Headaches, dizziness, nausea

GABA, gamma aminobutyric acid.

- A **diagnosis** requires **both** a history of **recurrent panic attacks** and a **pervasive fear** that the attacks will **recur**
- **History: recurrent panic attacks** that **occur without warning**, last up to 30 minutes, and consist of **extreme anxiety**, feelings of impending danger, chest pain, dyspnea, palpitations, nausea, dizziness, feelings of losing control, and chills or hot flashes
- **Physical examination:** tachycardia and diaphoresis during the attacks
- **Tests:** typically noncontributory but useful to rule out cardiac conditions
- **Treatment:**
  - SSRIs are considered the first-line therapy to reduce the frequency of panic attacks
  - Benzodiazepines or tricyclic antidepressants (TCAs) are considered second-line therapy
  - Psychotherapy may be useful for reducing the fear of recurrence between attacks and reducing the frequency of attacks
- **Outcomes:** the prognosis is excellent, with most patients having a significant reduction in the number of attacks after starting treatment
- **Why eliminated from differential:** despite the occurrence of multiple panic attacks, the close relationship of the patient's symptoms to social settings makes social phobia a better diagnosis

- **Specific phobia**
  - Fear of a particular **object**, **activity**, or **situation** that causes a patient to avoid the feared subject
    - Typically begins in childhood and cannot be associated with any medical comorbidity or substance use
  - **History:** occurrence of a panic attack when the feared subject is encountered, avoidance of contact with the feared subject, realization that behavior is irrational, possible syncope during panic attacks
  - **Physical examination:** typically noncontributory except in the presence of the feared subject (then consistent with a panic attack)
  - **Tests:** noncontributory
  - **Treatment:** psychotherapy is the cornerstone of treatment, with a focus on repeated graduated exposure, relaxation techniques, insight modification, and possible hypnosis
  - **Outcomes:** the prognosis is good, with the majority of patients being able to function normally; more specific phobias (e.g., snakes) tend to have a better response to treatment than more general ones (e.g., public places)
  - **Why eliminated from differential:** social phobia is essentially a form of specific phobia with a generalized fear of social interactions
- **Generalized anxiety disorder (GAD)**
  - Excessive, **persistent** anxiety that impairs a patient's ability to function
    - Occurs on the majority of days for **at least 6 months**
    - Typically begins in early adulthood and cannot be explained by medical comorbidities or substance use
    - **Diagnosis** requires **excessive anxiety**, **impaired ability to function**, and at least **three anxiety-related symptoms** for **at least 6 months**
  - **History:** restlessness or feeling on edge, inability to concentrate, insomnia, irritability, tenseness of muscles, sleep disturbances
  - **Physical examination:** possible tachycardia, tachypnea, tremor, or diaphoresis
  - **Tests:** typically noncontributory
  - **Treatment:**
    - SSRIs, serotonin–norepinephrine reuptake inhibitors (SNRIs), and buspirone are now considered the first line of therapy
    - Benzodiazepines are useful for the treatment of acute exacerbations
    - Psychotherapy is useful to improve insight into the overlying anxiety and to teach relaxation techniques
  - **Outcomes:** the prognosis depends on the level of impairment in daily function
  - **Why eliminated from differential:** the patient does not have persistent anxiety, and her symptoms occur in a particular situation (i.e., social interactions), so this diagnosis is unlikely

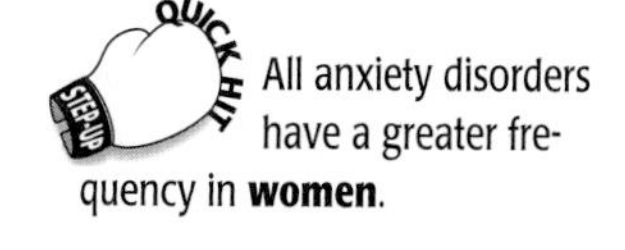

All anxiety disorders have a greater frequency in **women**.

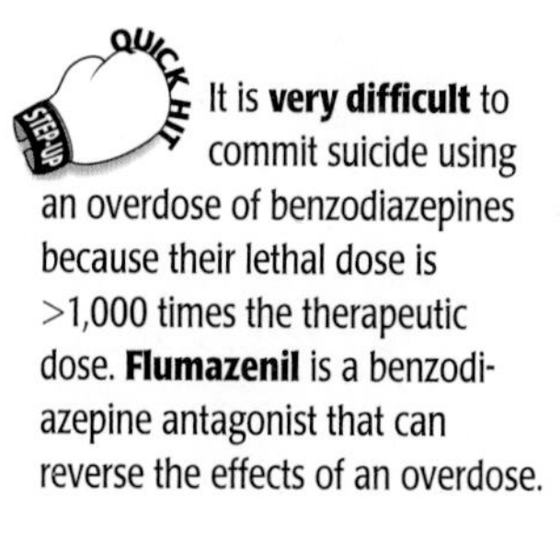

It is **very difficult** to commit suicide using an overdose of benzodiazepines because their lethal dose is >1,000 times the therapeutic dose. **Flumazenil** is a benzodiazepine antagonist that can reverse the effects of an overdose.

- **Schizoid personality disorder**
  - More thorough discussion in later case
  - **Why eliminated from differential:** the demonstrated ability to form some relationships and the presence of normal (albeit, excessive) emotion make this diagnosis unlikely
- **Avoidant personality disorder**
  - More thorough discussion in later case
  - **Why eliminated from differential:** although social phobia and avoidant personality disorder may be very similar in some regards, social phobia is a better diagnosis in this case because this patient is able to interact socially via some formats (i.e., email, Internet)

CASE 13-3 "I keep thinking about my partner"

A 26-year-old man presents to a psychiatrist on the request of his employer to be evaluated for repetitive intrusive thoughts. The patient is a police officer in a large city but has been unable to work for the past few months. He was in a good state of health until 3 months ago. At that time he and his partner were involved in a narcotics bust that ended violently in a shootout between the police and several drug dealers. Although the patient was unhurt in this incident, his partner, who was standing next to him at the time, was shot in the face and killed. The patient had difficulty performing his job after this incident. He says that he has a dream multiple nights per week in which the scene of his partner's death replays. He denies having any hallucinations. Whenever he hears gun shots or any other sudden noise, he becomes very anxious and feels like he is short of breath. He has been unable to hold a gun since the incident because it reminds him of his partner. He says that he constantly feels guilty that he did not save his partner's life. The patient says that he has had difficulty sleeping and frequently becomes angry at people for minor issues. He no longer exercises or goes out with friends because he feels that he lacks the energy to do so. Because he was unable to perform his job as a police officer, he was put on medical leave. His department is now trying to determine if he will ever be able to return to work. The patient says that he has a history of reflux disease for which he takes ranitidine. He smokes a half pack of cigarettes per day and has done so for 10 years. He drinks about ten beers per week. On the mental status examination, he appears well groomed. He is cooperative with questioning and answers all questions appropriately. The tone of his speech is low with decreased volume. He is able to complete his sentences completely without any abnormal structure. His affect is flat, and he displays little emotion. He is able to remain alert during the extent of the interview. He is oriented to his name, the current place, and the time. He is able to repeat the names of three objects spoken to him and can recall one of the objects several minutes later. The following vital signs are measured:

T: 98.6°F, HR: 85 bpm, BP: 130/80 mm Hg, RR: 15 breaths/min

Differential Diagnosis

- Major depressive disorder, dysthymia, posttraumatic stress disorder, adjustment disorder, bereavement, obsessive-compulsive disorder, schizophrenia, substance abuse

Laboratory Data and Other Study Results

- None performed

Diagnosis

- Posttraumatic stress disorder

Treatment Administered

- The patient was prescribed sertraline
- Psychotherapy was initiated, including group therapy with police officers and veterans who had witnessed traumatic events
- The patient was provided counseling regarding moderation of his alcohol intake

Follow-up

- Because of the inability to perform his job, the patient was placed on long-term disability
- Over time, the patient reported resolution of his nightmares and inappropriate responses to loud noises; by 18 months after the incident he felt that he would be able to return to work
- The patient returned to the police force 20 months after the incident, working initially at a desk job and later on patrol

Steps to the Diagnosis

- **Posttraumatic stress disorder (PTSD)**
  - A syndrome of anxiety symptoms that occurs following an **exposure to a significantly stressful event**
    - Symptoms begin within 3 months of the event
    - **Diagnosis** requires the patient to have been exposed to a **traumatic event**, to have **symptoms of reliving** the event, to **avoid situations** associated with the event, and to have symptoms of **increased arousal**
    - Symptoms lasting more than a 1 month are considered acute, and those lasting longer than 3 months are considered chronic
  - **History: vivid dreams** or **recurrent intrusive thoughts** about the event, avoidance of activity associated with the event, **anhedonia**, feelings of detachment, survivor guilt, social withdrawal, increased arousal (e.g., irritability, insomnia, difficulty concentrating)
  - **Physical examination:** possible disheveled appearance, exaggerated startle reaction
  - **Tests:** typically noncontributory
  - **Treatment:** SSRIs and MAOIs are the most commonly used medications to reduce feelings of anxiety and obtrusive thoughts; psychotherapy, particularly in a group setting or activity-directed therapy, is useful to teach coping skills
  - **Outcomes:** two thirds of patients will recover fully from the condition, although the average time for recovery is 3 years in treated patients and 5 years in untreated patients
  - **Clues to the diagnosis:**
    - History: history of traumatic event, recurrent dreams of the event, avoidance of gun use due to an association with the event, insomnia, irritability, anhedonia
    - Physical: flat affect, forgetfulness
    - Tests: none ordered
- **Major depressive disorder**
  - More thorough discussion in prior case
  - **Why eliminated from differential:** despite having several symptoms seen in major depressive disorder, the relation of the patients symptoms to a distinct traumatic event makes PTSD a better diagnosis
- **Dysthymia**
  - More thorough discussion in prior case
  - **Why eliminated from differential:** the patient's symptoms do not satisfy the time criteria for this diagnosis
- **Adjustment disorder**
  - Behavioral and mood changes that occur within 3 months of a **stressful event** (e.g., death of a loved one, assault, divorce) and causes **significant impairment** in the ability to function
    - Symptoms **begin within 3 months** of the event and **end within 6 months** of the conclusion of the event

- The symptoms are **generalized** and are not specific for situations associated with the stressful event
- **History: distress in excess** of what is expected for a given stressful event, difficulty concentrating, **self-isolation**, changes in sleep patterns, change in appetite
- **Physical examination:** noncontributory
- **Tests:** noncontributory
- **Treatment:** psychotherapy is the first-line treatment and is aimed at helping the patient cope with the stressful event; antidepressants may be considered in patients who do not respond to psychotherapy alone
- **Outcomes:** suicide rates and substance abuse are increased in patients with adjustment disorder
- **Why eliminated from differential:** the specificity of the patient's symptoms for the stressful event and elicitation of his symptoms by exposure to situations reminiscent of the event make PTSD a better explanation for his symptoms

- **Bereavement**
  - A natural period of mourning after the death of a loved one
    - The patient's ability to function is not impaired
  - **History:** sadness, repetitive thoughts about the recently deceased, difficulty concentrating, feelings of guilt, difficulty accepting the loss with an eventual acceptance, changes in sleep or appetite
  - **Physical examination:** noncontributory
  - **Tests:** noncontributory
  - **Treatment:** most cases will self-resolve; psychotherapy should be considered in longer-lasting cases
  - **Outcomes:** the prognosis is excellent, with almost all patients recovering; persistent symptoms are suggestive of adjustment disorder or another condition
  - **Why eliminated from differential:** the significant impact of the patient's symptoms on his life and the severe pervasive nature of his symptoms rule out his diagnosis
- **Obsessive-compulsive disorder (OCD)**
  - Significant recurrent **obsessions** (i.e., recurrent intrusive thoughts that are difficult to suppress and are recognized as being abnormal) and **compulsions** (i.e., repetitive behaviors performed in response to an obsession that are directed at reducing distress) that affect daily life and the ability to function
    - Typically begins in adolescence
  - **History:** recurrent obsessions and compulsions that affect the ability to function normally, obsessions and compulsions that consume a significant amount of time in daily life, awareness that behaviors are abnormal, feelings of an inability to control behaviors, worsening of abnormal behaviors in stressful situations
  - **Physical examination:** although there are no generalized physical findings, an examination may detect findings consistent with a particular compulsion (e.g., dry skin from constant hand washing, wounds from scratching or picking of skin)
  - **Tests:** typically noncontributory
  - **Treatment:**
    - SSRIs or SNRIs are considered the first-line pharmacologic therapy
    - Antipsychotics may be used in patients not responding to other medications
    - Behavioral psychotherapy is aimed at the recognition of obsessive thoughts and the conscious avoidance of the reflex compulsive behaviors
  - **Outcomes:** although 70% of patients will have a significant improvement in their symptoms, OCD tends to be a chronic condition with periodic exacerbations
  - **Why eliminated from differential:** although the patient is fixated upon the death of his partner, the lack of a compulsive behavior in response to these thoughts rules out this diagnosis

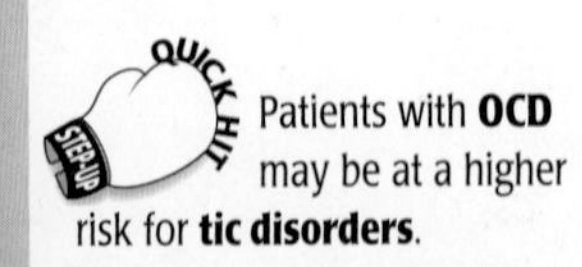

Patients with **OCD** may be at a higher risk for **tic disorders**.

- **Schizophrenia**
  - More thorough discussion in later case
  - **Why eliminated from differential:** although the patient has recurrent dreams and a flattened affect, he is not having any hallucinations or abnormalities in the processing of thoughts; furthermore, the distinct onset of his symptoms with the stressful event makes this diagnosis unlikely

- **Substance abuse**
  - More thorough discussion in later case
  - **Why eliminated from differential:** although the patient is consuming more than one alcoholic beverage per day, his alcohol and tobacco use are not the inciting force behind his intrusive thoughts and anxiety

CASE 13-4 "We found this guy harassing people"

A 48-year-old man is brought to a psychiatric emergency evaluation center by police after he was found yelling at people on the street. The police officers say that he was wandering on the sidewalk and approaching people demanding that they return his jacket. Several people contacted the police after feeling threatened. The officers say that they have seen the patient in the area for the past year and are aware of some erratic behavior, but are unaware of him threatening anyone previously. They say that he is homeless and lives underneath a bridge by the river. He has been seen wandering the area periodically asking for money but does not have a history of violence. The patient is resistant to speaking with others and requires much coaxing to answer questions. When the patient is asked by the psychiatrist on call why he was upset and accosting people, the man says that his jacket lets him "travel in time" and that the "bad people stole it." He then begins to talk about buying "apples for [his] elephant" and later that "the president is [his] father." When further questioned about his jacket, he is unable to describe the jacket or when he last had a jacket. He intermittently turns to his right side and speaks as if he was conversing with someone next to him, but no one is seated there. When asked if he hears voices, he does not respond but stares straight ahead. When asked if he is angry, sad, or happy, a similar response is offered. He is also unable to provide any information about any surviving family members, previous places of residence, or past medical history. He denies any substance use upon questioning. On the mental status examination, he is very disheveled and unkempt. He is dirty and smells bad. He is not very cooperative with questioning and requires encouragement to answer questions. He has little facial expression. The tone of his voice is low, and his words are not well articulated. He makes loose associations between different subjects as evidenced by the transition from talking about his jacket to talking about apples and the president. He displays little emotion during the interview, but becomes mildly agitated when talking about his jacket. Despite his lack of cooperation, he remains awake during the assessment. He knows his name but is not able to correctly name the day or place. When given the names of three objects, he is only able to repeat one named object and cannot recite any of them several minutes later. A physical examination detects no asymmetry of his face of lymphadenopathy. Auscultation of his heart, lungs, and abdomen is normal. He has no abdominal tenderness or masses. He has no pain with range of motion of his neck or any of his extremities. A neurovascular examination is normal in regards to all sensory and motor function. He has multiple bites and wounds on his skin in various stages of healing. The following vital signs are measured:

T: 98.4°F, HR: 72 bpm, BP: 138/86 mm Hg, RR: 18 breaths/min

Differential Diagnosis

- Schizophrenia, brief psychotic disorder, substance abuse, delusional disorder, schizoaffective disorder, schizophreniform disorder, bipolar disorder, dementia, stroke, brain tumor or abscess, encephalitis, vitamin B_{12} deficiency, hyperthyroidism, hypothyroidism, acute intermittent porphyria, syphilis, human immunodeficiency virus

Laboratory Data and Other Study Results

- CBC: WBC: 10.5, Hgb: 15.1, Plt: 372, mean corpuscular volume (MCV): 90 fL
- 10-electrolyte chemistry panel (Chem10): Na: 144 mEq/L, K: 4.2 mEq/L, Cl: 99 mEq/L, CO_2: 25 mEq/L, BUN: 20 mg/dL, Cr: 1.1 mg/dL, Glu: 99 mg/dL, magnesium (Mg): 1.6 mg/dL, calcium (Ca): 10.1 mg/dL, phosphorus (Phos): 4.2 mg/dL

- Liver function tests (LFTs): alkaline phosphatase (AlkPhos): 76 U/L, alanine aminotransferase (ALT): 41 U/L, aspartate aminotransferase (AST): 40 U/L, total bilirubin (TBili): 0.8 mg/dL, direct bilirubin (DBili): 0.5 mg/dL
- ESR: 9 mm/hr
- Folate: 5.1 mg/mL
- Vitamin B_{12}: 384 pg/mL
- Thyroid panel: TSH: 1.98 μU/mL, T_4: 7.6 μg/dL, free T_4 index: 7.0, T_3: 1.0 ng/mL, T_3 reuptake: 0.79
- Rapid plasma reagin (RPR): negative
- Human immunodeficiency virus enzyme-linked immunosorbent assay (HIV ELISA): negative
- Urine toxicology screen: positive for alcohol and tobacco
- Head CT: no focal masses, lesions, or sites of ischemia; normal cerebral and ventricular volume; no sites of hemorrhage

Diagnosis

- Schizophrenia

Treatment Administered

- The patient was convinced to consent to an inpatient psychiatric admission
- Risperidone was prescribed for the patient

Follow-up

- Following 2 weeks of risperidone use, the patient was more organized and was better able to perform personal hygiene
- He remained relatively unemotional, but did not become agitated during conversations and ceased discussing his former delusions
- The patient was able to disclose the names of local family members and was discharged to live at a relative's house 4 weeks after his admission
- During a follow-up appointment, the patient stated that he did not believe that he needed to continue taking his medicine; the patient was encouraged to continue his use of the risperidone and was cautioned about the problems of discontinuing antipsychotic medications
- Following this appointment, the patient was lost to follow-up; when the family was contacted, they said that patient had left their house and that they did not know his whereabouts

Steps to the Diagnosis

- Schizophrenia
  - A severe psychotic disorder that causes significant limitations in the ability to function
    - It is found at a significantly higher rate in the homeless and indigent populations because of the inability of those affected to function in society
    - Typically begins in late adolescence
    - **Diagnosis** requires the presence of **two or more significant psychotic symptoms** (i.e., delusions, hallucinations, disorganized speech, disorganized or catatonic behavior, or negative symptoms), the presence of the symptoms for **at least 1 month** within a 6-month period, and **impaired social function** for **>6 months**
  - **Risk factors:** family history, maternal malnutrition or illness during pregnancy
  - **History:**
    - **Positive** symptoms: **delusions**, **hallucinations** (usually auditory), **disorganized thoughts** and **behavior**, thought broadcasting (i.e., belief that others can read the patient's thoughts or that thoughts are being transmitted to others), ideas of reference (i.e., belief that hidden meanings are found in common items)

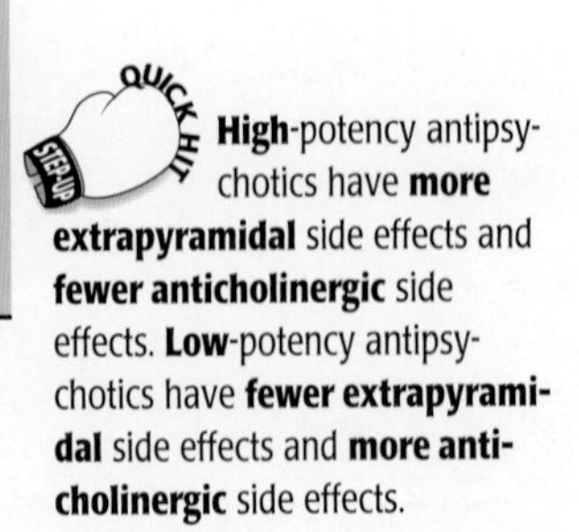

High-potency antipsychotics have **more extrapyramidal** side effects and **fewer anticholinergic** side effects. **Low**-potency antipsychotics have **fewer extrapyramidal** side effects and **more anticholinergic** side effects.

- **Negative** symptoms: **social withdrawal**, **flat affect** (i.e., displaying little emotional response to stimuli), apathy, anhedonia, lack of motivation
- **Cognitive** symptoms: attention deficits, inability to organize or form abstractions, poor memory
- Although the patient's baseline function is impaired, periodic psychotic exacerbations will occur with a further worsening of symptoms

- **Physical examination:** physical findings are consistent with the functional limitations of the disease and include poor hygiene, flat affect, bizarre behavior, interaction with perceived hallucinations, and inattentiveness
- **Tests:** typically noncontributory but useful to rule out other conditions
- **Treatment:**
  - **Antipsychotics** are the mainstay of therapy (Table 13-4)
  - Psychotherapy may be useful in teaching the patient how to recognize symptoms of the disease
  - Psychotic exacerbations frequently require inpatient treatment
- **Outcomes:**
  - The prognosis is generally poor, with a gradual deterioration in the ability to function over several years; over this time period symptoms generally wax and wane
  - **Positive** prognostic factors include a history of a comorbid mood disorder, predominantly positive symptoms, and good support systems
  - **Negative** prognostic factors include predominantly negative symptoms, neurologic abnormalities, and poor support systems
  - Many patients have a history of **substance abuse**, and this may cause other complications associated with the substance (e.g., HIV, cirrhosis)

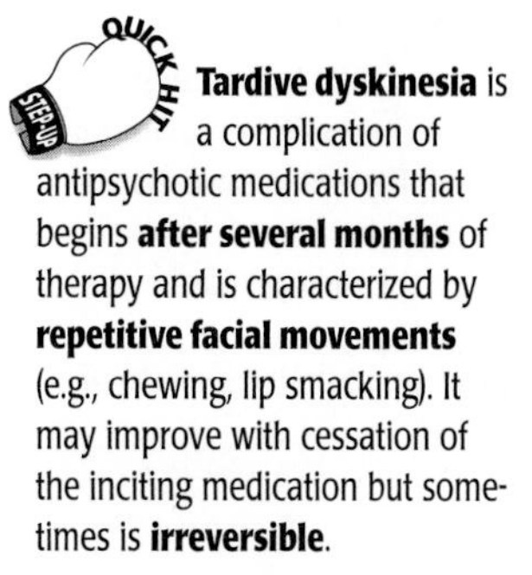

Tardive dyskinesia is a complication of antipsychotic medications that begins **after several months** of therapy and is characterized by **repetitive facial movements** (e.g., chewing, lip smacking). It may improve with cessation of the inciting medication but sometimes is **irreversible**.

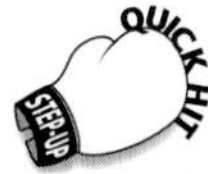

Neuroleptic malignant syndrome is an uncommon complication of antipsychotic medications that starts within **days** of usage and carries a high mortality rate. It is characterized by **high fever**, **muscle rigidity**, decreased consciousness, and an increased blood pressure and heart rate. It is treated by immediately **stopping** use of the drug and administering **dantrolene**.

TABLE 13-4 Antipsychotic Medications

Drug Type	Mechanism	Indications	Adverse Effects
Atypical antipsychotics (e.g., clozapine, risperidone, olanzapine, sertindole, quetiapine, ziprasidone, paliperidone)	Block **dopamine** and **serotonin** receptors	• **First-line** drugs for maintenance therapy for psychotic disorders • Clozapine is the most effective neuroleptic but is reserved for refractory psychosis due to the risk of agranulocytosis	Anticholinergic effects, weight gain, arrhythmias, seizures; **clozapine** carries a risk of **agranulocytosis;** the frequency and severity of side effects is significantly less than seen with traditional neuroleptics
Traditional high-potency (e.g., haloperidol, droperidol, fluphenazine, thiothixene)	Block **D_2 dopamine** receptors	• Strong positive symptoms • **Emergency control** of psychosis or agitation • Frequently second-line drugs for maintenance therapy	**Extrapyramidal effects** (e.g., dystonia, parkinsonism), **tardive dyskinesia, anticholinergic effects** (e.g., sedation, constipation, urinary retention, hypotension), confusion, sexual dysfunction, hyperprolactinemia, **neuroleptic malignant syndrome**, seizures, arrhythmias; least anticholinergic effects of traditional antipsychotics but highest rate of extrapyramidal effects
Traditional medium-potency (e.g., trifluoperazine, perphenazine)	Block **D_2** dopamine receptors	• Strong positive symptoms • Frequently second-line drugs for maintenance therapy • May be used in patients exhibiting significant extrapyramidal **and** anticholinergic side effects with other traditional neuroleptics	Similar to other traditional drugs; mix of moderate extrapyramidal and anticholinergic effects
Traditional low-potency (e.g., thioridazine, chlorpromazine)	Block **D_2** dopamine receptors	• Strong positive symptoms • Frequently second-line drugs for maintenance therapy	Similar to other traditional drugs; less extrapyramidal effects than more potent traditional antipsychotics but more anticholinergic effects

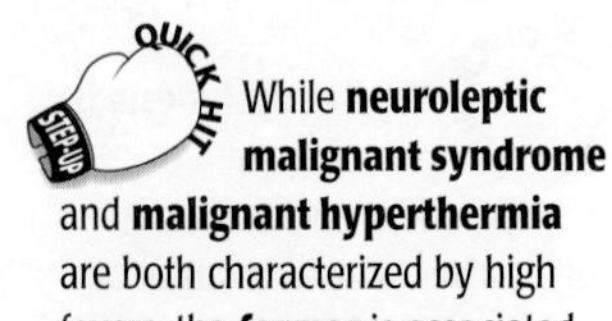

While **neuroleptic malignant syndrome** and **malignant hyperthermia** are both characterized by high fevers, the **former** is associated with **antipsychotic** use and the **latter** with **inhaled anesthetic** use.

- Medicine **noncompliance** is a common problem and complicates treatment
- Ten percent of cases will end in **suicide**
- **Clues to the diagnosis:**
  - History: bizarre behavior, history of homelessness and erratic behavior, loose associations, delusions, disorganized thoughts, poor memory
  - Physical: disheveled appearance, flat affect, interaction with hallucinations
  - Tests: noncontributory
- Brief psychotic disorder
  - More thorough discussion in Table 13-5
  - **Why eliminated from differential:** the patient's reported history of prior erratic behavior makes this diagnosis unlikely
- Schizoaffective disorder
  - More thorough discussion in Table 13-5
  - **Why eliminated from differential:** the predomination of psychotic features makes this diagnosis unlikely; in addition, the diagnostic criteria for schizophrenia are fulfilled, making this diagnosis unlikely
- Schizophreniform disorder
  - More thorough discussion in Table 13-5
  - **Why eliminated from differential:** because the patient's complete psychiatric history is unknown, it is difficult to fully rule out this diagnosis, but the report of prior strange behavior and chronic social disability makes schizophrenia a better classification for his presentation
- Delusional disorder
  - More thorough discussion in Table 13-5
  - **Why eliminated from differential:** the presence of multiple psychotic symptoms besides delusions rules out this diagnosis
- Bipolar disorder
  - More thorough discussion in prior case
  - **Why eliminated from differential:** although the patient's suboptimal cooperation and his active psychosis make a full assessment of his mood difficult, the predominance of his psychotic symptoms and the significant functional disability they place on him make schizophrenia a better diagnosis

TABLE 13-5 Psychotic Disorders Not Classified as Schizophrenia

Disorder	Description	Treatment
Schizophreniform	Symptoms similar to schizophrenia but **last >1 month and <6 months;** patients return to normal function following resolution of psychotic episode; two thirds of patients will go on to develop true schizophrenia in the future	Antipsychotics, psychotherapy
Schizoaffective	Presence of **mood disorder and psychotic symptoms** but not meeting the criteria for either diagnosis alone; diagnosis requires the presence of psychotic symptoms during a normal mood for more than 2 weeks	Combination of antipsychotics with mood stabilizers and/or antidepressants; psychotherapy is a useful adjunct
Delusional	Presence of one or more distinct **realistic delusions** lasting more than a month without any other psychotic symptoms; patient is able to function normally; **unrealistic delusions** are classified as **schizophreniform disorder or schizophrenia**	Antipsychotics, psychotherapy; SSRIs are helpful when delusions are of a somatic nature
Brief psychotic	**Sudden** onset of psychotic symptoms (possibly stress-related) that **last <1 month**	Psychotherapy or short-term antipsychotics; hospitalization is necessary if symptoms affect the ability to function
Shared psychotic (i.e., Folie à deux)	A **second patient** accepts and becomes involved in the preexisting delusions of the primary patient	Group psychotherapy, antipsychotics; the second patient's acceptance of delusions often wanes if separated from primary patient

SSRI, selective serotonin-reuptake inhibitors.

- **Dementia**
  - More thorough discussion in later case
  - **Why eliminated from differential:** because the patient's symptoms are not limited to cognitive dysfunction, this diagnosis is unlikely
- **Substance abuse**
  - More thorough discussion in later case
  - **Why eliminated from differential:** although this patient has been shown to use both alcohol and tobacco, the significant psychotic symptoms are better explained by a diagnosis of schizophrenia
- **Stroke/brain abscess/brain tumor**
  - More thorough discussion in Chapter 7
  - **Why eliminated from differential:** the negative head CT rules out these diagnoses
- **Vitamin B_{12} deficiency**
  - More thorough discussion in Chapter 6
  - **Why eliminated from differential:** the normal vitamin B_{12} level rules out this diagnosis
- **Hyperthyroidism/hypothyroidism**
  - More thorough discussion in Chapter 5
  - **Why eliminated from differential:** the normal thyroid panel rules out these diagnoses
- **Encephalitis**
  - More thorough discussion in Chapter 7
  - **Why eliminated from differential:** the absence of focal neurologic deficits and the absence of an effusion on the head CT make this diagnosis unlikely
- **Acute intermittent porphyria**
  - More thorough discussion in Chapter 6
  - **Why eliminated from differential:** the absence of neurologic deficits makes this diagnosis unlikely
- **Syphilis**
  - More thorough discussion in Chapter 11
  - **Why eliminated from differential:** the negative RPR rules out this diagnosis
- **Human immunodeficiency virus**
  - More thorough discussion in Chapter 6
  - **Why eliminated from differential:** the negative ELISA rules out this diagnosis

CASE 13-5 "I can't find a good relationship"

A 40-year-old woman presents to a psychiatrist because she feels that she is unable to maintain any committed relationships. She says that she wants help recognizing people who are not a good match for her. She says that she has fallen "head-over-heels" in love with several men, and that she has thrown herself full force into these relationships. In each case, the man was "bad for [her]" and the relationship ended in a serious argument. She has been in a couple of romantic relationships with women that have ended in a similar explosive way. She says that she typically has multiple sexual partners at a given time because "that's what gets men interested in you." She says that she "just can't find a good person." She says that she also has a difficult time making friends because she "always [manages] to find bad people." She has a few close friends that she says are "complete saints and are just like [her] in every way." She says that she has a new boyfriend who is "perfect" and is "exactly what [she] needs." She says that she is paying for private tennis and ski lessons because they are activities in which her new boyfriend is involved and "therefore, must be things [she] should be doing." Despite her excitement for this relationship, she is worried because of her previous negative relationships and wants "to know how to recognize if something is wrong." She is afraid that she may never find anyone to be in a long-term relationship because of her past experiences. She says that she has encountered a similar pattern in her work. She has changed jobs four times in the past 2 years because she cannot find "a good place to work." In her current job in an advertising agency she initially enjoyed it and spent long hours at work but now knows "that it is not a good place to work forever." She has called out of work several days in the past few months because she does not want to be at her current job. She feels that her difficulty with commitments stems from her childhood. She says that both of her parents traveled often and were not around much to take care of her brother and her. She feels that her parents never really knew her well. She feels that because of this upbringing she was "never taught to recognize the bad people in life." She denies being unhappy but is concerned about her love life. She denies having difficulty sleeping or eating. She adamantly denies ever having had auditory or visual hallucinations. She admits that she took a large amount of diazepam with considerable alcohol after the end of two different relationships and required treatment in an emergency department on each occasion. She says that she was not trying to commit suicide but wanted to "punish" her ex-lover in each case. She denies any current thought of suicide. She says that she has a medical history of irritable bowel syndrome that has responded well to eating small meals. She takes a multivitamin and uses a contraceptive vaginal ring for birth control. She says that she has two alcohol drinks each night to "help deal with the day." She denies other substance use. On the mental status examination, she is well groomed and dressed well. She is able to cooperate well with the entire interview. Her speech is articulate, and she is frequently expansive in her answers to questions. Occasionally she must be guided back to the direction of the question to get a clear answer. Her affect is variable, and she is both occasionally calm and emotional when talking about some past relationships. She remains alert during the entire interview. She is oriented to her name, the current place, and the time. She is able to repeat the names of three objects listed to her and is able to recall all three names later in the conversation. The following vital signs are measured:

T: 98.7°F, HR: 70 bpm, BP: 126/78 mm Hg, RR: 18 breaths/min

Differential Diagnosis

- Attention deficit hyperactivity disorder, borderline personality disorder, bipolar disorder, major depressive disorder, dysthymia, paranoid personality disorder, schizotypal personality disorder, histrionic personality disorder, narcissistic personality disorder, dependent personality disorder, substance abuse

Laboratory Data and Other Study Results

- None performed

Diagnosis

- Borderline personality disorder

Treatment Administered

- The patient was enrolled in psychotherapy designed to initially explore the patient's beliefs of why she was having difficulties in relationships and to help the patient gradually evaluate her actions and thought processes in relationships
- The patient was prescribed olanzapine

Follow-up

- The patient was initially suspicious of the pharmacologic prescription and refused to take the medication but agreed to participate in psychotherapy
- After some time in therapy, the patient became more agreeable to taking the prescribed medication
- The patient continued to have relatively tumultuous relationships with people but was better able to accept others' actions as not always being "bad" and was better able to realize not all of her actions were "good"

Steps to the Diagnosis

- **Borderline personality disorder**
  - A disorder of persistent abnormal behavior characterized by intense relationships with others, poor impulse control, and a skewed self-perception
    - **Personality disorders**
      - In general, these are all disorders of persistent behaviors that **deviate significantly** from what is considered the societal norm
      - They are typically manifested through the **interaction with others**
      - Behaviors tend to be **inflexible** and lead to an impairment of function
      - The abnormal behaviors begin in late adolescence and cannot be attributed to a medical comorbidity, substance use, or another psychiatric condition
  - **History:** findings are described in Table 13-6
  - **Physical examination:** a variable or emotional affect may be observed
  - **Tests:** typically noncontributory
  - **Treatment:** psychotherapy directed at addressing relationships with others is the primary treatment; antipsychotics, mood stabilizers, or SSRIs are also utilized in treatment
  - **Outcomes:**
    - Suicide and substance abuse are the most common complications
    - The response to medication is not as good as in full mood disorders or psychosis
    - Symptoms tend to be lifelong but become somewhat milder with age
  - **Clues to the diagnosis:**
    - History: unstable and intense relationships, splitting people into all good or all bad, impulsivity (e.g., sexual promiscuity, sudden commitments of time to learning tennis and skiing, daily alcohol use), dissociation from problems in relationships, multiple quasisuicidal attempts
    - Physical: variable emotional affect
    - Tests: none performed
- **Paranoid personality disorder**
  - More thorough discussion in Table 13-6
  - **Why eliminated from differential:** the multiple self-destructive activities and constant fear of being alone in this case are less consistent with this diagnosis
- **Schizotypal personality disorder**
  - More thorough discussion in Table 13-6
  - **Why eliminated from differential:** this diagnosis would be characterized less by a concern over relationships and more by a greater degree of quasipsychotic behaviors
- **Histrionic personality disorder**
  - More thorough discussion in Table 13-6
  - **Why eliminated from differential:** the self-destructive activities and explosive conclusions to relationships in this case are not typical of this diagnosis
- **Narcissistic personality disorder**
  - More thorough discussion in Table 13-6
  - **Why eliminated from differential:** the self-destructive activities and fear of being alone in this case are not typical of this diagnosis
- **Dependent personality disorder**
  - More thorough discussion in Table 13-6
  - **Why eliminated from differential:** the intensity of relationships would be much less in this diagnosis, and the patient would be expected to be resistant to ending any relationships
- **Attention deficit hyperactivity disorder**
  - More thorough discussion in later case
  - **Why eliminated from differential:** although the patient in this case has made some extremely impulsive decisions, impulsivity does not appear to be a problem with every single activity; likewise, inattentiveness and hyperactivity do not appear to be key features of her presentation
- **Bipolar disorder**
  - More thorough discussion in prior case

QUICK HIT: A patient who exhibits mild signs of a personality disorder but is able to function normally in society is said to have a **personality trait** and may not require treatment.

QUICK HIT: **Alcohol** and **tobacco** abuse are very common in patients with primary psychiatric diagnoses.

TABLE 13-6 Personality Disorders

Disorder	Characteristics	Treatment
CLUSTER A		
Paranoid	Persistent distrust of others' loyalty, others' actions are consistently interpreted as harmful or deceptive, reluctant to share information, frequent misinterpretation of comments, frequently bears grudges, perceives attacks on own reputation with an associated angry response, suspicions of partner infidelity	Supportive and nonjudgmental psychotherapy, low-dose antipsychotics
Schizoid	Inability to enjoy close relationships, social detachment, emotionally restricted, anhedonia, flat affect, lack of sexual interests, lack of close friends, indifferent to praise or criticism	Antipsychotics to initially resolve behavior, supportive psychotherapy focusing on achieving comfortable interactions with others
Schizotypal	Paranoia, ideas of reference, eccentric and inappropriate behavior, social anxiety, disorganized or vague speech, odd beliefs, relationships only with close relatives	Supportive psychotherapy focusing on recognition of reality, low-dose antipsychotics or anxiolytics
CLUSTER B		
Antisocial	Aggressive behavior toward people and animals, disregard for others' safety, destruction of property, illegal activity, pathological lying, irritability, impulsivity, risk-taking behavior, lack of responsibility, lack of remorse for actions; patients are typically older than 18 years and have a history of conduct disorder prior to 15 years of age; more common in men	Structured environment, psychotherapy with defined limit setting may be helpful in controlling behavior
Borderline	Unstable relationships, feelings of emptiness, fear of abandonment, poor self-esteem, impulsivity in self-damaging behaviors, mood lability, suicidal ideation or self-mutilating behavior, inappropriate irritability, paranoia, splitting (i.e., seeing others as either all good or all bad); much more common in women	Extensive psychotherapy employing multiple techniques combined with low-dose antipsychotics, SSRIs, or mood stabilizers
Histrionic	Dire need for attention, inappropriate seductive or theatrical behavior, emotional lability, exaggerated expression of emotions, dramatic speech, uses appearance to draw attention to self, easily influenced by others, believes relationships are more intimate than in reality	Long-term psychotherapy focusing on relationship development and limit setting
Narcissistic	Grandiosity, fantasies of success, manipulation of others, expectation of admiration, arrogance, sense of entitlement, believes self to be "special", lacks empathy, envious of others	Psychotherapy focusing on acceptance of shortcomings
CLUSTER C		
Avoidant	Fear of criticism and embarrassment, social withdrawal, unwillingness to interact with others without a certainty of being liked, fear of intimacy, poor self-esteem, reluctance to try new activities, preoccupied by fear of rejection, inhibited by feelings of inadequacy	Psychotherapy (initially individualized then group therapy later) focusing on self-confidence combined with antidepressants or anxiolytics
Dependent	Difficulty making decisions without the advice of others, fear of responsibility, difficulty expressing disagreement, difficulty in doing activities by self, going to excessive lengths to receive others' support, fear of being alone, requiring constant close relationships	Psychotherapy focusing on developing social skills and development of decisive behavior
Obsessive-compulsive	Preoccupied with details to the extent that the point of the activity is lost, perfectionistic, excessively devoted to work, inflexible in beliefs, miserly, difficulty working with others, hoarding of worthless objects, stubbornness	Psychotherapy focusing on accepting alternative ideas and working with others

SSRIs, selective serotonin reuptake inhibitors.

- **Why eliminated from differential:** the patient does not meet the criteria for major depression, and her extreme actions are more relationship-related and not independently periodic
- **Major depressive disorder/dysthymia**
  - More thorough discussion in prior case

  - **Why eliminated from differential:** the patient does not meet the depressive criteria for either of these diagnoses
- **Substance abuse**
  - More thorough discussion in later case
  - **Why eliminated from differential:** the patient's daily use of alcohol is somewhat concerning but appears to be more of a reaction to her personality disorder than a cause for her difficulties in relationships; toxicology screening should be seriously considered to rule out other substance use

CASE 13-6 "This man tried to kill his sister"

A 28-year-old man has recently been arrested for attacking his sister and is awaiting trial for assault and battery. Because of his odd behavior, a psychiatrist is called to evaluate the patient for a mental illness. Police records show that the patient lived in a basement apartment at his parents' house. He has been unemployed for 4 months but prior to that time he had worked as a dishwasher at a local restaurant. He was fired from that job because of getting into a fight with the manager over people secretly saying things about the patient. On the night of the assault, the patient's sister came to their parents' house for dinner. She tried to convince her brother to see fireworks that evening outside of town. When he refused to accompany her, she teased him about never leaving the house and being afraid of people. He became upset at these remarks. When the patient's sister grabbed the patient's arm and tried to drag him out of the house, the patient began punching his sister and continued to hit her after she let go of his arm. Their parents called the police, who had to restrain the patient from further attacking his sister. The patient was very agitated upon being removed from the house, but calmed down upon entering the holding cell at the police station. Since that time he has kept to himself, and has avoided speaking to other people unless necessary. In a conversation with the patient's sister, she confirms the details of the police report. She says that she thought it was best for the patient to "get out of the house for once" and never expected his violent response. She says that her brother started to become aloof during his last 2 years of high school. She says that he became extremely concerned with other people's perceptions of him. He attended a local college because he did not want to be far from home, but failed out in his second semester because he did not attend any classes. His sister says that he told his parents that everyone in class would look at him and would laugh at him behind his back. Since that time he has lived in his parents' basement. He has held low-level jobs on occasion, but these tend to be short-lived because of his perception that others are "looking down" on him. Much of the time he has been unemployed and supported by his parents. They tend to be overly protective of their son because of his eccentricities but feel powerless in how to help him feel more comfortable around people. His sister says that he is normally very tolerant of their parents and talks to them daily. She says that he is more hesitant to speak with her since she moved out of her parents' house, but that she is far better tolerated than nonrelatives. She says that her brother has no friends or relationships and spends much of his time watching television or playing on the computer. She is unaware of any medical problems that he has or medications that he takes on a regular basis. She is aware of a paternal uncle who was diagnosed with schizophrenia, but he had committed suicide prior to her birth. She says that her brother smokes cigarettes constantly, but she is unaware of any other substance use. When the patient is interviewed, he refuses to speak to the psychiatrist unless no one else is in the room. He is reluctant to speak until after the physician has reassured him that he is there to help the patient. The patient says that "everyone is out to get him" because "they know [his] secret." He refuses to explain what he means because "it would be too dangerous" for him. He says that he has "figured out this secret from watching television". He says that he refuses to watch news reports because "they spy on you" via the television. He feels that his parents were the only people he could trust prior to this incident. He also admits that he would become very anxious when leaving the house, so he tries to remain indoors as much as possible. He explains his attack on his sister only by saying "she became one of them." He denies wanting to hurt anyone else or himself, and says that he realizes that he could be incarcerated for his actions. He refuses to talk about any personal or family medical history. He admits to smoking cigarettes but denies other substance use. On the mental status examination, he appears clean but somewhat disheveled. His tone of speech is low, and he speaks quietly. Although he answers most questions, his answers tend to be rather vague and incomplete. He has no other abnormal patterns of speech. His affect is slightly flattened, but he does become more worried-appearing when talking about his "secret." He remains alert during the interview. He is oriented to his name, location, and the time. He is able to repeat the names of three listed objects and recalls all three objects several minutes later. He refuses physical examination. The following vital signs are measured:

T: 98.6°F, HR: 86 bpm, BP: 135/83 mm Hg, RR: 19 breaths/min

Differential Diagnosis

- Social phobia, delusional disorder, autism, schizotypal personality disorder, paranoid personality disorder, schizoid personality disorder, narcissistic personality disorder, avoidant personality disorder, major depressive disorder, substance abuse

Laboratory Data and Other Study Results

- Urine toxicology screen: positive for nicotine only

Diagnosis

- Schizotypal personality disorder

Treatment Administered

- The patient was enrolled in psychotherapy that focused on helping him discern reality from internal beliefs and on teaching him a means to cope with his perception of others
- Quetiapine was prescribed for the patient

Follow-up

- Although the patient agreed to participate in psychotherapy, he refused to use the antipsychotic medication
- Although charges were not pressed by his family members for the attack, the court ruled that the patient should receive inpatient psychiatric treatment
- Despite therapy, the patient did not significantly improve in his ability to interact with others and remained in the psychiatric facility

Steps to the Diagnosis

- **Schizotypal personality disorder**
  - More thorough discussion in Table 13-6
  - **Clues to the diagnosis:**
    - History: paranoia (e.g., worry of others' perceptions of him), ideas of reference (e.g., messages from the television), odd beliefs (e.g., "secret" ability), social anxiety and withdrawal, vague answers to questions, close relationships only with immediate family, family history of schizophrenia
    - Physical: flattened affect
    - Tests: noncontributory
- **Paranoid personality disorder**
  - More thorough discussion in Table 13-6
  - **Why eliminated from differential:** despite the important role of paranoia in this patient, the ideas of reference, odd beliefs, and social anxiety seen in this case are not characteristic of this disorder

- **Schizoid personality disorder**
  - More thorough discussion in Table 13-6
  - **Why eliminated from differential:** although social withdrawal and flattened affect are characteristic of this diagnosis, ideas of reference and odd beliefs are not typically demonstrated
- **Narcissistic personality disorder**
  - More thorough discussion in Table 13-6
  - **Why eliminated from differential:** grandiosity and personal fantasies may be seen in this diagnosis, but the social anxiety and withdrawal are not typical
- **Avoidant personality disorder**
  - More thorough discussion in Table 13-6
  - **Why eliminated from differential:** the ideas of reference, odd beliefs, and paranoia are not typically seen in this diagnosis
- **Social phobia**
  - More thorough discussion in prior case
  - **Why eliminated from differential:** the ideas of reference, odd beliefs, and paranoia are not typically seen in this diagnosis
- **Delusional disorder**
  - More thorough discussion in prior case
  - **Why eliminated from differential:** because isolated delusions are the main characteristic of this diagnosis, the other odd behaviors in this case rule it out
- **Autism**
  - A condition of severe impairment in interpersonal interactions and communication and unusual inflexible behaviors
    - Mental retardation is a common comorbid condition
    - Disease findings are usually exhibited prior to the age of 3 years
    - **Diagnosis** requires **six abnormal patterns** of interpersonal interactions including at least **two** types of **impaired social interactions**, **one** type of **impaired communication**, and **one** type of **restricted behavior**
  - **History:**
    - **Impaired social interactions:** impaired use of nonverbal behaviors, failure to develop peer relationships, failure to seek social interaction, lack of social reciprocity to others' attempts at interaction
    - **Impaired communication:** developmental language delays, poor initiation or sustenance of conversation, repetitive language, lack of imaginative or imitative play considered appropriate for age
    - **Restricted behavior:** inflexible routines, preoccupation with a restricted pattern of interest, repetitive motor mannerisms, preoccupation with parts of objects
  - **Physical examination:** findings are typically consistent with the abnormal behaviors (e.g., poor eye contact, mannerisms)
  - **Tests:** typically noncontributory, but appropriate testing is useful in ruling out other conditions
  - **Treatment:**
    - Behavioral, speech, and social psychotherapy involving peers and family members may help improve social interactions
    - Antipsychotics may be required to treat aggressive behaviors
    - Long-term supervision is usually required for these patients
  - **Outcomes:** the prognosis is generally poor with the majority of these patients never developing skills of social interaction and requiring lifelong care; patients with a milder form of the disease (i.e., Asperger disease) may be much more capable of functioning in society
  - **Why eliminated from differential:** although the social withdrawal and poor social interaction are consistent with this disease, the odd beliefs and ideas of reference make it an unlikely diagnosis
- **Major depressive disorder**
  - More thorough discussion in prior case

- **Why eliminated from differential:** some psychotic features may be seen in mood disorders, but the degree of social withdrawal and apparent lack of depressive characteristics make this diagnosis unlikely
- **Substance abuse**
  - More thorough discussion in later case
  - **Why eliminated from differential:** the denial of substance use beyond tobacco and the negative toxicology screen make this diagnosis unlikely

The following additional Psychiatry cases may be found online:

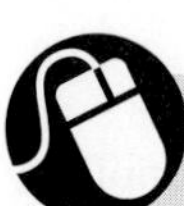

CASE 13-7 "It's so hot that I'm having a heart attack!"

CASE 13-8 "Our daughter has gotten so thin"

CASE 13-9 "My whole left leg is numb"

CASE 13-10 "My father isn't himself"

CASE 13-11 "My son is having problems in school"

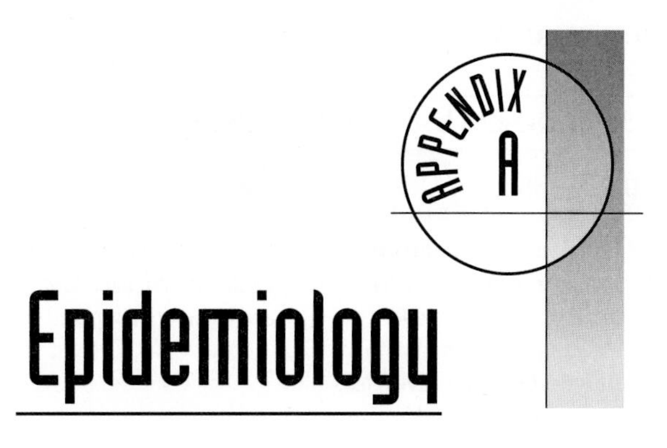

Epidemiology

RESEARCH STUDIES

- **Basic study requirements**
  - Subjects must be **representative** of the population examined
  - The **number** of subjects must be sufficient to detect statistical significance (i.e., adequate **power**)
  - Subjects must be able to give their **informed consent** to participation
  - Proper **control groups** are important to a study examining treatment efficacy
  - The interests of the patient take precedence over those of the study
    - Investigators must track data to look for potential risks to the subjects
    - An excessive amount of risk should lead to an early termination of the study
  - Subject **confidentiality** must be maintained
  - Human studies must be approved by an **institutional review board (IRB)**, and animal studies must be approved by an analogous animal review committee
- **Study design**
  - The chosen study design is based on the type of question proposed, the size of the affected patient population, the incidence of the disease or exposure in question, and the limitations of time and funding upon the study (Table A-1)
- **Study bias**
  - Biases in the design of a study or data interpretation will detract from the accuracy of the results (Table A-2)

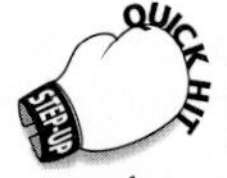

Investigator and observational bias may be avoided by **double-blinding** a study.

BIOSTATISTICS

- **Disease rates**
  - **Incidence:** the number of new cases that occurs within a certain time period in a population (i.e., the likelihood of developing that condition in that period of time)
    - 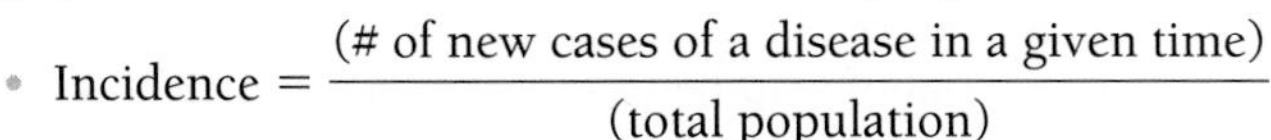
      $$\text{Incidence} = \frac{(\text{\# of new cases of a disease in a given time})}{(\text{total population})}$$
  - **Prevalence:** the number of individuals with a certain diagnosis at a given moment of time
    - $$\text{Prevalence} = \frac{(\text{\# of existing cases of a disease})}{(\text{total population})}$$
  - **Case fatality rate:** the percentage of individuals with a certain disease who die within a certain amount of time
    - $$\text{Fatality rate} = \frac{(\text{people who die from a disease in a given time})}{(\text{\# of cases of disease during given time})}$$
- **Disease-exposure associations**
  - **Relative risk (RR):** the risk of contracting a certain disease in a population with a common type of exposure (Table A-3)
  - $$\text{RR} = \frac{(\text{disease in exposed population})}{(\text{disease in unexposed population})} = \frac{A/(A + B)}{C/(C + D)}$$

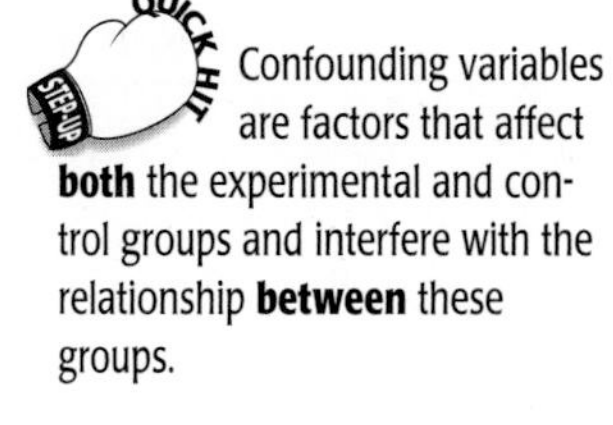

Confounding variables are factors that affect **both** the experimental and control groups and interfere with the relationship **between** these groups.

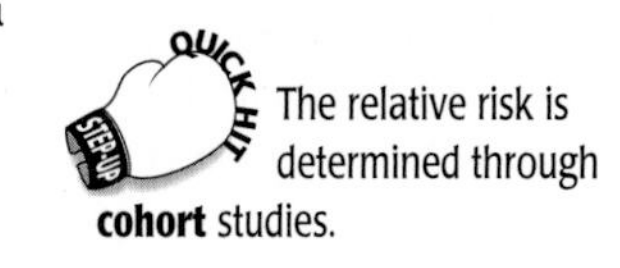

The relative risk is determined through **cohort** studies.

TABLE A-1 Study Designs Used in Clinical Research

Study Type	Description	Conclusions	Advantages	Disadvantages
Randomized clinical trial	• **Prospective comparison** of **experimental** treatment to **placebo** controls and **existing** therapies • **Double-blinded** to avoid bias • Patients **randomized** into study groups	Effectiveness of experimental treatment compared to controls and existing therapies	• **Gold standard** for testing therapies • May be controlled for several confounders	Often **costly** and **time consuming**, and patients may not be willing to undergo randomization
Cohort study	• Examines a group of subjects **exposed** to a given situation or factor • May be **prospective** (exposed group identified and followed over time) or **retrospective** (examines exposed group in whom disease has already occurred)	**Relative risk**	• Able to examine **rare exposures** • Can study multiple effects of exposure	May be costly and time consuming, and it is difficult to study rare diseases
Case-control study	• Retrospective comparison of patients with a **disease** to healthy controls; frequency of certain exposures in both groups is considered	**Odds ratio**	• May examine **rare diseases** or those with **long course** in short amount of time • Can study multiple types of exposure • May examine small group size	Susceptible to **recall** and **selection bias** and cannot determine disease incidence
Cross-sectional survey	• **Survey** of large number of people at one time to assess exposure and disease prevalence	Disease prevalence and a hypothesis for risk factors	• Can be used as an estimate for disease **prevalence** following exposure	Cannot be used to test hypotheses
Case series	• Report of characteristics of a disease by examining multiple cases	Hypothesis for risk factors	• May be easy to complete • Provides insight into poorly understood conditions	Cannot be used to test hypotheses
Meta-analysis	• **Pooling** of multiple studies examining a given disease or exposure	Depends on original study type	• Larger study size • Can resolve conflicts in literature	Unable to eliminate limiting factors in original studies

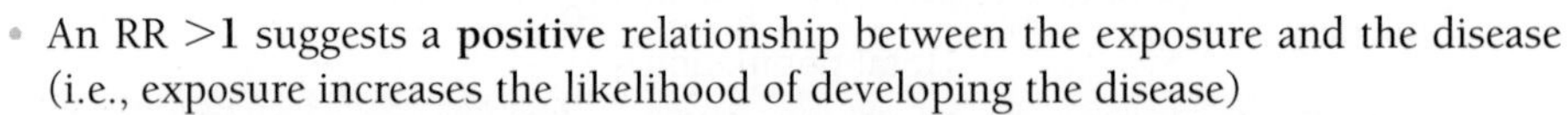

- An RR >1 suggests a **positive** relationship between the exposure and the disease (i.e., exposure increases the likelihood of developing the disease)
- An RR <1 suggests a **negative** relationship between the exposure and the disease (i.e., exposure decreases the likelihood of developing the disease)
- An RR **equal to 1** suggests **no** relationship between the exposure and the disease

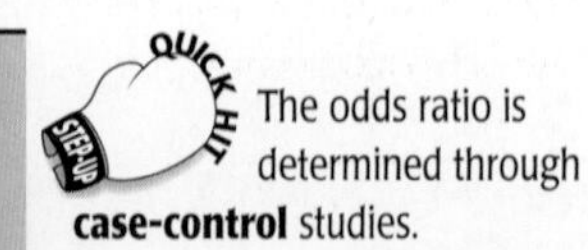

The odds ratio is determined through **case-control** studies.

- **Odds ratio (OR)**: the odds of having a history of a certain exposure among patients with a disease compared to those without the disease (Table A-3)
  - It is considered an estimate of the relative risk for that exposure
  - $OR = \frac{A/C}{B/D} = \frac{A \times D}{B \times C}$
- **Attributable risk (AR)**: the difference in the rates of a disease between exposed and unexposed populations
  - AR = (rate of disease in exposed population) − (rate of disease in unexposed population)
  - **Statistics of diagnostic tests**

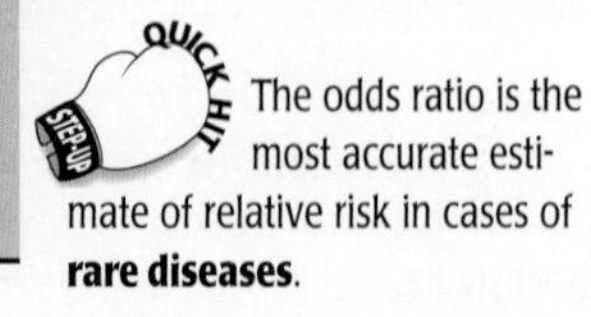

The odds ratio is the most accurate estimate of relative risk in cases of **rare diseases**.

TABLE A-2 Types of Bias in Clinical Studies

Type of Bias	Description	Consequences
Enrollment (selection)	**Nonrandom** assignment of subjects to study groups	Results of the study may not be applicable to the general population
Investigator	Subjective interpretation of the data by **investigator** deviates toward "**desired**" conclusions	Results of study will incorrectly resemble the proposed hypothesis
Lead-time	A screening test provides an **earlier diagnosis** in the studied group when compared to controls but has **no effect on time of survival**	The time from diagnosis to outcome increases because the earlier diagnosis causes the false appearance of an increased time of survival; the time from the beginning of the disease process to the outcome actually remains the same regardless of screening
Length	A screening test **detects** several **slowly** progressive cases of a disease and **misses rapidly** progressive cases	Effectiveness of screening test is overstated
Observational	Subjects may respond to subjective questions in a different way than normal because their **awareness** of the study changes their perception of the examined issue	Effectiveness of therapy is not accurately depicted by study group
Publication	Studies that show a difference between groups are **more likely to be published** than studies that do not show a difference	Data available for meta-analyses may not include studies that support the null hypothesis
Recall	Errors of memory within the subjects occurs due to **prior confounding experiences**	Patients with negative experiences are more likely to recall negative details
Self-selection	Patients with a certain **past medical history** may be more likely to participate in a study related to their condition	Subjects are not representative of the general population and introduce confounding variables

- **Sensitivity:** the probability that a screening test will be **positive in patients with a disease** (Table A-4)
  - Sensitivity $= \frac{A}{A + C}$
  - Most acceptable screening tests are >80% sensitive
  - A **false negative** is a negative test in a patient with the disease
  - The false negative rate is approximated by (1 − sensitivity)
- **Specificity:** the probability that a test will be **negative in patients without a disease** (Table A-4)
  - Specificity $= \frac{D}{B + D}$
  - Most acceptable confirmatory tests are >85% specific
  - A **false positive** is a positive test in a patient without the disease
  - The false-positive rate is approximated by (1 − specificity)

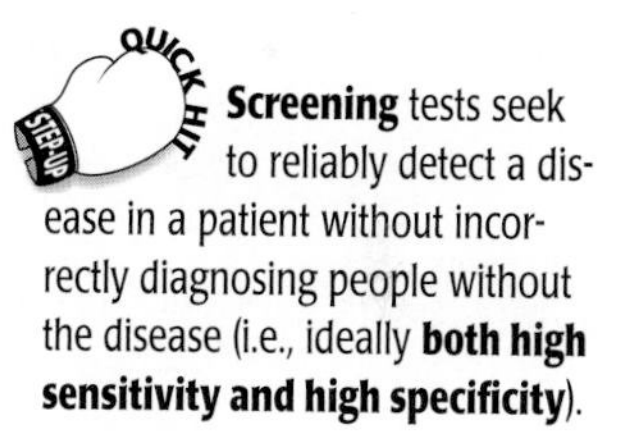

Screening tests seek to reliably detect a disease in a patient without incorrectly diagnosing people without the disease (i.e., ideally **both high sensitivity and high specificity**).

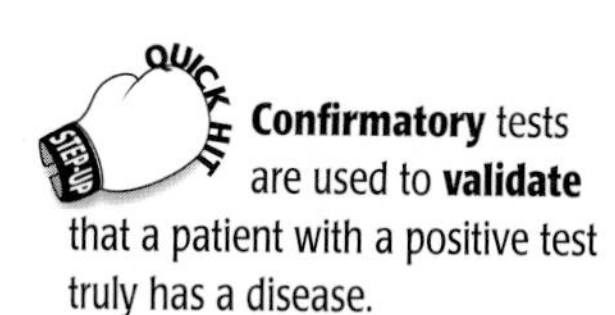

Confirmatory tests are used to **validate** that a patient with a positive test truly has a disease.

TABLE A-3 Calculation of Disease Risk

		Disease	
		Yes	No
Exposure	Yes	A	B
	No	C	D

Relative risk (RR) $= \frac{A/(A + B)}{C/(C + D)}$; Odds ratio (OR) $= \frac{A/C}{B/D} = \frac{A \times D}{B \times C}$

TABLE A-4 Analysis of Diagnostic Tests

		Disease	
		Yes	No
Test	Positive	A	B
	Negative	C	D

Sensitivity $= \frac{A}{A + C}$; Specificity $= \frac{D}{B + D}$; Positive predictive value (PPV) $= \frac{A}{A + B}$;

Negative predictive value (NPV) $= \frac{D}{C + D}$

QUICK HIT: A disease with a **high** prevalence will be associated with a high **positive** predictive value in a screening test.

QUICK HIT: A disease with a **low** prevalence will be associated with a high **negative** predictive value in a screening test.

- **Positive predictive value (PPV):** the probability that a patient with a positive test has the disease of interest (Table A-4)
    - $PPV = \frac{A}{A + B}$
- **Negative predictive value (NPV):** the probability that a patient with a negative test does not have the disease of interest (Table A-4)
    - $NPV = \frac{D}{C + D}$
- **Likelihood ratios:** the odds of having a positive test result in patients with a disease compared to those without it (i.e., positive likelihood ratio; PLR) or the odds of having a negative test result in patients with a disease compared to those without it (i.e., negative likelihood ratio; NLR)
    - Used to measure the performance of a diagnostic test while eliminating the test's dependence on the disease prevalence
    - Positive likelihood ratio (PLR) $= \frac{(\text{sensitivity})}{(1 - \text{specificity})}$
    - Negative likelihood ratio (NLR) $= \frac{(1 - \text{sensitivity})}{(\text{specificity})}$
- **Accuracy:** the performance of diagnostic tests, considering only the number of true positive and true negative results
    - $\text{Accuracy} = \frac{A + D}{A + B + C + D}$

- **Error in studies**
    - **Null hypothesis:** the hypothesis that there is **no** association between the exposure and a disease or the treatment and a response
    - **Alternative hypothesis:** the hypothesis that there **is** an association between the exposure and a disease or the treatment and a response
    - **Type I error:** the null hypothesis is rejected although it is true (i.e., **false positive**)
    - **Type II error:** the null hypothesis is not rejected although it is false (i.e., **false negative**)
    - The risk of an error occurring decreases with an increasing sample size (i.e., increasing study power)
- **Significance:** the statistically detectable difference between two sample groups
    - **Probability value (*P* value)**
        - The chance of a type I error occurring for a given result
        - If $P < 0.05$, the null hypothesis can be rejected (i.e., there is a significant relationship between the groups)
    - **Confidence interval (CI)**
        - A range of values (e.g., relative risk, odds ratio, objective data) calculated in a study and the likelihood that the true result falls within that range

  - Most commonly listed as a 95% CI (i.e., there is a 95% chance that the true result falls within the study-derived range)
  - If the CIs for a measure in two sample groups overlap, the likelihood that the measure is statistically different between the groups is low
  - If the CI for a calculated relative risk or odds ratio include 1.0 within its range, the risk of exposure is not significant
- **Power**: the ability of a study to detect an actual difference between two groups
  - Studies with insufficient power may state two groups are equal when they are actually significantly different (i.e., occurrence of a type II error)

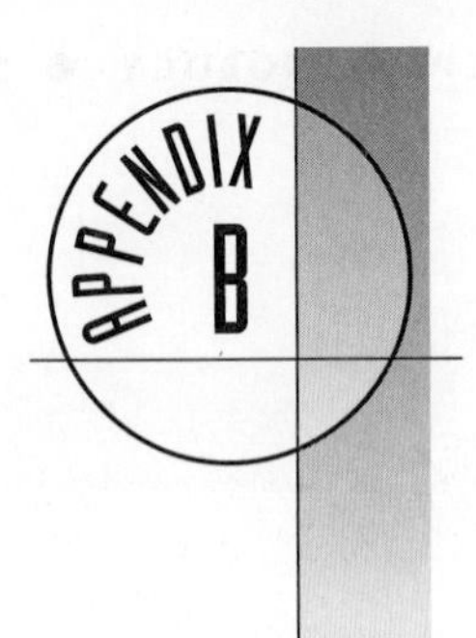

Ethics

QUICK HIT: Confidentiality should be maintained in **adolescents** seeking treatment for **sexually transmitted diseases (STDs)** or **pregnancy** (a point that may need to be clarified with parents).

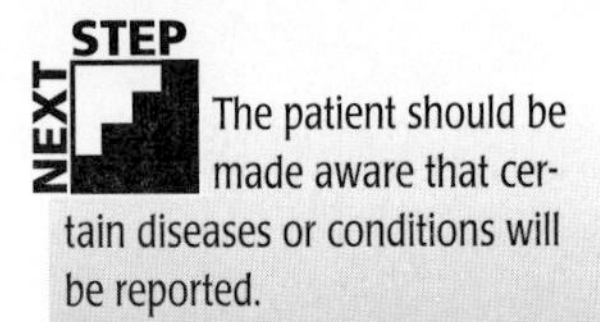

The patient should be made aware that certain diseases or conditions will be reported.

QUICK HIT: A **competent** patient may change his or her mind regarding accepting therapy **at any time**.

PATIENT RIGHTS

- Confidentiality
  - All information regarding the patient must be kept **private** between the **physician** and the **patient**
    - All patient records and billing must be designed to maintain confidentiality
    - The exchange of patient information may only occur between providers involved with the care of that patient
  - Confidentiality may be forgone in some circumstances
    - The patient gives the physician **permission** to share information with designated parties (e.g., family members)
    - The patient carries a **legally reportable disease** (e.g., human immunodeficiency virus [HIV], tuberculosis [TB], syphilis)
    - The patient is **homicidal** or **suicidal**
    - The patient has sustained a **penetrating wound** from an assault
    - The patient is an **adolescent** with a condition that is potentially harmful to him or herself or others
- Public reporting
  - **By law**, a public health department must be notified of cases of certain **STDs** or other transmissible diseases (e.g., **HIV**, hepatitis, Lyme disease, food-borne illness, meningitis, rabies, and **TB**)
  - Impairments in driving ability, **child abuse**, and **elder abuse** must be reported to authorities (exact legal requirements vary from state to state)
- Informed consent
  - **Prior to any procedure or therapy**, the patient must be made aware of the indications, risks, and potential benefits of a proposed treatment, any alternative treatments and their risks, and the risks of refusing treatment
  - Informed consent (including parental consent in the case of a minor) is not required for emergent therapy (i.e., **implied consent**)
  - If a patient is not capable of making a decision for a nonemergent procedure, a designated surrogate decision maker is required
- Full disclosure
  - Patients have the right to be made aware of their medical status, prognosis, treatment options, and medical errors in their care
  - If a family requests that a physician withhold information from the patient, physicians must deny the request unless it is determined that disclosing information would significantly harm the patient

MEDICAL DECISION MAKING

- Competency
  - A **competent** patient is entitled to make all decisions regarding his or her medical care
  - **Requirements for competency**
    - The patient cannot be currently psychotic or intoxicated

        - The patient must have an **understanding** of his or her **medical situation**
        - The patient must be capable of making decisions that are in agreement with his or her history of values
    - Medical decisions for **nonemancipated minors** (i.e., younger than 18 years) are made by a minor's parents unless legally ruled to be not in the best interests of the child
    - **Emancipated minors** (e.g., pregnant, married, financially independent) may make their own decisions
- **Durable power of attorney**
    - Legal documentation that designates a **second party** (e.g., family member) **as a surrogate decision maker** for medical issues (not valid in all states)
    - The designated individual should be able to make decisions **consistent with the patient's values**
- **Living will**
    - A written document that details a patient's wishes in specific medical situations (e.g., resuscitation, ventilation, extraordinary maintenance of life)
    - The **patient** is responsible for creating the definitions of his or her own living will
    - It may be more stringent than a durable power of attorney to solidly define the patient's wishes

QUICK HIT: Parents' decisions regarding their children may be legally **overruled** if they are considered **harmful** to the children.

END-OF-LIFE ISSUES

- **Do-not-resuscitate orders (DNR)**
    - A type of advanced directive document that details care in cases of coma, cardiac arrest, severe dementia, and terminal illness
    - A DNR may object to all nonpalliative therapies or may only restrict use of specific therapies (e.g., ventilation, cardiopulmonary resuscitation, feeding tubes, antibiotics)
    - A **physician** writes a DNR in correspondence with the patient's wishes (may be outlined in a living will)
- **Life support**
    - Competent patients may request to have supportive measures withdrawn at any time (including through a living will)
    - Physicians are able to remove respiratory care in cases in which there is **no living will** and the patient is **incapable** of voicing a decision if both the **family** and the **physician** believe that removal of care is **consistent** with **what the patient would want**
- **Physician-aided death**
    - Physician-assisted suicide occurs when a physician **supplies** a patient with a means of ending his or her life but is not directly responsible for the death
    - Euthanasia is the **active administration by a physician** of a lethal agent to a patient in order to cause death and eliminate suffering from a condition
- **Death**
    - **Brain death** is defined as the irreversible **absence** of all brain activity (including the brainstem) in a patient lasting more than 6 hours
        - The absence of cranial nerve reflexes (e.g., gag, corneal, and caloric reflexes)
        - Apnea off of a ventilator for a duration considered sufficient to produce a normal hypercarbic drive
        - The absence of hypothermia or intoxication
        - The absence of brainstem-evoked responses, a persistent isoelectric EEG, or absent cerebral circulation on vascular imaging studies
        - A patient's appearance cannot be explained by a medical condition that mimics death
    - **Cardiac death** is considered the inability to restore a spontaneous heartbeat in an asystolic patient
    - Either brain death or heart death may be used to define formal patient death, but both are not required
    - **Hypothermic** patients must be warmed to a normal body temperature before death can be declared

QUICK HIT: Physicians are not required to supply therapies that are irrational for the current condition or when the maximum reasonable therapy has already failed.

QUICK HIT: The absence of electroencephalogram (EEG) activity does **not** define brain death but may help prompt a brain death work-up

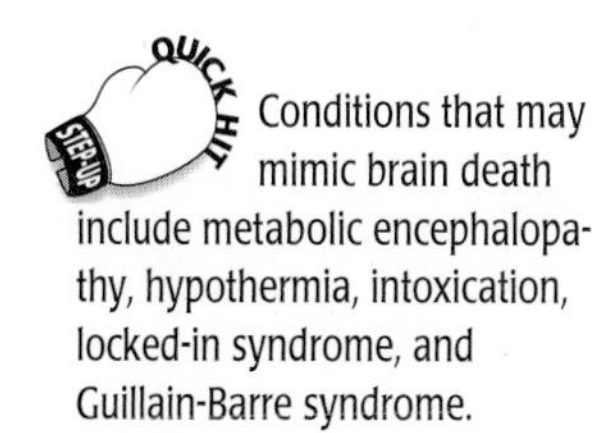

QUICK HIT: Conditions that may mimic brain death include metabolic encephalopathy, hypothermia, intoxication, locked-in syndrome, and Guillain-Barre syndrome.

- Organ donation
  - Patients may declare themselves as organ donors prior to death (e.g., living will, designated on driver's license)
    - Patients and their families may define exactly which organs may be donated
  - Hospitals receiving payments from Medicare are required to approach the family of the deceased regarding organ donation
  - Organs may be judged unsuitable for donation in cases of widespread or uncured **neoplasm**, **sepsis** or blood-borne infection, compromised organ function, organ-specific infection or disease, hypothermia, age >80 years, hemoglobinopathy, or **prolonged ischemia**

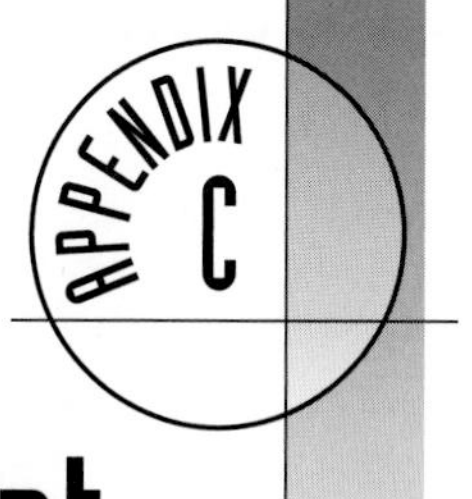

Pediatric Development

PEDIATRIC PHYSICAL GROWTH

- Weight
  - **Rate of weight gain**
    - Body weight decreases for the first few days after birth
    - The birth weight is regained by 2 weeks after delivery
    - The child's weight should **double** by 4 months, **triple** by 1 year, and **quadruple** by 2 years
    - Annual weight gain should be approximately **5 pounds** between 2 and 13 years of age
    - Inadequate weight gain may be due to **poor food intake**, chronic vomiting or diarrhea, **malabsorption**, neoplasm, or congenital diseases (e.g., cardiac, endocrine)
  - Weight below the 5th percentile suggests **failure to thrive**
  - **Childhood obesity** (weight over the 95th percentile) is associated with increased rates of sleep apnea, hypertension (HTN), slipped capital femoral epiphysis, precocious puberty, skin infections, social dysfunction, and diabetes mellitus
- Height
  - **Rate of height gain**
    - The child's height should increase by **50%** by 1 year after birth, should **double** by 4 years, and should **triple** by 13 years of age
    - The annual increase in height should be 2 inches per year between 2 and 13 years of age
  - Greater-than-normal height may be associated with familial tall stature, precocious puberty, acromegaly, hyperthyroidism, Klinefelter syndrome, Marfan syndrome, or obesity
  - Lower-than-normal height may be associated with familial short stature, neglect, Turner syndrome, constitutional growth delay, chronic renal failure, asthma, cystic fibrosis, inflammatory bowel disease, immunologic disease, growth hormone deficiency, hypothyroidism, glucocorticoid excess, skeletal dysplasias, or neoplasm
- **Head circumference**
  - **Rate of increase**
    - Approximately 5 cm of growth occurs by 3 months after birth, an additional 4 cm by 6 months, an additional 2 cm by 9 months, and an additional 1 cm by 1 year
  - **Macrocephaly** may be associated with cerebral metabolic diseases (e.g., Tay-Sachs, maple syrup urine disease), neurocutaneous syndromes (e.g., neurofibromatosis, tuberous sclerosis), hydrocephalus, increased intracranial pressure, skeletal dysplasia, acromegaly, or intracranial hemorrhage
  - **Microcephaly** may be associated with fetal toxin exposure (e.g., fetal alcohol syndrome), chromosomal trisomies, congenital infection, cranial anatomical abnormalities, metabolic disorders, or neural tube defects
- **Cumulative growth abnormalities**
  - A child with normal fetal growth, an initially normal growth rate, and a delayed onset of inadequate growth following birth has a **postnatal** cause of the growth abnormality
  - Growth that is **abnormal from the time of birth** suggests a **prenatal** onset (e.g., genetic abnormalities, intrauterine pathology)

MNEMONIC

Causes of short stature may be remembered by the mnemonic **ABCDEFGHIJKL**: **A**buse, **B**ad cancers, **C**hromosomal (Turner), **D**elayed growth (constitutional), **E**ndocrine (growth hormone deficiency, hypothyroidism), **F**amilial short stature, **GI** disease (IBD, celiac), **H**eart (congenital disease), **I**mmune disorders, **J**oint and bone dysplasias, **K**idney failure, **L**ung disease (asthma, cystic fibrosis).

- Growth that is low-normal in range but eventually becomes closer to the mean suggests **constitutional growth delay**
- Growth that is **consistently low-normal** suggests genetic short stature
  - A comparison to the parents' growth histories will help make this diagnosis
- Other symptoms and physical signs are useful for determining the cause of the growth abnormality
- Growth should be assessed and recorded on a growth chart at **each health visit** to confirm normal patterns and to catch abnormalities early in their process

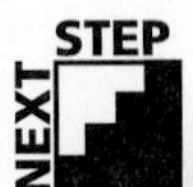

Ages for developmental milestones are **guidelines**. It is normal for milestones to occur at an appropriate **range of ages**, and parents should be reassured that milestones occur within such a range and not at concrete ages.

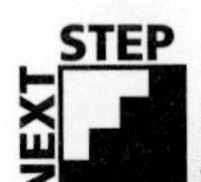

Be sure to collect a thorough **family history** while assessing growth or developmental delays in order to help distinguish a **hereditary** cause from an **environmental** one.

PEDIATRIC DEVELOPMENTAL MILESTONES

- Schedule of milestones
  - **Social**, **physical**, and **intellectual** achievements are reached by children at characteristic ages (Table A-5)
  - The absence of delay of milestones may suggest developmental delays
    - Some delays are hereditary, but the presence of multiple or persistent delays is concerning for pathologic process (e.g., mental retardation, genetic disorders, language or hearing impairments, child abuse, psychiatric disease)
    - The persistence of **infantile reflexes** beyond 6 months of age may suggest a central nervous system abnormality
- Adolescence
  - A period of **rapid physical**, **psychosocial**, and **sexual** growth during the second decade of life
  - **Psychosocial issues**
    - Early adolescence (i.e., 10 to 13 years old) is typified by concrete thinking and early independent behavior

TABLE A-5 Important Developmental Milestones During Childhood

Age	Social/Cognitive	Gross Motor	Fine Motor	Language
2 months	Social smile	Lifts head 45°	Eyes follow object to midline	Coos
4 months	Laughs Aware of caregiver Localizes sound	Lifts head 90°	Eyes follow object past midline	
6 months	Differentiates parents from others Separation anxiety	Rolls over Holds self up with hands Sits	Grasps/rakes Attempts to feed self	Babbles
9 months	Interactive games	Crawls	Grasps with thumb	First words
12 months		Pulls to stand Walks with help	Pincer grasp Makes tower of 2 blocks	~5- to 10-word vocabulary
18 months	Parallel play	Walks well Walks backwards	Makes tower of 4 blocks Uses cup or spoon	10- to 50-word vocabulary 2-word sentences
2 years	Dresses self with help	Runs Climbs stairs (initially 2 feet/step, then 1 foot/step)	Makes tower of 6 blocks	50- to 75-word vocabulary 3-word sentences
3 years	Magical thinking	Climbs/descends stairs	Makes tower of 9 blocks Able to draw circle (O)	
4 years	Plays with others	Hops on 1 foot	Able to draw line image (+), later able to draw closed line drawing (Δ)	250+ word vocabulary 4-word sentences
6 years	Able to distinguish fantasy from reality	Skips	Draws a person	Fluent speech

- Middle adolescence (i.e., 14 to 16 years old) is typified by the emergence of **sexuality** (i.e., sexual identity, sexual activity), an increased **desire for independence** (i.e., conflict with parents, need for guidance, self-absorption), and abstract thought
- Late adolescence (i.e., 17 to 21 years old) is typified by an increased self-awareness, an increased confidence in one's own abilities, a more open relationship with one's parents, and cognitive maturity
- Adolescents are at an increased risk for **risk-taking behaviors** (e.g., drug use, unprotected sexual activity, violence), **depression**, **suicidal ideation**, **homicide**, and **eating disorders**
- It is important to consider both the psychological and emotional issues of these patients in addition to their medical issues during routine office visits
  - Patient issues should be approached in a **nonjudgmental** fashion

CHILDHOOD HEALTH MAINTENANCE

- **Well-child visits**
  - Periodic physician visits are important during childhood to assess **growth** and **developmental milestones**, provide **vaccinations**, **screen** for certain disease processes, and provide **anticipatory guidance** (Table A-6)
    - Screening tests should be performed to address common medical concerns (e.g., vision, hearing, dentition, diseases in high-risk populations)
    - Anticipatory guidance should address **nutrition**, **development**, **daily care**, **accident prevention**, and **behavioral issues**

QUICK HIT: Some teaching methods that maximize the communication of important information during a visit are **repetition**, **positive reinforcement**, limitation of the number of topics discussed, and not focusing on minor points.

TABLE A-6 Screening Performed and Anticipatory Guidance Discussed during Regular Childhood Health Visits

Visit	Screening	Nutrition	Daily Care	Accident Prevention	Behavioral Issues
Newborn/ 1 week	Phenylketonuria, hypothyroidism, genetic metabolic disorders (maple syrup urine disease, cystic fibrosis, etc.) in high-risk patients, hearing, visual mobility and reflexes	Breast or bottle feeding	Crying, sleep position, bathing	Smoke detectors, baby furniture, car seats	Parent-child interaction
1 month	Visual mobility and reflexes	Breast or bottle feeding, fluoride supplements	Sleep, bowel and bladder habits	Sun exposure	Importance of close contact
2 months	Visual mobility and reflexes		Sleep, bowel habits	Close supervision, risks due to ability to roll over	
4 months	Visual mobility and reflexes	Solid foods, fruits and vegetables	Teething	Keeping small objects out of reach	Vocal interaction
6 months	Visual mobility and reflexes	Cup training, daily caloric needs, finger foods, avoidance of milk or juice at bedtime	Shoes	Preparation for increased mobility ("child-proofing" the house), electrical socket covers, stair and door gates	Stranger anxiety, separation anxiety
9 months	Hgb/Hct; visual mobility and reflexes	Iron supplementation, self-feeding, spoon training	Tooth care, favorite toys	Aspiration risks	Communication, discipline

(continued)

TABLE A-6 Screening Performed and Anticipatory Guidance Discussed during Regular Childhood Health Visits (*Continued*)

Visit	Screening	Nutrition	Daily Care	Accident Prevention	Behavioral Issues
12 months	Visual mobility and reflexes, lead exposure, PPD in high-risk areas	Bottle weaning, eating at table, whole cow's milk		Poisoning risks, stair safety, burns	Speech, rules, positive reinforcement
15 months	Hgb/Hct, visual mobility and reflexes	Family meals			Toilet training, temper tantrums, punishment, listening to parent read
18 months	Visual mobility and reflexes	Reinforcement of utensil use	Nightmares, bedtime regimens	Supervised play, dangerous toys	Discipline, "terrible 2s", toilet training, games
2 years	Lead exposure, visual mobility and reflexes	Avoiding unhealthy snacks, encouraging eating during meals	Transition from crib to bed, toothbrush training		Toddler independence, explanation of body parts, early play with other children
3 years	Visual acuity, cholesterol (if family history of high cholesterol or CAD)	Healthy diet	Regular sleep schedule, television limitation	Water safety, animal safety	Day care or babysitters (earlier if both parents work), play with other children, reinforce consistent toileting, conversation
4 years	Hearing, lead exposure, visual acuity, PPD (if high-risk group), urinalysis	Meals as time for family bonding	Self dental care	Pedestrian and bicycle safety, car seat or seat belt, dangers of strangers, guns, fires, poisons, teach phone number	Chores, interactions at day care or preschool, school preparation
6 years	Lead exposure, visual acuity	Avoidance of excess weight, obesity prevention counseling	Exercise, hygiene, school activities	Swimming	Allowance, encourage learning and development, reading
10 years	Hearing, visual acuity			Hazardous activities, drug use (including alcohol and tobacco)	Friends, sexual education, puberty, responsibility
12 years	Hearing, visual acuity, PPD (if high-risk group), Pap smear only if sexually active (girls)		Adequate sleep, school and extracurricular activities	Sexual responsibility	Body image, privacy issues
14 years and older	Hearing, Hgb/Hct (girls), visual acuity, STD screening (if sexually active)	Weight maintenance	School and activities	Risk-taking behavior, driving, sexual responsibility	Dating, sexuality, goals, careers, independence issues

Note: Anticipatory guidance from **prior** visits should be **reviewed** when appropriate.

CAD, coronary artery disease; Hgb/Hct, hemoglobin and hematocrit; PPD, purified protein derivative of tuberculin (TB test); STD, sexually transmitted disease.

TABLE A-7 **Vaccination Schedule and Contraindications During Well-Child Health Visits (2008 Recommendations)**

<table>
<tr><th></th><th colspan="11">Age</th></tr>
<tr><th>Vaccine</th><th>Birth</th><th>1 mo</th><th>2 mo</th><th>4 mo</th><th>6 mo</th><th>12 mo</th><th>15 mo</th><th>18 mo</th><th>24 mo</th><th>4–6 yr</th><th>11–12 yr</th></tr>
<tr><td>HepB[1]</td><td>HepB</td><td colspan="2">HepB</td><td></td><td colspan="4">HepB</td><td></td><td></td><td></td></tr>
<tr><td>Rota[2]</td><td></td><td></td><td>Rota</td><td>Rota</td><td>Rota</td><td></td><td></td><td></td><td></td><td></td><td></td></tr>
<tr><td>DTaP[3]</td><td></td><td></td><td>DTaP</td><td>DTaP</td><td>DTaP</td><td></td><td colspan="2">DTaP</td><td></td><td>DTaP</td><td>Td</td></tr>
<tr><td>Hib[4]</td><td></td><td></td><td>Hib</td><td>Hib</td><td>Hib</td><td colspan="2">Hib</td><td></td><td></td><td></td><td></td></tr>
<tr><td>PCV[5]</td><td></td><td></td><td>PCV</td><td>PCV</td><td>PCV</td><td colspan="2">PCV</td><td></td><td></td><td></td><td></td></tr>
<tr><td>IPV[6]</td><td></td><td></td><td>IPV</td><td>IPV</td><td colspan="4">IPV</td><td></td><td></td><td></td></tr>
<tr><td>MMR[7]</td><td></td><td></td><td></td><td></td><td></td><td colspan="2">MMR</td><td></td><td></td><td>MMR</td><td></td></tr>
<tr><td>VZV[8]</td><td></td><td></td><td></td><td></td><td></td><td colspan="2">VZV</td><td></td><td></td><td>VZV</td><td></td></tr>
<tr><td>HepA[9]</td><td></td><td></td><td></td><td></td><td></td><td colspan="4">HepA × 2</td><td></td><td></td></tr>
<tr><td>MCV4[10]</td><td></td><td></td><td></td><td></td><td></td><td></td><td></td><td></td><td></td><td></td><td>MCV4</td></tr>
<tr><td>HPV[11]</td><td></td><td></td><td></td><td></td><td></td><td></td><td></td><td></td><td></td><td></td><td>HPV × 3</td></tr>
</table>

[1]Hepatitis B (HepB); contraindications: allergy to yeast or anaphylaxis following prior dose

[2]Rotavirus (Rota); contraindications: anaphylaxis following prior dose

[3]Diptheria, tetanus, acellular pertussis (DTaP); tetanus booster (Td) given in adolescence; contraindications: encephalopathy or anaphylaxis following prior dose

[4]*Haemophilus influenzae* type b (Hib); no contraindications

[5]Pneumococcal vaccine (PCV); contraindications: anaphylaxis following prior dose

[6]Inactivated polio vaccine (IPV); contraindications: pregnancy (or pregnant female at home) and anaphylaxis following prior dose

[7]Measles, mumps, rubella (MMR); contraindications: pregnancy (or pregnant female at home), immunocompromise, thrombocytopenia, hematologic or solid neoplasm, anaphylaxis following prior dose

[8]Varicella zoster vaccine (VZV); contraindications: allergy to neomycin, anaphylaxis following prior dose, immunosuppression, pregnancy (or pregnant female at home), moderate or severe illness

[9]Hepatitis A (HepA); given in two doses at least 6 months apart; contraindications: anaphylaxis following prior dose

[10]Meningococcal vaccine (MCV4); possible rare association with Guillain-Barré syndrome

[11]Human papilloma virus vaccine (HPV); given as three doses over 6-month period

- Vaccinations should be administered at the appropriate visits according to the recommended schedule (Table A-7)

QUICK HIT: The first dose of hepatitis B vaccine is typically administered shortly after birth before the infant leaves the hospital.

QUICK HIT: *Haemophilus influenzae* type b (Hib) vaccine is **unnecessary** in previously unvaccinated children **older than 5 years** because of the low risk of severe infection at this age and older. **Asplenic** children should **always** receive Hib and pneumococcal vaccines regardless of their age.

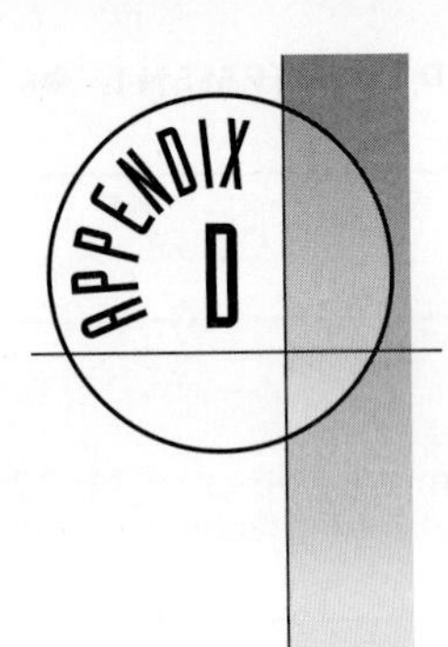

Traumatology

MECHANISMS OF INJURY

- **Blunt trauma:** contusion of local structures and induction of a significant local inflammatory response
- **Penetrating trauma:** the penetrating object (e.g., bullet, sharp object) damages tissue in path of its trajectory and causes indirect damage from fragmented bone and external objects
- **Acceleration-deceleration injuries** (e.g., falls, motor vehicle crashes): injury occurs secondary to shearing forces in tissues due to sudden changes in momentum and sudden forces applied to tethered portions of organs (e.g., aortic arch, mesentery)

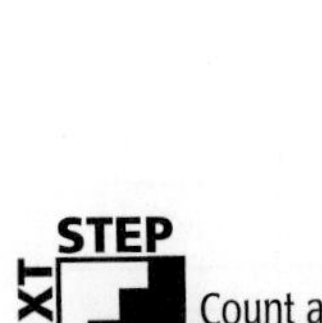

Count and pair all entrance and exit gunshot wounds to suggest a number of insulting bullets and to deduce a path for each bullet.

ASSESSMENT OF THE TRAUMA PATIENT

- The primary assessment must be performed in an organized manner to detect all life-threatening injuries and to judge their severity
- The initial assessment focuses on the **ABCs**
  - A secure **airway** must be established
  - **Breathing** is confirmed, and adequate oxygenation (e.g., supplemental oxygen, ventilation) is secured
  - Adequate **circulation** is confirmed, adequate vascular access is secured, and bleeding is controlled
- The **secondary** assessment consists of a highly detailed examination performed to detect all wounds, fractures, signs of internal injury, and neurologic insult
- The Glasgow coma scale (GCS) and the revised trauma score (RTS) are used to objectify injury severity (Tables A-8 and A-9)
- **Head trauma**
  - Trauma may cause direct injury or secondary injuries though intracranial bleeding
  - Cerebral damage may be at the point of insult (i.e., **coup**) or on the opposite side of the head (i.e., **contrecoup**)
  - The physical examination should include assessments of the level of consciousness, papillary light reflex, and oculocephalic reflex
  - A **head and cervical spine computed tomography (CT)** should be performed on every patient with suspected head trauma
  - Management should focus on maintaining cerebral perfusion, decreasing excessive intracranial pressure, and stabilizing spinal instability
- **Neck trauma**
  - Because of the multiple vascular, neurologic, gastrointestinal (GI), and respiratory structures, injuries can quickly become life-threatening
  - The physical examination should include assessments of perfusion, airway patency, and neurologic injury
  - X-ray and CT of the neck, Doppler ultrasound (US), esophagogastroduodenoscopy (EGD), bronchoscopy, and angiography are tests that should be considered in the proper clinical scenarios

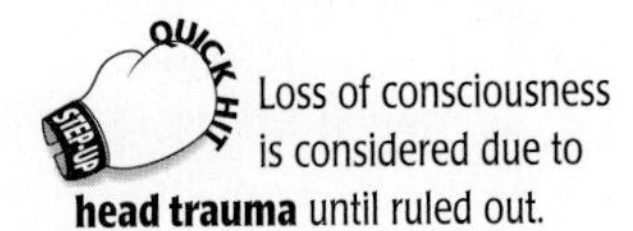

Loss of consciousness is considered due to **head trauma** until ruled out.

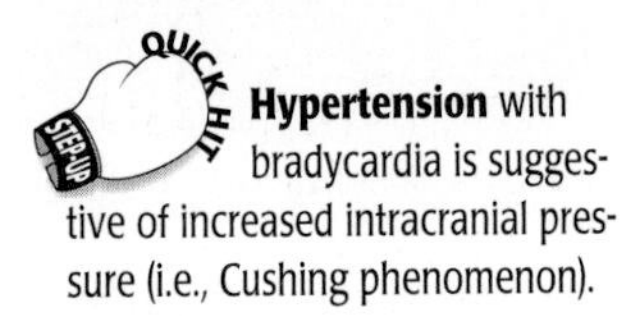

Hypertension with bradycardia is suggestive of increased intracranial pressure (i.e., Cushing phenomenon).

MNEMONIC

Key points of the neurologic examination for suspected head trauma may be remembered by the **12 Ps**: **P**aired ocular movement, **P**apilledema, **P**aralysis, **P**aresthesias, **P**atellar and other reflexes, **P**ee (incontinence), **P**ressure (blood and intracranial), **P**sychological (mental) status, **P**tosis, **P**ulse rate, **P**upils (size, symmetry, reflexes), **P**yramidal signs (abnormal movements).

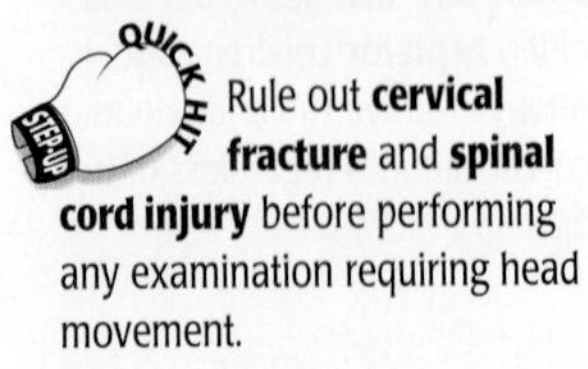

Rule out **cervical fracture** and **spinal cord injury** before performing any examination requiring head movement.

TABLE A-8 Glasgow Coma Scale[1]

Category	Condition	Points
Eye opening	Spontaneous	4
	To voice	3
	To pain	2
	None	1
Verbal response	Oriented	5
	Confused	4
	Inappropriate words	3
	Incomprehensible	2
	None	1
Motor response	Obeys commands	6
	Localizes pain	5
	Withdraws from pain	4
	Flexion with pain	3
	Extension with pain	2
	None	1

[1]Total score is calculated by adding the component score for each category.
12+: minor brain injury with probable recovery
9–11: moderate severity requiring close observation for changes
8 or less: coma; 8 after 6 hours associated with 50% mortality

- Management should focus on maintaining cerebral perfusion, maintaining airway patency, stabilizing spinal injuries, and treating any contamination of surrounding structures by esophageal perforation
- Chest trauma
  - Injuries can occur to the lungs, heart, and GI system
  - **Aortic injury**, **pneumothorax**, and **cardiac injury** (e.g., perforation, tamponade) are the most emergently life-threatening injuries
  - The physical examination should focus on clinical signs of injury to the major vascular structures, heart, and lungs
  - Chest x-ray (CXR), chest CT, EGD, bronchoscopy, and angiography are potential useful tests to be considered if the patient is stable
  - Management should focus on immediate stabilization of life-threatening injuries
- Abdominal trauma
  - Injuries can occur to the abdominal viscera and abdominal vascular structures

QUICK HIT: Sites of significant (>1,500 mL) blood loss frequently not found by physical examination include blood left at the **injury scene, pleural cavity** bleeding (seen with CXR), **intra-abdominal** bleeding (seen with CT or US), **pelvic** bleeding (seen with CT), and bleeding into the **thighs** (seen on x-ray).

TABLE A-9 Revised Trauma Score[1]

Coded Value[2]	Glasgow Coma Scale Score	Systolic Blood Pressure	Respiratory Rate
4	13–15	>89	10–29
3	9–12	76–89	>29
2	6–8	50–75	6–9
1	4–5	1–49	1–5
0	3	0	0
RTS = 0.9368 (GCS coded value) + 0.7326 (SBP coded value) + 0.2908 (RR coded value)			

GCS, Glasgow coma scale; RR, respiratory rate; RTS, revised trauma score; SBP, systolic blood pressure.
[1]RTS of 4 or greater is associated with 60% survival.
[2]Coded value is assigned to each measurement individually.

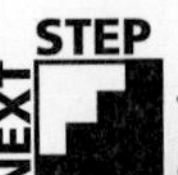

The **hemodynamically unstable** blunt trauma patient should be taken to the **operating room** and not to radiology.

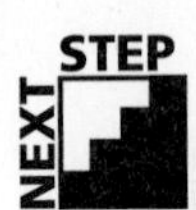

A Foley catheter should **never** be placed in a patient with a **suspected urethral rupture** (e.g., blood seen at the urethral meatus, high-riding prostate on rectal examination) to avoid further urologic injury unless performed under cystoscopic guidance.

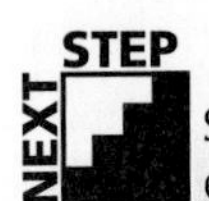

Serial neurovascular examinations should be performed following any type of treatment for an extremity to detect an evolving or iatrogenic neurologic injury.

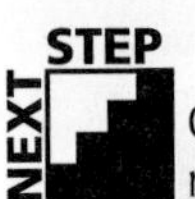

Criteria that should be met in posttraumatic pregnant females prior to discharge are contractions **no more frequent** than **every ten minutes**, **no vaginal bleeding**, **no abdominal pain**, and a **normal fetal heart tracing**.

QUICK HIT: A physician who has due cause to suspect child abuse but does not report it or act to protect the child **may be held liable** for subsequent injury or mortality.

- Physical examination should look for signs of peritoneal irritation and peritoneal perforation
- Abdominal CT and the **focused abdominal sonography for trauma (FAST)** examination are the best means of detecting injury
- **Exploratory laparotomy** is required for any penetrating injury, retroperitoneal vascular injury, or in an unstable patient with an intraperitoneal vascular injury

- **Genitourinary and pelvic trauma**
  - Injury may occur to the kidneys or lower urinary system
  - Physical examination should look for signs of urologic bleeding (e.g., blood at the urethral meatus) and should include a pelvic examination in women
  - Pelvic CT, retrograde urethrogram, or intravenous pyelogram should be considered to rule out urologic disruptions
  - Disruption of the urologic tract must be treated surgically
- **Extremity trauma**
  - Injury may involve **bones**, **vasculature**, **soft tissues**, or **nerves** in the extremities
  - The physical examination should focus on the detection of gross instability and neurovascular deficits
  - X-ray, CT, and MRI are the principal tools for detecting injuries
  - Immediate management should focus on the stabilization of bony injuries and the maintenance of perfusion
- **Trauma in expectant mothers**
  - **Trauma** is the leading cause of nonobstetric maternal death
    - Inferior vena cava (IVC) compression by the uterus makes pregnant women more susceptible to **poor cardiac output** following injury
    - **Superior displacement of the bowel** by the uterus decreases the risk of GI injury from lower abdominal trauma but increases the risk of GI injury from upper abdominal or chest trauma
  - Although the risk of fetal death is low with minor injuries, it increases significantly in high-energy trauma
  - Any trauma increases the risk of **abruptio placentae**
  - The assessment must consider both the mother and the fetus
  - Management should prioritize the needs of the **mother**

ABUSE AND SEXUAL ASSAULT

- Abuse of anyone may be **physical**, **emotional**, **sexual**, or **exploitative**
- **Child abuse**
  - **Neglect** is the most prevalent form of child abuse and constitutes the **failure to provide** the physical, emotional, educational, and medical needs of a child
  - **Concerning findings** during the assessment of an injured child include an injury inconsistent with the history, vague details, discrepancies in the history, delays in seeking treatment, a lack of parental concern, evidence of multiple injuries in various stages of healing, and injuries pathognomonic for abuse (e.g., rib fractures, femur fractures in nonambulatory children, burns in the shapes of objects)
  - The treating physician has an **obligation** to report any suspected cases of child abuse to the legal child-protective services
  - All suspected cases should be **well documented**
- **Spousal/partner abuse**
  - Patients may present with vague complaints (e.g., chronic headaches, abdominal pains)
  - **Concerning findings** during the assessment include an injury inconsistent with the history, vague details, inconsistencies in the history, delays in seeking treatment, evidence of multiple injuries in various stages of healing, a hypervigilant partner, and recurrent sexually transmitted diseases (STDs)
  - The patient should be interviewed **without** the partner present
  - The initial approach should focus on the **immediate safety of the patient**

- Patients should be provided with information on safety plans, escape strategies, legal rights, and shelter locations, but the victim should not be forced into any action
- Reporting of this type of abuse is **nonmandatory**

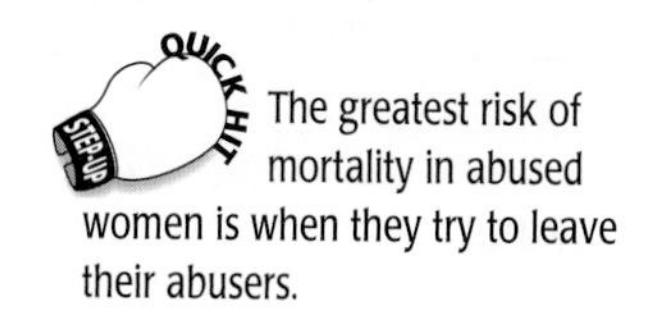

The greatest risk of mortality in abused women is when they try to leave their abusers.

- **Elder abuse**
  - Considered to be abuse in a patient >60 years old that occurs at the hands of a caregiver
  - The concerning findings are similar to those seen in child and partner abuse
  - The physician should contact social services to facilitate placement of the patient in a safe environment
  - Reporting of this type of abuse is **mandatory**
- **Sexual assault**
  - **Nonconsensual** sexual activity with physical contact
    - Nonconsensual, forced intercourse is **rape**
  - Victims may be children or adults
  - A **detailed history** must be collected and thoroughly documented
  - The examination should focus on the entire body with particular attention paid to the genitals, anus, and mouth to look for signs of assault
  - In cases of rape, all injuries must be well documented and vaginal fluid and pubic hair should be collected for evidence (i.e., **rape kit**)
  - Oral, vaginal, and penile fluid specimens should be tested for STDs
  - Pregnancy testing should be performed to look for incidental conception occurring during assault
  - The careful and well-documented collection of all details and evidence is important to future follow-up and legal action
  - Referral to **social support systems** and **counseling** is very important

Another health care worker (chaperone) must be present when a sexual examination is performed, and the patient should be made to feel as comfortable as possible with the history and physical examination.

TOXICOLOGY

- **Treatment principles**
  - The initial evaluation must focus on determining the **type of poison** involved
  - Patient history, witness input, and clues found near the patient (e.g., empty bottles of medications, other medications) will help in making diagnosis
  - **Therapies for poisoning**
    - Induced vomiting: chemical induction of vomiting to empty the stomach of its contents; it is rarely performed because it is only useful in the initial 1 to 2 hours after ingestion and is contraindicated in caustic agents
    - **Activated charcoal:** absorbs substances and blocks their systemic absorption but is not as useful in cases of ingested metals or alcohol
    - Gastric lavage: suction drainage and saline lavage of the gastric contents via a nasogastric tube; it carries similar limitations to induced vomiting and must be performed within the initial hour of ingestion for much benefit
    - **Antidotes:** chemicals that reverse or inhibit an ingested poison's activity
    - Diuretics: may help in cases where increased urination helps remove toxin (e.g., salicylates, phenobarbital)
    - Dialysis or exchange transfusion: used in cases of severe symptoms or when other treatments are unsuccessful
    - Supportive care is routinely administered including airway stabilization, IV hydration, cardiac support, and anticonvulsant therapy when appropriate
- **Ingested poisons**
  - May occur in children from the accidental ingestion of cleaning products, medications, or personal care products
  - May occur in elderly patients from an accidental repeat dosing of usual medications
  - May be intentional (i.e., suicide attempt)
  - Identification of the ingested poison is important to dictating treatment (Table A-10)

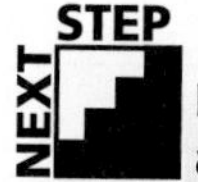

Beware of the alcohol abuser that comes into the emergency department **fictitiously** saying that he has ingested ethylene glycol and needs ethanol for treatment; check for sweet breath and perform a toxicology screen before administering ethanol.

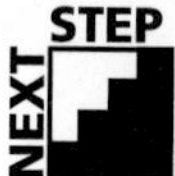

Organophosphates may also be absorbed through the **skin,** so all contaminated clothing must be removed from patients with this type of poisoning.

TABLE A-10 Common Poisons and Their Antidotes

Substance	Symptoms	Treatment
DRUGS		
Acetaminophen	Nausea, hepatic insufficiency	N-acetylcysteine
Anticholinergics	Dry mouth, urinary retention, QRS widening on the ECG	Physostigmine
Benzodiazepines	Sedation, respiratory depression	Flumazenil
β-blockers	Bradycardia, hypotension, hypoglycemia, pulmonary edema	Glucagon, calcium, insulin, and dextrose
Calcium channel blockers	Bradycardia, hypotension	Glucagon, calcium, insulin, and dextrose
Cocaine	Tachycardia, agitation	Supportive care
Cyanide	Headache, nausea, vomiting, altered mental status	Nitrates, hydroxocobalamin
Digoxin	Nausea, vomiting, visual changes, arrhythmias	Digoxin antibodies
Heparin	Excessive bleeding, easy bruising	Protamine sulfate
Isoniazid	Neuropathy, hepatotoxicity	Vitamin B_6
Isopropyl alcohol	Decreased consciousness, nausea, abdominal pain	Supportive care
Methanol	Headache, visual changes, dizziness	Ethanol, dialysis
Opioids	Pinpoint pupils, respiratory depression	Naloxone
Salicylates	Nausea, vomiting, tinnitus, hyperventilation, anion gap metabolic acidosis	Charcoal, dialysis, sodium bicarbonate
Sulfonylureas	Hypoglycemia	Octreotide and dextrose
Tricyclic antidepressants	Tachycardia, dry mouth, urinary retention, QRS widening on the ECG	Sodium bicarbonate, diazepam
Warfarin	Excessive bleeding, easy bruising	Vitamin K, FFP
INDUSTRIAL CHEMICALS		
Caustics (e.g., acids, alkali)	Severe oropharyngeal and gastric irritation or burns, drooling, odynophagia, abdominal pain, symptoms of gastric perforation	Copious irrigation (do not induce emesis or attempt neutralization), activated charcoal
Ethylene glycol	Ataxia, hallucinations, seizures, sweet breath	Ethanol, dialysis
Organophosphates (e.g., insecticides, fertilizers)	Salivation, lacrimation, miosis, vomiting, diarrhea, increased urination, paralysis, decreased consciousness	Atropine, pralidoxime, supportive care
METALS		
Iron	Nausea, constipation, hepatotoxicity	Deferoxamine
Lead	Peripheral neuropathy, anemia	EDTA, dimercaprol
Mercury	Renal insufficiency, tremor, mental status changes	Dimercaprol

ECG, electrocardiogram; EDTA, ethylenediamine tetraacetic acid; FFP, fresh frozen plasma.

TABLE A-11 **Common Types of Venomous Bites and Stings**

Type of Bite	Symptoms	Treatment	Complications
Snake (e.g., rattlesnake, copperhead, water moccasin, coral snake)	Pain and swelling at the bite, progressive dyspnea, toxin-induced DIC	Immobilize the extremity and cleanse the wound **Antivenin** is likely required	Effects are more severe in children Increased mortality without prompt treatment
Scorpion	Severe pain and swelling at bite, increased sweating, vomiting, diarrhea	Antivenin, atropine, phenobarbital	Acute pancreatitis, myocardial toxicity, respiratory paralysis
Spider (e.g., black widow, brown recluse)	Abdominal pain, wound pain, vomiting, jaundice, DIC	Black widow: calcium gluconate, methocarbamol Brown recluse: dexamethasone, colchicine, dapsone	DIC Brown recluse bites are more severe
Mammals	Pain and swelling at bite, penetrating trauma depending on the size of bite	Saline irrigation, debridement, tetanus and rabies prophylaxis, antibiotics for infection	Infection (e.g., staphylococci, *Pasteurella multocida*, rabies virus)
Human	Pain and swelling at bite, tender local lymphadenopathy	Saline irrigation, broad coverage antibiotics, surgical debridement, thorough documentation	High incidence of infection with primary closure or delayed presentation

DIC, disseminated intravascular coagulation.

- **Venomous bites and stings**
  - Poisonous bites can come from snakes (e.g., rattlesnake, copperhead, coral snake), spiders (e.g., black widow, brown recluse), or other less frequently encountered animals (e.g., scorpion)
  - The venom in these bites may contain neurotoxins, cardiotoxins, or proteolytic enzymes that can potentially be fatal
  - The treatment of a poisonous bite depends on the causative animal (Table A-11)

MNEMONIC

The symptoms of organophosphate poisoning can be remembered by the mnemonic **DUDE SLOP**: **D**iarrhea, **U**rination, **D**ecreased consciousness, **E**mesis, **S**alivation, **L**acrimation, **O**cular miosis, **P**aralysis.

QUICK HIT

Body packing involves ingesting a large number of drug-filled latex and/or wax packets for the purpose of smuggling them; rupture of a packet may cause a massive overdose effect from a large quantity of the drug.

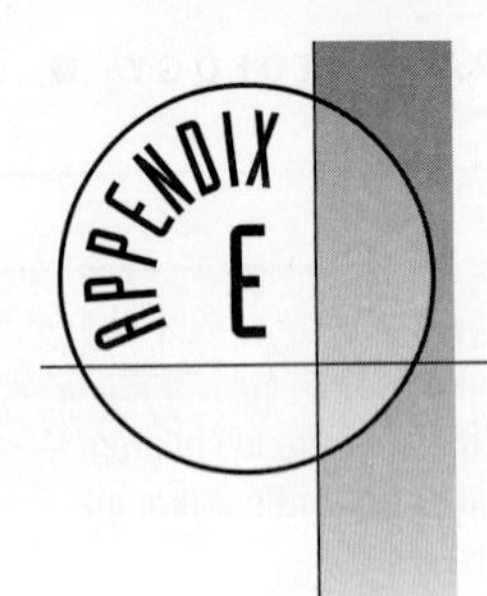

Normal Lab Values

Hematology

Test	Normal Range	Units
CD4 count	800–1,500	cells/mL
Free erythrocyte protoporphyrin	16–36	μg/dL
Haptoglobin	83–267	mg/dL
Hematocrit		
Female	34–48	
Male	40–52	%
Hemoglobin		
Female	12.0–16.0	
Male	13.5–17.5	g/dL
Hemoglobin A_2	2.0–3.3	%
Hemoglobin F	<2.0	%
Immunoglobulins		
IgA	80–350	mg/dL
IgD	0.3–3.0	mg/dL
IgE	0.002–0.2	mg/dL
IgG	620–1,400	mg/dL
IgM	45–250	mg/dL
Mean corpuscular hemoglobin concentration	31–36	g/dL
Mean corpuscular volume	80–100	fL
Platelets	150–400	1,000 units/μL
Reticulocyte count	0.5–2	%
White blood cells	4.0–11.0	1,000 cells/μL

Serum Chemistry

Test	Normal Range	Units
Adrenocorticotropin hormone		pg/mL
Morning (0800)	25–100	
Afternoon (1800)	<50	
Alanine aminotransferase	9–52	U/L
Albumin	3.5–5.8	g/dL
Aldosterone		ng/dL
Female	5–30	
Male	6–22	

Serum Chemistry (*Continued*)

Test	Normal Range	Units
Alkaline phosphatase	35–125	U/L
Ammonia	9–33	μmol/L
Amylase	0–140	U/L
Aspartate aminotransferase	14–36	U/L
Bilirubin, direct	0.0–0.4	mg/dL
Bilirubin, indirect	Total bili.–direct bili.	mg/dL
Bilirubin, total	0.0–1.2	mg/dL
Brain natriuretic peptide	0–99	pg/mL
Minimal heart failure	100–299	
Mild heart failure	300–599	
Moderate heart failure	600–899	
Severe heart failure	900+	
CA125	<35	U/mL
Calcium	8.5–10.5	mg/dL
Calcium, ionized	1.00–1.25	mmol/L
Carbon dioxide	22–30	mEq/L
Ceruloplasmin	27–37	mg/dL
Chloride	97–107	mEq/L
Cholesterol, total	<200	mg/dL
High density lipoprotein	>40	
Low density lipoprotein	<130	
Cortisol		μg/dL
Morning (0800)	5–23	
Afternoon (1600)	3–15	
C-reactive protein	0.1–0.9	mg/dL
Creatine kinase	20–315	U/L
Myocardium fraction	0.0–5.0	ng/mL
Creatinine	0.8–1.3	mg/dL
D-dimer	0–300	ng/mL
Erythrocyte sedimentation rate	0–25	mm/hr
DHEA		ng/mL
Female	1.4–8.0	
Female (post-menopausal)	0.3–4.5	
Male	0.5–5.5	
Estradiol		pg/mL
Pre/post cycle	20–60	
Midcycle	100–500	
Post-menopausal	10–30	
Ferritin	9–120	ng/mL
Fibrinogen	200–400	mg/dL
Folate	3.0–17.0	ng/mL
Follicle-stimulating hormone		U/L
Prepubertal	<5	
Pre-/postcycle	4.6–22.4	
Midcycle	13–41	
Postmenopausal	30–170	

(*continued*)

Serum Chemistry (*Continued*)

Test	Normal Range	Units
Glucose	70–99	mg/dL
Growth hormone	0–4	ng/mL
Hemoglobin A1c	4.0–6.0	%
Human chorionic gonadotropin		U/L
Nonpregnant	<5	
3 weeks pregnant	5–50	
6 weeks pregnant	1,080–56,500	
9–12 weeks pregnant	25,700–288,000	
13–16 weeks pregnant	13,300–254,000	
17–24 weeks pregnant	4,060–165,400	
25–40 weeks pregnant	3,640–117,000	
Postmenopausal	<9.5	
Iron	37–170	μg/dL
Lactate	0.3–2.3	mEq/L
Lactate dehydrogenase	313–618	U/L
Lead	<10	μg/dL
Lipase	23–300	U/L
Luteinizing hormone		U/L
Prepubertal	<5	
Pre-/postcycle	3–30	
Midcycle	75–150	
Postmenopausal	30–130	
Magnesium	1.3–2.5	mg/dL
Osmolality		mOsm/kg
Serum	275–295	
Plasma	285–295	
Parathyroid hormone	10–55	pg/mL
Phenylalanine	<3	mg/dL
Phosphorus	2.5–5.0	mg/dL
Potassium	3.5–5.3	mEq/L
Prolactin		ng/mL
Male	2–18	
Female (nonpregnant)	2–29	
Female (pregnant)	10–300	
Prostate-specific antigen	0.0–4.0	ng/mL
Protein, total serum	6.1–8.5	g/dL
Sodium	133–143	mEq/L
Thyroid stimulating hormone	0.40–4.00	μU/mL
Thyroxine	4.5–12.5	μg/dL
Free T_4 index	3.5–14.6	
Transferrin	200–400	mg/dL
Triglycerides	<150	mg/dL
Triiodothyronine	0.7–1.7	ng/mL
T_3 reuptake	0.77–1.17	
Troponin-I	0.0–0.4	ng/mL

Serum Chemistry (*Continued*)

Test	Normal Range	Units
Urea nitrogen, blood	10–20	mg/dL
Vitamin B_{12}	193–982	pg/mL
Vitamin D 1, 25-dihydroxycholecalciferol	25–45	pg/mL
Vitamin D 25-hydroxyvitamin D_3	15–80	ng/mL

Arterial Blood Gas

Test	Normal Range	Units
pH	7.35–7.45	
Oxygen	75–100	mmHg
Carbon dioxide	35–45	mmHg
Bicarbonate	22.0–26.0	mEq/L
Base excess	–3.0–3.0	mEq/L
Oxygen saturation	94.0–99.0	%
Carboxyhemoglobin Toxicity Lethality	0–2.3 >20 >50	%

Sweat Chemistry

Test	Normal Range	Units
Chloride	3–35	mEq/L
Sodium	10–40	mEq/L

Urine Chemistry

Test	Normal Range	Units
Calcium	100–250	mg/day
Chloride	<8 110–250	mEq/L mEq/day
Copper	15–30	µg/day
Cortisol	10–100	µg/day
Creatinine	800–2,800	mg/day
Osmolality	80–1,300	mOsm/kg
pH	4.5–8.0	
Porphobilinogen	0–2.0	mg/day
Potassium	<8 35–85	mEq/L mEq/day
Protein	1–15 0–150	mg/dL mg/day
Sodium	10–40 15–25	mEq/L mEq/day
Specific gravity	<1.030	

Stool Chemistry

Test	Normal Range	Units
Osmolality	~ 290	mOsm/kg
pH	6.1–7.9	

Coagulation

Test	Normal Range	Units
Prothrombin time	10.4–13.2	sec
Partial thromboplastin time	21.8–32.5	sec
INR	Dependent on PT	

Cerebral Spinal Fluid

Test	Normal Range	Units
Glucose	40–70	mg/dL
Opening pressure	50–100	mm H_2O
Protein	20–45	mg/dL
White blood cells	<5	cells/μL

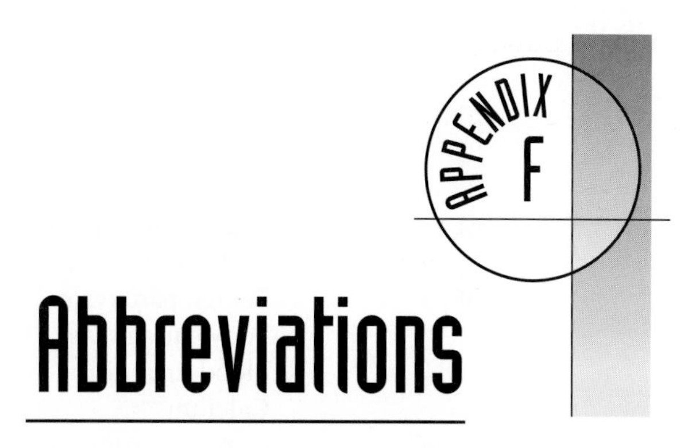

Abbreviations

%	Percent
°F	Degrees Fahrenheit
AAA	Abdominal aortic aneurysm
A-a gradient	Alveolar-arterial gradient
ABC	Airway, Breathing, Circulation
ABG	Arterial blood gas
ABI	Ankle-brachial index
AC	Assist-control ventilation
ACA	Anterior cerebral artery
ACE-I	Angiotensin-converting enzyme inhibitor
ACL	Anterior cruciate ligament
ACTH	Adrenocorticotropic hormone
ADH	Antidiuretic hormone
ADHD	Attention-deficit/hyperactivity disorder
ADP	Adenosine diphosphate
Afib	Atrial fibrillation
Aflutter	Atrial flutter
AI	Apnea Index
AICA	Anterior inferior cerebellar artery
AIDS	Acquired immune deficiency syndrome
α-IFN	α-interferon
AlkPhos	Alkaline phosphatase
ALL	Acute lymphocytic leukemia
ALS	Amyotrophic lateral sclerosis
ALT	Alanine aminotransferase
AML	Acute myelogenous leukemia
ANA	Antinuclear antibodies
APUD	Amine-precursor-uptake and decarboxylation
AR	Aortic regurgitation
ARB	Angiotensin receptor blocker
ARDS	Acute respiratory distress syndrome
ARF	Acute renal failure
AS	Aortic stenosis
ASA	Aspirin
ASCA	Anti-saccharomyces cerevisiae antibodies
ASCH	Atypical squamous cells, cannot exclude HSIL
ASCUS	Atypical squamous cells of undetermined significance
ASD	Atrial septal defect
AST	Aspartate aminotransferase
ATN	Acute tubular necrosis
AV	Arteriovenous or atrioventricular
AVM	Arteriovenous malformation
AXR	Abdominal x-ray
Bicarb	Bicarbonate

BMI	Body mass index
BNP	Brain natriuretic peptide
BP	Blood pressure
BPH	Benign prostatic hypertrophy
bpm	Beats per minute
BPPV	Benign paroxysmal positional vertigo
BSA	Body surface area
BUN	Blood urea nitrogen
Ca	Calcium
CABG	Coronary artery bypass grafting
CAD	Coronary artery disease
CAH	Congenital adrenal hyperplasia
cANCA	Cytoplasmic antineutrophil cytoplasmic antibodies
CBC	Complete blood cell count
CEA	Carcinoembryonic antigen
CF	Cystic fibrosis
CFTR	Cystic fibrosis transmembrane conductance regulator
Chem10	10-electrolyte chemistry panel
Chem7	7-electrolyte chemistry panel
CHF	Congestive heart failure
CI	Confidence interval
CICU	Cardiac intensive care unit
CIN	Cervical intraepithelial neoplasia
CK	Creatine kinase (a.k.a. creatine phosphokinase)
CKD	Chronic kidney disease
CK-MB	Creatine kinase myocardial component
Cl	Chloride
CLL	Chronic lymphocytic leukemia
cm	Centimeter
CML	Chronic myelogenous leukemia
CMT	Charcot-Marie-Tooth disease
CMV	Controlled mechanical ventilation
CN	Cranial nerve
CNS	Central nervous system
CO	Cardiac output
CO_2	Carbon dioxide
Coags	Coagulation panel
COPD	Chronic obstructive pulmonary disease
CPAP	Continuous positive airway pressure
CPPD	calcium pyrophosphate dehydrate deposition
CPRS	Complex regional pain syndrome
Cr	Creatinine
CRP	C-reactive protein
CSF	Cerebral spinal fluid
CT	Computed tomography
CVA	Cerebrovascular accident
CXR	Chest x-ray
DBili	Direct bilirubin
DCIS	Ductal carcinoma *in–situ*
DDAVP	Demopressin acelate
DDH	Developmental dysplasia of the hip
DES	Diffuse esophageal spasm
DEXA	Dual energy x-ray absorptiometry
DHEA	Dehydroepiandrosterone
DI	Diabetes insipidus
DIC	Disseminated intravascular coagulation
DIP	Distal interphalangeal

DKA	Diabetic ketoacidosis
dL	Deciliters
D_{Lco}	Diffusing capacity of lungs
DM	Diabetes mellitus
DMSA	2,3-dimercaptosuccinic acid
DNR	Do-not-resuscitate
DTR	deep tendon reflex
DVT	Deep vein thrombosis
EBV	Epstein-Barr virus
ECG	Electrocardiogram
ECMO	Extracorporeal membrane oxygenation
ECT	Electroconvulsive therapy
EDTA	Ethylenediamine tetraacetic acid
EEG	Electroencephalogram
EF	Ejection fraction
EGD	Esophagogastroduodenoscopy
ELISA	Enzyme-linked immunosorbent assay
EMG	Electromyography
EMT	Emergency medical technician
EPO	Erythropoietin
ERCP	Endoscopic retrograde cholangiopancreatography
ERV	Expiratory reserve volume
ESR	Erythrocyte sedimentation rate
EtOH	Ethyl alcohol
FAP	Familial adenomatous polyposis
FAST	Focused abdominal sonography for trauma
FDG-PET	Fluorodeoxyglucose positron emission tomography
Fe	Iron
$FEF_{25\%-75\%}$	Forced expiratory flow rate from 25%–75% of functional vital capacity
FENa	Fractional excretion of sodium
FEV_1	Forced expiratory volume in 1 second
FFP	Fresh frozen plasma
FH	Familial hypercholesterolemia
Fio_2	Fraction of inspired oxygen
fL	Femtoliters
FNA	Fine needle aspiration
FRC	Functional reserve capacity
FSH	Follicle-stimulating hormone
FTA-ABS	Fluorescent treponemal antibody absorption
FVC	Functional vital capacity
g	Grams
G6PD	Glucose 6-phosphate dehydrogenase
GABA	γ-aminobutyric acid
GAD	Generalized anxiety disorder
GBM	Glioblastoma multiforme
GBS	Group B streptococcus
GCS	Glasgow coma scale
GERD	Gastroesophageal reflux disease
GGT	Gamma glutamyl transpeptidase
GH	Growth hormone
GHB	Gamma hydroxybutyrate
GI	Gastrointestinal
Glu	Glucose
GnRH	Gonadotropin-releasing hormone
H_2O	Water
HAART	Highly active antiretroviral treatment
HAV	Hepatitis A virus

HbA1c	Hemoglobin A1c
HBV	Hepatitis B virus
hCG	Human chorionic gonadotropin
HCO_3^-	Bicarbonate
HCTZ	Hydrochlorothiazide
HCV	Hepatitis C virus
HDL	High-density lipoprotein
HDV	Hepatitis D virus
HEV	Hepatitis E virus
Hgb	Hemoglobin
HgbCO	Carboxyhemoglobin
HHNC	Hyperosmolar hyperglycemic nonketotic coma
HIDA	Hepatic iminodiacetic
HIT	Heparin-induced thrombocytopenia
HIV	Human immunodeficiency virus
HLA	Human leukocyte antigen
HNPCC	Hereditary nonpolyposis colorectal cancer
HOCM	Hypertrophic obstructive cardiomyopathy
HPV	Human papilloma virus
hr	Hours
HR	Heart rate
HSIL	High grade squamous intraepithelial lesion
HSV	Herpes simplex virus
HTN	Hypertension
HUS	Hemolytic uremic syndrome
IBD	Inflammatory bowel disease
Ibili	Indirect bilirubin
IBS	Irritable bowel syndrome
IC	Inspiratory capacity
ICP	Intracranial pressure
ICU	Intensive care unit
I + D	Incision and drainage
Ig	Immunoglubulin
IMV	Intermittent mandatory ventilation
INH	Isoniazid
INR	International normalized ratio
IPF	Idiopathic pulmonary fibrosis
IRB	Institutional review board
IRV	Inspiratory reserve volume
ITP	Idiopathic thrombocytopenia purpura
IUD	Intrauterine device
IUGR	Intrauterine growth restriction
IV	Intravenous
IVC	Inferior vena cava
IVDA	Intravenous drug abuse
IVDU	Intravenous drug use
IVF	Intravenous fluids
IVIG	Intravenous immunoglobulin
IVP	Intravenous pyelogram
JRA	Juvenile rheumatoid arthritis
JVD	Jugular venous distention
K	Potassium
kg	Kilograms
KOH	Potassium hydroxide
L	Liters
LAD	Left anterior descending artery
LBBB	Left bundle branch block

LBO	Large bowel obstruction
lb	Pounds
LCIS	Lobular carcinoma *in situ*
LDH	Lactate dehydrogenase
LDL	Low-density lipoprotein
LES	Lower esophageal sphincter
LFT	Liver function test
LH	Luteinizing hormone
LMWH	Low molecular weight heparin
LSD	Lysergic acid diethylamide
LSIL	Low grade squamous intraepithelial lesion
LVH	Left ventricular hypertrophy
MAC	*Mycobacterium avis* complex
MAOI	Monoamine oxidase inhibitors
MAP	Mean arterial pressure
MAT	Multifocal atrial tachycardia
MCA	Middle cerebral artery
MCL	Medial collateral ligament
MCP	Metacarpophalangeal
MCV	Mean corpuscular volume
MEN	Multiple endocrine neoplasia
mEq	Milliequivalents
mg	Milligrams
Mg	Magnesium
MGUS	Monoclonal gammopathy of undetermined significance
MHA-TP	Microhemagglutination assay for antibodies to treponemes
MI	Myocardial infarction
MICU	Medical intensive care unit
min	Minutes
mL	Milliliters
MLF	Medial longitudinal fasciculus
mm	Millimeters
mm Hg	Millimeters of mercury
mmol	Millimoles
MMR	measles, mumps rubella vaccine
MMSE	Minimental status examination
mOsm	Milliosmoles
MR	Mitral regurgitation
MRA	Magnetic resonance angiography
MRI	Magnetic resonance imaging
MRSA	Methicillin-resistent *S. aureus*
MS	Mitral stenosis
MSH	Melanocyte-stimulating hormone
MSSA	Methicillin-sensitive *S. aureus*
Na	Sodium
NCS	Nerve conduction study
ng	Nanograms
NICU	Neonatal intensive care unit
NMDA	N-methyl-D-aspartate
NPH	Neutral protamine Hagedorn (insulin)
NPO	Nulla per orem (i.e., nothing by mouth)
NPV	Negative predictive value
NSAID	Nonsteroidal anti-inflammatory drug
O_2	Oxygen
OA	Osteoarthritis
OCD	Obsessive-compulsive disorder
OCP	Oral contraceptive pill

OR	Odds ratio
pANCA	Perinuclear antineutrophil cytoplasmic antibodies
PAO_2	Alveolar oxygen pressure
PaO_2	Arterial oxygen pressure
PAPP-A	Pregnancy-associated plasma protein A
PBC	Primary biliary cirrhosis
PCA	Patient-controlled analgesia
PCA	Posterior cerebral artery
PCO_2	Partial pressure of carbon dioxide
PCOS	Polycystic ovary syndrome
PCP	Primary care provider
PCR	Polymerase chain reaction
PDA	Patent ductus arteriosus
PE	Pulmonary embolism
PEA	Pulseless electrical activity
PEEP	Positive end-expiratory pressure
PEFR	Peak expiratory flow rate
PET	Positron emission tomography
PFT	Pulmonary function test
pg	Picograms
Phos	Phosphorus
PICA	Posterior inferior cerebellar artery
PICC	Peripheral indwelling central catheter
PID	Pelvic inflammatory disease
PIP	Proximal interphalangeal
Plt	Platelets
PMDD	Premenstrual dystrophic disorder
PMN	Polymorphonuclear cells
PMR	Polymyalgia rheumatica
PMS	Premenstrual syndrome
PO_2	Partial pressure of oxygen
PPD	Purified protein derivative
PPI	Proton pump inhibitor
PPV	Positive predictive value
PRBC	Packed red blood cells
PROM	Premature rupture of membranes
PSA	Prostate-specific antigen
PSC	Primary sclerosing cholangitis
PSVT	Paroxysmal supraventricular tachycardia
PT	Protime
PTA	Percutaneous transluminal angioplasty
PTCA	Percutaneous transluminal coronary angioplasty
PTH	Parathyroid hormone
PTSD	Posttraumatic stress disorder
PTT	Partial thromboplastin time
PTU	Propylthiouracil
PTX	Pneumothorax
PUD	Peptic ulcer disease
PVC	Premature ventricular complex
PVD	Peripheral vascular disease
RA	Rheumatoid arthritis
RAST	Radioallergosorbent testing
RBBB	Right bindle branch block
RBC	Red blood cell
REM	Rapid eye movement
RF	Rheumatoid factor
RHD	Rheumatic heart disease

RPR	Rapid plasma reagin
RR	Relative risk
RR	Respiratory rate
RSD	Reflex sympathetic dystrophy
RSV	Respiratory syncytial virus
RTS	Revised trauma score
RV	Residual volume
RVH	Right ventricular hypertrophy
SBO	Small bowel obstruction
SCFE	Slipped capital femoral epiphysis
SCID	Severe combined immunodeficiency syndrome
sec	Seconds
SIADH	Syndrome of inappropriate antidiuretic hormone secretion
SIMV	Synchronized intermittent mandatory ventilation
SLE	Systemic lupus erythematosus
SNF	Skilled nursing facility
SNRI	Serotonin–norepinephrine reuptake inhibitor
SPECT	Single-positron emission computed tomography
SPEP	Serum protein electrophoresis
SSRI	Selective serotonin reuptake inhibitor
STD	Sexually transmitted disease
SV	Stroke volume
T	Temperature
TAH-BSO	Total abdominal hysterectomy and bilateral salpingo-oophorectomy
TB	Tuberculosis
TBG	Thyroid-binding globulin
TBili	Total bilirubin
TCA	Tricyclic antidepressant
TEE	Transesophageal echocardiogram
TEN	Toxic epidermal necrosis
TENS	Transcutaneous electrical nerve stimulation
TIA	Transient ischemic attack
TIPS	Transjugular intrahepatic portal-caval shunting
TLC	Total lung capacity
TMP-SMX	Trimethoprim-sulfamethoxazole
TNF	Tumor necrosis factor
TPN	Total parenteral nutrition
TRH	Thyrotropin-releasing hormone
Trig	Triglycerides
Trop-I	Troponin I
TSH	Thyroid-stimulating hormone
TSIs	Thyroid-stimulating immunoglobulins
TTP-HUS	Thrombotic thrombocytopenic purpura-hemolytic uremic syndrome
TURP	Transurethral resection of the prostate
TV	Tidal volume
U	Units
UA	Urinalysis
UC	Ulcerative colitis
UPEP	Urine protein electrophoresis
URI	Upper respiratory infection
US	Ultrasound
UTI	Urinary tract infection
VDRL	Venereal Disease Research Laboratory test
Vfib	Ventricular fibrillation
VIP	Vasoactive intestinal peptide
V/Q scan	Ventilation-perfusion scan
VSD	Ventricular septal defect

Vtach	Ventricular tachycardia
vWF	von Willebrand factor
VZV	varicella zoster vaccine
WBC	White blood cells
WPW	Wolff-Parkinson-White syndrome
XRT	X-ray therapy
μg	Micrograms
μL	Microliters
μmol	Micromoles
μU	Microunits

Index

Note: Page numbers followed by f indicate figure; those followed by t indicate table.